# THE
# SHALAKYA TANTRA
*Diseases of Eye, Head & E.N.T.*
(2 Vols. bound in One)

*By*

**Dr. Dingari Lakshmana Chary**
*B.A. M.S., M.D., (Ph.D.)*

CHAUKHAMBA SANSKRIT PRATISHTHAN
DELHI

# THE SHALAKYA TANTRA

*Publishers :*

## CHAUKHAMBA SANSKRIT PRATISHTHAN

38 U. A., Bungalow Road, Jawahar Nagar
Post Box No. 2113, Delhi 110007
Phone : (011) 23856391, 41530902
E-mail : cspdel.sales@gmail.com
Website : www.chaukhambabooks.in

© **All Rights Reserved**
ISBN : 978-81-7084-175-3
Reprint : 2017
Pages : II+VIII+398 (Part I) ⎫ Bound in one
 10+410 (Part II) ⎭ with Coloured Plates
Price : ₹ 625.00


*Also can be had from :*
CHOWKHAMBA VIDYABHAWAN
Chowk (Behind The Bank of Baroda Building)
Post Box No. 1069
Varanasi 221001

✳

CHAUKHAMBA SURBHARATI PRAKASHAN
K. 37/117 Gopal Mandir Lane
Post Box No. 1129
Varanasi 221001

✳

CHAUKHAMBA PUBLISHING HOUSE
4697/2, Ground Floor, Street No. 21-A
Ansari Road, Darya Ganj
New Delhi 110002

Printed by :
A. K. Lithographers, Delhi

आयुर्वेद के आदि प्रवर्तक

भगवान          धन्वन्तरि

आविर्भूव कलशां दक्षहस्तेन वाचः        पीयूषपूर्णममृतं कलशं सुराणाम्
भगवान जीर्ण जनता जनित प्रशंसो,        धन्वन्तरिः भवभयहरण भवनिकाय भूयात्

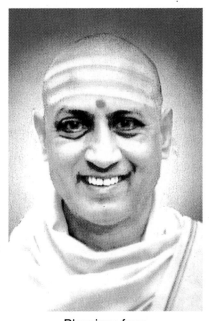

Blessings from
**H.H. Sh. Shivakumar Swamiji**
The Chairman
C.S.S. N.K.J. Ayurvedic Medical College, Bidar.

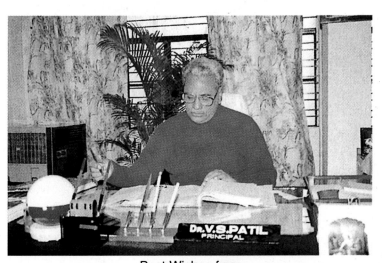

Best Wishes from
**Prof. V.S. Patil**
Principal
C.S.S. N.K.J. Ayurvedic Medical College, Bidar.

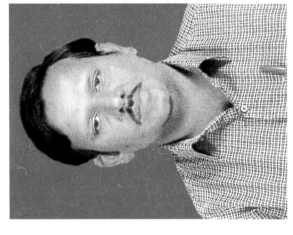

The Author
**Dr. Dingari Lakshmana Chary**
B.A.M.S.; M.D.; (Ph.D)
Date of Birth : 26-01-1962
B.A.M.S. 1979-1985 (Kakatiya University
M.D. 1986 TO 1989 (Osmania University
Ph.D - from 1998 (Pune University)
Working as HOD of Shalya Shalkya Department,
N.K.J. Ayurvedic Medical College, Bidar.

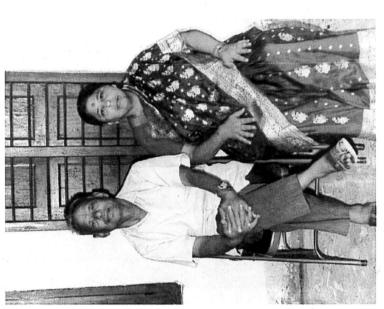

Late Shri Dingari Venkata Charyulu
Late Smt. Dingari Venkata Ramanamma

# FORE WORD

The Shalakya Tantra is an important Branch of Ayurveda dealing with the diseases of E.N.T. and eye, written by Dr. D. Lakshmana Chary. B.A. M.S; M.D; (Ph.D) Shalakya, in English language is based on the syllabus contents of B.A.M.S. degree course. This book is helpful not only to the students of Ayurveda but also to the teachers of Shalakya Tantra.

The work of Dr. Chary is really appreciable. He has taken great pains to compile and collect the various scholarly commentaries and tried to compare and contrass them to elucidate the real interpretation for better understanding of the subject. His work is the need of the hour, particularly for the students of south where the books in English Language are very few. This work fullfils the long felt need of the students.

I welcome this publication on "Shalakyatantra" subject and congratulate the young author for this onerous task which he completed energitically and patiently. I wish him all success and hope that he will continue to write many more books on various subjects in future with this experience, I feel honoured to write this foreword for the book brought out by Dr. Chary who was my student. I wish him success in all his future endeavour.

With love and blessings

**Prof. Dr. V.S. PATIL**
G.C. I.M; M.D (B.H.U)
Principal,
N.K.J. Ayurvedic Medical College,
Bidar, Karnataka.

# PREFACE

It is my great privilege and pleasure to undertake the work of writing the book "Shaalakya Tantra" in two volumes. It is by the grace of God Dhanvanthari alone that my book has been uninterruptedly completed.

Since there has been no book of its kind in English furnishing the fullest information about Shalakyatantra, I have made a bold attempt to venture on it keeping in view the C.C.I.M. syllabus of final B.A.M.S. Students. The success of my work fully depends upon its utility to many a student.

I express my sincere gratitude to H.H. Sri Sri Sri Shivakumar Swamiji, the presedent, C.S.S;N.K.J. Ayurvedic Medical College, Bidar, for providing me the best opportunity to serve in his esteemed Medical Institution. It is he who has been the source of my inspiration to bring out this book.

I offer my heartfelt thanks to the Principal, Dr. V.S. Patil for giving me the most Valuable suggestions from time to time. It is kind of him to write the foreword to my book.

I owe a great deal to Dr. V.V. Doiphode, the principal Tilak Ayurvedic Mahavidyalaya, Pune and the Dean of faculty of Ayurveda Pune University Pune, for extending his utmost co-operation for my Ph.D. work and I am profusely thankful to the Director P.G. Section Dr. Purchure and the Joint Director Dr. D.P. Puranic for rendering their invaluable help to me.

I whole heartedly thank here Dr. S.M. Sathye who is giving me the very good guidance for my Ph.D. work.

I also wish to record my unfailing thankfulness to the Professors, the Readers, the Lecturers of N.K.J. Ayurvedic Medical College, Bidar and Tilak Ayurveda Mahavidyalaya Rastapet, Pune for their best encouragement in my endeavour.

I. Sincerely acknowledge and place on record the direct and Indirect help and guidance of the authors of modern text books on ophthalmology and E.N.T. whose views presentations and illustrations are very much helpful to me in bringing out the book.

Last but not the least I thank Printers of the book and all others who helped me in completing the book as desired

Yours Sincerely
**Dr. D. LAKSHMANA CHARY**
M.D. (Ph.D) Shalakya
H.O.D. of Shalya Shalakya Dept.
N.K.J. Ayurvedic Medical College,
Bidar, Karnataka.

# Contents

CANAL OF SCHLEMM

CONJUNCTIVA

CORNEA

ANTERIOR CHAMBER

CILIARY BODY

IRIS

POSTERIOR CHAMBER

LENS

ORA SERRATA

ZONULE (SUSPENSORY) LIGAMENT

VITREOUS

HYALOID CANAL

RETINA

CHOROID

SCLERA

MACULA

OPTIC NERVE HEAD

CENTRAL ARTERY OF RETINA

CENTRAL VEIN OF RETINA

OPTIC NERVE

## बाल आंजनेय स्वामि (शेषु) प्रसन्न

## गणेश स्तुति

शुक्लाम्बरधरं विष्णुं शशिवर्णम चतुर्बुजम्
प्रसन वदनम ध्ययेतसर्व विघ्नोपशांतये

## धन्वंतरि प्रार्थन

नमामि धन्वंतरि मादिदेवम
सुरा सुरैर्वन्दित पाद पद्मम्
लोके जारा रुग्भय मृत्युनाशम
दातार मीशं विविधौशधीनाम

रागादि रोगा: सहजा: समूला
येनाशु सर्वे जगातोप्यपास्त:
तमेक वैद्यं शिरसा नमामि
वैद्याग मझांश्चा पितामहादीन

1

# INTRODUCTION TO AYURVEDA

Ayurveda is the science of life, it is the God gifted very ancient and the first medical science which was memorised and composed by the originator Brahma (Swayambhoo) and considered it as the branch of Atharvana veda (Upaveda to atharvana veda and treated it as panchama veda). It is explained as 3 principled (3 sutra Hethu - Linga-Aushada) and 8 branched medical science (Astanga Ayurveda)

Ayurveda is the first and the Oldest medical science, existing since or before the human creation. It is aimed to1) Protect the health by giving the knowledge of preventive health principles,2) Protect or cure the diseases by explaining the differrent types of treatment-procedures and principles (Maintanence of health and correction of ill health Swasthasya swastha rakshanam-aaturasya vikara prashamanam)

The Eight branches of Ayurveda are

| | | |
|---|---|---|
| 1) | Kaya Chikitsa | (General Medicine) |
| 2) | Balaroga Chikitsa | (Paediatrics) |
| 3) | Graha roga Chikitsa | (Demonology) |
| 4) | Urdwanga roga Chikitsa | (E.N.T., Ophthalmology) |
| 5) | Shalya Chikitsa | (Surgery) |
| 6) | Visha Chikitsa | (Toxicology) |
| 7) | Rasayana Chikitsa | (Rejuvenative therapy) |
| 8) | Vajee karana Chikitsa | (Aphrodisiacs) |

Among the Astangas, Urdwanga Chikitsa or shalakya chikitsa or uttamanga chikitsa or jathrurdwa roga chikitsa or E.N.T. and ophthalmology is explained as the best for existing in the shiras which is the Seat for all the vital organs (Prana, Indria, Marma etc.)

The shalakya tantra gives the detailed discription of the diseases of the following parts 1) Ear diseases 2) Nose diseases 3) Throat diseases (Lips - Teeth, Gums Tongue Palate Throat proper etc) 4) Eye diseases and 5) Shiro rogas. All these are sensory organs seated in the shiras so only this branch of the medicine is given prime importance among the 8 branches of Ayurveda Again in this branch ophthalmology (Netra roga vigyana ) is having utmost importance because eye is the organ for visual sensation, if vision is lost merely every thing is lost - A blind man, though rich cannot enjoy the world, so only it is explained that " Sarvendrianam Nayanam Pradhanam".

## आयुर्वेद निरुक्ति

हिताहितं सुखं दु:खं आयु: तस्य हिताहितम
मानंच तच्या यत्रोक्तं आयुर्वेद स उच्यते


## अष्टाङ्गायुर्वेद

काय बाल ग्रहोर्ध्वांङ्ग शल्य दंष्ट्राजरावृषान
अष्टावङ्गानि तस्याहुश्चिकित्सायेशु


## उत्तमांग या शिर:

प्राणा : प्राणभृतां यत्र श्रिता: सर्वेन्द्रियाणि च।
यदुत्तमांगमंगानां शिरस्तदभिधीयते॥

चरक

सर्वेन्द्रियाणि येनास्मिन् प्राणा येन च संश्रिता: ।
तेन तस्योत्तमांगस्य रक्षायामादृतो भवेत् ॥

वाग्भट


## शालाक्यतन्त्र की निरुक्ति

शलाकया यत्कर्म क्रियते तच्छालाक्यम्।
शालाकाया: कर्म शालाक्यम्, तत्प्रधानं तन्त्रमपि शालाक्यम् ॥

डल्हण

शालाक्यं नामोर्ध्वजत्रुगतानां श्रवण नयन वदन
घ्राणादिसंश्रितानां ध्याधीनामुपशमनार्थम

सु.सू.1

## नेत्र-शारीर

विद्याद् द्वयङ्गुल-बाहुल्यं स्वांगुष्ठोदरसम्मितम् ।
द्वयङ्गुलं सर्वत: सार्ध भिषङ्नयन-बुद्बुदम् ॥
सुवृत्तं गोस्तनाकारं सर्वभूतगुणोद्भवम् ।

(सु. उ. 1-10)

## नेत्र का पांचभौतिकत्व

पलं भूवोग्निंतो रक्तं वातात् कृष्णं सितं जलात्।
आकाशादश्रुमार्गाश्च जायन्ते नेत्रबुद्बुदे ॥

(सु. उ. 1-11)

## कृष्णमण्डल-दृष्टि मण्डल प्रमाण

नेत्रायामत्रिभागन्तु कृष्ण मण्डलमुच्यते
कृष्णात् स्प्तमिमिच्छन्ति दृष्टि दृष्टि विशारदाः

(सु. उ. 1 – 12,13)

## नेत्रभाग

मण्डलानि च सन्धींश्च पटलानि च लोचने ।
यथाक्रमं विजानीयात् पंचषट् च षडेव च ॥

(सु. उ. 1/14)

## नेत्रमंडल

पक्ष्मवर्त्मश्वेतकृष्णदृष्टीनां मण्डलानि तु ।
अनुपूर्वेंतु ते मध्याश्चत्वारोत्या यथोत्तरम् ॥

(सु. उ. 1-15)

## नेत्रसन्धि

पक्ष्मवर्त्मगतः सन्धिर्वर्त्मशुक्लगातोपरः ।
शुक्लकृष्णगातस्त्वन्यः कृष्णदृष्टिगतोपरः ॥
तथा कनीनकगतः षष्टश्चापाङ्गः स्मृतः ।

(सु. उ. 1-16)

## नेत्रशारीरःपटल

द्वे वर्त्मपटले विद्याच्चत्वार्यन्यानि चाक्षिणिक्
जायते तिमिरं येषु व्याधिः परमदारुणः ॥

(सु. उ. 1/17)

तेजो जलाश्रितं बाह्यं तेष्वन्यत् पिशिताश्रितम्
मेदस्तृतीयं पटलमाश्रितं त्वस्थिचापरम्॥
पंचमांशसमं दृष्टेस्तेषां बाहुल्यमिष्यते ॥

(सु. उ. 1/18)

5

## नेत्र का बन्धन

सिराणां कण्डराणां मेदस: कालकस्य च ॥

गुणा: कालात् पर: श्लेष्मा बन्धनेक्ष्णो: सिरायुत: ॥

(सु. उ. 1/19)

## नेत्ररोग की साधारण सम्प्राप्ति

सिरानुसारिभिर्दोषै विगुणैरूर्ध्वमागतै: ॥

जायन्ते नेत्रभागेषु रोगा: परमदारुणा: ॥

(सु. उ. 1/20)

सर्वरोगनिदानोक्तैरहितै: कुपिता मला: ।

अचक्षुष्यैर्विशेषेण प्राय: पित्तानुसारिण: ॥

सिराभिरूर्ध्वं प्रसृता नेत्रावयवमाश्रिता: ।

वर्त्मसन्धिं सितं कृष्णं दृष्टिं वा सर्वमाक्षिवा ॥

वग्भट

## नेत्र रोगों के पूर्वरूप

तत्राविलं ससंरम्भमश्रुकण्डूपदेहवत् ॥

गुरूषातोदरागाद्यैर्जुष्टं चाव्यक्तलक्षणै: ॥

सशूलं वर्त्मकोषेषु शूकपूर्णाभमेव च ॥

विहन्यमानं रूपे वा क्रियास्वक्षि यथापुरा ॥

दृष्ट्वैव धीमान् बुध्येत दोषेणाधिष्टितं तु तत् ॥

(सु. उ. 10)

## नेत्र रोग का निदान

उष्णाभितप्तस्य जलप्रवेशाद्दूरेक्षणात् स्वप्नविपर्ययाच्च ॥

प्रसक्तसंरोदनकोपशोककक्लेशाभिघातादतिमैथुनाच्च ॥

शुक्तरणालाम्लकुलत्थमाषनिषेवणाद्वेगविनिग्रहाच्च ॥

स्वेदादथोधूमनिषेवणाच्च छर्देर्विघाताद् वमनातियोगात् ॥

वाष्पग्रहात् सुक्ष्मनिरीक्षणांच नेत्रविकारान् जनयन्ति दोषा: ॥

(सु. उ. १ म अ.)

उष्णाभितप्तस्य जलप्रवेशाद्दूरेक्षणात् स्वप्नविपर्ययाच्च ॥

स्वेदाद् रजो धूमनिवेषणाच्च छर्देर्विघाताद् वमनातियोगात् ॥

6

शुक्राणालाम्बुकुलत्थमाषाद्विण्मूत्रवातागमनिग्रहाच्च ॥

प्रसक्तस्रंरोदनशोकतापाच्छिरौरभिघातादतिशीघ्रयानात् ॥

तथा ऋतुनां च विपर्ययेण क्लेशाभितापादतिमैथुनाच्च ॥

वाष्पग्रहात् सूक्ष्मनिरीक्षणाच्च नेत्रे विकारं जनयन्ति दोषाः ॥

भावमिश्रा

यथाः– उष्णाभितप्तस्य जलप्रवेशाद्

दूरेक्षणात् स्वप्नविपर्ययाच्च ।

स्वेदाद्रजोधूमनिषेवणाच्च

छर्देविघाताद् वमनातियोगात्

द्रवान्नपानातिनिषेवणाच्च

विण्मूत्रवातक्रमनिग्रहाच्च ।

प्रसक्तस्रंरोदनशोकतापा

च्छिरोरभिघातादतिमद्यपानात्

तथा ऋतुनांचविपर्ययेण

क्लेशाभितापादतिमैथुनाच्च ।

वाष्पग्रहात् सूक्ष्मानिरीक्षणाच्च ।

नेत्रे विकारांजनयन्ति दोषाः ।

योगरत्नाकर

# नेत्र रोग संख्या

नव सन्ध्याश्रयास्तेषु वर्त्मजास्त्वेकविंशतिः ।

शुक्लभागे दशैकश्च चत्वारः कृष्णभागजाः ॥

सर्वाश्रयाः सप्तदश दृष्टिजा द्वादशैव तु ।

बाह्यजौ द्वौ समाख्यातौ रोगौ परमदारुणौ ॥

भूय एतान् प्रवक्ष्यामि सङ्ख्यारूपचिकित्सितैः ॥

## The Ancient Literary references of Shalakya Tantra :-

1)    Rujashwa & Kanwa were treated for the blindness by the Ashwini Kumaras - Rugveda 1-116-9 to 16 shlokas.
2)    Paravruja was treated for the blindness by Indra. Rugveda-1-111-8.
3)    Nahusha was treated for the deafness by Ashwini kumaras Rugveda 1-116-16.
4)    Dadeechi got shira sandhanam by Ashwini kumaras.
5)    Shiro mardana (in shira shoola) ref:- paraskara guhya sutra.
6)    In shukla yajurveda samhitha mukha pakam (stomatitis), Arma (pterigium etc.) are explained.
7)    Description of Netra shareeera in brhadaranyaka is as follows.

Raktha Raji- Adhipathi (protector) Rudra

| Jala            | " | Parchanna |
|-----------------|---|-----------|
| Kaneenika       | " | Surya     |
| Shukla Mandala  | " | Chandra   |
| Krishna mandala | " | Agni      |
| Ado varthma     | " | Pruthwi   |
| Urdwa varthma   | " | Akasha    |

8)    Atharvana vedic references

    a)    Description of different parts of shalakya (E.N.T. Eye)
    b)    Description of Nava Dwaras.
    c)    Description of Karna shoola.
    d)    Discription of Gandamala-manyaja 55 types and galaja 77 types.
    e)    Krimi (of Ear, Eye, dantha, mukha)-shodhana with apamarga.
    f)    Synonyms of Netra given as chakshu - Chakshmani-Netra Akshi etc.

9)    Description, usage, utility of Anjanas explained in Ithareya brahmana.
10)   In Chakshushyopanishath 40 to 45 mantras are explained for the improvement of vision through suryopasan.
11)   The references are also available from vishnu purana, Agni purana, Geetha, Ramayan and Maha Bharath etc.

By the above references it is obvious that the science of shalakya tantra (medical & surgical) is existing since time of vedas.

# Description of Shalaka - Shalakya tantra:-

Neither charaka nor sushrutha defined the word " Shalakya ", but Dalhana has given the meaning as, Shalakayah yath karma kriyathe taccha shalakyam " shalaka is an instrument used frequently in the diagnostic and treatment procedures of this branch so only it is named as shalakya and the science (tantram) is named as shalakya tantram (" Trayathe anena ithi Tantram - the science that protects the body is explained as tantram.)

Shalaka is an instrument used to pierce or to cut the Netra patalas (Tunics of eye ball ) Though it is mentioned as Netra patalas it is also applicable to the ear nose and throat (Shivadasa Sena)

The science that deals with the discription and treatments of shravana (ear), Nayana (eye), vadana (mouth) and ghrana (Nose), which are situated above the Jathru (Greeva moola or Akshakasti or clavicle ) is named as shalakya tantra.(Sushrutha)

Synonyms   (1)    Shalakya Tantram
           (2)    Urdwanaga Chikitsa
           (3)    Jathru Urdwa Chikitsa
           (4)    Utthamanga Chikitsa.

(1)    Shalakya Tantra
It is the science in which " Shalaka " is used frequently for the diagnosis as well as treatment of ear nose throat and eye diseases, which are seated above the Clavicle.
(2)    Urdwanga or Jathru Urdwa Chikitsa :- It is the science that deals with the organs seated above the Jathru /clavicle ) so only named as Jathru Urdwachikitsa or Urdwanga Chikitsa.
(3)    Utthamanga Chikitsa :- Shiras (Head) is explained as Utthamangam for the existence of pranas Indrias and its belongings in it, so only shalakya Chikitsa is named as Utthamanga Chikitsa.

While describing the importance of uttamanga, vagbhata compared the shiras to the root of tree and body to the stem of the tree. If the root is nourished tree survives, if not destroys, like wise if the head is protected health is maintained, if not death follows. So only it is advised to protect the shiras against the injuries and diseases and it is explained as utthamanga chikitsa.

" The specialists of shalakya is known as shalakini or shalaki ".

# Availability of Shalakya literature in Ayurvedic Samhitas:-

The original text books of shalakya (nimi tantra or others) are not available, from the following books we get the shalakya literature references:-

## 1) Sushrutha references :-

(a)  **Sushrutha utthara stana** 1 to 26 chapters.
Netra, karna, Nasa and shiro rogas explained.
(he has written this by following Nimi tantram only)

(b)  **Sushrutha Nidana :-** and chikitsa 22nd chapter,
Mukha rogas explained

(c)  **Sushrutha Sthana:-** 16 Chapter explained Karna chedana, Bandhana, Sandhana ; Nasa-ostha sandhana, description of karna etc.

## 2) Charaka references :-

a) **Sutra Stana**  In 17th Chapter explained about shiro rogas and in 18 chapter explained about upajihwaka, Gala Shundi, Rohini.

b) **Chikitsa Stana**  In 11th chapter, Dantha mukha chikitsa, 26th Chapter, Nasa shiro mukha. Karna netra chikitsa. Discription of pindi bidalaka and anjana and abhishyanda

c) **Siddhi Stana**  In 2. 9 chapters, shirovirechana Shiro vasti, Shankhaka, Arthavabhedak, ananthavatha - Lakshanas & Chikitsa ex plained eye diseases are 94 according to him.

3)  Vagbhata utthara stanam  - 8 to 24 chapters - detailed.explanation is given like in Sushrutha utthara sthanam. According to vagbhata eye diseases are 95. We get the shalakya references from the following also:

Bhavaprakash,                                 Sarangadhara samhitha

Madhava Nidana                               Chakradatta, Vangasena
Gadanigraha                                    Hareetha samhitha
Yogaratnakar                                   Basava rajeeva (Telugu)
Vaidya Chinthamani                          Dhanvanthari, etc.,

# Shalakya tantra Acharya Rishies :-

Perfect history of shalakya tantram is not available," Videhadipa"  The king of Videha or Tirahutadipa, " Nimi or Janaka or Videha" got the Authority on Shalakya tantram, who wrote " Videha tantra " or " Nimi tantra " - But the original book is not available

Among the existing books, only in Sushrutha utthara sthanam we get much more matter related to shalakya and Sushrutha himself mentioned That " he followed Nimi tantram" while writing the shalakya part of susrutha utthara stanam.

By sushrutha's above words it is clear that Nimi is the authentic for shalakya. In addition to Nimi the following rishies (Saints) also worked and wrote the books on shalakya tantram. they are. Karala, Bhadraka, - Kankayan Garghya, Galava, Shaunaka, Chakshushyena, Chakshyushya, Bhoja, Bhrugu, Sathyaki, Krishnathreya, etc., the above references were mentioned in the commentories of sushrutha and charaka (By Dalhana and Chakrapani etc.) Neither the books nor the specific history is available now.

## NIMI

The names, Nimi-Videha - Janaka are controvercial, whether they are one or different, the majority accepts as one and called by different names. References Related to the identity of Nimi-Janaka-Videha.

1)      a) Videhadipa - the king of videha means - janaka,
        b) Videhapida keerthitha - itthi Nimi praneetha (Dalhana) Dalhana Commented that Janaka is known as Nimi.

2)      a) In charaka sutra stana 26th chapter - Nimi is explained as the king of videha.
        b) In charaka chikitsa 26th chapter, while giving the classfication of eye diseases, he said eye diseases are 76 according to videha.
        c) In charaka shareera, 6th chapter Janaka is explained as the king of videha.
        In above 3 references the same person is called by 3 names ( syn onyms) (Nimi Janaka videha)

3)      According to Gireendhranath (Historian) the above 3 persons were different, not one.

4)      As per Ramayan and puranas Nimi is the king of videha, mithi, is his son Janaka is mithi's son - So Nimi is the first person of the generation and janaka is the last one.

        " According to above discription above 3 were different."

5)      According to Bauddha grantha " Majja Manikaya ", Nimi is the last person of his generation. and Karala janaka is his son.

6)      As per kashyapa samhitha - siddhi stanam - 116 - page Janaka is named as the king of videha.

7)      As per Astanga Sangraha - Indu commentory - uttarastana 126 and 314 pages - Janaka is mentioned as the king of videha.

8) Videhadipa keerthitha - Nimi Praneetha - videha vachanath these 3 words are generally used by the commentators - That indicates they are one but called differently.

9) As per Brahma vyvartha purana, Janaka is the disciple of lord Surya.

10) According to shalihothri samhitha - Ist part 104 page Janaka and videha were explained as different persons.

11) In Gada nigrah he used the names of Nimi and videhadipa, word as synonyms so it is very difficult to conclude whether Nimi Janak and videha are one or different. But majority accepts that they are one.

## Nimi's period :-

1) He Studied shalakya (Ayurveda) from Indra, along with Aathreya, Kashyapa, Dhanwanthari, Alambayan. So Nimi and above Acharyas were of same period.        A.S. Sutra Stana 2nd page.

2) In Chaithra ratha vanam - In a Meeting he participated along with Athreya, Kankayan etc.     Cha-Sutra Stana 26 Chapt.3-7 Pages.

3) In Alochana gosti he participated along with varyovid and Kankayan Kashyapa Samitha sutra, 27 Page.

4) He Lived 200 yrs before Maha Bharatha Yuddham (Baudha Jathaka Kathas)

5) He lived 320- 350 years before Dhanwanthari (puranas).

6) Because of Vashista Abhishapa he lost his body so they were( Nimi and Vashista) of same period.

7) Nimi (the king of Ayodya and ) vikukshi shashada, pururava were of same period.

Because of inperfect history, it is not possible to fix the time of Nimi.

**A story related to Nimi :-** (Reference) Bhagavatha Navama Scanda (9th Scanda) Trayodasha Adyaya (13th chapter)

Once the king of videha - Nimi - proposed to conduct a yagyam along with Brahmins. He asked Rajarshi vashista to be as purohith to complete the yagyam. But because of previous appointment with Indra (Deva Raja) he got ready to go to heaven and said to Nimi to wait upto his arrival. Vashista did late so Nimi Completed the yagyam with other Brahmins. After his arrival Vashista heard the news, got angry and cursed Nimi to lost his body. Devatas were pleased with Nimi's yagyam and blessed him for rebirth. But Nimi refused to enter into his old body, then devates told him to stay in the eye lids of the people. The opening and closing of eye lids is termed as Nimesha, it is derived from the word Nimi for his presence in the eye lids.

12

For taking rebirth he is called as Janaka. His dead body was undergone Manthama so he got named as Mithi, he lost his body by vashista Abhishapa and remained without body so he was named as Videha. (king of Videha) By staying in eye lids and performing Nimeshana kriya (opening and closing of eye lids) he is named as Nimi .

**2nd story :-** Once videha raja-Rajarshi Janaka Conducted Alambha yagya along with Brahmins - Bhagavan Amshumali cursed him to lost his sight - Janaka did Tapas, Lord surya was pleased and taught Chakshurveda (Science of Opthalmology) to Janaka, like that Shalakya tantra was brought to earth.

## Other Rishies who worked on Shalakya

1) **Kankayana tantram : -** It is not available now, the book reference is given by Dalhana.
   1) He attended the meeting which was arrranged by Dhanwantari (Dalhana )
   2) He is the Doctor of Bahleka (Bahleeka Bhishak) (Charak)
   3) He had so many disciples (Gadanigraha Ist part 103 Page)
   4) He Participated in the meeting (Panditha sabha)along with Nimi, Bhoja etc. which was conducted near by Himalayas (Himavath Parvatha Parshwa).
   5) The Medicine Kankayana vati might be his remedy.
   6) He was at Romapada assembly (Aasthana vaidya) (Palakapya Hastyayurveda)
   7) 4 yogas were mentioned by him  - (reference History of Indian medicine 2nd part - 465/466 pages)

2) **Karala Tantra :-** Written by A) Karala Bhadra or a) Karala bhatt, It is not available, the book reference is given by Gireendhranatha Mukhopadyaya and Shri, Gananada sena. He is also named as Karala Janaka Ref: (Shalihothra) According to him Netra rogas are 96 (Ref : Chakrapani), Nimi was his teacher. (Ref:- Astanga Sangraha Sutra Sthana)

3) **Garghya :-** In the History Garghya name reference is available at different places, and identity is very difficult.
   1) He attended the maha rishies meeting which was arranged near by Himalayas.
   2) He was in the assembly of Romapada (Palakapya Hastyayurved).
   3) Kashyapa, panini and yask mentioned his name .
   4) Garghya, Galava Nimi, Kankayan were of same period (Dalhan)
   5) He is the author of shalakya tantra (Harishastri in A. Hrudaya).
   6) He is also expert in vastu and vyakarana.

13

**4)    Galava :-** 1) He also attended the Rishies assembly (gathering) which was conducted near by Himalayas.2)He has written the Shalakya tantra, Sarvaloka Chikitsa, Rigveda Krama patha, Shiksha pranayana,Vyakarnana, KamaShastra etc.3)He is the disciple of Dhavanthari (Dalhana's reference)

**5)    Sathyaki :-** 1) Dalhana mentioned his name as the author of shalakya text.2) His name is famous - He introduced the coucching system of treatment for cataract, even now this method is practising by some people in north India.(The tradition is known as sathyakeeya sampradaya or Sathiye. 3) According to him Netra rogas are. 80.4) He is the brother of Lord ShriKrishna and friend of Arjuna. 5) He mentioned shirah kampa as incurable disease.


**6) Chakshushyena tantram : -** The reference is given by Gananatha sena and Shrikantha as it is a book on Shalakya tantra.


**7)    Bhoja :-** He worked on shalya and shalakya, book is known as Bhoja samhitha or Bhoja prabandha, the references are given by Gayadasa and Dalhana.

**8)    Bhrugu Tantra :-** The Book is not available now, his yogas are present in the available shalakya books for the treatment of Timira, shukra, etc.

**9)    Krishnathreya :-** Son of Atri and Chandrabhaga, Because of different references the exact identity is difficult. The reference is given by Srikantha datta and shivadasa sena. These people mentioned so many yogas of Atreya, in their texts.

**10)   Shaunaka Tantram :-** The Book is not available, His name is famous in the history but the perfect identity is difficult as the author of shalakya text.1) According to chakrapani & Dalhana he is known as the author of Shalakya text.2) He attended the rishi parishad which was conducted at near by Himalayas.3) He is the author of the book Bhriha.devatha.4) His shalakya references available in Sushrutha Shareera 3-32 (Dalhana commentory ) charaka sutra 11th chapter (Chakrapani. comm) Shaunaka, Bhadra Shaunaka, madra Shaunaka etc names available in the History. Acharya Gananatha sena said that above people are not one they are separate individuals.

" Neither Nimi Tantra Nor other books available.

# NETRA SHAREERAM
## (Anatomy of eye - Ayurvedic aspect )

**Synonyms :-** Netra, Nayana, Chakshu, Akshi, Netra Golaka, Nayana budbuda, Akshi golaka, Drusti, Linga etc.

**Netra uthpathi : -** It is gyanendria adhistanam meant for rupa grahanam (for the perception of vision) .

1) Indrias derived from atma, in particular Netra Indriam derived from agni maha bhuta <u>Sushrutha.</u>

2) Satwa guna + Raja guna + Agni bhutha = Chakshurendriam <u>(A.H)</u>

3) Drusti is formed by the essence of Kapha, Raktha and Panchamaha bhutas. Shukla Mandalam - by the essence of Kapha (Pithruja) Krishna Mandala by Raktha (Mathruja), and Drusti mandala By both <u>(A.Sangraha).</u>

4) Drusti formed by the essence of pancha maha bhutas with agni bhuta predominence.

| | | |
|---|---|---|
| Mamsa | - | By pruthwi maha bhuta |
| Raktha | - | Agni |
| Krishna Mandalam | - | Vayu |
| Swetha Mandalam | - | Jala |
| Ashru Margam | - | Aakasha |

Anatomical words of Netra available in old Samhitas:-

Pakshma (eye lashes), varthma (eye lids), swetha mandala (Sclera - bulbar conjunctiva), Krishna Mandal ( Cornea - iris ), Drusti mandala (pupil - Lens - retina), Pakshma Varthma sandhi (Lid Margins), Krishna drusti sandhi (Pupillary margin), Kaneenika sandhi ( inner canthus) Apanga sandhi (outer canthus), Patala (Tunics,) Ashru Pinda (Lacrimal gland), Ashru Sira (Lacrimal Ducts), Ashru Vahini (L. Canaliculi ) Netra nadi (Optic nerve).

## TRANSLATED WORDS AVAILABLE IN LATEST BOOKS

Sautrika Patala (Fibrous coat), Raktha vahini maya ranjitha patala (Vascular layer), Nadi Patala (Nervous Layer), Bahya patala (Sclera), Krishnamandala, (Cornea), Taramandalam (Iris), Madhya Patala (Choroid), Sandhana mandalam or Tanthu samuha (Cilliary body), Sandhana peshi (Cilliary muscle), Kaneenika Sankochaka (constrictor Pupillae), Kaneenika Vispharaka (Dilator Pupillae) poorva jala maya rasa Khanda (Anterior chamber), Jalamaya rasa or Tejorasa (Aqueous humour), Pashchima khanda (Posterior chamber), Sandra medo drava (Vitreous humour), Drusti peetha (Macula Lutea), Nadisheersha (optic disc), drusti vithana or Drusti patal (Retina), Bhru (eye brow), Tala bandhan (Suspensary ligament) Drusti Patalantharbhaga (ora serrata), Netracchada or varthma (eye lids), Ashru dwara (punctum), Ashrunala (Lacrimal canaliculi), Ashru aashaya (lacrimal sac), Ashru pinda (Lacrimal gland), Nasa gatha Ashru vahika (Naso Lacrimal duct).

**Note : -**    1to 6, Translated names for extra ocular muscles and
7to 10    "    "    Nerves, they are
1)    Bahyasta sarala or sarala bahir netra chalani or bahir darshini
(Lateral rectus Muscle).
2)    Antasta sarala or Saralantar netra chalani or Antar darshini
(Medial rectus muscle).
3)    Urdwasta sarala or sarala urdwa netra chalani or adho darshini
(inferior rectus).
4)    Urdwasta vakra, vakrodwa netra chalani or vakrordwa darshini
(superior oblique muscle).
5)    Adhasta vakra or vakradho netra chalani or vakradho darshini (inferior oblique muscle) 6) Druk nadi (optic nerve) 7) Netra Chestani nadi (Oculo motor nerver) 8) Katakshinee nadi (Trochlear nerve) 9)Tridhara nadi (Trigeminal nerve)

## Netra Shareer :-

Nayana budbudam (eye ball) is almost in round shape and resembles the teet of a cow (Go sthanakram) it is formed by the essence of Panchamaha bhutas (Pancha bhutha prasadajam) with Agni bhutha predominence.

## Netra pramanam :-

"I angula =Breadth of thumb (individuallly)(Swa angustodara Sammitham) Bahulyam =2 angulas and sarvatah pramana 2 1/2 angulas and the commentry is as follows but not confirmatory
1)    Bahulayam of Netra :-
or
Agra pashchath pramanam
or                                    Dwi angulas
Antah pravesha pramanam        =    (Two angulas)
or
Antero Posterior diameter (some authors)

2)    Sarvatah Pramanam
Aayama and Visthara
a) Aaayama or
Poorva Pashchima Pramanam or =    2-1/2 angulas
Antero Posterior diameter or        (Dalhana 3-1/2 angula
Vertical diameter

b) Visthara or
Utthara dakshina pramana or    =    -do-
Horizontal diameter

**Note** :- Discription of Natra sharera having controversy, Ex. some authors discribed the aayam - visthara means circumference of eye ball, and the distance between kaneenika to apanga.

3.     **Krishna mandalal pramanam**
(Netraayama tri bhaganthu krishna mandalamucchyathe)

A)     = $\underline{Netra\ Aayama} = 5/2/3 = 5/6$ angulas
             3

(B)          Dwi yava pramanam (Dalhana)

4)           **Drustimandala Pramanam :-**

a)     (Krishnaath saptha micchanthi drusti)
       $\underline{Krihsna\ mandala\ pramanam}$
                   7
       $= 5/6/7 = 5/42$ angulas (S.U. 13)

b)     (Navama stharakamsho drusti )
       $\underline{Krihsna\ Mandala\ pramanam}$
                   9
       $5/6/9 = 5/54$ angulas (SU, sutra)

c)     Masura dala pramanam

d)     Artha masura dala pramanam (Sarangadhara teeka)

5)     **Patala pramanam :-**
       $\underline{Drusti\ pramanam}$
                   5          (Pancha mamsha samam drusti)
       $5/42/5 = 1/42$ angulas

Eye ball is formed by the essence of pancha mahabhutas, the following parts are formed by the corresponding bhutha predominence.

| Part of the eye | Bhutha predominence |
|---|---|
| 1) Mamsa | Pruthwi maha bhutha |
| 2) Raktha | Agni       " |
| 3) Krihsna  Mandalam | Vayu       " |
| 4) Swetha mandalam | Jala       " |
| 5) Ashru margam | Aakasha    " |

### Parts of Nayana budbuda (eye ball)

| | | | |
|---|---|---|---|
| 1) Mandala | Circles of eye ball | - | 5 |
| 2) Sandhies | Junctions of   " | - | 6 |
| 3) Patalas | tunics of       " | - | 6 |

# NETRA MANDALA

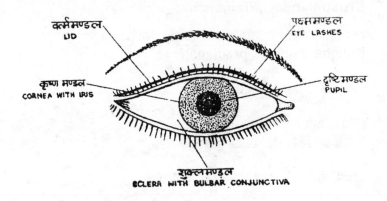

कर्ममण्डल
LID

पक्ष्ममण्डल
EYE LASHES

कृष्ण मण्डल
CORNEA WITH IRIS

दृष्टि मण्डल
PUPIL

शुक्लमण्डल
SCLERA WITH BULBAR CONJUNCTIVA

# NETRA SANDHI

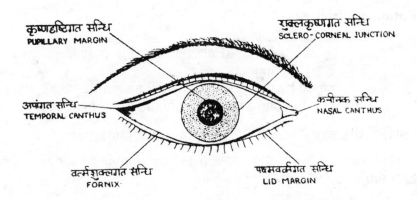

कृष्णदृष्टिगत सन्धि
PUPILLARY MARGIN

शुक्लकृष्णगत सन्धि
SCLERO-CORNEAL JUNCTION

अपांगगत सन्धि
TEMPORAL CANTHUS

कनीनक सन्धि
NASAL CANTHUS

वर्त्मशुक्लगत सन्धि
FORNIX

पक्ष्मवर्त्मगत सन्धि
LID MARGIN

## A) Mandalas

Five in number, having circular form, arranged in " anu purva " order (From with out to inwards) Ex. Pakshma mandalam is the outer most part and the drusti mandalam is the most interior part.

1) Pakshma mandalam    -    Circle of eye lashes
2) Varthma mandalam    -    circle of eye lids
3) Swetha or Shukla Mandam - Sclera and bulbar conjunctiva.
4) Krishna Mandalam  - Cornea and Iris

(Infact cornea is colour less fresh and transparant, but appears black due to the iris which is exactly behind)

5) Drusti mandalam  - (pupil - lens - Retina.)
1) It is in the size of masura dala   2) Formed with the pancha maha bhutas
3) Having vivara Akruthi (circular or hole like)
4) Shines like khadyotha (Spark like)  5) Covered by a layer infront
6) Cool things or items are helpful or suitable.

**Note :-** Detailed description is given at Drusti rogas.

**B) Sandhies : -** Junctions betweeen mandalas, 6 in number, they are
1) Pakshma varhtma sandhi -(Lid margins) junction between eye lid and eye lashes.
2) Varthma shukla sandhi  - Fornix (superior & inferior) originally it is the fold of conjunctival sac, but appears to be sandhi of varthma and shukla mandala (If we take palpebral conjuctiva the internal lining of varthma as varthma, and shukla mandala as bulbar conjunctiva its juction is exactly the fornix).
3) Shukla Krishna sandhi - (Limbus) sclero corneal junction.
4) Krishna drusti sandhi  - exact identity is not possible, but can be taken as pupillary margin. 5) Kaneenika sandhi - inner canthus, It is the junction of 2 lids at Nasal side (nasa sameeepa sthitha sandhi (Dalhana), 6) Apanga sandhi - outer canthus. It is the junction of 2 lids at temporal side. (Bhru pucchantha sthitha sandhi) (Dalhana)

**c) Patalas :-**  2      varthma patalas (eye lids)
          4      Akshi patalas
    Total   6

**Netra patalas :-** It is the site for the dreadful disease timira (immature cataract) and Linganaasha (Mature cataract) exact correlation is not possible to patalas. But can be understood asthe tunics of eye ball which are responsible for the refraction (Refractive media).

**Ist patala :-**   Tejo jalaashrayam

        **Tejo :-**        Alochaka pittashraya Rakthadhathu.

        **Jala :-**        Twak aashraya rasa dhathu.

      The cornea + aqueous humour which is the Ist layer of Refractive media can be correlated to the Ist patala.

(Teja - bright transparant cornea, Jala - Transparant, watery aqueous humour)

## 2nd Patala

### PISHITHAASRITHAM (musclular layer)

      The second layer of eye ball, Iris, cilliary body and (choroid) which is behind the cornea can be compared to 2nd patala, probably for containing cilliary muscle constrictor and dilator pupillae muscles, which are responsible for accommodation, contraction and dilatation of pupil.

## 3rd Patala :-

### MEDO AASHRITAM (Fatty Layer)

It is the layer, that should be interior to musclular layer, for the correlation different opinions present, they are as follows.

a) Lens is explained as 3rd patala for its position next to uvea (2nd layer).

b) Vitreous is explained as 3rd patala for appearing like medas (fat).

c) Lens, and vitreous together explained as 3rd patala by most of the authors.

## 4th Patala :-

### ASTI PATALA (Bony layer)

      Exact correlation is not possible, different opinions are here under.

a) Some authors explained Lens as Asti Patala because of its solid appearence and gving seat for the dreadful disease timira (Videha said that Timira vyadhi is patalashritha vyadhi)

b) Some authers named it as Akshi patala and told Retina as 4th patala which is responsible for rupa garahanam ( Visual perception)

c) Some authors explained the 4 patalas as the tunics of lens which is the seat for Timira vyadhi (Cataract).

**Note :-** Some sanskrit Commentators counted the number from interior to exterior as

| | | |
|---|---|---|
| Asti Aashraya | | Ist patala |
| Medo | " | 2nd patala |
| Mamsa | " | 3rd patala |
| Tejo Jala | " | 4th Patala |

      It is opposite to the previous explanation. Because of the different opinions, exact correlation and conclusion of patalas is not possible.

**Vagbhata :-** He has not mentioned the number of sandhies, and not explained the pakshma mandala in mandalas.

**Bhavamishra :-** He has not explained the number of sandhies.

**Sarangadhara :-** First mentioned the sandhies as 4 and the 5th Kaneenika sandhi explained during the discription of the disease and left the 6th Apanga sandhi (5 sandhies explained).

**Yogarathnakar :-** He explained just like Sushrutha but counted the Netra Patalas as 4 (he left the 2 Bahya Patalas)

## Netra Kriya Vigyan

| Indriartham | Gyanendriam | Predominent Bhutamsha |
|---|---|---|
| Shabda | Experienced by   Shravan indriam | Akasha |
| Sparsha | "                           Twak        " | Vayu |
| Rupa | "                           Nayana   " | Agni |
| Rasa | "                           Jihwa      " | Jala |
| Gandha | "                           Ghrana   " | Pruthwi |

One Indiriam receives its specific Indriartham only - because of common bhutha predominence between them.

**Ex**. eye (Nayanendriam) Receive Rupam because of Tejo predominence.
For perception of Indriartham by Indrias the following things are needed.

Aatma -        Manas        -        Indrias -        Indriarthas

If this chain is interrupted, objects are not received

**Ex.:-** In the absence of concentration (Anya manas while thinking some thing else), a person can't identify the things though he has observed.

Aatma along with manas stimulates the Alochaka pitta which resides in the eye, by that external objects are focussed and stimulus carried through the vata vahini srotas and with the Interference of Indria bhudhi (Darshana Bhudhi) only the objects are visualised and distinguished accordingly.

## NETRA GUHA (Orbit)

**Synonyms :-** Shrungataka, Bhruchakra , Akshikuta ,Netra guha

### Contents of shrungataka (orbit) according to Ayurvedic science.

1) Eye ball (Netra)
2) Eye lids (Varthma)
3) Veins arteries nerves (Sira, damani, Nadi)
4) Kosha - (Sacs :- conjunctival sac & Lacrimal sac etc)
5) Ashruvaha shrotas (Lacrimal gland and Lacrimal apparatus.)

Clear discription is available about the Lacrimal secretion and its flow in samhitas.

1) Lacrimal fluid is secreted by Ashru pinda (L.gland)

2) Through sira (Ashru pranalika) (Jala vahini) the fluid reaches Netra sandhi (Videha) or varthma shukla sandhi (Vagbhata) (i.e. fornix)

3) From Netra sandhi the fluid collects in the Kaneenika sandhi (inner canthus) From here the fluid is eliminated out

## CONTENTS OF ORBIT THAT BINDS THE EYE BALL

Eye ball is fixed properly in the orbit by the following contents.

1)    Sira (Veins arteries and Nerves)

2)    Kandara (Tendons and Ligaments)

3)    Meda - orbital fat

4)    Kalakasti - Fascia that is attached to the bony cavity

5)    Sleshma bandana - especially the eye ball is supported by the orbital fat.

## ANATOMY OF ORBIT (AKSHI GUHA - NETRA GUHA)

The orbits are a pair of pyramidal cavities, situated one on each side of nose, it appears like dathura flower. Orbits are formed by the combination of following 7 bones

1)    Frontal bone (Lalata asthi )        2) Sphenoid bone (Jathukaasthi)

3)    Ethmoid bone (Bharbharaasthi)        4) Maxilla (Urdhwa Hanu asthi)

5)    Palatal bone (Talu asthi)        6) Lacrimal bone (Ashru asthi)

7)    Malor bone or zygomatic bone (Gandaasthi.)

**Measurements of orbit :-** Antero posteriorly -5 to 8 cm. Vertically (at base) and Horizontally (at base) 4 c.m.

**Parts of orbit :-**        1) Base 2) Apex 3) Roof (Superior wall) 4) Floor (inferior wall ) (5) Medial wall) 6) Lateral wall.)

**1) Base :-** It is known as orbital margin, quadrangular in shape directed forwards. laterally and slightly downwards.

Formed above by        1) Supra orbital margin of frontal bone

Laterally by        1) Frontal process of zygomatic (mainly)
2) Zygomatic process of frontal (partly)

Inferiorly by        1) Zygomatic bone (Lateral half)
2) Maxilla (Medial half)

Medially by    1) Anterior Lacrimal crest of the frontal process of maxilla.
2) Medial end of the supra orbital margin of frontal.

**2)      Apex :-** It corresponds to the optic canal which is behind and towards medially, it is at the medial end of the superior orbital fissure.

**3)      Roof** :- Triangular and concave, separates the orbital cavity from an terior cranial Fossa.

**Formed by :**   a) Orbital plate of frontal bone, infront
                  b) Under surface of lesser wing of sphenoid, behind

**It contains :-** 1) Lacrimal fossa for the orbital part of Lacrimal gland.
                   2) Trochlear spine or fossa -Gives attachment to superior oblique muscle of orbit.
                   3) Optic canal  - transmits optic nerve (Drusti nadi) and oph thalmic artery.
                   4) A common tendinous ring gives origin to intra ocular muscle

**4)      Floor :-** Formed by 1) Orbital plate of maxilla (mainly)
                     2) Orbital plate of zygomatic bone, antero laterally
                     3) Orbital Process of palatine bone, posterio medially

It separates the orbital cavity from maxillary air sinuses.

**It contains :-** 1) Infra Orbital groove and canal for the Transmission of infra orbital vessels and nerves.2) Upper opening of Naso Lacrimal canal at antero medial angle 3) A small depression, lateral to the upper opening of Lacrimal canal gives origin to inferior oblique muscle of orbit.

**4) Inferior orbital fissure:-**Lies between the floor and lateral wall posteriorly. It transmits 1) Maxillary division of Trigeminal nerve (5th cranial nerve) 2)Zygomatic nerve 3) Branches of spheno Palatine ganglion 4) Infra orbital artery 5) Branches from inferior ophthalmic vein to the pterigoid venous plexus.

**5) Medial Wall :-** QuadriLateral in shape, medial walls of the two orbital cavities are almost parallel to each other.

Formed by (from before backwards)
1) Frontal process of maxilla.               2) Lacrimal bone
3) Orbial plate of the labrynth of ethmoid bone.    4) Body of sphenoid.

It separates the orbital cavities from ethmoidal air sinuses and the anterior part of sphenoid air sinuses.

**It contains :-** 1) Lacrimal groove for lacrimal sac, this groove separates the orbital cavity from Nasal cavity.

2) Anterior lacrimal crest of the frontal process of maxilla gives attachment to medial palpebral ligament, lacrimal fascia and gives attachment to orbicularis oculi.

3) Posterior lacrimal crest of the lacrimal bone gives attachment to lacrimal fascia and gives origin to lacrimal head of orbicularis oculi.

4) Anterior and posterior ethmoidal foramina for the transmission of corresponding vessels and nerves.

**6) Lateral Wall :-** It is the thickest of all parts of orbit and separates the orbital cavity from middle cranial fossa, formed by 1) orbital surface of the frontal process of zygomatic bone infront 2) orbital surface of the greater wing of sphenoid, behind.

**Contains :-** 1) Openings for zygomatico facial and zygomatico temporal nerves. 2) A small tubercle, lower to the superior orbital fissure, gives origin to intra ocular muscles of the orbit.

3) Superior orbital fissure lies between lateral wall and roof posteriorly, gives transmission for 3rd (Netra chestanee nadi, oculomotor) 4th (Katakshinee nadi-Trochlear Nerve, 6th (Netra parshwaki Nadi-Abducent nerve) and Ist part of trigeminal nerve). Ophthalmic vein, recurrent lacrimal artery, sympathetic fibres from cavernous sinus and cilliary ganglian.

**In Brief :-** The follwing openings (foramina) Present in <u>orbit</u>
1)      Optic foramina for optic Nerve
2)      Superior orbital (foramina) Fissure for 3,4,5 (Ist division) and 6th cranial nerves.
3)      Inferior orbital (Foramina) fissure for 2nd divison of 5th cranial nerve.
4)      Anterior and posterior ethmoidal foramina for corresponding vessels and nerves.
6)      Lacrimal canal
7)      Openings for zygomatico temporal and zygomatico facial nerves.
8)      Supra orbital fissure
9)      Infra orbital fissure      for corresponding vessels and nerves.

## Contents of orbits
1) Eye ball and intra orbital part of optic nerve
2) Tenon's capsule (it forms a socket in which eye ball moves, it extends from limbus to the attachment of optic nerve.)
3) Extra ocular muscles for the movement of eye ball in different directions
    (4 Recti muscles and 2 oblique muscles).
4) Lacrimal gland and lacrimal sac.
5) Ophthalmic artery with its branches.
6) 3rd, 4th, 5th (ist and 2nd branches only ) and 6th cranial nerves
7) Branches from carotid and cavernous plexus of sympathetic.
8) Cilliary ganglian 9) Orbital fat and fascia
        (Description will be given at relevent chapters).

24

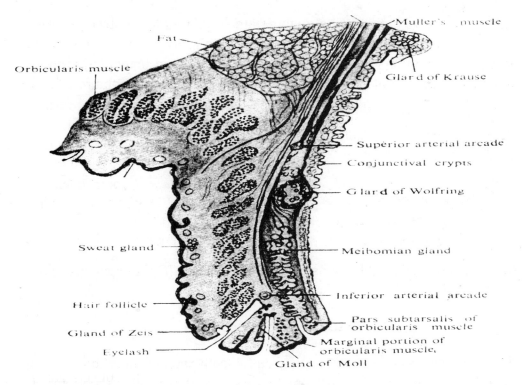

Fig. 10-4. Vertical section through th

Labels on figure: Müller's muscle, Fat, Gland of Krause, Orbicularis muscle, Superior arterial arcade, Conjunctival crypts, Gland of Wolfring, Sweat gland, Meibomian gland, Inferior arterial arcade, Hair follicle, Pars subtarsalis of orbicularis muscle, Gland of Zeis, Marginal portion of orbicularis muscle, Eyelash, Gland of Moll

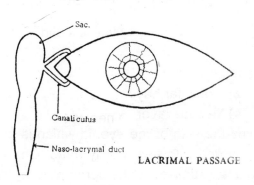

Sac.

Canaliculus

Naso-lacrymal duct

LACRIMAL PASSAGE

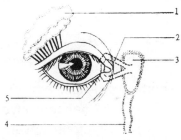

1
2
3
5
4

Lacrimal system:
1—lacrimal gland, 2—lacrimal duct, 3—lacrimal sac, 4—naso-lacrimal duct, 5—lacrimal punctum

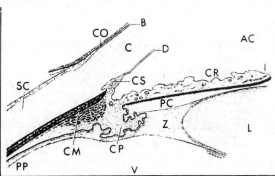

The region of the angle of the anterior chamber: AC, anterior chamber; B, Bowman's membrane; C, cornea; CM, ciliary muscle, CO, corneal epithelium; CP, ciliary processes; CR, iris crypts; CS canal of Schlemm; D, Descemet's membrane; I, iris; L, lens; PC, posterior chamber; PP, pars plana of ciliary body; SC, sclera; V, vitreous; Z, zonule of Zinn

25

The above mentioned structures are supported in the orbit by orbital fat. The periosteum lining the bony walls of the orbit is called peri orbitan; infront the orbital base is partially closed by a septum extending from the upper and lower orbital margins to the tarsal plates known as septum orbitale.

Arterial supply - Ophthalmic artery branch of Internal carotid artery.

**Veins :-** Drain into ophthalmic veins

**Nerve Supply**
**Motor:-**

| | | |
|---|---|---|
| Superior rectus muscle | - | 4th cranial neve |
| Lateral rectus muscle | - | 6th cranial nerve |
| rest of 4 muscles | - | 3rd cranial nerve |

**Sensory :-** Ist and 2nd divisions of Trigeminal Nerve (Ophthalmic nerve and maxillary nerve)

## Anatomy of eye lids

The eye lids are mobile tissue curtains placed infront of the eye ball, for protective functions, formed from before backwards by skin (Anterior part), loose connective tissue, muscle, tarsal plate, fascia and conjunctiva (posterior part). the eye lashes are attached to its margins, the lids contain glands, blood vessels, lymphatics and nerves.

The parts of eye lid can be divided like the following :
1) Cutaneous layer 2) Muscular Layer
3) Fibrous Layer 4) Mucous layer
1) Cutaneous layer :- It contains the skin of the eye lid which is extremely delicate, highly elastic and is covered with fine downy hairs. On looking straight or upwards a horizontal fold is visualised in the upper eyelid. Underneath the skin is the loose areolor tissue with no fat and is loosely attached to its underlying muscle and permits for easy accumulation of oedematous fluid or for the extravasation of blood underneath the skin.

2) Muscle layer :- Underneath the skin and cutaneous tissue is the muscle layer which consist of

a) Orbicularis oculi muscle :- It is an oval sheat of concentric muscle fibres, it covers the lids and the orbital margins.By contraction of this, the lids are firmy closed it is supplied by zygomatic nerve branch of facial nerve.

26

b) Levator palpebrae superioris - Present only in upper lid. Arises from the apex of orbit, passes underneath the roof and is inserted into the skin, upper parts of tarsus, fornix, conjunctiva and mid points of lateral and medial orbital margins. It is helpful for raising the upper lid (opening of eye ) and is supplied by upper division of occulomotor nerve (3rd cranial )

## 3rd Palpebral muscle of Muller :-

These are sheets of plain muscles one on each lid, in the upper lid the muscle arises from the surface of levator palpebre superioras and is inserted in to the upper margin of the tarsal plate. In the lower lid muscle arises from the fascial sheath of the inferior rectus and is inserted in to tarsal plate. It is supplied by cervical sympathetic.

**3) Fibrous layer :-** underneath the Orbicularis Muscle is the fibrous layer. consist of.

**a) Septum orbitale :-** it is a thin membrane of connective tissue extending from the proximal border of tarsal plate to the periosteum around the orbital margin. It is perforated by vessels and nerves entering the lids from the orbit.

**b) Tarsal plate :-** It is a thin plate of dense connective tissue one in each eye lid. Larger in upper lid, smaller in lower lid. It is present in betweeen muscle layer and mucous layer and responsible for its firmness.
Its connections to orbit.:-

It is connected to the lateral walls of orbit by medial and lateral tarsal ligaments and to the upper and lower borders of orbit with an aponeurotic fibrous layer known as palpebral fascia.The plate contain numerous meibomian glands (Sebacious glands) secretes oily secretion on to the lid margin.

4) Palpebral conjunctiva is thin, vascular and closely adherent to the tarsus.

## Glands of the eye lids :-
There are 3 types of glands in th eye lids.

**1)     Meibomian glands :-** Elongated glands, vertically placed in the tarsus and also known as tarsal glands, 30 to 40 glands in upper lid and 20 to 30 glands In the lower eye lid these are modified sebaceous glands, Secret oily secretion and opens to the lid margin just infront of its sharp posterior border.

**2) Glands of zeis :-** These are sebaceous glands developed as out growths of the epithelial wall of the hair follicles of the eye lashes, situated on the lid margin and opens into the follicles of the eye lashes.

**3) Glands of Moll :-** These are modified sweat glands, lie between the cilia on the lid margin, ducts open either into ducts of zeis or into follicles of cilia, and not directly on to the the surface of lid margin.

**Lid margin : -** It is the Anterior thick border of eye lid, the Anterior margin is rounded from which eye lashes originates and posteriorly sharp margin present. In betweeen anterior margin and openings of the meibomian glands there is a grey line konwn as inter marginal sulcus, Lid margins unite medially and laterally and form medial canthus and lateral canthus, at medial canthus a rounded space knwon as lacus lacrimalis, is present which is occupied by a small reddish elevation known as caruncle .

**Eye lashes :-** Stouter than hair and are arranged in 2 to 3 rows in upper lid and 1 to 2 rows in lower lid, the roots are deeply embeded in the connective tissue of the lid margin, upper lid lashes are curved forwards and upwards and lower lid eye lashes are downwards and forwards.

**Arterial supply :-**
1) Lacrimal Palpebral branches of ophthamic artery.
2) Facial artery
3) Superficial temporal artery
4) Infra Orbital artery.

**Venous drainage :-**
1) Opthalmic vein
2) Temporal vein
3) Facial vein

**Lymphatic drainage :-**
Outer half drains into pre auricular lymph glands, inner half drains into sub maxillary lymph glands.

**Sensory nerve supply :-**
Ist - 2nd branches of trigeminal nerve

**Motor** (1) Orbicularis oculi supplied by branches of facial nerve.
(2) Levator palpebre superioris Supplied by the branches of oculo motor.
(3) Palpebral muscle of muller supplied by the nerves derived from cervical sympathetic.

# LACRIMAL APPARATUS

The Lacrimal apparatus consits of a secretory portion (the lacrimal gland,) and an excretory portion which collects the tears and drains them into the nose.

**1)** **Lacrimal gland :-** It is a serous gland situated at the upper and outer part of the orbit, in a depression of the orbital plate of frontal bone known as the fossa for lacrimal gland. Anteriorly the gland is deeply divided into two upper orbital part, and lower palpebral part (Situated beneath the outer part of the upper conjuctival fornix), the ducts of the Lacrimal glands are about border of the tarsal plate of the upper lid.The histological structure resembles the salivary gland

## Accessory Lacrimal glands:-

The small glands exactly resembles the lacrimal glands.
1) Glands of krause :- About 20 in upper lid and 8 in lower lid deeply situated in the conjuctiva near the lateral part of fornix.
2) Glands of wolfring :- Few in number, situated near the upper border of the tarsal plate.

## Blood Supply :-

Arterial Supply : -     Lacrimal branch of ophthalmic artery and infra orbital branch of maxillary artery.
Venous drainage   :-   Lacrimal vein that opens into superior ophthalmic vein.
Lymphatic draiage :-  Conjunctival & palpebral lymph nodes pass into pre auricular lymph nodes.

## Nerve supply
1) Sensory :- Lacrimal branch of the ophthalmic division of trigeminal nerve.
2) Sympathetic :- Carotid plexus of cervical sympathetic
3) Motor :- Facial Nerve

## Lacrimal Passage

it consists of
1) Lacrimal puncta (Upper - Lower) 2) Lacrimal canaliculi (upper - lower)
3) Lacrimal sac -1  4) Naso Lacrimal duct -1

1) Lacrimal puncta :- 2 small openings one on each lid margin, 6mm from inner canthus, visible when lids are slightly everted.

2) Canalicul :- 2 in number, starts from puncta as a tubular passage 1-2mm verticle portion, and 6 to 7 mm horizontal protion. The two (upper - lower) Canaliculi open into the Lacrimal sac.

3) Lacrimal sac:- 13mm long and 6mm wide sac, situated in the lacrimal fossa, 2 canaliculi open at its lateral wall, inferiorly it is continuous with naso Lacrimal duct.

4) Naso Lacrimal duct:- Continuation of the sac, moves downwards and ends in the inferior meatus of the Nose.

**Arterial supply:** -(1) Palpebral branches of ophthalmic artery

2) Angular branch of facial artery.

3) Infra orbital & spheno palatine branches of internal maxillary artery .

**Venus return:-** Above into angular and infra orbital veins, below into pterigoid plexus and internal maxillary vein.

**Lymphatic drainage:-**Drains into sub maxillary lymphnodes.

**Nerve supply :-** Nasocilliary nerve & anterior superior alveolar nerve.

**Sympathetic :-** Sympathetic nerves in the orbit.

## LACRIMAL PASSAGE

Lacrimal glands secret the lacrimal fluid

Through Lacrimal ducts drains into Superior fornix of conjunctival sac

By gravity it comes to Inferior fornix of conjunctival sac and collects at Lacrimal Lake of inner canthus,

Then through Puncta enters into Lacrimal Canaliculi

From both canaliculi it opens into Lacrimal Sac

Through Naso Lacrimal duct enters into Inferior meatus of Nose. Like this the lacrimal fluid finally reaches the nose and evaporated by the heat of inhaled air.

## CONJUNCTIVA

Conjunctiva is a thin layer of mucous membrane which lines the under surface of eye lids and is reflected on to the anterior part of eye ball, forming a sac called conjunctival sac. It is named differently according to site they are

1) Palpebral conjunctiva

    a) Marginal      b) Tarsal    c) orbital

    a) Marginal   -   Lid margin to sulcus subtarsais.

    b) Tarsal     -   Conjunctiva that covers the tarsal plate

    c) Orbital     -   rest of the conjuctiva that covers the eye lid.

2) Fornix, Fold of conjunctiva formed by the reflection of the mucous membrane from the lid to the eye ball.

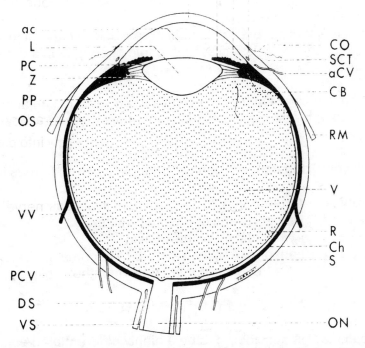

C I a CS

ac
L
PC
Z
PP
OS

VV

PCV

DS
VS

CO
SCT
aCV

CB

RM

V

R
Ch
S

ON

Diagram of a longitudinal section of the eyeball: a, angle of anterior chamber; ac, anterior chamber; aCV, anterior ciliary vessel; C, cornea; CB, ciliary body; Ch, choroid; CO, ocular conjunctiva; CS, canal of Schlemm; DS, dural sheath; I, iris; L, lens; ON, optic nerve; OS, ora serrata: PC, posterior chamber; PCV, posterior ciliary vessel; PP, pars plana; R, retina; RM, rectus muscle; S, sclera; SCT, sub-conjunctival tissue; V, vitreous; VS, vaginal sheath; VV, vortex vein; Z, zonule

EXAMINATION OF THE EYES AND THE VISUAL FUNCTIONS

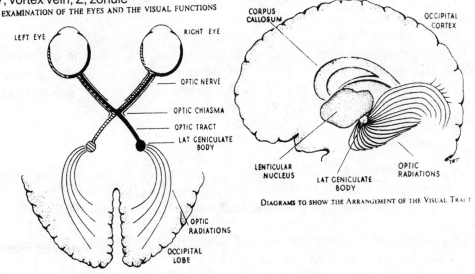

LEFT EYE
RIGHT EYE

OPTIC NERVE
OPTIC CHIASMA
OPTIC TRACT
LAT GENICULATE BODY

OPTIC RADIATIONS

OCCIPITAL LOBE

CORPUS CALLOSUM
OCCIPITAL CORTEX

LENTICULAR NUCLEUS
LAT GENICULATE BODY
OPTIC RADIATIONS

DIAGRAMS TO SHOW THE ARRANGEMENT OF THE VISUAL TRACT

3) Bulbar conjunctiva - It covers the anterior part of eye ball upto the limbus.
4) Conjunctiva of the Limbus
Conjunctiva that covers the Limbal area ( Sclero corneal junction)
5) Plica semilunaris - It is a crescentric fold of conjunctiva at inner canthus.

(The marginal Tarsal and Limbal conjunctiva firmly fixed to subjacent tissues and Bulbar, orbital, fornix conjunctiva loosely attached to the underlying tissues.)

**Histology** :-
1) Epithelial layer 2) substantia propria a) adenoid layer  b) fibrous layer.

**Arterial supply :-** Anterior and posteior conjunctival vessels.
**venous :-** Palpebral and ophthalmic veins.
**Lymphatic :-** Lymphatic channals of skin
**Nerve supply :-** sensory - a) cilliary nerve, b) Lacrimal nerve c) supra & infra trochleor nerves d) sympathetic plexus.

## ANATOMY OF EYE BALL

Eye ball may be considered to be a highly differentiated end organ of optic nerve, which is a sensary nerve, eye balls are two, and placed in a quadrilateral bony cavity known as orbit. It is  slightly assymmetrical sphere

**Topography of eye ball**
Antero posterior diameter
        or                          -    24.15mm (outer)
Sagittal diameter                    24.12mm (inner)

Transvers diameter         -      24.13 mm
Vertical diameter           -      24. 48 mm
Circumference               -      74.91 mm
(Dimensions are 1/2 mm less in ladies)
weight of the eye ball        7.5 grams
Volume of the eye ball        6.5 cc

Eye ball is merely a round structure consisting of an inelastic wall with a cavity inside, the wall is formed of 3 coats or tunics, they are
1) Outer fibrous coat, (2) middle vascular coat, 3) Inner nervous coat.

**1) Fibrous coat :-** It is outer inelastic supporting membrane of eye ball.
a) Anterior 1/6th part, transparent cornea .
b) Posterior 5/6th part, opaque sclera.

**a) Cornea :-** It is the clear, colourless smooth, transparent, anterior 1/6th part of outer fibrous coat, looks elliptical anteriorly and circular posteriorly, its curvature is not uniform, central part is (4 mm) in spherical, thinner, optical zone and the flattened, thicker part is peripheral zone.

| | | |
|---|---|---|
| Horizontal diameter | 11.7 | mm |
| Vertical diameter | 10.6 | mm |
| Radius of anterior curvature | 7.8 | mm |
| Radius of posterior curvature | 6.8 to 7 | mm |

Thickness

| | |
|---|---|
| Peripherally | 1.1 mm |
| Centrally | o.6 mm |

**Micro anatomy of cornea :-**
Cornea is composed of five layers from out to inwards

1) Epithelial membrane          (2) Bowman's membrane
3) Substantia propria (Stroma)   (4) Descemet's membrane
5) Endothelial membrane.

**1) Epithelium :-** It is regarded as the continuation of bulbar conjunctiva. 1/10 of the total thickness of cornea (50 to 100 u) stratified squamous in structure, superficially flattened, middle polygonal, deeper columnar cells and are arranged paralelly in uniform order thus prevents the admission of water salts, respiratory gases into the substantia propria (Self repairing zone)

**2) Bowman's membrane :-** It is a thin homogenous membrane, separates the epithelium from substantia propria, Once destroyed it cannot be regenerated. Thickness is 10 to 14 u.

**3) Substantia propria - (Stroma)**
The thickest of all layers, 9/10th of corneal thickness, may be regarded as forward continuation of sclera, stroma comprises of regularly, equidistantly arranged thin fibres of collagen, by this regularity of stromal components only the transparancy of cornea is maintained.

**4) Descemets membrane :-** 6 u in thickness, it is thin elastic membrane, separates stroma from endothelium. It is very resistant to infection and it can regenerate if destroyed.

**5) Corneal endothelium :-** It is a single layer of hexagonal cells, aimed to control the stromal hydration.

**Blood supply :-** Cornea proper is Avascular except 1-2 mm of its periphery (from circum corneal arterial plexus (derived from anterior ciliary arteries.)

**Nutrition to cornea:** (1) From circum corneal plexus
2) Diffusion from aqeous humour (3) from tears.

**Nerve supply :-** Corneal tissue is the most sensitive of all the body tissues.
1) Long cilliary nerves, the branches of Naso ciliary of Trigeminal nerve, gives
60 to 80 minute branches those spread from limbus to cornea, the fibres are
non medullated for optical reason.

**Sclera :-** Sclera forms the posterior 5/6th part of fibrous wall of eye ball. It is
pale white, strong, opaque and slightly elastic layer which maintain the contour (shape) of the eyeball
Its average thickness is 1mm. It is made up of bundles of collagenous fibres
with connective tissue corpuscles, it is covered by tenon's capsule and episcleral tissue, 4 recti muscles are inserted into sclera infront of the equator
and 2 obliqe muscles behind the equator of the eye ball.

The inner surface of sclera is separated from choroid by a potential space
called **supra choroidea**. Sclera gives 2 openings one Anteriorly (to join with
cornea) and another one posteriorly the **Lamina cribrosa,** for the exit of
optic nerve at posterior opening 2/3 of slcera continued as dural sheet of
optic nerve, 1/3 mixes with choroidal tissue, Sclera is perforated by many
vessels (a) Long posterior cilliary arteries (b) short posterior ciliary arteries
(c) Anterior ciliary arteries (d) Veinae verticose (6) Long and short ciliary
nerves. Though sclera traversed by many blood vassels, has a little vascular
supply, but episcleral tissue contains more blood supply.

**c) Limbus :-** It is a transition zone between cornea and sclera. It is about
1mm wide, epithelium is thick, upto 10 or more layers, stroma losts its regular arrangement here, The marginal vascular plexus derived from anterior
ciliary vassels, channel of schlemm present in the Limbus. The medial boundary of Limbus is formed by scleral spur and trabecular mesh, through the
pores of trabecular mesh only it communicates with anterior chamber, al-
lowing the usual drainage of aqueous from anterior chamber to general circulation to maintain normal intra ocular pressure. (18 to 24 mm Hg)

## 2)VASCULAR LAYER (Uveal Tract)

It is second or middle layer of eye ball, highly vascular, supplies nutrition to
the 3rd layer (Retina). It is termed as uveal tract. Formed of 3 parts (1) Iris,
(2) Ciliary body, (3) Choroid.

Iris and cilliary body or together called as Anterior Uvea, The Choroid is called as posterior Uvea. Anatomically above 3 parts are continuous and so the disease of one part easily spreads to the another.

**a) Iris :-** It is a circular, pigmented diaphragm hanging in between cornea (Anteriorly) and lens (posteriorly ) with central perforation (pupil). Iris divides anterior compartment of eye ball into two (a) Anterior chamber (the chamber betweeen iris and cornea) (b) Posterior chamber (the chamber between iris and Lens), its peripheral part is attached to the Anterio medial part of ciliary body.

It is made up of 4 layers from out to inwards.
1) Layer of endothelium (2) Iris stroma (3) Muscular layer
(constrictor pupillae -dilator pupillae) (4) Layer of pigments
Anterior surface of Iris is uneven and shows many crypts and fissures.

Spinctor pupillae or constrictor pupillae muscle is made up of circular fibres, situated close to the pupillary margin, supplied by Oculomotor nerve responsible for the constriction of pupil. Dilator pupillae muscle consists radial fibres extending from cilliary body to pupillary margin supplied by the cervical sympathetic nerves which is responsible for the dilatation of pupil.

**Pupil :** It is the circular central perforation of the iris about 3 to 4mm in diameter, large in young and smaller in the aged, It regulates the amount of light admitted into the eye, it becomes small (Contracted) in day time or in bright illumination and becomes big (dilated) at nights and in dim illumination, with the Action of constrictor pupilae and dilator pupillae muscles only constriction and dilatation of pupil takes place.

**Blood Supply :-** Greater vascular ring of iris formed by posterior and anterior ciliary arteries, gives branches to ciliary body and iris, the branches of iris converge at pupillary margin and form small circle of iris.

**Nerve Supply**   1)   oculomotor nerve
                   2)   Naso ciliary branch of ophthalmic division of
                        Trigeminal nerve
                   3)   Sympathetic nerve.

**b) Ciliary body :-** It is the middle part of vascular coat, Triangular in cross section with its base directed forwards and medially, the Apex becomes continuous with the anterior part of choroid . From the middle of the base the Iris arises. The lateral part of the base forms a part of the angle of anterior chamber.

Outer aspect of triangle contain ciliary muscle with 3 types of muscle fibres (meridional, radial and circular) in the Anterior half of inner surface contain 60 to 70 longitudinal folds knowon as ciliary process - secretes aqueous humour. Inner surface of cilliary body is covered by 2 layers of cubical epithelium to which fibres of suspensory ligament of Lens is attached.

**Blood supply :-**    Greater ring of iris
                    (Formed by Anterior and posterior ciliary arteries)

**Nerve Supply :-**    Sensory - Trigeminal nerve branches.
**Motor :-**    Oculomotor nerve.

**c) Choroid :-** Choroid forms the major portion of uveal tract posteriorly, lying in between sclera and retina, starting from posterior limit of ciliary body (at the level of ora serrata) to the opening of optic nerve. It consists of connective tissue with pigment contain chromatophores. outer surface is separated from retina by an elastic "Bruch's membrane".

Choroid can be divided into 5 layers as follows:

1)    Lamina supra Choroidea
        (attached to sclera by loose connective tissue)

2)    Layer of large vessels.

3)    Layer of middle sized vessels.

4)    Layer of choroidal capillaries.

5)    Lamina vitrea or bruch's membrane.

| | | |
|---|---|---|
| Function | : - | To give nourishment to retina and vitrious. |
| Blood Supply | :- | Short posterior ciliary arteries. |
| Venous return | :- | 4 vortex veins. |
| Nerve Supply : | :- | Trigeminal nerve branches. |

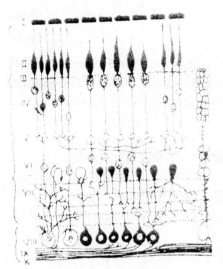

**Different layers of Retina**

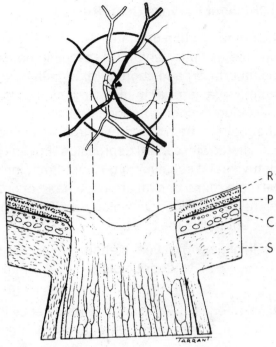

Physiological cup: R, retina; P, pigmentary epithelium; C, choroid; S, sclera

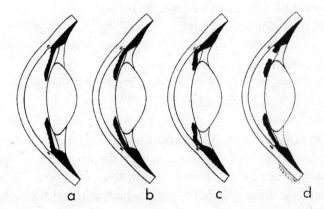

The anterior chamber and its angle. (a) in a normal eye with a wide angle; (b) in an eye with a narrow angle; (c) physiological iris bombe with a semi-dilated pupil; (d) restoration of the patency of the angle after peripheral iridectomy

## b) 3rd layer Nervous Coat (Retina)

The retina is a thin delicate membrane, contains a layer of nerve fibres, that continue as optic nerve. It is placed in between hyaloid membrane of vitreous (internally) and choroid (externally), It extends upto the Anterior end of choroid (ora serrata) in the living eye it is transparent and have faint purple-red colour, becomes opaque and white immediately after death. At the posterior pole of the retina presents a yellow spot, called macula lutea, 1-2 mm in diameter with central depression (Fovea centralis), this is the area of maximum visual discrimination, About 3mm innner side to the posterior pole of eye, pale round or oval area, the head of optic nerve (optic disc)present with central depression (physiological pit or cup) here the blood vessels of retina enter and leave the eye ball.

| The thickness of retina is about | 0.5 mm |
| Near optic disc | 0.2 mm |
| at equator | 0.1 mm |

retinal arteries have no anastomosis hence in occlusion of central artery there is no compensatory collateral circulation and so blindness results.

### Micro anatomy of retina :-
8 layer of nervous elements. 2 layers of supporting tissue (Fibres of muller) Blood supply :- 1 to4 layers have no direct blood supply, derive nutrition by diffusion from chorio capillaries, remaining from central artery branches of ophthalmic artery.

**Venous drainage :-** 1 to 4 vortex veins, remaining central veins, cavernous sinus.

### The layer of retina from out to inwards :-
1)    Layer of pigment epithelium :-
       Single layer of hexagonal cells, contains melanin pigment and resting on bruch membrane.
2)    Layer of rods and cones - the end organs for visual sensation.
3)    External limiting membrane
4)    Outer nuclear layer :- consisting of arborizations of the axons of the rods and cones nuclei and dendrites of the bipolar cells.
5)    Outer plexiform layer :- Consisting of arborizations of the axons of the rods and cones nuclei and dendrites of the bipolar cells.
6)    Inner nuclear layer :- Bipolar cells which are rod bipolars connecting with rods, cone bipolars connecting with cones associated elements which are two types a) Horizontal cells b) amacrine cells.

They inter connect different cells with one another.

7) Inner plexiform layer :- consisting of arborization of the axons of bipolar cells with the dendrites of ganglion cells.

8) Layer of ganglion cells    :- Consisting of large ganglion cells

9) Nerve fibres layer        :- Consisting of axons of ganglion cells.

These fibres are non medullated and are continued as optic nerve fibres.


10)    Internal limiting membrane
       1 to 8  stops at  optic disc
       9 is continued as optic nerve

## Rods  - Cones

There are the organs for visual sensation, cones are 7 millions and rods are 75 to 170 millions. At fovea centralis cones are tightly packed, here cones density is about 150000/mm2 -out side the macula cones density is 5000/mm2 and gradually becomes negligible towards periphery. Rods are absent at fovea centralis, appears from 0.1 mm of fovea and having greatest density 160000/mm$^2$. from 5mm of fovea. Rodes are sensitive to low illumination responsible for night vision (scotopic vision,) cones are sensitive to bright illumination responsible for day light and colour light (Photophic vision.)

## Visual Pathway :-

The long fibres originating from all ganglian cells of retina meet together and form as optic nerve and come out of the eye ball through Lamina cribrosa. The both optic nerves (left & Right) form optic chiasma, here the fibres from nasal half of each retina crosses to join the optic tract of opposite and the fibres from temporal half of retina proceeds to the same side . The two optic tracts from chiasma moves out wards backwards, wind round the cerebri to end in the lateral geniculate bodies.From which new fibres for the optic radiation originates, the optic radiations on either sides pass through the posterior portion of the internal capsule and end in the calcarine cortex surrounding the calcarine fissure in the occipital lobe, which is also known as visual cortex.

## CAVITY OF EYE BALL

The cavity of eye ball is divided into two compartments by crystalline lens with its suspensory ligament - a small anterior and large posterior compartments. Anterior compartment further divided into two chambers by the Iris, anterior chamber and posterior chamber, it contains aqueous humour.

**Posterior Compartment :-** Contains transparent jellly like structure known as vitreous humour, which separated from retina by hyaloid membrane, gives support to the interior of eye and helps in the formation of retinal images properly, Avascular so no inflammatory changes occurs, only possibility of degenerative changes.

## ANTERIOR CHAMBER

### Boundaries

| | | |
|---|---|---|
| Anteriorly | - | Endothelial layer of cornea |
| Posteriorly | - | Cilliary body - Iris - Pupillary aperture |

**Normal Depth:-**      2.5 mm (in central part)

It s angle and depth having importance in the maintanence of normal intra ocular pressure.

### Posterior Chamber

| | | |
|---|---|---|
| Boundaries | - | Anteriorly Iris |
| Posteriorly | - | Lens supensary ligament |
| Laterally | - | Ciliary body. |

**Aqueous humour :-** From ciliary process of ciliary body aqueous is diffused into posterior chamber.

Clear, watery alkaline fluid, density slight more than water,
volume in Anterior chamber  is      0.25 cc
Volume in posterior chamber is      0.06 cc

**Composition :-** It consists mostly water and all the minute traces of the diffusible constituents of plasma, the protein content is negligible and sodium Ascorbic acids are in higher concentration

## AQUEOUS CIRCULATION

Aqueous circulation is having important role in the maintanence of normal intra ocular pressure (Normal pressure 16 to 23 mm Hg)

It is secreted from the blood in the cilliary process of ciliary body. enters into posterio chamber, via pupil it enters into Anterior chamber, moves towards the  angle of Anterior chamber, from here   through the pores (Spaces of fontanna) of trabecular mesh enters into schlemm's canal of limbus. Then through the Aqueous Veins,episcleral veinous plexus, absorbs into general circulation.

# LENS

Lens is a transparent, biconvex structure with rounded border (equator), the main function is to converge the light rays to form image on retina properly, anterior surface is less convex than posterior surface, it is kept in its position by suspensory ligaments or zonule which is extending form ciliary body, its position is posterior to iris and anterior to vitreous, it is made up of Lens fibres and enclosed in an elastic capsule.

Lens axis deviates from visual axis by about $4^0$, underneath the lens capsule there is a single layer of cubical epithelium from which the lens fibres are developed and arranged concentrically around the axis like the scales of an onion. Central part of lens which is hard is known as nucleus and peripheral part which is soft is known as cortex.

Axial diameter        3.5 to 4mm  -  equatorial diameter  8 to 10 mm
weight of lens approx  0.2 grams  - Volume of Lens approx -      0.163 ml

**Parts : (1) Capsule -** (a) zonular lamellae or pericapsular layer to which suspensory ligament is attached  (b) Capsule proper.

**(2) Subcapsular epithelium  -** It is a single layer of epithelium from which the Lens fibres are developed and it  is situated underneath the anterior capsule only.

**(3) Lens (fibres) substance :-** Lens fibres are developed from sub capsular epithelium and arranged concentrically arround the axis like the scales of an onion, centrally placed cells known as nucleus and peripherally placed cells known as cortex. Lens fibers while moving from equator to Anterior and posterior poles coverge at a point and form sutures, cortical sutures are multi radiated and nucleus sutures are tri  radiated, Anteriorly  Y shaped and posteriorly inverted Y shaped. Lens fibres doesn't exfoliate collected even from foetal life and are tightly burried at the nucleus.

Embryonic fibres            In the interior nucleus
Foetal fibres
Infantile fibres          } Arranged from interior to
Adult fibres              Exterior gradully.

So only by age the lens nucleus becomes hard flat (due to tightly crushed lens fibres at nucleus) hypermetropic with increased density, so only lens appears as grey, it is a physiological process, ultimately causes lental sclerosis.

## Chemical Composition

63% to 69% water     35 to 36% proteins    crystallines albuminoid
1% lipoids, in organic ions, carbo hydrates, ascorbic acid, glutathione and amino acids.

# NETRA ROGA SAMANYA NIDANAM
### (Common aetiology of eye diseases)

Nidana means **"Roga karana"** (The cause of the disease)

Sushrutha, Vagbhata, Bhavamishra, Yogaratnakara, Dalhana, Saranga- dhara, etc. Acharyas given the list of roga karanas which are practically observed by them, they are as follows :-

## 1) Ushnabhitapthasya jala praveshath:-

Exposing, or drinking cool water immediately after exposing to heat, because of immediate opposite exposures the eye muscles affects and causes the eye diseases.

## 2) Doorekshanath :-
(Looking at the very distant objects regularly for a long time)

Eye can visualise the things upto some distance without any strain, by seeing the very distant objects for a long time, the accommodative capacity of eye will be distorted, leads to eye disorders

## 3) Swapna viparya yaashcha :- Abnormal sleeping habits.
Diwa swapna   -  Day Sleeping causes kapha vitiation
Nishi Jagara   -  Night orousal causes vata and  pitta vitiation.
and produces Hyperamia, watering of eyes, oedema, eye strain and headache etc.

## 4) Prasaktha samrodhana :- (Continuous weeping), It causes excessive stimulation to Lacrimal gland, by that the gland secrets more fluid that washes away the nutrients and bacterio static activity of conjunctival sac so that conjuctival sac and Lacrimal apparatus looses the stamina against the diseases, finally it causes xerosis and the diseases of Lacrimal apparatus.

## 5) Kopa  (Excessive anger)pitta vitiates and causes pitta vikaras in the eye.

## 6) Shoka ( grief ) vata vitiates and causes vataja netra vikaras in the eye

## 7) Klesha  - stress - suffering - pain:- Physical & mental exhaustion, vitiates both shareera and manasa doshas, leads to eye diseases.

**8) Abhighaatha :-** Minute irritative injuries or contusion injuries or perforating injuries causes a great loss to the eye, If proper care is not taken blindness follow immediatley.

**9) Ati Maithunna** - indulging more sexual intercourse it causes dhathu kshya and eye diseases.

**10) Shuktha Aaranala, amla, Kulutta, masha**
 If taken excessively causes netra vikaras because the above things are sandhana davyas having the following bad qualities

| Shuktha Aaranal Amla | Having the alcoholic properties which are quite Opposite to ojas |

**Kuluttha :-** Kashaya rasa, Katuvipaka; if taken for a long time vitiates and causes rakthaja pittaj disorders of eye

**Masha :-** Guru madhura snigda - if taken for a long time causes kaphaj disorders of the eye.

11) Adharaneeya vega dhaarana (Vegaavarodha) Suppressing natural urges

It produces udavartha vyadhi that causes eye strain and other vataja eye disorders.

**12) Atisweda :-** Excessive fomentation or sudation to the eye :-
(Swedana Karma is conttra indicated to the eyes, if necessary mrudu sweda is suggested with perfect care) it causes pittaj Rakthaj disorder of eye

**13) Dhooma nisevanath :-** the eye either exposing to smoke or by smoking the tobaco (Tobaco amblyopia causes visual disordes, partial or total blindness)

**14) Chardhir vighatath** - Suppressing the vomiting urge leads to udavartha vyadhi that causes eye strain and visual problems. Suppressing vomiting leads to Kusta eye lesions etc.

**15) Vamanathi yogath :-** Indulging excessive vamana therapy. (Vamana ati yoga ) Produces complication like protrusion of eye ball (Akshnor vyavruthi) and Retinal or sub conjunctival haemorrhages etc.

**16 Bhashpa grahath :-** Suppressing the tears produces ashruja udavartha in which doshas obstructed in the ashru vaha srotas and causes eye disease.

**17) Sukshma nireeksha nath :** observing the minute things regularly causes Strain to the cilliary muscles and lens results in visual problems.

**Additonal points by Bhavamishra :**

18) **Rajo dhooma nisevanath** :- Exposing to dust smoke causes pricking injury or foreign body sensation in the eyes.

19) **Athi sheeghgra Yaanath :-** Quick walking - it causes discomfort and strain to the body and eyes.

20) **Ruthunancha viparyayena** :- Not following the health principles of Ruthucharya.
   Taking hot things in ushna ruthu - pittavitiates
   Taking cool things in sheetha ruthu - Kapha vitiates

21) **Shiro Abhitapa :-** Head exposing to the hot produces Rakthaja and pittaja disorders of eye.

**Additional points by yogarathnakar**

22) **Ati dravanna panam:-** taking more liquid diet -Causes hypo vitaminosis leads to eye disorders

23) **Atimadya panam :-** Excessive intake of alcohlic preparations causes ojo kshaya and visual disorders.

**Additional points by Dalhana;**

24) **Avaak shira shayanam :-** Sleeping by putting the head in the down ward position than body. (cervical, Brachial neuralgia)

25) **Ucchitha shira shayanam :-** sleeping by putting the head in the up ward position than body. (cervical, Brachial neuralgia)

26) **Jwara abhitapa :-** Due to high fever or sun stroke, head including eyes are afffected and causes the eye diseases.

**Additional points from Hareetha samhitha.**

27) Excessive intake of ushna, Kshara, katu rasa, food or drugs, causes eye diseases.

**Additional points by Sarangadhara**

28) **Bhaaswara vasthu veekshanam ;-** The eye exposing to bright things - causes, Timira and other eye diseases.

29) **Midhyaahara vihara causes eye diseases,**

**Additional point by Vagbhata.:-**

30) **Pada peedana:-** (Not wearing the chappals) foot massage with hot oils or hot water, causes eye diseases.

**The Above causes can be grouped as follows :**
a) Doshaja        b) Aganthuja
a) 1) Shareera doshaja karana. 2) Manasa doshaja Karana.

1) Shareera dosaja karanas, Ex midhyaahara vihara, vegavarodha, swapna viparyaya - ruthu viparyaya, etc.

2) Manasa doshaja Karanas - kopa, shoka, klesha, etc.

     b) Aganthuja karanas

1) Instrumental      Penetrating injuries
                       Contusion injuries

2) Injury to eye by dust particles, Foeign bodies, bhaaswara vasthu veekshanam etc.

3) Injury to eye due to the factors those causes eye strain.
           1) ushnabhitapthasya jala praveshaath (Sudden opposite exposures)
           2) Doorekshanath (Seeing the very distant objects)
           3) Bhashpa graha (Suppressing the tears)
           4) Sukshma nireeekshana. (Seeing the minute very nearer objects)

## Demonstration of netra Nidana according to
## Sushrutha's Classification (7 types of classification)

It can be implied to the netra nidana as follow :

1)      Adibala pravruttha vyadhies (hereditory disorders)
2)      Janmabala pravruttha vyadhies (Congenital disorders)
3)      Doshabala pravruttha vyadhies (Bodily & mental disorders)
4)      Kala bala pravruttha vyadhies (Seasonal a) Normal b) abnormal)
5)      Swabhaavabala pravruttha vyadhies (Degenerative disorders)
6)      Daiva bala pravruttha vyadhies (Traumatic injury due to exposure of Bright and spiritual things)
7)      Sanghatha bala pravruttha vyadhies (Traumatic disorders)

     1 to 5 -      Doshaj
     6 & 7 -      Aaganthuja disorders.

## Description :

1) Adi bala pravruttha vyadhies (Hereditory disorders)
The diseases which are carried to their generation due to beeja dosha (Sperm -ovum) are grouped under this classification, Ex. - Night blindness (Nakthandhya).

2) Janma bala pravruth vyadhies (Congenital disorders) arises due to (1) Malnutrition to pregnant lady (dauhrudaapachara Krutha)
Ex. Micro cornea or Megalo cornea or Kerato conus, congenital myopia or Hypermetropia Congenital cataract, ptosis, congenital dacryo cystitis, etc.

3) Dosha bala pravruttha vyadhies

| Shareera - | Amashaya gatha | Manasa - | Rajo doshaja |
| | Pakwashaya gatha | | Tamo doshaja |

The diseses which arises due to dosha vitiation can be grouped under this classification.

4) Kala bala pravrutha vyadhies

a) Vyapanna       -       Diseases arises due to Vikrutha ruthu
Ex. Abhjshyandha (abnormal seasonal changes)

b) Avyapanna       -       Diseases arises due to prakrutha ruthu
(Common seasonal changes).

5) Swabhava bala pravrutha vyadhies (Degenerative changes)
a) Kalaja       - Normal changes by age.
ex:- Presbyopia - Senile Cataract, Arcus senilis

b) Akalaja       - earlier changes due to some pathology.
Ex:  cataract in adults (Diabetic cataract), Visual problems in children etc.

6) Daiva bala pravruttha vyadhies

Diseases arising due to observing the bright light or graha or Devata etc. (Divya Tejo moorthi drashana) Ex : cataract or blindness which arises due bright things exposure, can be grouped under this.

7) Sanghatha bala pravruttha vyadhies (Traumatic disorders)

Shastra krutha           Instrumental injuries
Vyala krutha             animated injuries
Injury of any origin causes eye diseases quickly - if proper care is not taken blindness may follow.

**Modern  - classification :**

1) Prenatal :-  - Hereditary (Adibala pravruttha)
                 - Congenital (janmabala pravruttha)

**2) Post Natal :**
a) Physical injuries
b) Chemical injuries                  Doshabala
c) Mechanical  injuries                  &
d) Parasitic Injuries               Sanghatha bala

e) Degenerative disorders (Swabhava bala Pravruttha vyadhies)
f) New growths, Cysts, Tumours, abscess, etc. Dosh bala pravruttha and Sanghatha bala pravruttha.

## Samaanya poorva rupam of netra rogas :-

A) Samanya poorva rupa (common features of poorva rupa)
B) Visesha poorva rupa (Specific features for every disease).
Poorva rupam or Avyaktha rupam - partial manifestation of the diesease, if it is suppressed in this stage the diseases can be controlled easily

### Samanya poorva rupa :

Prior to the manifestation of the disease, most of the diseases of eye having the following signs and symptoms.

1)   Aavila          -    Dirty eye with discharges (Malayuktham)
2)   Sa samrambha -    Angry look with watering of eyes.
3)   Kandu          -    Itching sensation
4)   Upadeha        -    Sticking of eye lids due to organised discharges
5)   Guru           -    Heavyness of lids (in kapha predominence)
                         (chemosis of lids)
6)   Uusha               Burning sensation (in pitta predominence)
7)   Toda                Pricking pain (In vata predonimnce)
8)   Raga                Hyperaemia (red eyes in Raktha predominence)
9)   Shoola in varthma kosha pain in the eye lids
10)  Shooka poornabham - Foreign body sensation.
11)  Vihanya manam rupam - Visual diturbance
12)  Kriya haani - Difficulty in opening closing the lids and improper
     visualisation.

By observing the above symptoms it can be understood that Dosha dooshya sammurchana has completed and the disease is going to arise, If ,proper medication is given inthis stage it is very easy to control the dosha vitiation or manifestation of disease

### Samanya samprapthi of netra rogas :-
According to sushrutha :-The vitiated vatadi doshas propogates through the channels of sira - damani towards the utthamangam (Shiras-Head) and into the eyes and produces dreadful diseases in the eyes.

### 2) According to vagbhata
The vitiated vatadi doshas associated with pitta dosha, propogates through the Channels of sira - damani towards shiras and enter in the parts of the eye like varthma, sandhies, shukla mandala, krishna mandal, drustimandala to the all parts, and produces dreadful diseases in the eyes.
3) In traumatic lesion first disease occurs later doshas vitiates.

# CLASSIFICATION OF EYE DISESES

| | | |
|---|---|---|
| 1) | According to Sushrutha and Yogaratnakar | 76 diseases |
| 2) | According to Vagbhata and Darangdhar | 94 diseases |
| 3) | According to Charaka and Karala | 96 diseaes |
| 4) | According to Bhavamishra | 78 diseases |
| 5) | According to Satyakee | 80 diseases |

## CLASSIFICATION OF EYE DISEASES ACCORDING TO SUSHRUTA AND VAGBHATA

| | | Sushrutha | Vagbhata |
|---|---|---|---|
| | | 76 | 94 |
| 1) | Sandhi gatha | 9 | 9 |
| 2) | Vartma gatha | 21 | 24 |
| 3) | shukla gatha | 11 | 13 |
| 4) | Krishna gatha | 4 | 5 |
| 5) | Sarvaja | 17 | 16 |
| 6) | Drustigatha | 12 | 27 |
| 7) | Bahya | 2 | |
| | **Total** | 76 | 94 |

# NETRA ROGA VARGEEKARANA
## (Classifications of eye diseases)

**1) According to doshas :-**

a) Vatika netra rogas 10     (b) Paithika netrarogas    10

c) Kaphaj    "     13     (d) Rakthaja "       16

e) Sannipathaj "    25     (f) Bahya   "        2

$$(a) \quad (b) \quad (c) \quad (d) \quad (e) \quad (f)$$
$$10 + 10 + 13 + 16 + 25 + 2 = \underline{76}$$

a) Vatika netra rogas -10

| Sadhya - (curable) | 5 | 1) Vatika Abhishyandha, 2) Vatika Adhimanda, 3) Shushkakshipaka, 4) Anyatho Vata 5) Anila Paryaya, (1 to 5 sarvagatha rogas) |
|---|---|---|
| Yapya - | 1 | Vatika kacha, (1- Drustigatha roga) |
| Asadhya - (incurable) | 4 | 1) Gambheerika (Drustigatha), 2) Hathadhimanda (Sarvagat), 3) Nimesha (varthma gatha), 4) Vata hatha varthma (Varthma roga). |
| **Total** | **10** | |

b) Paithika netra rocgas - 10

| Sadhya (curable) | 6 | 1) Paithika abhisyanda 2) paithika adhimanda, 3) Amladyushitha (1 to 3 sarvagatha), 4) shukthika (Shukla gatha), 5) Dhoomadarshi, 6) Pitta vidhagdha drusti (5 and 6 Drusti gatha). |
|---|---|---|
| Yapya | 2 | 1) Parimlayi kacha, 2)Neela kacha(1 to 2-Drustigatha roagas) |
| Asadhya (incurable) | 2 | 1) Paithika jala srava (1-sandhigatha), 2) Hraswajaadya (1-sarvagatha) |
| **Total** | **10** | |

c) Kaphaj netra rogas -13

| Sadhya | 11 | 1) Shleshmaja upanaha, 2) Krimi grandhi (1 to 2-sandhi gatha), 3) Klinnavarthma, 4) Lagana, 5) Phothaki (3 to 5 varthmagatha), 6) Shuklarma, 7) Pishtaka, 8) Balasa Graditha (6 to 8 shukla gata), 9) Kaphaj abhishyanda, 10) Kaphaj adhimantha.(9 & 10 sarvagata) 11) Shleshma vidagdha drusti (1-drustigatha), |
|---|---|---|
| Yapya | 1 | 1) Kaphaj kacha - (1- Drustigatha) |
| Asadhya | 1 | 1) Kaphaj netra srava (1 Sandhigatha) |
| **Total** | **13** | |

## D) Rakthaja netra roga -16, They are as follows

| Sadhya (Curable) | 11 | 1) Parvani (1 sandhi gatha roga), 2) Klista varthma, 3) Anjana Namika (2 and 3 varthma gatha), 4) Sirajala, 5) Arjuna, 6) Shonitarma(4-5-6 shukla gatha), 7) Avrana shuka (1krishna gatha), 8) Rakthaja Abhishyandha, 9) Rakthaja, Addhimanda, 10) Sirothpatha, 11) sira harsha (8 to 11 sarva gatha), |
|---|---|---|
| Yapya | 1 | 1) Rakthaja Kacha (1Drustigatha) |
| Asadhya Incurable | 4 | 1) Rakthaj srava (1 sandhigatha), 2) Shonitharsha (1- Varthma gatha), 3) Ajakajatha 4) Savrana shukla (3 and 4 krishna gatha), |
| **Total** | **16** | |

## e) Sannipathaja netra rogas - 25, They are as follows

| Sadhya - (Curable) | 19 | | 1) Uthsangini, 2) Kumbheeka, 3) varthma sharkara, 4) Arshovarthma, 5) Shushkarsha , 6) Arbuda, 7) Aklinna varthma, 8) Varthma avabandha, 9) Bahala varthma, 10) shyava varthma, 11) Bisa varthma, 12) varthma Kardama (1to12 varthmaja rogas)13) Sashopha Akshipaka 14) Ashopa Akshi paka (13 and 14 Sarvaja), 15) Puyalasa (1sandhija), 16) Prastariarma, 17) Adhimamsaja arma, 18) Snayuarma, 19) sira Pitika (16 to 19 shukla gatha), |
|---|---|---|---|
| Yopya - | 2 | = | 1) Pakshma kopa (Sandhigatha) 2) Sarvaja Kacha (Drustigatha-1) |
| Asadhya - (incurable) | 4 | = | 1) Puyasrava 2) Alaji (2 sandhigatha) 3) Nakulandhya (1 Drusti Gatha) 4) Akshi Pakathyaya l1 Krishna gatha) |
| **Total** | **25** | | |

## 7) Bahyaja netra rogas- 2, They are as follow:-

| Asadhya (incurable) | 1) Sanimitthaj Linganasha 2) Animitthaj Linganasha |
|---|---|

II. Classification of eye diseases according to shareera
(Vitiated parts of eye ball)

a) Sandhigatha      -      9
b) varthma gath     -      21
c) Shuklagatha      -      11
d) Krishna gatha    -      4
e) Drustigatha      -      12
f) Sarvagatha       -      17
g) Bahya                   2

| Total | 76 |
| --- | --- |

**a) Sandhigatha rogas - 9 they are -**
1) Puyalasa (2) upanaha, (3.4.5.6.)
4 types of netra srava
(7) Parvani 8) Alaji (9) Krimi grandhi

**b) Diseases of Varthma Mandal  -21 :-** They are

1) Uthsangini (2) Kumbheeka (3) Phothaki (4) Varthma sarkara (5) Arsho varthma (6) shushkarsha (7) Anjana namika (8) Bahala varthma (9) Varthmaavabhandha (10) Klishta varthma (11) Varthma Kardama (12) Shyava varthma (13) Praklinna varthma (14) Aklinna Varthma (15) Vatahatha varthma (16) Arbuda (17) Nimesha (18) Shonitharsha (18) Lagana (20 ) Bisavarthma (21) Pakshma Kopa.

**c)  Diseases of Shukla Mandala  -11** They are

1)Prasthari arma (2) Shuklarma (3) Kshathaja Arma (Shonitharma) 4) Adhimamsarma (5) snayu arma (6) shukthika (7) Arjuna (8) Pistaka  (9) Sirajala (10) Sira Pidaka (11) Balasa graditha.

**d) Diseases of Krishna Mandal 4 ,** they are
1) Savrana shukla 2) Avrana shukla 3) Ajaka jatha 4) Akshi pakathyaya

**e) Diseases of Drusti mandal -12,** They are

| | |
| --- | --- |
| 1) Vataja Linganasha | 7) Pitta vidhagdha drusti |
| 2) Pittaja Linganasha | 8) Kapha vidhagdha drusti |
| 3) Kaphaja Linganasha | 9) Hraswajadya |
| 4) Rakthaja Linganasha | 10) Nakulandhya |
| 5) Sannipathaj Linganasha | 11) Dhcomadarshi |
| 6) Parimlayi | 12) Gambheerika |

**f) Sarvaja netra rogas - 17,** They are

1) Vataja Abhisyanda
2) Pittaja Abhisyanda
3) Kaphaja Abhishyanda
4) Rakthaja Abhishyanda

5) vatika adhimanda
6) Pittaja Adhimanda
7) Kaphaja Adhimanda
8) Rakthaja Adhimanda

9) Sashopha Akshi Paka
10) Ashopha Akshi paka
11) Shushkakshi paka

12 Hathaadhimanda
13 Anila paryaya
14) Anyatho vatha
15) Siroth path
16) Siraharsha
17) Amla dyushitha

**g) Bahya - 2**

1) Sanimittaj Linganasha
2) Animittaja Linganasha

III) Classicfication of eye disease according to sadhya- Asadhyatha.

1) Sadhya    -    52    Diseases
2) Yapya     -    7     "
3) Asadhya   -    17    "

**Total  76    "**

a) Sadhya - 52 :    Vataj 5, Pittaj 6, Kaphaj 11, Rakthaj 11, Sarvaja 19,
b) Yappya  7   :    vataj 1, Pittaj 2, Kaphaj 1, Rakthaja 1, Sarvaja 2,
c) Asadhya 17 =    Vataj 4, Pittaja 2, kaphaj 1, Rakthaj 4,  sarvaja 6.

## IV) CLASSIFICATION OF EYE DISEASES ACCORDING TO THE TREATMENT PRINCIPLE (KARMAANUSARA)

**a) Chedhya vyadhies - 11,**  They are

1) Prasthari arma    2) Shuklarama      3) Raktharma
4) Adimamsarma       5) Snayuarma       6) Sirajala
7) Sira Pitika       8) Arsho Varthma   9) Shushkarsha
10) Arbuda           11) parvani.

**b) Bhedhya Vyadhies - 5,** they are

1) Anjana namika    2) Langana 3) Bisa varthma
4) Krimi grandhi    5) Shleshmopanaha

## C) Lekhya vyadhies -9, They are

1) Uthsangini 2) Kumbheeka 3) phothaki 4) Varthma sharkara 5) Bahala varthma 6) Varthmaava bandha 7) Shyava varthma 8) Varthma Kardama 9) Klista Varthma

## d) Vydhan Sadya vyadhies -15 , They are

1) Sirothpatha 2) Sira harsha 3) Sashopha Akshipaka 4) Ashopha akshipak (5) (6) (7) (8) Abhishyanda 4 types (9) (10) (11) (12) Adhimanda 4 types (13) anyatha vatho 14) Anila Paryaya (15) puyalasa

## e) Ashastra krutha vyadhies - 12, They are

1) Shushkakshi paaka 2) kapha vidhadga drusti
3) Pitta vidhagdha drusti 4) Amladyushitha 5) Aavrana shukla 6) Shukthika 7) Arjuna 8) Pistak 9) Praklinna Varthma 10) Aklinna varthma 11) Balasa Graditha 12) Dhuma darshi $\pm$ 2 Bahya rogas.

## f) Asadhya vyadhies -15 , They are

1) Hathadimanda 2) Nimesh 3) Gambheerika 4) Vatahath Varthma 5) Hraswajadya 6) Pitta jala srava 7) Kaphaja srava 8) Rakthaja srava 9) Ajakajatha 10) Shonitharsha 11) Savrana shukram 12) Puyasrava 13) Nakulandhy 14) Akshi Pakatyaya 15) Alaji + 2 bahyarogas.

## g) Yapya rogas -7

1)   Vatika kacha
2)   Pittika Kacha
3)   Kaphaja Kacha
4)   Rakthaja kacha
5)   Tridoshaja kacha
6)   parimlayi kacha
7)   pakshma kopa.

# DISEASES OF NETRA SANDHIES (SANDHIGATHA ROGA)

9 diseases are explained, they are

1) Puyalasa            -            Acute Dacryo cystitis

2) Sleshmopanah    -            Lacrymal cyst or Iris cyst

(3) (4) (5) (6)  4 types of netra srava - Epiphora or chronic dacryocystitis

7) Parvani              -            Phlyctenular conjunctivitis

8) Alaji                   -            Advanced stage of phlyctenular conjunctivitis

9) Krimi grandhi      -            Blepharitis

> **Note :** 1) Among the 9 diseases, 5 diseases (4 types of netra srava and alaji) are asadya
>
> 2) 4 diseases (puyalasa - upanaha, parvani, krimigranthi) are sadya rogas

## 1) PUYALASA (ACUTE DACRYOCYSTITIS)

It is sannipataja vyadana sadya vyadhi, affected sandhi is kaneenika sandhi (inner canthus)

**Clinical features :-**

1) A suppurative cyst (pakwa shoha - sushrutha; vrana shopha - vagbhat ) develops at kaneenika sandi, it is spreading type of cyst.

2) The cyst discharges foul sticky and purulent secretion.

3) Severe pricking pain, angry look, restlessness, etc. are present

**Note :** By the above acute inflammatory features, it can be corelated to acute dacryo cystitis

**Treatment :**

1)      Shareera shodhana

2)      It is vyadana sadya vyadhi (Raktha mokshana)

3)      upanaha sweda at the lesion  4)    Vrana shopha chikitsa

5)      Chakshushya lepas      6)  Anjana

a) Kaseesa saindhava lavana, Aardraka + honey

b) Above drugs + fine powders of Loha bhasma and tamra bhasma

**According to modern**

a) Incision and drainage of lacrimal abscess

b) Excision of lacrimal sac (Dacryo cystectomy)

c) Dacryo cysto rhinostomy

## 2) UPANAHA
## ( Lacrimal cyst or Iris cyst)

It is kaphaja, Bhedana sadhya vyadhi The affected sandhi is Drusti sandhi (Vagbhata has not mentioned the name of the affected sandhi)

**Description:-** of Sushruth -

A painless, non suppurative, bigger cyst originates in the drusti sandhi and have only itching sensation at the lesion.

**Description of vagbhata :-**

A painless, non suppurative, bigger, deep rooted, soft sticky, same coloured cyst develops and contain itching sensation, is explained as upanaha.

Note. : Exact corelation is not possible, drusti identity itself not clear so confirmation of drusti sandhi is also difficult. But most of the authors explained it as lacrimal cyst or Iris cyst .

**Chikitsa It is bhedhana sadhya vyadhi :-** (but according to modern excision is the treatment principle.)
**A) Sushrutha**

1) Bhedhana and then prathisarana with pippali, madhu and Saindhava lavana.
2) In bigger and painless upanaha " Bhedhana - Lekhana - Pratisarana"
3) In rakthanu bandhi upanaha Pracchana and Prathisarana has to do.

**B) Vagbhata :-**1) Sweda with Hot water
2) Bhedana with vreehi mukha shastra
3) Lekhana with mandalagra shastra
4) Pratisarana with pippali, madhu, Saindhava lavanam
5) Cleaning with hot water
6) Applicationof ghee + honey and bandaging.
7) After 5 days, bandage should open and Aschyotana has to do with the decoction of patra parta, and Aamalaki

**C) Yogaratnaker :-**

1) Chedana with mandalagra shastra (Four sided excision).
2) Pratisarana with pippali saindhava lavana and madhu

# सन्धिगत रोग

पूयालसः सोपनाहः स्त्रावाः पर्वणिकालजी ।
कृमिग्रन्थिश्च विज्ञेया रोगाः सन्धिगता नव ॥

## 1. पूयालस

पक्वः शोफः सन्धिजः संस्त्रवेद् यः
सान्द्रं पूयं पूति पूयालस सः

सु. उ.2 अ

पूयालसो व्रणः सुक्ष्मः शोफसंरम्भपुर्वकः
कनीनसन्धावाध्मायी पूयास्त्रावी सवेदनः ॥

अ. हृ. उ. 10 अ

## 2. उपनाह

ग्रन्थिनल्पा दृष्टिसन्धावपाकः
कण्डूप्रायो नीरजस्तूपनाहः ॥

सु. उ. 2 अ

कफेन शोफस्तीक्ष्णाग्रः क्षारबुद्बुदकोपमः ।
पृथुमूलः स्निग्धः सवर्णो मृदुपिच्छिलः ॥
महानपाकः कण्डूमानुपनाहः सनीरुजः ।

अ. हृ. उ. 10. अ

## 3 से 6) नेत्रस्त्राव सम्प्राप्ति और लक्षण

गत्वा सन्धीनश्रुमार्गेण दोषाः कुर्युः स्त्रावन् रुग्विहीनान् कनीनात् ।
तान् वैस्त्रांवान् नेत्रनाडीमथैके तस्या लिङ्गं कीर्तयिष्ये चतुर्धा॥
पाकः सन्धौ संस्त्रवेद् यश्च पूयं पूयास्त्रावो नीरुज स प्रदिष्टः ॥
रक्तास्त्रावः शोणितोत्थः सरक्तमुष्णं नाल्पं संस्त्रवेन्नातिसान्द्रम् ।
पीताभासं नीलमुष्णं जलाभं पित्तास्त्राव संस्त्रवत् सन्धिमध्यात् ॥

सु. उ. 2 अ.

''अश्रुस्त्रावः सिरा गत्वा नेत्रसन्धिषु तिष्ठति ।
ततः कनीनकं गत्वा चाश्रु कृत्वा कनीनके ॥
ततः स्त्रवत्यथास्त्रावं यथादोषमवेदनम्''-

विदेह

56

## वाग्भट

वायुः कृद्धः सिराः प्राप्य जलाभं जलवाहिनीः ।
अश्रु स्रावयते वर्त्मशुक्लसन्धे: कनीनकात् ॥
तेन नेत्रं सरुग्रागशोफं स्यात् स जलास्रवः ॥

अ. हृ. उ. 10. अ

## कफस्राव

कफात् कफास्रवे श्वेतं पिच्छिलं बहलं स्रवेत

अ. हृ. उ. 10. अ

## रक्तस्राव

रक्ताद् रक्तास्रवे ताम्रं बहूष्णं चाश्रुसंस्रवेत् ।

## पूयस्राव

पूयास्रवे मलाः सास्रा वर्त्मसन्धे: कनीनकात् ।
स्रावयन्ति मुहुः पुयं सास्रं त्वङ्मांसपाकतः ॥

अ. हृ. उ. 10. अ

## 7. पर्वणी

ताम्रा तन्वी दाहशूलोपपन्ना रक्ताज्ज्ञेया पर्वणी वृत्तशोफा ।


वर्त्मसन्ध्याश्रया शुक्ले पिटिका दाहशूलिनी ।
ताम्रा मुद्गोपमा भिन्ना रक्तं स्रवति पर्वणी ॥

अ. हृ. उ. 10. अ

## 8. अलजी

जाता सन्धौ कृष्णशुक्ले अलजी स्यात् तस्मिन्नेव ख्यापिता पर्वलिङ्गं :

सु. उ. 2 अ.

कनीनस्यान्तरलजी शोफोरुक्तोददाहवान् ।

अ. हृ. उ. 10. अ

## 9. कृमिग्रन्थि

कृमिग्रन्थिर्वर्त्मन: पक्ष्मणश्च कण्डू कुर्युः क्रिमयः सन्धिजाताः ।
नानारूपा वर्त्मशुक्लस्य सन्धौ चरन्तोंऽतर्नयनं दूषयन्ति ॥

सु. उ. 2 अ.

अपांगे वा कनीने वा कण्डूपक्ष्मपोटवान् ॥
पूयास्रावी कृमिग्रन्थिर्ग्रन्थिः कृमियुतोर्तिमान् ॥

57

# 4 TYPES OF NETRA SRAVA
## Chronic dacryo-cystitis - Epiphora - Lacrimation

The vitiated doshas by vitiating Ashruvaha srotas causes painless Netra srava through Kaneenika sandhi. It is also Known as Netra nadi

Netra sravas are 4 types.

1) Kapha or shleshma srava  2) Pitta srava  3) Raktha srava
4) Pooya srava or sannipataja srava. (No vataja srava)

**Note : -** Vagbhata in Astanga sangrah has mentioned Jala srava by the vitiation of vata so he explained jala srava instead of pittaja srava.

1) Kapha srava    :-  Painless, whitish, sticky and solid eye discharge
2) Raktha srava   :-  Semi solid, bulk, hot and blood stained eye discharge
3) Pooya srava    :-  Pus discharge comes due to suppuration of twak
   (Tridoshaja )        Mamsa and Raktha
4) Pitta srava    :-  a) Yellowish or bluish, Hot, watery eye discharge
                      (Vagbhata mentioned jala srava instead of pitta srava)

   **(b) Jala srava :-** watery discharge due to vitiation of vata in varthma shukla sandhi, and kaneenika sandhi associated with pain, redness and oedema .

**Note :-** Netra sravas can be compared to chronic dacryocystitis, epiphora etc

**Treatment :-** 4 types are Asadhyam, but can be tried like the following
1) Grahi Shodhana rasayan yogas 2) Sira vyada 3) Prakshalan with (a) In kaphaja Srava, Madhu + triphala kashaya (b) Pitta and Rakthaja srava, Ghritha + Triphala Keshaya 4) Anjan :-Triphala varthi anjana 2) Babbula patra concentrated decoction

## 7) PARVANI : PHLYCTENULAR CONJUNCTIVITIS (P. KERATITIS)
It is Rakthaja, chedana sadhya vyadhi, The affected sandhi is shukla krishna sandhi. (Vagbhata - varthma shukla sandhi)

**Description :- Sushrutha**
A small, nodular, (Vrutha shopa), copper coloured (red colour) nodule or Shopha Arises in shukla Krishna sandhi by the vitiation of raktha dosha, it associate with pain and burning sensation.

**Vagbhata :-** A small, round, copper coloured pitica (follicle or nodule) resembling the mudga, originates in varthma shukla sandhi - associated with pain and burning sensation - if the nodule (pitica) is excised it bleeds.

**Chikitsa :-** 1) Swedana 2) Chedhana like arma and 3) Residue has to scrape by Lakhana or pratisarana with saindhava lavana + madhu etc drugs.

## 8) ALAJI
### Advanced condition of Phlyctenular Conjunctivitis (P. Keratitis)

It is the advanced stage of parvani in which all the symptoms appear. More severely than parvani, affected sandhi is krishna shukla sandhi. According to sushrutha and "Kaneenika sandhi" according to vagbhata, it is a deep rooted infection with more pain, and burning and said to incurable disease

## Comparision

| Parvani | Alaji |
|---|---|
| 1) Smaller nodule | Bigger nodule |
| 2) Superficial lesion | Deep rooted lesion |
| 3) Raktha doshaj | Sanni pathaja (Tridoshas |
| 4) Vedana + (mild) | Vedana + + + (Severe) |
| 5) Daha + (mild) | daha +++ (Sever) |
| 6) Sadhya Vyadhi (curable) | Asadhya vyadhi (incurable) |
| 7) Simple lesion | Complicated lesion. |

## Phlyctenular Conjunctivitis (Parvani alaji)

It is a type of allergic conjunctivitis in which one or more small nodules develops on limbal conjunctiva

**Predisposing factors - Pathology :-**

1) Under nourished children with enlarged lymph glands of neck
2) Un hygienic surroundings
3) Endogenous toxins like Tuberculois, infected tonsil adenoids may cause the disease.
4) Section of phlycten show triangular area of infiltration, the apex of the triangle being towards the deeper layers

**Symptoms :-** Discomfort irritation lacrimation of the eye, conjunctival discharge and photophobia

**Signs :-** Small greyish nodule appear near the limbus with peripheral hyperaemia

**Treatment :-** 1) Cause should be treated. (T. B, Tonsils, Adenoids etc.)
2) Precautions of corneal ulceration
3) Treatment principles of conjunctivitis should follow.

# KRIMIGRANDHI (BLEPHARITIS)

Yogaratnakar called it as Jantha grandi

It is kaphaja Bhedan Sadhya vyadhi affected sandhi is "Pakshma varthma " "sandhi" (eye lids margins) but according to vagbhata affected sandhi is "Kaneenika and Apanaga Sandhi " (inner and outer canthus).

**Description** :- Different types of Micro organisms, parasites, maggots etc, by vitiating pakshma varthma sandhi (kaneenika - apanga sandhi by vagbhata) Produces smaller cysts, on the eye lid margin the infection(Krimi) spreads. into the varthma shukla sandhi and interior of eye. The associated symptoms are 1) Irritation 2) discomfort. 3) itching sensation 4) Burning sensation 5) Falling of eye lashes 6) Purulent secretion from the lesion (eye lid margin)

**Treatment (chikitsa):-** a)Swedan 2) Bhedan 3) Prathisaran with Saindhava lavan + madu 4) Anjan with the varthi prepared with triphala, tuttha, kaseesa and saindhava lavana.

**Note :-** It is corelated to Blepharits (Inflammation of lid margin), it need only anti inflammatory treatment but not incision and drainage (Bhedan) like above If pustules are formed, those should be drained.

## WATERING OF EYE (NETRA SRAVAS)
## (EPIPHORA  - LACRIMATION)

**a) Epiphora :** -Means watering of eyes due to obstruction to out flow of  tears through lacrimal apparatus into inferior meatus of nose
b) Lacrimation means watering of eyes to excessive secretion of tears.

**Causes of epiphora**
1) Stenosis of the punctum, particularly the lower punctum either Congenitally or Acquired 2) Evertion  of the lower punctum due to laxity of orbicularis occuli muscle as in old age, facial paralysis and ectropion. 3) Obstruction in Lacrimal canaliculi due to calculus or infection by Fungus etc. 4) obstruction in the sac due to tumour of the sac or following removal of the sac.5) Obstruction in the naso- Lacrimal duct due to chronic dacryo cystitis, nasal polyp, maxillary antrum tumour which is pressing on the duct.

**Causes**

1) Reflex causes :- (a) Due to sensory stimulation of the structures of the eye ball.

eg :- corneal foreign body, corneal ulcer, Keratitis, exposure to dust, smoke or irritant gasses.

(b) Due to stimulation of optic nerve, eg : Exposure to " bright light ." etc

(c) Due to stimulation of the sensory nerves of the eye muscles.
    eg :- Eye strain.

(d) Due to stimulation of the nasal mucosa. eg: Nasal catarrh.

2) Action of parasympatho mimetic drugs eg:- Pilocarpine and physostigmin.

3) Diseases of Lacrimal gland

4) Emotional & Psychical effects.

# Dacryocystitis (Puyalasa or puya srava)

It is the inflammatory condition of the Lacrimal sac

**Dacryo Cystitis :-**    - 1) Congenital (in the new born)

- 2) Primary    { Chronic / Acute

-3) Secondary    { in Adults / in Infants.

## I) Congenital dacryocystitis :-

This condition is due to failure in canalization of Naso Lacrimal duct, the lumen being blocked by epithelial debris

**Signs :-** (1) Epiphora (Watering of eye)

2) Muco purulent discharge through punctum by pressing over the sac area.

3) Slight distention of Lacrimal sac

4) The discharge is sterile at first later becomes infected

**Symptoms :-** Discomfort, watering , foul sticky discharge at inner canthus

**Treatment :-** 1) Sharp pressure over the sac area, 5 to 6 times a day to evacuate the pus and has to put antibiotic drops, 2) By gentle pressure over sac area may force the sac contents down, thus the patency of Naso Lacrimal duct is achieved.

3) Probing of Naso Lacrimal duct has to do, if delayed causes cicatrical obliteration of duct

## II) Chronic primary dacryocystitis

**Predisposing factor :-** Stricture of Naso Lacrimal duct due to narrowing of bony canal assocaited with inflammed nasal mucosa, Hypertrophied inferior turbinate, deviation of Nasal septum and by the pressure of the Nasal polyp etc.

**Exciting factor :-** Infection of stagnated sac contents by the pneumo coccus, streptococcus and staphylo coccus.

**Pathology :-** Because of stagnation of sac contents followed by the infection, the sac epithelium thickens and becomes atonic, the sac contents are at first watery, later on mucoid, afterwards become muco purulent.

**Symptoms :-** Epiphora and discomfort at inner canthus.

**Sign :-** Can be discribed in 3 stages

1) **Catarrhal State ;-** Watering of eye, conjunctival hyperaemia at affected inner canthus, little regurgitation of fluids through punctum by pressing over the sac area, on syrenging fluid regurgitates with flakes of mucus through punctum, no local swelling on the sac area is found.

2) **mucocele stage :-** Watering of eyes, conjunctival hyperaemia
Swelling of sac area with no tenderness, mucoid material comes through punctum when pressed over the sac area and some times both lacrimal caniliculi may be blocked and sac contents are retained (No regurgitation through punctum) Known as encysted mucocele.

3) **Pyocele or suppurative stage :-** epiphora, increased conjunctival hyperaemia, mucopurulent discharge comes through punctum when pressed over the sac area.

**Complications :-** Actue dacryocystitis, corneal ulcer, chronic conjunctivitis

**Treatment : -** 1)Probing the Naso lacrimal duct and syringing the sac with antibitic solution like pencillin 50000 units /cc of distilled water, if the disease is not controlled, surgical correction has to do by following method.
1) Dacryocystectomy (Sac is removed, life long epiphora remained).
2) Dacryo cystorhinostomy (medial wall of the sac is anastomosed with the mucous membrane of the middle meatus of nose)

## ACUTE PRIMARY DACRYOCYSTITIS

It is an acute suppurative inflammation of Lacrimal sac, commonly observed as a complication of chronic dacryocystitis (some times occur spontaneously )

**Causative agents :-** Strepto coccus haemolyticus, pneumo cocus and staphylo coccus aureus.

**Patholoy :-** The sac get full with frank pus, infection also spreads to periphery and causing pericystitis, finally lacrimal abscess forms, that bursts on the skin and cause Lacrimal fistuia, as soon as pus drained out the inflammation subsides.

**Symptoms :-** Severe pain, hot sensation over the sac area, fever and watering of eye.

**Signs :-** 1) Marked swelling, tenderness, hot and redness over the sac area
(2) oedema of eyelids (3) No regurgitation of sac contents through punctum
(4) chemosis of conjunctiva (5) Enlargement of sub maxillary lymphglands
(6) Formation of Lacrimal abscess, that may burst and cause lacrimal fistula
(7) Patient feels comfort after pus discharge. 8) If the condition is not treated
it recurs after some time with complications.

**Complications :**
1) Osteomyelitis of Lacrimal bone
2) Lacrimal fistula may open into nose
3) Orbital cellulitis (4) Facial cellulitis
5) Cavernous sinus thrombosis

**Treatment**

**a) Before abscess Formation**
1) Hot compress over the sac area
2) Systemic and Local Broad spectrum antibioics.
3) Analgesic 4) Symptomatic treatment

**b) When Abscess formed**
1) Vertical incision over sac area to drain the pus 2) Dacryo-cystectomy

**c)After fistula formation**
1) Excision of Fistulous passage
2) Dacryo cystectomy or dacryo cystorhinostomy

**Secondary Dacryocystitis**
**In infants :-** due to tuberculosis or syphilitic affections of surrounding bones.

**In adults :-**   a)   Trachoma
                   b)   Tuberculous or Syphilitic affections
                   c)   Leprosy.

**Treatment :-** Causative diseases should be treated, local and symptomatic
treatment should give.

## BLEPHARITIS (KRIMI GRANTHI)

It is the Inflammatory condition of the eye lid margins (Sub Acute or chronic
inflammation)

Predisposing factors :-

1) External irritants - Exposure to dust, smoke and cosmetics
2) Eye strain due to refractive error.
3) Un hygienic conditions.
4) nature of the skin. (Seborrhoea - Allergic factors (eczema)
5) Excessive - carbhoydrates in take.

6) Septic focus - From peripheral inflammatory conditions like chronic dacryo-cystitis, chronic conjunctivitis.

7) Parasitic infection:- eye lashes are covered with black nits of the pediculis pubis and the lid margin becomes red and irritable

8) Exciting causes are infection with coagulase positive staphylo coccus.

# TYPES

A) Squamous Blepharitis (B) Ulcerative Blepharitis.

| Squamous Blepharitis | Ulcerative Blepharitis |
|---|---|
| 1) It is not essentially infective condition, but caused by metabolic causes, un hygienic factors eye strain and seborrhoea of the scalp | 1) It is an infective condition caused by coagulase positive Staphylo coccus - in which Suppurative inflammation of the Ciliary follicle with glands of zeis and moll is observed. |
| 2) Scales formation (like dandruff) on the lid margin. | 2) Yellowish crusts deposited ulcers with pus points seen. |
| 3) on removing the scales hyperaemia appears, no Ulceration. | 3) on removing the crust small ulcers with pus points are seeen. |
| 4) Falling of eye lashes seen - but quickly replaced without distortion | 4) Falling of eye lashes seen does not replaced, if replaced, become misdirected. |

## Complications :-

1) Madarosis falling of eye lashes or scanty eye lashes
2) Trichiasis - Misdirection of eye lashes (hardening of eye lashes)
3) Tylosis - Hypertrophy of lid margin.
4) Ectropion - Evertion of lid margin.

**Treatment :-** A) Local1) Removal of scales or crusts, application of 3% sodabicarb, lotion (2) Local & systemic antibiotics (3) after healing of ulcer hydro cortisone 1% ointment has to use as Antiallergic (4) Treatment of the complications.

B) General :- 1) Improvement of general health, giving of vitaminous food, removal of septic focus and correction of refrective errors.

# SANDHI GATHA ROGAS

Total diseaes == 9
Curable == 4
Incurable == 5

| S.No. | name of the disease | Treatment |
|-------|---------------------|-----------|
| 1) | puyalasa | Vyadana sadya |
| 2) | Sleshmopanaha | Bhedana sadya |
| 3) | Parvani | chedana sadya |
| 4) | Krimi grandhi | Bhedana sadya |
| 5) | | |
| 6) | | |
| 7) | 4 types of | Asadya |
| 8) | Netra sravas, | (in curable) |
| 9) | Alagi | |

# DISEASES OF NETRA SANDHI

| Sl. No. | Name of the disease Modern name | Vitiated dosha Affected sandhi | Clinical feature | Treatment Principles |
|---|---|---|---|---|
| 1) | Puyalasa (Acute dacryocystitis) | Tridoshas Kaneenika sandhi | Foul sticky pus discharge From a cyst ot Kaneenika | Vyadan Sadya |
| 2) | Upanaha or sleshmopanaha or Iris cyst | Kaphaj Drustic sandhi | A painless bigger non Suppurative cyst with itching sensation | Bhedan Sadya Vyadhi |
| 3) | Kaphaj netra Srava | kaphaj Karneenika Sandhi | Painless whitish sticky Solid eye discharge | Asadya |
| 4) | Raktaj Netra Srava | Raktaj Kaneenika | Semi solid, bulk, hot Asadya Blood stained eye discharge | |
| 5) | Puya srava | Tridosha Kaneenika | Foul sticky pus discharge from the eyes | Asadya |
| 6) | a) Pitta srava (Sushrutha) b) Jala srava (Vagbhata) (4 types of sravas can be corelated to epiphora , | Pitta kaneenika Vataj Kaneenika | Yellowish or bluish, hot Watery eye discharge. Watery eye discharge chronic dacryocystitis | Asadya Asadya |
| 7) | Parvani (Phlyctenular conjunctivitis | Raktaja a) Shukla krishna sandhi (sushruth) b) Varthma shukla sandhi (Vagbhat) | A small red noduler growth with pain and burning Sensation | Chedan Sadya vyadhi |
| 8) | Alaji Advanced stage of phlyctenular conjunctivits | Tridosha a) shukla Krishna sandhi (sushrutha) karneeni ka (vagbhat) | Features same as above but more severa | Asadya |
| 9) | Krimi granthi (Blepharitis) | Kaphaj a) Pakshma varthma sandhi (sushruth) b) Kaneenika apang (vagbhat) | Small cysts formation with pain itching Burning disceomfort and falling of eye Lashes | Bhedan Sadya vyadhi |

# वर्त्मगत रोग

उत्सङ्गिन्यथ कुम्भीका पोथक्यो वर्त्मशर्करा ।
तथार्शोवर्त्मशुष्कार्शस्तथैवाजंननामिका ॥

बहलं वर्त्म यच्चापि व्याधिर्वर्त्मावबन्धकः ।
क्लिष्टकर्दमवर्त्माख्यौ श्यावर्त्म तथैव च ॥

प्रक्लिन्नमपरिक्लिन्नं च वर्त्मवातहतं यत् ।
अर्बुदं निमिषश्चापि शोणितार्शश्च यत् स्मृतम् ॥

लगणो बिशनामा च पक्ष्मकोपस्तथैव च ।
एकविंशतिरित्येते विकारा वर्त्मसंश्रयाः ॥

सु. उ. 3 अ.

# वर्त्मगत रोगी की सम्प्राप्ति

पृथग्दोषाः समस्ता वा यदा वर्त्मव्य पाश्रयाः ।
सिरा व्याप्यावतिष्ठन्ते वर्त्मस्वधिकमूर्च्छिताः ॥

विवर्ध्य मांसं रक्तं च तदा वर्त्मव्यपाश्रयान् ।
विकाराजनयन्त्याशु, नामतस्तान्निबोधत ॥

## 1. उत्सङ्गिनी

अभ्यन्तरमुखी बाह्योत्सङ्गोधो वर्त्मनश्च या ॥
विज्ञेयोत्सङ्गिनी नाम तद्रूपपिडकाचिता ॥

सु. उ. 3 अ.

## 2. कुम्भीकपिड़का या कुम्भीका

कुम्भीकबीजप्रतिमाः पिड़का यास्तु वर्त्मजाः ।
आध्मापयन्ति भिन्ना याः कुम्भीकपिड़कास्तुताः ॥

(सु. उ. 3/10)

## 3. पोथकी

स्राविण्यः कण्डूरा गुर्व्यो रक्तसर्षपसान्निभाः ।
पिड़काश्च रुजावत्यः पोथक्य इति संज्ञिताः ॥

(सु. उ. 3/11)

## 4. वर्त्मशर्करा

पिडकाभि: सुसूक्ष्माभिर्घनाभिरभिसंवृता ।
पिडका या खरा स्थूला सा ज्ञेया वर्त्मशर्करा ॥

(सु. उ. 3/12)

## 5. अर्शोवर्त्म वा वर्त्मार्श

एर्वारु बीज प्रतिमा: पिडका मन्दवेदना: ।
सूक्ष्मा: खराश्च वर्त्मस्थास्तदर्शोवर्त्म कीत्त्यैते ॥

(सु. उ. 3/13)

## 6. शुष्कार्श

दीर्घोंकुर: खर: स्तब्धो दारुणो वर्त्मसम्भव: ।
व्याधिरेष समाख्यात: शुष्कार्श इति संज्ञित: ॥

(सु. उ. 3/14)

## 7. अंजननामिका

दाहतोदवती ताम्र पिड़का वर्त्मसम्भवा ।
पृथ्वी मन्दरुजा सूक्ष्मा ज्ञेयासांजननामिका ॥

(सु. उ. 3/15)

## 8. बहलवर्त्म

वर्त्मोपचीयते यस्य पिड़काभि: समन्तत: ।
सवर्णाभि: समाभिश्च विद्याद् बहलवर्त्म तत्

(सु. उ. 3/16)

## 9. वर्त्मावबन्ध वा वर्त्मबन्ध

कण्डूमताल्पतोदेन वर्त्मशोफेन योनर: ।
न समं छादयेदक्षि भवेद् बन्ध: स वर्त्मन:

(सु. उ. 3/17)

## 10. क्लिष्टवर्त्म

मृद्वल्पवेदनं ताम्रं यद् वर्त्म सममेव च ।
अकस्माच्च भवेद्रक्तं क्लिष्टवर्त्म तदादिशेत् ॥

(सु. उ. 3/18)

## 11. वर्त्मकर्दम

क्लिष्टं पुन: पित्तयुतं विदहेच्छोणितं यदा ।
तदा क्लिन्नत्वमापन्नमुच्यते वर्त्मकर्दम: ॥

(सु. उ. 3/19)

## 12. श्याववर्त्म

यद् वर्त्म बाह्यतोन्तश्च श्यावं शूनं सवेदनम् ।
दाहकण्डूपरिक्लेदि श्याववर्त्मेति तन्मतम् ॥

(सु. उ. 3/20)

## 13. क्लिन्नवर्त्म

अरुजं बाह्यत: क्लिन्नं स्रवत्यपि ।
कण्डूनिस्तोदभूयिष्टं क्लिन्नवर्त्म तदुच्यते ॥

(सु. उ. 3/21)

## 14. अक्लिन्नवर्त्म वा पिल्ल

यस्य धौतानि धोतानि संबध्यन्ते पुन: पुन: ।
वर्त्मान्यपरिपक्वानि विद्यादक्लिन्नवर्त्म तत् ॥

(सु. उ. 3/22)

## 15. वातहत वर्त्म

विमुत्कसन्धि निश्चेष्टं वर्त्म यस्य न मील्यते ।
एतद्वातहतं विद्यात् सरुजं यदि वारुजम् ॥

(सु. उ. 3/23)

## 16. अर्बुद

वर्त्मान्तरस्थं विषमं ग्रन्थिभूतमवेदनम् ।
विज्ञेयमर्बुदं पुंसां सरक्तमवलम्बितम् ॥

(सु. उ. 3/24)

## 17. निमेष वा निमिष

निमेषणी: सिरा वायु: प्रविष्टो वर्त्मसंश्रया:
चालयत्यतिवर्त्मानि निमेष: स गदो मत: ॥

(सु. उ. 3/25)

## 18. शोणितार्श

छिन्नाश्छिन्ना विवर्धन्ते वर्त्मस्था मृदवोङ्कुरा: ।
दाहकण्डुराजोपेतास्तेर्श:शोणितसंभवा ॥

(सु. उ. 3/26)

## 19. लगण

अपाक: कठिन: स्थूल ग्रन्थिर्वर्त्मभवोरुज: ।
सकण्डू: पिच्छिल : कोलप्रमाणो लगणस्तु स: ॥

(सु. उ. 3/27)

## 20. बिसवर्त्म

शूनं यद् वर्त्म बहुभि: सुक्ष्मैश्छिद्दै: समन्वितम् ।
बिसमन्तर्जल इव बिसवर्त्मेति तन्मतम् ॥

(सु. उ. 3/28)

## 21. पक्ष्मकोप

दोषा: पक्ष्माशयगतास्तीक्ष्णाग्राणि खराणि च ।
निर्वर्त्तयन्ति पक्ष्माणि तैर्घुष्टं चाक्षि दूयते ॥

(सु. उ. 3/29)

## वाग्भट अनुसार

पक्ष्म तथा वर्त्म के २४ रोग–

....चलस्तत्र प्राप्य वर्त्माश्रया: सिरा: ।
सुप्तोत्थितस्य कुरुते वर्त्मस्तम्भं सवेदनम् ॥
पांसुपूर्णाभनेत्रत्वं कृच्छ्रोन्मीलनमश्रु च ।
विमर्दनात्स्याच्च शम: कृच्छ्रोन्मीलं वदन्ति तत् ॥
चालयन्वर्त्मनी वायुर्निमेषन्मेषणं मुहु: ।
करोत्यरुढ निमेषोसौ वर्त्म यत्तु निमील्यते ॥
विमुक्तसन्धि निश्चेष्टं हीनं वातहतं हि तत् ।
कृष्णा: पित्तेन बह्वयोन्तर्वर्त्म कुम्भीकबीजवत ॥
आध्मायन्ते पुनर्भिन्ना: पिटिका: कुम्भीसंज्ञिता: ।

सदाहक्लेदनिस्तोदं रत्ताभं स्पर्शनाक्षमम् ॥
पित्तेन जायते वर्त्म, पित्तोत्क्लिष्टमुशन्ति तत् ।
करोति कण्डुं दाहं च पित्तं पक्ष्मान्तमास्थितम् ॥
पक्ष्मणां शातनं चानु पक्ष्मशातं वदन्ति तम् ।
पोथक्य: पिटिका: श्वेता: सर्षपाभा घना: कफात्॥
शोफोपदेहरुक्कण्डूपिच्छिलाश्रुसमन्विता: ।
कफोत्क्लिष्टं भवेद्वर्त्म स्तम्भक्लेदोपदेहवत्॥
ग्रन्थि: पाण्डुररुक्पाक: कण्डुमान कठिन: कफातू ।
कोलमात्र: स लगण: किंचिदल्पस्ततोपि वा ॥
रक्तं रक्तेन पिटिका तत्तुल्यपिटिकाचिता ।
उत्सङ्गाख्या तथोत्क्लिष्टं राजिमत्स्पर्शनाक्षमम्॥
अर्शोधिमांसं वर्त्मान्त: स्तब्धं स्निग्धं सदाहरुक ।
रक्तं रक्तेन तत्स्रावि छिन्नं छिन्नं च बर्धते ॥
मध्ये वा वर्त्मनोन्ते वा कण्डूसा रुग्वती स्थिरा ।
मुद्गमात्रासृज ताम्रा पिटिकांजननामिका ॥
दोषैर्वर्त्म बहि: शूनं यदन्त: सूक्ष्मखाचितम् ।
सस्रावमन्तरुदकबिसाभं बिसवर्त्म तत् ॥
यद्वर्त्मृोत्क्लिष्टमुत्क्लिष्ट मकस्मान्म्लानतामियात् ।
रक्तदोषत्रयोत्क्लेशाद् वदन्त्युत्किलष्टवर्म तत् ॥
श्याववर्त्म मलै: सास्रै. श्यावं रुक्क्लेदशोफवत् ।
शिलष्टाख्यवर्त्मनी शिलष्टे कण्डूश्वयथुरागिणी ॥
वर्त्मनोन्त: खरा रूक्षा: पिटिका: सिकतोपमा: ।
सिकतावर्त्म कृष्णं तु कर्दमं कर्दमोमम् ॥
बहलं बहलैर्मांसै: सवर्णैश्चीयते समै: ।
कुकूणक: शिशोरेव दन्तोत्पत्तिनिमित्तत: ॥

स्यात्तेन शिशुरुच्छूनताम्राक्षा वीक्षणाक्षमः ।
सवर्त्मशूलपैच्छिल्यः कर्णनासाक्षिमर्दनः ॥
पक्ष्मोपरोधे सङ्कोचो वर्त्मनोर्जायते तथा ।
खरतान्तमुखत्वं च लोम्नामन्यानि वा पुनः ॥
कण्टकैरिव तीक्ष्णाग्रैर्घृष्टं तैरक्षि शूयते ।
उष्यते चानिलादिद्विडरुपाहः शान्तिरुद्घृतैः ॥
कनीनके बहिर्वर्त्म कठिनो ग्रन्थिरुन्नतः ।
ताम्रः पक्वोस्रपूयास्रुद् अलज्या ध्मायते मुहुः ॥
वर्त्मान्तर्मांसपिण्डाभः श्वयथुर्ग्रथितोरुजः ।
स्रास्रौः स्यादर्बुदो दोषैर्विषमो बह्यतश्चलः
चतुर्विंशतिरित्येते व्यधयो वर्म संश्रयाः

# VARTHMA ROGAS
## (Diseases of eye lids)

**NIDANA :-**

Vitiated vatadi doshas individually or togetherly localise in the vessels of varthma, vitiates twak, raktha, mamsa and medas and causes different types of diseases in the eye lids:

1) Varthma rogas according to Sushruth are 21
2) Varthma rogas according to Vagbhata are 24

**Sushrutha -21**

| | | |
|---|---|---|
| 1) Uthsangini | 2) Kumbheeka | 3) Pothaki |
| 4) Vartma sharkara | 5) Arsho varthma | 6) Shushkarsha |
| 7) Anjana namika | 8) Bahala varthma | 9) Varthmaavabandha |
| 10) Varthma Kardama | 11) Klistra varthma | 12) Shyava Varthma |
| 13) Praklinna varthma | 14) Aklinna varthma | 15) Vata hatha varthma |
| 16) Varthma arbuda | 17) Nimesha | 18) Shonitarsha |
| 19) Lagana | 20) Bisa varthma | 21) Pakshma kopa. |

Vagbhata -24 diseases :-
Among 24, 15 are as like Sushruta's diseases,    they are

**Serial numbers** - 1,2,3,4, (called it as Sikatha varthma), 5 (called it as varthmarsha), 7.8. 10. 12. 15. 16, 17, 19, 20, 21 (Pakshmoparoda).
The Extra 9 diseases are : 1) Alaji 2) Pakshma shaatha 3) Kruchronmeelana 4) Kukunaka 5) Shlishta varthma 6) Uthklista 7) Uthklishta varthma 8) Kaphothklista 9) Pittothklista.

## 1) UTHSANGINI (SUSHRUTHA)  -  UTHSANGA (VAGBHATA)

(Chalazian cyst - or meibomian cyst or Tarsal cyst)
" It is varthmaja - Tridoshaja lekhana sadhya vyadhi "

**Signs - symptoms :-**

One or multiple cysts originates commonly in the lower eye lid, if multiple cysts present the bigger cyst is encircled with others. (multiple chalazia.)

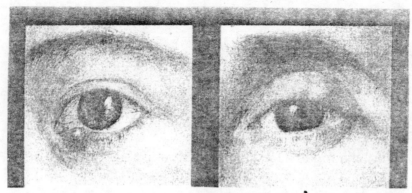

Stye (External Hordeolum)          Chalazian (Internal Hordeolum)

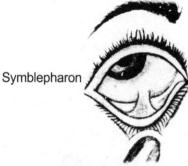

Symblepharon

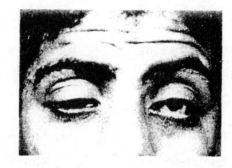

Congenital ptosis, more marked on the right side.
Note the wrinkling of the forehead in the attempt
to open the eye. (By courtesy of Kamel.)

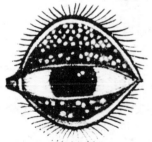

Follicles in trachoma

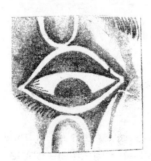

Conjunctival Concertions

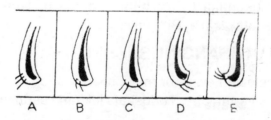

Section of the upper eyelid showing normal and
abnormal positions of tarsus and eyelashes. A-
Normal eyelid; B-Trichiasis; C-Distichiasis; D-
Entropion; E-Ectropion (May and Worth

74

**Description :**

**a) Abhyanthara Mukhi :-** The Cyst opens toward the internal surface of eye lid (towards palpebral Conjunctiva)

**Bahya uthsanga :-** Cystic swelling is seen through the skin of eye lid

**c) Adho Varthma :-** Commonly originates in the lower eye lid

**d) Kathina :-** Hard Cyst
e) Manda vedana - with slight pain

**f) Sraveth sraavam Kukkutanda rasopama :-** Discharges fluid resembling egg yolk After suppuration or after incision,

**Vagbhath ;-** Red pitica arises due to raktha vitiation, among them a big pitica is encircled with the small piticas. He called it as uthsang.

**(Summary :-** One or multiple cystic swellings originates commonly in lower eye lid, swelling appears through the skin of eye lid but cyst opens towards palpebral conjunctiva, it flows egg yolk like fluid after suppuration or incision, is known as Uthsangini).

**Chikitsa : -** Lekhana Sadhya Vyadhi
Pitica if bigger Non suppurative (Apakwa) chedhana followed by Lekhana has to do pitica if smaller suppurative (pakwa) Bhedhana followed by Lekhana has to do.

**After pradhana karma :-** (Pashchath Karma)
1)   Swedanam and 2) Prathisarana has to do with manashila kaseesa shunti maricha pippali rasanjana saindhava lavana + madhu, after 5-10 minutes, 3) prakshalana with Lukewarm water, then 4) Ghritha sekam & Bandhanam (Vranopachara has to do)

2)   **Lagana** (Sushrutha)   or   **Nagana** (Bhava mishra)
                                      or   **Alagana** (others)

## CHALAZIAN CYST - MEIBOMIAN CYST - TARSAL CYST.

it is varthmaja Kaphaja Bhedan Sadhya Vyadhi.

## Description :-

A small cystic swelling, resembling kola phala (Badari phala), originates in the eye lids, which is hard (kathima), stout (Sthula), painless (Avedanam ), Sticky (Pischila), with itching sensation and doesn't suppurate (Apkwam).

Vagbhata mentioned it is white in colour and occurs due to the vitiation of kapha dosa.            " Bhavamishra called it as nagana"

**" It is also a cystic swelling or hard tumour of meibomian glands of eye lids "**

**Chikitsa:-** Bhedhana Sadhya vyadhi and prathisarana should do with gorochana, Yavakshara, neela tuttha pippali + Madhu - and has to treat like Vrana (Ulcer)

**Note : -** 1) If the gland is bigger Bhedhana, kshara Karma and Agni Karma has to do.

2) Being the non suppurative cyst the treatment should be chedan lekhan and pratisaran instead of Bhedana (Others)

## 3. BAHALA VARTHMA  (MULTIPLE CHALAZIA)

It is varthmaja Rakthaja Lekhana Sadhya vyadhi

## Description :-

Hard - (kathina), same coloured and same sized papules originates in the eye lid completely and causes the eye lid thicker, is known as Bahala varthma.

**Chikitsa :-** Lekhana Sadhya Vyadhi.
**1)Murudu Sweda 2) Pracchana 3) Lekhana and 4) Pratisarana**
After 5 to 10 minutes 5) Ushnodaka prakshalana 6) Ghritha sekam and Bandhana, has to do
(Pratisarana dravyas are Manashila, Kaseesa, Shunti, Marcha, Pippali, rasanjana, Saindhava lavana + madhu)

**Note ;-** Specific site of the disease is not mentioned so it can be correlated to muliple chalazia or follicular conjunctivitis  or A  form of trachoma

## CHALAZIAN CYST OR MEIBOMIAN CYST OR TARSAL CYST

It is a chronic inflammatory granuloma of meibomian gland. (Tarsal glands)

**PATHOLOGY:-** The staphylococcus is the commonest organism that enters into meibomian gland through its duct, as a result of low grade infection, the glandular tissue of the gland is replaced by granular tissue, leads to enlargement of the gland- the glandular secretion is jelly like (Fatty). If more then one cyst develops it is called as multiple chalazia.

**AETIOLOGY:-** Low grade infection often associatas with refractive errors.

**SYMPTOMS :-** Slight heavyness, pain or irritation
(The symptoms depending on the size of the cyst)

**SIGNS:-** 1) Small cystic or hard swelling, in the size of a pea, on the eye lid, a little distance away from the lid margin.
2) Swelling is fixed to the tarsus. skin is free with no signs of inflammation.
3) Tarsal conjunctiva is velvety or purple.
4) If the duct is affected the swelling is seen at the lid margin.
5) If it is secondarily infected called as internal Hordeolum.

**Treatment :-**
1)      A very small chalazian may under go resolution.
2)      Hot fomentation is suggestive.
3)      Antibiotics Local as well as systemic, (Sulfonamides- chloremphenicol)
4)      Bigger chalazian should be incised vertically under local anaesthesia and granulation tissue should be scooped out.
5)      Very hard chalazia (comming at canthus) should be exicsed (very rare).
6)      The bigger and recurrently arising cyst has to send for Histology to elicit the carcinoma (rare).

### 4) KUMBHEEKA PITICA (SUSHRUTHA)
### Kumbhee Pitica (Vagbhata)
### (Stye or zeis gland cyst or External Hordeolum).

It is **varthmaja sannipathaja Lekhana Sadhya vyadhi.**

**Description :-** Small papules (cysts) resembling the seeds of pomegranate fruit (Kumbheeka beeja Sadrusha pitica) originates in the eye lid margin (Varthmantha pitica), suppurates (get pakwam), discharges the fluid and bulges again (Admapayanthi bhinna).

**Vagbhata :-** Called it as Kumbhee pitica that originates in varthma due to vitiation of pitta dosha, the colour of pitica is RED AT FIRST AND THEN BECOMES BLACK.

77

**Chikitsa :-** Lekhana sadhya vyadhi.

A) Sushrutha's Treatment principle is like Uthsangini.

B) Vagbhata's Treatment principle is as follows :- 1) Lekhana 2) pratisarana 3) sekam with Aamalaki yastimadu, patola kwatha and ghritha.

**Note :** - 1) If is the cystic swelling of zeis gland that develops at the eye lid margin, known as multiple stye or External Hordeolum

2) Some body has commented it as chalazian (meibomian cyst ) if so that may be marginal chalazian cyst that occurs at lid margins due to obstruction of duct of meibomian gland.

## 5) ANJANA NAMIKA

### (Multiple stye or zeis gland cysts or External Hordeolum)

It is varthmaja Rakthaja Bhedana Sadhya Vyadhi.

**Description : -** Small (Sukshma), copper coloured (Tamra varna red colour) piticas (follicles) originates in the eye lid, the patient experiences daha (burning sensation ) Toda (Pricking pain) and manda ruja (slight pain).

**Vagbhata :-** Sthira (fixed), mudga pramana, Tamra varna (Red) piticas (follicles), originates either inthe middle or in the margin of eye lid, due to vitiation of raktha dosha and exihibits the symptoms like daha (Burning), toda (Pricking Pain) and kandu (itching sensation). It is explained as Anjan namika.

**Chikitsa :-** It is Bhedhana Sadhya vyadhi.
**Treatment Principle :-**
    1) Mrudu Sweda
    2) Bhedhana
    3) Pratisarana with Ela Tagara, manasila, saindhava lavana + madhu).

**Note :-**It can be compared to multiple stye (zies gland cyst) but vagbhata mentioned it' s Location as, not only margin of lid - but also middle of the eye lid if so it can be correlated to Chalazian also .

### EXTERNAL HORDEOLUM OR STYE   OR   ZEIS GLAND CYST

It is a suppurative inflammation of the follicle of the eye lash including the glands of zeis.

The Causative agent is **coagulase positive staphylococcus.** Common in the adults, often occurs in crops, frequently associated with constipation and un corrected refractive errors, diabete's malnutrition (low socio econmic status.

**Symptoms :-** Acute pain in the lid margin, Heavyness and burning sensation.

**Signs :-** (1) Swelling, redness, marked oedema of effected lid margin.

2)      Congestion and chemosis of neighbouring conjunctiva.
3)      Finally a white pus point appears on the lid margin at the base of one of the cillia , indicates suppuration of the gland.
4)      Enlargement of pre auricular lymph nodes.

**Treatment :-**
1)      Hot compression to hasten suppuration
2)      Broad spectrum antibiotics local/systemic (sulfa drugs or Ampicillin)
3)      Pulling of affected cilia to drain the pus, if not a tiny Horizontal incsion should give at the affected area to drain the pus.
4)      Treating the neighbouring inflammatory conditions.

## 6) POTHAKI
### (Trachoma - follicular conjunctivitis)

It is **Varthmaja kaphaja Lekhana Sadhya vyadhi**
Multiple piticas (follicles) resembling **Raktha sarshap beeja** originates in varthma due to the vitiation of kapha dosha, associated symptoms are srava (Lacrimation,) Kandu (itching sensation), Gurutwa (heavyness of eye lid ) and Ruja (Pain).
**Vagbhata :** Hard follicles resembling the seeds of
**Swetha sarshapa** Originates in varthma due to the vitiation of kapha dosha. Associate symptoms are shopha (oedema), pischila srava (Sticky exudation), Vedana (pain), Kandu (itching) and Upadeha. (Membrane formation) due to collection of exudates
**Note :-** In the primary condition, follicles appears red (Raktha sarshapa), afterwards the colour changes into white (Swetha sarshap) so above two types of descriptions are not opposite.

**Chikitsa :** It is Lekhana sadhya vyadhi, Sushrutha suggested.

**1) Pracchana 2) Lekhana 3) Pratisaran 4) Prakshalan**
**5) Seka and bandan 6) After Pracchan Lekhana The prathisarana** has to do with fine powders of manashila, kaseesa, shunti, maricha, pippali, Rasanjan, saindhava lavana + madhu, after 5 to 10 minutes prakshalana with luke warm water, then seka with ghrita and Bandhana, is advised.

**Other Seka yogas :-** 1) Decoctions of khadhira, phalasha shigru twak.
2) Decoction of haridra, Daru haridra, Triphala, Yastimadu + madhu.

3)      Aashchyotan with extracts of Aamra patra, jambu patra. etc.

4)      Aaschyotan with  Triphala, Khadhira + madhu.

5)      Anjana with vidanga,Laksha, Daru haridra, Gyrika, Haritala, Manashila + Madhu.

**Note : -** If the diease is not controlled with above treatments Lekhana has to do again.

## TRACHOMA

It is a kind of Keratoconjunctivitis (spontaneous affection of Keratitis and conjunctivitis ) . It is a chronic contagious disease

**Causative organism :-** is chalamydia or Bedsonia group of organism (it is not a true virus, occupies an intermediate portion betweeen smaller bacteria and true virus and if affects the epithelium of cornea and conjunctiva produces inclusion bodies known as hallberstaedter prowazek (H.P. inclusion bodies).

It is common in the poor and in the dusty weather. Incubation period is 6 to 12 days, infection spreads by contamination with the conjunctival discharge through fingers, towels and flies etc.

**Pathology :-** Conjunctival changes are mostly seen in tarsal and fornix conjunctiva, marked congestion is seen, epithelium shows degenerative changes and the superficial cells exfoliate, in addition to degeneration there is **proliferation with papillary formation.** Submucoid tissue shows diffuse infiltration of lymphocytes which later on become aggravated to form follicles.

**Corneal changes :-** Pannus formation  - cellular infitration of lymphocytes which invades the epithelium with corneal vascularisation leads to Superficial keratitis, corneal opacities, pannus formation, and other complications.

**Symptoms :-** Lacrimation, foreign body sensation, stickyness of eye lids (muco purulent discharge).

**Signs :-** Mac callan stages of trachoma (4 stages) Ist, 2nd stages :- corneal conjunctival changes explained in pathology.

**3rd stage** :-  Stage of cicatrization,  It Starts when healing starts. Follicles Atrophied, pannus retrogresses leaving opacities behind, scaring starts (horizontal white lines across the tarsus and palpebral conjunctiva, the line is known as cicatrical line of arlt).

4th stage : stage of complications :- Entropeon, Trichiasis, xerosis of con-junctiva, corneal opacities - corneal ulcer, chalazian etc.

**Diagnostic criteria :-** (1) Conjunctival papillary formation.
2) Pannus on cornea 3) Cicatrization of palpebral conjunctiva
Treatment 1) painting with CuSo4 if no corneal ulcer, painting with Ag No$_3$ if ulcer present. 2) Oral Local antibiotics 3) Atropine 1 % ointment if cornea is involved.

## 7.VARTHMA SHARKARA   (LITHIASIS CONJUNCTIVAE)

It is **Varthmaja Sannipathaja** Lekhana sadya vyadhi, multiple small hard follicle is encircle with so many small follicles, is discribed as varthma Sharkara.

**Vagbhata :-** explained it in the of name of **Sikatha Varthma** in which multiple small follicles resembling the sand particles are observed.

**Chikitsa  - Lekhana** and pratisarana.

Like uthsangini and Kumbheeka.

(It can be compared to Lithiasis conjunctiva or a form of trachoma.)

**Lithiasis Conjunctivae:-** Minute hard yellow spots on palpebral conjunctiva, it occurs due to accumulation of epithelial cells and inspissated mucosa in depressions, it  never become calcareous but causes severe foreign body sensation.

## 8) ARSHOVARTHMA
A form of trachoma

It is varthmaja **Sannipathaja** chedan Sadhya vyadhi, pain full, small rough piticas (follicles or nodules) resembling the Ervaru beeja (kakadi beeja - cucumbar seeds) originates in the internal surface of the eye lid, is known as Arshovarthma (It develops on the - external aspect of eye )

**Vagbhata** called it as varthmarsha, in which vitiated **Raktha dosha**  pro-duces painful, burning rigid, oily red coloured masses (adimamsa) in the in-ternal aspect of eye lid. The masses recurs even after excision

**Chikitsa** 1) Swedana 2) Chedhana 3) pratisarana with saindhava lavana, kaseesa and pippali 4) the residual part - should be burnt with shalaka,
5) If the residual part further remained, kshara pratisarana should be advised.

# 9) SHUSKARSHA
(Polyp of the palpebral Conjunctiva)

It is varthmaja Sannipathaja Chedan Sadhya Vyadhi.

A Lengthy, hard, rigid, troublesome, polyp (ankura) develops in the internal surface of the eye lid.

**Chikitsa : -** Chedhan Sadhya Vyadhi, like varthmarsha.

## 10) VARTHMA BANDHA OR VARTHMAAVABANDHA
### (Imperfect closure of eye lids following
### inflammatory swelling or Angio neurotic oedema)

It is varthmaja Sannipathaja Lekhana sadhya vyadhi. It is condition in which Imperfect closure of eye lids occur due to varthma shopha, associated with kandu (itching sensation) and alpa-toda (Slight pricking pain) - is known as varthma bandha.

**Chikitsa :-**   1) Lekhana - shotha hara chikitsa
                2) Pracchana & Lekhana Pratisarana

## 11) KLISTA VARTHMA (Allergic Conjunctivitis)

It is varthmaja Rakthaja lekhana sadhya vyadhi:
The eye lids suddenly becomes soft, coppery red coloured with negligible pain, is known as klista varthma.

Videha explained that it is due to kapha and Raktha Vitiation in which the eye lids suddenly become red like japa pushpa (Hibiscus flower)

**Chikitsa** 1) Nidana Parivarjana (avoiding the allergic causes)
2) Lekhana and pratisaran 3) pracchana Lekhana and Pratisarana

## 12. Varthma Kardama
It is varthmaja Sannipathaja Lekhana Sadhya vyadhi.
If klista varthma get burnt by pitta dosha, klinnatwa or Ardhratha or Exudation increases, that is known as Varthma Kardama.
Klista Varthma (Raktha + Kapha) + pitta  =     Varthma Kardama
                                         (Kapha + Raktha + Pitta)

**Note :** It is secondary to Klista varthma in which more exudation or sticky lacrimation is observed.

**Chikitsa :** 1) Lekhana 2) Vrana shotha Chikitsa 3) Abhishyanda Chikitsa. should give.

## 13) SHYAVA VARTHMA
### (Inflammatory Condition of eye lid)

It is sannipathaja lekhana Sadhya vyadhi. the eye lid completely (externally - Internally) inflames and become blackish (Shyama varna)

**Signs & Symptoms :** - Blackish discolouration of eye lids with pain, burning, itching, discharge and oedema

Vagbhata explained that it is due to the vitiation of Tridosha and Raktha dosha.

**Chikitsa :-** Lekhana Sadya vyadhi a) Lekhana b) Pratisarana
c) Vrana or shothahara Chikitsa

## 14) PRAKLINNA VARTHMA OR KLINNA VARTHMA
### (A form of Blepharitis or allergic conjunctivitis)

It is varthmaja, Kaphaja, Ashastra Krutha, Sadhya vyadhi.

A Painless swelling (of external aspect) of eye lid, assoicated with itching pricking pain and sticky exudation (some body explained it as " pilla vyadhi")

**Chikitsa - Aushadha Sadhyam - (Asastra Kruth)**
1) It can be treated by medicines it self 2) Anjana Prepared with Triphala or phalasha pushpa or apamarga, rasa kriyanjan should prepare in copper vessel 3) Varthi anjan with kaseesa, samudraphena, Rasanjan , jathi pushpa + honey (yoganjan) 4) Srotonjan + honey 5) Vamshi moola kept in copper vessel, Triphala phalasha pushpa and apamaraga rasakriyaanjan 6) Amalaki phala swarasa Aashchyotan or rasakriya anjan 7) Abhishyanda chikitsa

## 15) AKLINNA VARTHMA
### (Ankyloblepharon;Symblepharon ; Blepharo - phimosis)

It is sannipathaja Ashastra krutha, sadhya vyadhi - it is also named as " pilla vyadhi" Though there is no inflammation, and discharge, and the eye lids are perfectly cleaned, the eye lids sticks together is known as Aklinna varthma.

**Chikitsa :-** Aushadha Sadhyam - Ashastra Krutam
1) It can be treated by medicines it self 2) anjana like praklinna varthma 3) Anjan with tuttha, kajjali which is kept in copper vessel and in ghee. 4) Anjana with Samudra phena, Lavan, Shankha, mudga, & sweta maricha

## ANKHYLOBLEPHARON

It is a condition where the lid margins Adhere together, it usually associate with symblepharan

a)      1) Congenital       2) Acquired.            b) 1) Partial   2) Total

**Treatment :-** Surgical separation of lids or lid margins.

83

## 2) Symblepharon

It is a condition in which the lid becomes adhered to the eye ball (Adhesion between palpebral conjunctiva and bulbar conjunctiva). It is due to rawness of the conjunctival surfaces Ex:- in burns & Ulcerative conditions, and in membranous conjunctivitis.

**Treatment :-** operative separation

## Blepharo Phimosis

It is a condition in which the palpebral fissure of the eye is diminished without adhesion, it is usually congenital, and observed at the inner and outer canthus.

### 16. VATA HATHA VARTHMA
(Lagophthalmos  - ptosis)

It is varthmaj vataja Asadhya Vyadhi.

A)      According to the description of sushrutha, the disease can be compared to Lagophalmos.

**Description: -** Due to vitiation of vata, the Kaneenika apanga and varthma shukla sandhi are paralysed so that the person can't able to close his eye lids properly, (pain may exist or not.) **"Varthma yasya na meelyathe"**

B)      According to the description of vaghata and **Yogaratnaker,** the disease can be compared to the **ptosis. " Varthma yathu nimeelyathe "**
        The kaneenika apanga and the varthma shukla sandhis are paralised when the lids are closed, so the person can't able to open his eye lids (eye lids dropped)

**Chikitsa - Asadhya** (Tarpan snehan Anjan etc, can try for the strengthening of muscles and nerves)

#### LAGOPHTHALMOS :

It is a condition in which the eye lids cann't  be closed properly when the eyes are closed. (Improper closure of eye lids)

**Causes :-** (1) Congenital abnormalities of lid. 2) Paralysis of orbicularis oculi muscle (facial nerve palsy) 3) Cicatrical contraction of eye lid (trachoma), ectropion or proptosis are the causes commonly  observed.

**Treatment of Lagophthalmos:-**

1)      Application of ointment to keep the cornea moist, if not lead to exposure keratitis. 2) Tarsorraphy operation to narrow the palpebral aperture.
3). Cause should be treated.

# PTOSIS

it is a condition in whcih the eye lids are dropped below its normal position (3rd cranial nerve palsy)

a)     Unilateral or bilateral

b)     Partial or total

**Causes :-** (1)  Congenital maldevelopment of levator palpebrae superioris muscle.

2)     Congenital weakness of superior rectus muscle.

3)     Acquired ptosis due to **paralysis** (partial or total) of 3rd cranial nerve (oculomotor)

4)     Paralysis of cervical sympathetic nerves that supplies to muller muscle.

5)     Lack of support of upper eye lid, as in case of micro ophthalmos, shrunken eye ball etc.

6)     Due to increased weight of upper eye lid as a result of Oedema - Hypertrophy - tumour, etc.

7)     Trauma to levator muscle, etc.

**Symptoms :-** If the dropping of eye lid covers the pupil the only visual disturbance occurs.

**Sign :-**1)     Lid covers most of the cornea (abnormal)

2)     Palpebral fissure get narrowed.

3)     To see the objects, head should be tilted back to draw the lids upwards.

**Treatment :-** Congenital ptosis, only by operative correction.

a)  If muscle action is existing the length of the muscle should be reduced.

b)  If levator muscle's action is abolished but superior rectus muscle is normal this muscle is attached to the anterior surface of upper tarsal plate.

c)  If above two muscles are inactive, The frontalis muscle is attached to tarsal plate, by which the lid moves along with contraction of frontalis

**Acquired ptosis -** Cause should be treated.

## 16) VARTHMA ARBUDA
### (Benign Tumour in the eye lid)

It is varthmaja, sannipathaja, sadhya vyadhi, a painless (Avedanam), irregular (Vishamam) , red (Saraktham) cystic swelling (Grandhi) develops by hanging from the internal surface of the eye lid, is explained as Varthma Arbuda.

**Vagbhata** used the word " Mamsa Pindhabha shotha" instead of grandhi.
**Chickitsa : Chedhana** sadhya vyadhi.

**Treatment Principle :**

1) Swedana 2) chedhana 3) prathisarana with the fine powders of lavana, kaseesa and pippali 4) The residual part should be burnt with shalaka 5) if any residue remained again that should be scraped out by the application of kshara (prathisarana).

**Note:-** It is a curable disease so it can be corelated to benign tumour of eye lid

## 17) NIMESHA
### (Blinking of eye lids)

It is varthmaja, vataja, Asadhya vyadhi. Vitiated vata enters the nimeshani sira and Sandhies of varthma - Causes painless, abnormal and increased movements of eye lids (Repeated opening and closing of lids)
**Chikitsa :-** Asadhya vyadhi.

### BLINKING OF EYE LIDS.

For the movement (physiologically) of eye lids.
Orbicularis oculi-(Facial Nerve supply)
Superior rectus    -    (Oculomotor nerve) and
Levator palpebrae superioris   (Oculomotor nerve) are responsible.

1)    Either due to congenital anomalies of above nerves or
2)    Reflex stimulations of cervical sympathetic nerves or
3)    Sensory stimulation of the branches of Trigeminal nerve (Foreign bodies - inflammatory Focus ( conrneal ulcer etc.)
4)    Excessive stimulation of retina for exposing to dazzling light etc
5)    Hysteria.

In above conditions we can see the vigorous movements of eye lids (Blepharo spasm) But in modern science there is no diseases for the abnormal vigorous movements of eye lids.

# TUMOURS OF EYE LIDS

Benign tumours (Varthma Arbuda)

**1) Papilloma :-** There is a vascular mesodermal core surrounded by proliferated epithelium, rarely becomes malignant

**2) Xanthelasma :-** presence of xanthelasma cells in the subepithelial layers of the skin of eye lid

**3) Molluscum contagiosum :-** It contain Molluscum bodies which are oval highly refractile and derived from degeneration of the epithelial cell

**4) Angiona :-** Small localised nodule either capillary or cavernous in nature

**5) Simple melanoma :-** it affects the epidermis or the dermis of eye lid.

## Malignant tumours
### (Shonitharsha)

**1) Epithelioma :-** Derived from the epithelial cell of the skin of eye An ulcerative nodule develops at the lid margin

**2) Rodent ulcer :-** A small nodule covered by a crust which drops off at times to allow a small amount of serosanguineous discharge malignant but does nut metastasise.

**3) Malignant Melanoma :-** A slowly progressive pigmented lesion and invades the epidermis to form intra epiderma melanoma

Note : - **Benign tumours :-** not complicative need excision to controle the disease Malignant tumour complicative, need surgery and Radio therapy to treat the disease completely.

## 19) SHONITHARSHA
(Malignant tumour of eye lids (carcinoma of eye lid)

It is rakthaja Asadhya Vyadhi (Vata Raktaja - videha) in which red (tamra varna), soft - (mrudu) Mamsankuras (Granulation tissue or polypoidal mass) originates in the eye lids - Associated with pain (painless according to some authors ) Burning sensation and itching sensation. It recurs even after excision

**Treatment** - Asadhya. (in curable)
(Chemotherapy and radiation therapy may give some result in the treatment of carcinoma.

## 20) BISA VARTHMA
(Porous oedema of eye lid)

It is Tridoshaja sadhya Vyadhi,
The skin of the eye lid is inflammed due to the vitiation of Tridoshas, and causes multiple small holes and oozing of inflammatory exudations through the varthma like in pot, so only known as Bisa varthma.

**Chikitsa :** 1) Bhedhana sadhya vyadhi.2) Pratisaran with saindhava, lavan, kaseesa, pippali, pushpanjan, manahshila, Ela and honey. (In general anti inflammatory treatment is given, if abscess is formed Bhedhana (Incision and drainage) is suggestive

## 21) PAKSHMA KOPA (SUSHRUTHA), OR PAKSHMOPARODA (VAGBHATA)
(Trichiasis with entropion)
It is sannipathaja **YAPYA** vyadhi.

The vitiated doshas by vitiating the roots of cilia (eye lashes) causes the eye lashes hard sharp and misdirected (Trichiasis), with inverted Ilidmargin (entropion ) The hard sharp misdirected cilia prick and injures the cornea (Akshi Shotha) and produces severe complications
" Teekshnagrani Kharanicha ". (Sharp and hard eye lashes)
" Nirvarthayanthi pakshmani " (eye lashes with lid margin is inverted).

88

**Vagbhata :-**

a)      Romnaamanyani Va punah (Additional Production of mis shaped cilia) (upa pakshma mala - Distichiasis )

b)      Tiirakshi shoyathe (eye becomes inflamed due to pricking of cilla to cornea etc.)

(soft eye lashes becomes sharp, eye lid margin is inverted so sharp cilia pricks or injures the cornea and produce corneal complications)

**Chikitsa :** 1) Sannipathaja yapya vyadhi
2) Shastra Karma 3) Agni Karma, 4) kshara Karma, 5) Aushada karma
(4 types of treatments)

**a) Shastra karma**
1)      Sneha karma (Oleation)
2)      utthana Shayanam (Sleeping on back)
3)      eye has to close (Shut)

2 parts from the base, 1 part from margin of eye has to leave and cut the remaining middle part of skin of eye lid in the yava shape, suture it with Horse hair, apply ghritha + madhu for healing  The sutured horse hair should tie to the fore head (lalatha bandhanam), after 5 days sutures has to remove and apply the gyrica churna for perfect healing.

**2 and 3rd Methods (Shastra and Agni Karma)**
        If the disease is not controlled with shastra karma,kshara, Agni karma has to do.
4)      Aushada Chikitsa.

        Cut the misplaced eye lashes and apply the essence (Gandham) of hareertaki or Tuvaraka phala

**As per Yoga ratnakar :-**
        The cilia are burnt with loha shalaka and apply the anjana (Pushpakaseesa got bhavana in Tulasi swarasa which was kept in copper vessel for 10 days has to use as anjana).

        If the disease is not controlled by above treatments, Rechana, Aashchyotan, dhoom, nasya, lepa, Anjana, etc. should do.

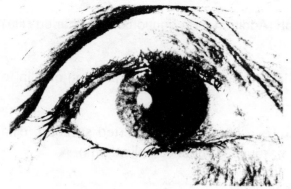
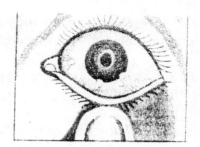

Phlyctenular
conjunctivitis

Spastic entropion. The lid margin is partially curled
in and the lashes sweep the cornea

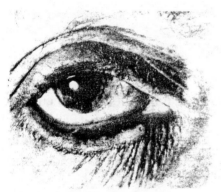

Eversion of the punctum in a case of
senile ectropion

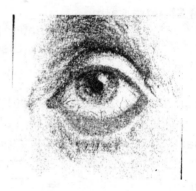

Ectropion

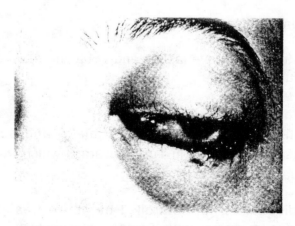

Orbital cellulitis, (By courtesy of Jarrett.)

# ENTROPION

Inversion of the (Rolling in) eye lid margin with its lashes is called entropion.

**Types :-** 1) cicatrical entropion  - due to cicatrical contraction of the conjunctiva and tarsus, typically found in trachoma, burns and in injuries of conjunctiva

**Treatment :- Tarsectomy**.

2) Spastic entropion   - Due to spasm of orbicularis oculi muscle, commonly found in the old, atrophy or absence of eye ball and prolonged bandaging

**Treatment :-** (Alcoholic injection to eyelid muscle (Wheeler's operation)

**Signs & Symptoms:-**

Corneal lesions, pain watering of eye photophobia congestion, blurred vision and foreign body sensation

# ECTROPION

Eversion of the (Rolling out) eye lid margin is known as ectropion

**Types :-**

1) spastic ectropion  - seen in children with acute conjunctivitis, associated with blepharospasm

2)      Cicatrical ectropion  -  following wounds, burns, Operative scars of eye lid.

3)      Paralytic ectropion  - Especially in lower eye lid due to facial paralysis

4)      Senile ectropion   -  lower eye lid affects due to laxity of the skin and muscles  in the old

**Clinical features :-**

Watering of the eye, conjunctival congestion, exposure Keratitis etc.

**Treatment :-** 1) spastic types -  proper bandaging

2) Cicatrical types   -  Excision of the scar and skin grafting

3) Paralytic and

4) Senile types Plastic repair of the lower eye lid due to laxity of the skin and muscles.

# TRICHIASIS
## (Pakshma kopa)

This is a condition in which varying number of eye lashes are inverted (misdirected) causes injury to cornea and produce so many complications.

**Causes:-**
1) Congenital districhiases.
2) Spastic entropion,like in trachoma.
3) Blepharitis (ulcerative type )
4) Membranous Conjunctivitis (in diphtheria)
5) Scars due to injuries,operations, burns etc.
6) External hordeolum (stye)
7) Any other destructive diseases of lid margins.

**Symptoms:-**
1)Foreign body sensation  (irritation) 2) Pain 3) conjunctival congestion 4) reflex blepharospasm 5) lacrimation 6) opacities and vascularisation of cornea 7) Corneal ulcers 8) photophobia.

**Treatment:-**
1) Misdirected cilia has to remove by epilation.
2) Destruction of hair follicle by diathermy or electrolysis
   (Galvano current is  passed to the root of cilia by fine platinum needle.
3) plastic surgery.

# ADDITIONAL DISEASES OF VAGBHATA

## 1) Kruchronmeelana
( Difficulty in opening the eyes ( Blepharo spasm)
Vitiated vata enters the eye lids of sleeping person and causes difficulty to open the eye lids.

**Associated symptoms are:-**
Pain, Foreign body (Sandy) sensation, watering of eyes and feels happy by rubbing the eyes.

**Chikitsa:-**
Vatha hara chikitsa 1) swedana, 2) vasti 3) Snigda nasya 4) snigda dhooma 5) Snigda Anjana 6) The medicated ghee prepared with Draksha kalka + purana ghritam+ sugar.

**2)      Alaji :-** A hard, red, cystic swelling develops on the external eye lid near Kaneenika sandhi, it suppurates, discharges the blood stained pus then gland bulges again. It can be compared to **External Hordeolum ( stye) or lacrimal abscess.**

**Chikitsa:-** Like vrana shotha chikitsa.

**3) Pakshma shaatha:-** ( Madarosis)
The vitiated pitta by vitiating the eye lid margins, causes burning sensation itching sensation and falling of lashes is known as pakshma shatha (congenital or Acquired, partial loss or Total loss of eye lashes)

**Chikitsa :-**
1)      Canalisation of roots of cillia.
2)      Jalaukavacharana at lid margins.
3)      Vamana with milk and sugar cane juice
4)      Nasya with the ghee prepared from Madhura sheetha Aushadha
5)      Anjana with pushpa kaseesa churna, get bhavana in Tulasi swarasa and preserved in copper vessel for 10 days,
4)      **Uthklista varthma -** (allergic conjunctivitis.)
          Because of tridosha + Raktha vitiation the eye lid becomes dry (Atrophic changes)
**Chikitsa** - Abhishyandhi Chikitsa.

**5)      Uthlista**
          Eye lid becomes tender due to vitiation of rakta and is congested with follicles and capillary net formation.

**Chikitsa -** Shothahara chikitsa

**6)      PittothKlista Varthma :-**
Because of pitta vitiation the eye appear red and tender and is associated with pain, discharge and burning sensation.

**Chikitsa :-** 1) Madhura ghritha snehana, and sira vyadhana, 2) rechan with trivrutha, 3) Lekhana, 4) Yastikashaya prakshalana 5) Dugda sechana.

## 7) KAPOTHKLISTA VARTHMA

Because of kapha vitiation the lid becomes rigid with sticky discharge and the lid margins sticked together.

**Chikitsa :-**    Lekhana and pratisarana with kaseesa manahshila pippali Rasanjan + madhu,

Then vaman, Anjana, nasya, dhooma pana - Kaphahara therapy should give.

## 8) KUKUNAKA

(Ophthalmia Neonatorum or Acute conjunctivitis of infants.)

It is an eye lid disorder of children, arises during dentation period (Danthod bhava janya vikara) due to stanya dosha or prakopa

**Signs, and symptoms :-** Akshi shotha (oedema of eye ball ) - Tamrakshi (red eyes), prakasha asahishnutha (photophobia), pain in the lids, sticky discharge from eye, itching sensation in the nose ear and eye (child is used to rub the above parts).

**Sushrutha :-** Considered the disease as varthma roga (under Abhishyanda) but not counted separately

**Chikitsa :-**
1) Raktha mokshana with Jalauka.
2) Lekhana with shephalika leaf.
3) Trikatu + madhu - pratisarana. (Local application)
4) Vamana with(Apamarga beeja, maricha, saindhava lavan, madhu+ stanya)
5) If the child cann't able to take the medicine it should be given to mother.
6) Parisheka with The decoctions of amra, Jambu, Aamalaki, ashmanthaka leaves
7) Ashchyotana with Triphala ghritha, Guduchi ghritha etc.
8) Varthi Anjan :- Manashila, Maricha, shankha, rasanjan, saindhava lavana, guda, madhu etc.
9) Varthi Anjan with murva yasti madhu, Amra twak - Satwam.
10) Gutikanjan with trikatu, palandu, Yastimadhu, Saindhava lavana, Laksha, gyrika with madhu.
11) Varthi Anjan with Nimba patra, Yastimadhu, Daru haridra, Tamra bhasma, lodhra + madhu.
12) Choornanjan :- Kanthaloha bhasma + ghritha or madhu or dugda.

**Medicine to dhatri**

1)    Sneha panam (with medicated ghritha)
2)    Vaman with pippali, sarshapa, saindhavlavan, yashtimadhu,
3)    Rechan with the decoction of Hareetaki pippali draksha
4)    Application of Musta, Haridhra, Daruharidra, pippali, to the breast
5)    Gritha + sarsapa - dhoopam
      (Varthma :- Lekhana - Raktha mokshan, parisheka, etc. should do)

## 9 SHISTA VARTHMA

The two eye lids sticked together with itching sensation, redness and oedema

**Treatment :-** Anti Inflammatory treatment.

## KUNCHANA
( Bhavamishra - Yogaratnakar.)

The vitiated vatadi doshas causes varthma sankocha (Blepharo spasm) and the patient can not able to see the things.

It can be compared to blepharospasm in which the eye lids forcibly closed. due to reflex stimulus

**Congenital abnormalties of eye lids.**

**1) Coloboma of eye lid :-** Triangular notching (Gaping) at the eye lid margin with out eye lashes and glands.

**2) Epicanthus :-** A perpendicular fold of the skin runs from the root of nose to the inner end, of the lower eye lid, concealing the medial canthus and caruncle. It causes difficulty in opening of eye lids and convergent squint.

**3) Distichiasis :-** Misdirected extra row of eye lashes which causes corneal lesions etc.

**4) Ptosis :-** Drooping of the upper eye lid, Usually due to paresis or maldevelopment of levator muscle

## Inflammatory rare lesions of eye lids.

1) Syphilis of the eye lids :- A primary chancre occasionally occurs on one of the eye lids with pre auricular and submaxillary adenitis. skin rashes seen in secondary stage, gummatous tarsitis and nodules resembling chalazia forms on eye lid

**Treatment :-** Controling of the primary disease.

2) **Phthiriasis palpebrum :-** Eye lashes are covered with black nits of the pediculus pubis, eye lids become red and irritable

**Treatment :-**

1)Cleanliness at the lesion 2)Application of Ammoniated mercury.

3)    **Vaccinia of the eye lids: -** a virus infection causes an ulcer covered with greyish exudate or crust at the lid margin with lymph adenitis.

4)    **Herpes simplex or Febrilis :-**Occurs on the eye lids aswell as lips and nose, in the course of febrile    affections.

5)    **Herpes zoster ophthalmicus:-** Unilateral herpetic eruptions of the skin of eye lid along with the ophthalmic branch of Trigeminal nerve.

6)    **Dermatitis of eye lid** :- inflammation of the skin of the eye lid which is spread from scalp, face etc.

**Treatment :-**

1) Cleanliness  of the affected site

2) Controlling the peripheral lesions

3) Local application of hydrocortisone ointment.

**7) Oedema of eye lids  -** It is due to

1) Trauma

2) inflammation

3) systemic - renal and cardiac disorders

4) Non inflammatory (angio neurotic oedema )

arises due to allergic causes, emotional factors and hormonal disturbances etc.

## Sushruta's Classification of varthma roga

| S.No. | Name of the disease | | | | Treatment |
|---|---|---|---|---|---|
| | (Total disease s | = | 21 | | |
| | Asadya | = | 3 | | |
| | yapya | = | 1 | | |
| | Ashastra Kruth | = | 2 | | |
| | Shastra sadya | = | 15 | | (9 Lekhan - 3 bhedan and 3 chedan sadya vyadhies) |

| 1) | Vata hata varthma | |
|---|---|---|
| 2) | Nimesha | } Asadya |
| 3) | Shonitarsha | |

| 1) | Pakshma Kopa | Yapya |
|---|---|---|

| 1) | Praklinna Varthma | |
|---|---|---|
| 2) | Aklinna Varthma | } Ashastra Krutha |

| 1) | Utsangini | |
|---|---|---|
| 2) | Kumbheeka | |
| 3) | Varthma sharkara | 9 Lekhan |
| 4) | Pothaki | Sadya vyadhies |
| 5) | Varthmaavabandha | |
| 6) | Bahala varthma | |
| 7) | Shyava varthma | |
| 8) | Varthma Kardama | |
| 9) | Klishta varthma | |

| 10) | Lagana | |
|---|---|---|
| 11) | Anjana namika | } 3 Bhedan |
| 12) | Bisa Varthma | Sadya vyadhies |

| 13) | Arsho varthma | |
|---|---|---|
| 14) | Shuska arsha | } 3 Chedan |
| 15) | Arbuda | sadya Vyadhies |

97

## Vagbhata's Classification of varthma roga

|  | Total diseases | 24 |
|---|---|---|
|  | 3 diseases | Asadya |
|  | 1 " | Yapya |
|  | 1 " | Aushada sadya (Ashastra Kruth) |
|  | 19 diseases | shastra sadya |

| | | | |
|---|---|---|---|
| 1) | Nimesha | | |
| 2) | vata hatha Varthma | | 3 - Asadya |
| 3) | Varthma Arsha | | |
| 1) | Paksmopa rodha | - | 1 Yapyam |
| 1) | Krichronmeelan | - | 1 Aushada sadyam |
| 1) | Arbuda | - | 1 Chedan |
| 1) | Paksha shatha | - | 1 Kuttana with needle like instrument |
| 1) | Utsangini | | |
| 2) | Anjana namika | | |
| 3) | Alaji | | |
| 4) | Bisa varthma | | 6 diseases |
| 5) | Lagana | | Bhedan sadya |
| 6) | Kumbheeka | | |
| 1) | Pothaki | | |
| 2) | Shyava varthma | | 11. Lekhan |
| 3) | Sikatha Varthma | | sadya Vyadhies |
| 4) | Slista varthma | | |
| 5) | Kukunak | | |
| 6) | Babala varthma | | |
| 7) | Kardama varthma | | |
| 8) | Ithklista varthma | | |
| 9) | Pittoth Klista varthma | | |
| 10) | Kaphoth Klista varthma | | |
| 11) | Rakthoth Klista varthma | | |

## DISEASES OF EYE LIDS (VARTHMA ROGAS)

| S.No. | Name Modernname | Clinical features | Treatment Principle |
|---|---|---|---|
| 1) | Utsangini (Chalazian or meibomian cyst) | One or multiple hard cysts commonly Originate in Lower eye lid, swelling Appears through the skin but pus point is internally, discharges egg yolk like secretion, occurs by the Vitiation of Tridoshas | 1) Lekhan Sadya vyadhi <br><br> 2) Pratisaran (chedana and Bhedana according to the condition) |
| 2) | Kumbheeeka (zeis cyst or Stye) | Small papules resembling the seeds of pomegranate fruit develops at the lid margin, cyst discharges the pus and bulges again it occurs by the vitation of Tridosha (Sushruth), pitta dosha (Vagbhat) | 1) Lekhan <br> 2) Pratisaran <br> 3) Sadya vyadhi |
| 3) | Pothaki (Trachoma) | multiple follicles resembling Raktha sarshapa beeja, originates in varthma By the vitiation of **kapha dosha** (Su), follicles resembling swetha sarshapa originates in varthma (Vagbhata) | 1) Lekhan <br> 2) Pratisaran <br> 3) Sadya vyadhi |
| 4) | Varthma Sharkara (Lithiasis conjunctivae) or Varthma Sikatha (Vagbhat) | Multiple hard small follicles resembling sugar or sand particles develops in varthma, the bigger follicle is encircled by smaller follicles, it is Tridoshaja Vyadhi. | 1) Lekhana <br> 2) Pratisaran <br> 3) Sadya vyadhi |
| 5) | Arsho Varthma (A form of Pratisaran Trachoma) | Painful small rough follicles resembling Ervaru beeja, develop in eye lid by the Vitiation of **Tridosha** (Sushruth), **Rakta** (Vagbhat) | 1) Chedana <br> 2) <br> 3) Sadya vyadhi |
| 6) | Shuska arsha (Polyp of the Palpebral conjunctiva) | A lengthy hard rigid polyp develops in the internal surface of eye lid by the Vitiation of Tridoshas | 1) Chedan <br> 2) Pratisaran <br> 3) Sadya vyadhi |

| 7) | Anjana namika (Stye or zeis cyst) | Small red coloured follicles originates in the eye lid with pain burning sensation by the vitiation of **Raktha dosha** | 1) Bhedana<br>2) Pratisaran<br>3) Sadya vyadhi |
|---|---|---|---|
| 8) | Bahala Varthma (multiple Chalazia) | Hard same coloured same sized papules Originates in the eye lid, make it thicker by the vitiation of **Rakta dosha** | 1) Lekhana<br>2) Pratisaran<br>3) Sadya vyadhi |
| 9) | Varthma bandha (imperfect Closure of eye lid due to oedema) | Imperfect closure of eye lid due to Varthma shopha, associated with itching and slight pain. it occurs by the vitiation of **Tridoshas** | 1) Lekhana<br>2) pratisaran<br>3) Sadya vyadhi |
| 10) | Klista varthama (Allergic conjunctivitis) | The eye lids suddenly become soft, red and painful by the vitiation of **rakta (Rakta + Kapha) dosha** | 1) Avoid the cause<br>2) Pracchana<br>3) Lekhana<br>4) Pratisaran<br>5) Sadya vyadhi |
| 11) | Kardama Varthma (inflammed eye lid with Conjunctivitis) | klista varthma get burnt by pitta dosha and causes more exudation than klista Varthma . The vitiated doshas are **Rakta Kapha and pitta** | 1) Lekhan<br>2) Vrana Chikitsa<br>3) Abhishyanda Chikitsa<br>4) Sadya Vyadhi |
| 12) | Shyava varthma (Inflammed eye lid) | Eye lid becomes black due to **Tridosha vitiation,** clinical features are pain, burning, itching and oedema | 1) Lekhana<br>2) Pratisaran<br>3) Sadya vyadhi |
| 13) | Praklinna Varthma (Allergic Conjunctivitis) | Painless swelling of the eye with Itching sensation and sticky exudation It occurs by the vitiation of **Kapha dosha** | 1) Ashastra kruta<br>2) Kaphaj Abhishyand aushada Chikitsa |
| 14) | Aklinna Varthma (Ankylo-blepharm Symblepharon | Though there is no inflammation, no discharge and the eye lids are cleaned, the lids sticks together, it is by the Vitiation of **Tridoshas**. | 1) Ashastrakrutha<br>2) Abhishyanda Aushada chikitsa |

| 15) | Vata hata varthma (Logophthalmos, Ptosis) | Due to vitiated **vata** the apanga, the Kaneenika and varthma shukla sandhies are paralised and causes difficulty in opening and closing the eye lids | 1) Asadya |
|---|---|---|---|
| 16) | Varthma arbuda (Benign tumour) | A painless, irregular red cystic swelling developed by hanging from the internal surface of eye lids, by the vitiation of **Tridoshas** | 1) Chedan 2) Pratisaran 3) Sadya vyadhi |
| 17) | Nimesha (Blinking of eye lids) | Vitiated **vata** enters the nimeshani siras, sandhies of varthma and causes pain less abnormal movement of eye lids | Asadya |
| 18) | Shonitharsha (carcinoma of eye lid) | Raktaj or vata raktaj disorder in which a red, soft - granulation tissue develops in varthma, recurs even after excision | Asadya |
| 19) | Lagana (Chalazian or meibomian cyst) | A small cystic swelling resembling kola phala, develops in eye lid, which is hard stout, pain less, sticky with itching sensation, by the vitiation of **kapha dosha** | 1) Bhedan 2) Pratisaran 3) Sadya vyadhi |
| 20) | Bisa varthma (Porous oedema of eye lid) | Due to tridosha vitiation the eye lid inflammes and causes multiple small holes, like in pot through which inflammatory exudates oozes. | 1) Bhedana 2) Pratisaran 3) Sadya vyadhi |
| 21) | Pakshmakopa (Trichiasis with entropion) | The vitiated tridosha vitiate the roots of cilia and causes the eye lashes hard sharp and misdirected with inverted lidmargin, causes injury to cornea | 1) Aushada Chikitsa 2) shastra Karma 3) Agnikarma 4) Ksharakarma 5) Yapya vyadhi |

# शुक्लगत रोग

## अर्म

प्रस्तारि शुक्ल क्षतजाधिमांस – स्नायर्म संज्ञा: खलु पंच रोगा: ।

स्यु: शुक्तिका चार्जुनापिष्टको च

जालं सिराणां पिड़काश्चया:स्यु: ॥

रोगा बलासग्रथितेन सार्ध

मेकादशम्क्ष्णो: खलु शुक्लभागे ॥

(सु॰ उ॰ 4/3 अ॰)

## 1. प्रस्तारि अर्म

प्रस्तारि प्रथितमिहार्म शुक्लभागे

विस्तीर्ण तनु रुधिरप्रभं सनीलम् ॥

(सु. उ. 4 अ:)

मृद्वाशुवृद्ध्यरुड़ू मांसं प्रस्तारि श्यावलोहितम् ॥

प्रस्तार्यर्म मलै: सासै:

(अ॰ हृ॰ उ॰ १० अ:)

## 2. शुक्लार्म

शुक्लाख्यं मृदु कथयन्ति शुक्लभागे

सश्वेतं सममिह वर्धते चिरेण ।

(सु उ 4/4)

कफाच्छुक्ले समंश्वेतं चिरवृद्ध्यधिमांसकम् ।

शुक्लार्म

(अ:हृ:उ:१०अ:)

## 3. लोहितार्म या क्षतजार्म

यन्मांसं प्रचयमुपैति शुक्लभागे

पद्माभं तदुपदिशन्ति लोहितार्म ॥

(सु॰ उ॰ 4/5)

शोणितार्म समं श्लक्ष्णं पद्माभमधिमांसकम् ॥

(अ:हृ:उ:१०अ:)

## 4. अधिमांसार्म

विस्तीर्ण मृदु बहलं यकृत्प्रकाशं
श्यावं वा तदधिकमांसजार्म विद्यात् ॥

(सु॰ उ॰ 4/6)

शुष्कासृक्पिण्डवच्छयावं मन्मांसं बहलं पृथु॥
अधिमांसार्मतद्

(अ:हृ:उ:१०)

## 5. स्नाय्वर्म

शुकलेयत् पिशितमुपैति वृद्धिमेतत्
स्नाय्वर्मेत्यभिपठितं खरं प्रपाण्डु॥

(सु॰ उ॰ 4/6 अ॰)

स्नावार्म स्नावसन्निमम् ॥

(अ:हृ:उ:१०)

## 6. शुक्तिका या शुक्ति

श्यावा: स्यु : पिशितनिभाश्च बिन्दवो ये
शुक्तयाभा: सितनयने स सुक्तिसंज्ञ: ॥

(सु॰ उ॰ 4/7 अ॰)

पित्तं कुर्यात् सिते बिन्दुनसितश्याव पीतकान्॥
मलाक्तादर्शतुल्यं वा सर्व शुक्लं सदाहरुक्।
रोगोयं शुक्तिकासंज्ञ: सशकृद्भेदतृड्ज्वर: ॥

(अ:हृ:उ:१०)

## 7. अर्जुन

एको य: शशरुधिरोपमस्तु बिन्दु:
शुक्लस्थो भवति तमर्जुनं वदन्ति ॥

(सु॰ उ॰ 4/8 अ:)

नीरुक् श्लक्ष्णोर्जुन बिन्दु: शशलोहितलोहित:

(अ:हृ:उ:१०अ॰)

## 8. पिष्टक

उत्सन्नः सलिलनिभोथ पिष्टशुक्लो बिन्दुर्यो भवति सपिष्टक: सुवृत्त: ॥

(सु॰ उ॰ 4/8 अ॰)

बिन्दुभिः पिष्टधवलैरुत्सन्नैः पिष्टकं वदेत् ।

(अ:ह:उ:१०अ:)

## 9. सिराजाल

जालाभः कठिनसिरो महान् सरक्तः
सन्तानः स्मृत इह जालसंज्ञितस्तु ॥

(सु॰ उ॰ 4/8)

सिराजाले सिराजालं बृहद्रक्तं घनोन्नतम्

(अ:ह:उ:१०अ:)

## 10. सिरापिड़िका

शुक्लस्याः सितपिड़का: सिरावृता या-
स्ता विद्धदसितसमीपजा: सिराजा: ॥

(सु॰ उ॰ 4/9 अ॰)

तद्दाह-घर्षवन्ता: सिरावृता:
कृष्णासन्ना: सिरा संज्ञा पिटिका सर्षपोपमा:

(अ:ह:उ:१०अ:)

## 11. बलासग्रथित

कांस्याभो भवति सितोम्बुबिन्दुतुल्य
स ज्ञेयोमृदुररुजो बलासकारख्य: ॥

(सु॰ उ॰ 4 अ॰)

शोफस्त्वरुज: सवर्णोवहलोमृदु:
गुरु:स्निग्धोम्बुबिन्द्वा भो बलासग्रथितं स्मृतम् ॥

(अ:ह:उ:१०अ:)

# DISEASES OF SHUKLA MANDALA

### (Diseases of sclera and bulbar conjunctiva)

11    diseases according to Sushrutha,

13    "        "        "        Vagbhata.


they are


1)    Prasthari arma

2)    Shukla arma

3)    Kshathaja arma                    -5 types of arma.

4)    Adimamsa arma

5)    Snayu arma

6)    Shukthika

7)    Arjuna

8)    Pistaka

9)    Sira jala

10)    Sira pidaka

11)    Balasa graditha.

**(Sushrutha)**


1 to 11 are common according to Sushrutha and Vagbhata, the other extra two diseases of Vagbhata are


12)    Sirothpatha  13) Sira harsha.(But these 2 Diseases are explained by Sushrutha in Sarvagatha rogas.)

# ARMA (PTERIGIUM)

" Iyarthi gacchathi ithi Arma "

The Gradually spreading extra membrane in shukla mandala (Mamsa Vruddhi) is Known as Arma

It is of 5 types, they are
1) Prasthari arma 2) Shukla arma 3) Kshataja Arma 4) Adimamsa arma 5) Snanu arma

## 1) PRASTHARI ARMA {progressive Pterigium}

It is sannipathaja, chedana sadya, vyadhi in which spreading type of membrane formed on shukla mandala

**Sushrutha :-** Thin spreading, Reddish blue coloured membrane formed in shukla mandal

**Vagbhat :-** a soft, quickly spreading, blackish, red, painless membrane formed by the vitiation of tridosha and Raktha dosha

**Treatment :-** Chedan sadya vyadhi (Excision of the arma)

## 2) SHUKLA ARMA :- (progressive Pterigium)

It is kaphaja chedan sadya vyadhi, in which a slowly growing, soft pale white coloured membrane develops on shukla mandala.

**Treatment :-** Chedan (Excision) Sadya vyadhi

## 3) KSHATAJA ARMA OR LOHITARMA OR SHONITHARMA
### (pterigium- Melanoma - Haemangioma)

It is raktaja chedan sadya vyadhi, in which soft red coloured membrane (Resembling the colour of Lotus flower) Develops on shukla mandala

**Treatment:** - Chedan (Excision ) Sadya vyadhi

## 4) ADHIMAMSA ARMA

It is sannipathaj chedan sadya vyadhi in which a soft thick widely spreading chocolate coloured (yakruth varna) membrane develps on shukla mandala

**Treatment :** - Chedan (Excision) Sadya vyadhi

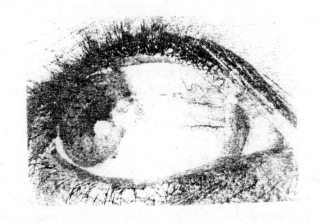

Pterygium

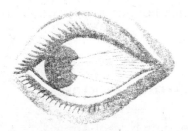

Pterygium - progressive stage.

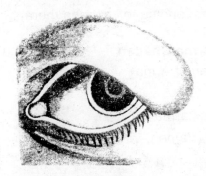

Pinguecula

## 5) SNAYU ARMA

It is sannipathaja chedan sadya vyadhi in which a hard wide yellow coloured membrane resembling "Snayu" develops in shukla mandala.

**Treatment :-** Chedan (Excision ) Sadya vyadhi

**Note :-** Among 5 types of Arma

a) Snayu arma and adhimamsaja arma are thicker wide with snayu and mamsa so chedana is advised b) But prasthari shukla kshataj arma are advised to treat with Lekhana anjanas as like in Avrana shukla or lekhana therapy for having thin and smaller membrane development on shuklamndala in white or blue or red or in brown colour.

1) In thin membranous Arma  - Lekhana Therapy (Prasthari, Shukla, and Kshataja arma 2) Thick fibrous membranous arma (Adhimamsa and Snayu Arma ) has to do.

## Indications of Arma Chedan

1) Thicker wider spreading type of Arma
2) Arma like the thick Skin
3) When spreading on to the krishna mandala
4) Snayu and mamsaja Arma
5) When arma not responding to Lekhana theraphy

### Poorva Karma to Arma Chedan
(Pre excision regimen of Arma)

1) Sneha and sweda karma
2) Shareer shodhan (Vaman, Virechan, vasti etc.)
3) Shiro Shodhan by Nasya Karma
4) Giving of oleus substanas to eat  or drink
5) Lavan pratisaran to disintegrate the tissue of the arma.

**Pradhan Karma** (Method of excision therapy)

Patient is asked to see towards Apanga (outer canthus) and eyelids should open widely

1) Sthanika mrudu sweda ( Local light fomentation)
2) Separation of arma from the floor with Badisha (Hook)
3) Clear separation of Arma from the floor with a thread
4) Elevation of Arma with muchundi (forceps)
5) Arma is separated and cut at the krishna mandala then the flap is lifted to wards kaneenika sandhi and 3/4 th part is cut with mandalagra shastra by leaving the 1/4 th part as residue to prevent from the complications like Nadivrana Raktha srava Drustinash etc.

The residue should be scraped with the application of lekhan anjanas, afterwards .

**Pashchath karma**   (post excision regimen) :-

1)    Pratisaran with yavakshar, shunthi, maricha, pippali and lavan
2)    Mrudu sweda
3)    Ghritha sechan
4)    Cheen bandan  (eye bandage)
5)    After 3 to 5 days bandage should open to observe the healing process
6)    Vrana ropan chikitsa  (wound healing therapy)
7)    Treatment of the complications, if any. .

After the excision of arma if pain is associated that should be treated with medicated milk prepared with  1) Aamalaki, yastimadu and milk Honey Aashchyotan has to do.

1)    The decoction of karanja beeja as eye drops)
2)    Application of (Shiro and netra lepa) yastimadu + Kamal Kesar + milk + ghee
3)    The residual Part of Arma should be scraped by the application of Lekhana anjanas

**Signs of Proper excision:-**

1)    Getting of Normal colour and vision.
2)    Painless Movements of eye ball
3)    Relief from pain, oedema, ulceration, discomfort and other inflammatory signs and symptoms.

**Aushadhi Chikitsa of arma :-**

(Prasthari arma, shukla arma and Kshataja arma)

1)    All the lekhana anjanas mentioned for Avrana shula
2)    Krishnadi puta Paka :- Maricha, Loharaja, Tamra, shankha, vidruma, saindhava lavan, srotoanjan kaseesa + Dadhi.
3)    Pippalyadi gutikanjan :- Pippali, triphala ,laksha, Lohachurna, Saindhava lavan + Brungaraja swarasa
4)    Marichadi lepa - maricha, Vibheetaki + Haridra swarasa
5)    Pushpadi rasakriya  - yashada pushpa, rasanjan, sita, dadhi, samudra phena, Shankha, saindhava lavan, gyrika, manashila, maricha + madhu.

Arma can be compared to the pterigium, a disease that occurs due to sub conjunctival degeneration, in which a triangular layer develops underneath the bulbar conjunctiva towards cornea in Horizontal meridian, develops either form inner canthus or outer canthus and spreads towards cornea.

| Psuedo Pterigium | Pterigium |
|---|---|
| 1)    Inflammatory lesion | 1) Degenerative lesion |
| 2)    Probe can be passed underneath the membrane | 2) Probe Cannot be passed |
| 3)    Can develop in any Meridian | 3) Develops only in Horizontal meridian |
| 4)    Stationary | 4) Stationary or progressive |
| 5)    Can occur in any age | 5) only in adults |

**Pterigium :-**

It is a triangular fold of Conjunctiva, encroaching the cornea in the horizontal meridian, in the palpebral fissure, either from the nasal side or from the temporal side of the bulbar conjunctiva or from both the sides It is due to degenerative changes in the subconjunctiva tissue

It consist of head, neck and a body

**Types :-** a)    Progressive pterigium       2) Non Progressive pterigium or Atrophic Pterigium

Progressive pterigium progresses in the cornea in the level of Bowman's membrane, which is destroyed.

b) Atrophic or Non- progressive pterigium. It is very thin with little vascularity, doesn't spread upto cornea (Stationery)

**Symptoms :-** No symptom appears unless it reaches the pupillary area. Occasionally there may be diplopia due to restricted movements of eye ball (Slight discomfort may present).

**Treatment of pterigium :-**

Stationary pterigium require no treatment, but in progressive pterigium surgery is conducted (1) Mc Reynold's transplantaion method (2) Excision of entire pterigium . (The Residual part is turned to 6 clock position and mattress suÿÿves are given to control the recurrence)

## 6) SHUKTHIKA OR SHUKTHI
### (Xerosis or xerophthalmia)

It is pittaja Aushada sadya Vyadhi, Shukla mandala is spread with blackish white (shyava varna) Patches or dots, like in jala shukthi.

**Vagbhata** has given little more description as follows :

1) Eye appears dirty as the mirror with dust particles. 2) Blackish white or yellowish dots spread in shukla mandal.3) The Patient have pain, burning sensation in the eye and also associate with diarrhoea thirst and fever

**Treatment :**
1)      It is Ashastra krutha vyadhi (has to treat with medicines only)
2)      It should be treated like pittaja Abhishyanda vyadhi or Amladyushitha
3)      The treatment principle is oral a) administratin of Triphala ghritha or Tilwak ghritha or purana ghritha  for Virechana, b) Application of sheeta Anjanas like

a) Vydoorya, spatika, pravala, muktha, shankha, Raupya, swarna bhasma (Anyone or few of ) + madhu as Anjanam. b) phalasha pushpa swarasa + Honey c) Rasakrianjan with yastimadu, Daruharidra and Rasanjan d) Lodra Drakha, Sharkara, kamala, yastimadu + Stanya e) Samudraphena + stanya f) Amalaki phala swarasa + ghritha g) Rasanjan + Stanya or madhu or ghritha

## XEROSIS OR XEROPHTHALMIA
### (Shukthika)

It is a degenerative condition characterised by dry lustreless condition of conjunctiva.

**Causes :-**

1) Local diseases of conjunctiva, ex trachoma, pemphigus, membranous conjunctivitis, Extensive burn of conjunctiva
2) Chronic exposure of Conjunctiva to dust and smoke due to Lagophthalmos, ectropion etc.
3) Nutritional diisturbances - especially Vitamin A deficiency
4) Exposure to chemicals, toxins etc.

**Note :-**

If it is neglected it may cause kerato malacia (degeneration of Corneal epithelium) corneal ulcer, Panophthalmitis etc.

**Treatment ;-**

1) Liquid paraffin drops in eyes  2) Improvement of general health
3) Oral administration of vitamin A through food or medicines
4) Deep intra muscular injection of vit. A 100000 units once a week (according to the neccssity)

## 7) Arjuna
( Sub conjunctival haemorrhage or mole or melanoma)

It is rakthaja Sadhya vyadhi in which red coloured dot or patch (Red colour as the blood of rabbit ) Originates in shukla mandala.

**Vagbhata : -** Description is same as above but added the following words, soft painless red coloured dot in shukla mandala. (mole-melanoma commonly congenital - No need of treatment, traumatic lesions of conjunctiva like sub conjunctival haemorrhage, hamangioma need treatment

**Treatment :-**
1) Ashastra Kruth (Should treat with medicines only)
2) Traumatic subconjunctival haemorrhage naturally disappears within 7 days.
3) should treat like pittaja or Rakthaja Abhishyanda

**4) Seka or Anjana:-** With Ikshurasa, madhu, sugar, ksheera, Rasanjan, Yastimadhu, Saindhava lavana (few of the drugs.)

**5) Aaschyotan :-**
 Sugar, Yastimadhu, madhu, sour things Nimburasa, saindhavalavana, Badari phala, Amla, Dadima (with few of the drugs)

6)      **Anjanas :-**
a)      Shankha + Sugar + madhu + Samudra phena.
b)      Shankha or spatika or pravala or yastimadhu + madhu,
c)      Rasanjan + madhu
d)      Kaseesa + madhu
e)      Saindhava lavana + madhu + Nirmali phala
f)      Lekhana Anjanas.
g)      Samudraphena, swetha maricha, manashila + mathulunga swarasa.
h)      Kukkutanda twak, Lashuna,Trikatu, Ela, Karanja, beej.

## 8) PISTAK (Pinguecula)

It is Kaphaja Sadhya vyadhi in which shukla mandala is spread with white round and fresh papules (nodular eruptions, whitish like Rice flour and fresh like water ) (Bhava Mishra described, it is due to kapha + vata vitiation)
**Treatment :**
1) Ashastrakrutha vyadhi. (Should be treated with medicines only )
2) Treatment can be given like kaphaja Abhishyanda Vyadhi except Raktha mokshana therapy.

**3) Mahaushadadi Anjan:-** Prepared with Shunti, pippali, musta, swetha maricha, saindhava lavana (equally) and grinded with mathulunga swarasa.
4) Kantakari (Varthaka) or shigru or Indravaruni or patola or kirathatiktha, or amalaki.

Any of the above durgs (fruits) after pakwa, the seeds should be removed and fill the fruit capsule with pippali and sauveeranjan. Kept it for 7 days after that the medicine should be collected and grinded with mathulunga rasa and used as Anjana.

## 9) SIRA JALA
(Haemangioma of the sclera or scleral staphyloma or congestion)

It is rakthaj chedan sadya vyadhi in which a hard big red coloured capillary net appears in shukla mandala, is known as siraajala
**Treatment:-**
**Like Arma Vyadhi**
a) In soft thin Smaller capillary net treatment is application of the Lekhan anjana or lekhana therapy.b) In Hard thick bigger Capillary net, Treatment is chedan and pratisaran Like in **"Arma"** (3/4th part should cut with mandalagra shastra and the residue (1/4 ) Should treat by the application of Lekhan anjanas).

## 10 SIRA PIDIKA (EPISCLERITIS - SCLERITIS)

It is sanni pathaja chedan sadya vyadhi, in which a white nodule encircled with capillary net is seen near the Krishna mandal (Limbal area ) - (Sushrutha).

A nodule (resembling the Sarshapa beeja) encircled with capillary net is observed near krishna mandalam. Associated with Burning and foreign body sensation (Vagbhata)

**Treatment** :- Like sirajala (Like Arma)

## BALASA GRADITHA
(Pinguecula, episcleral Rheumatoid nodule, parinauds conjunctivitis)

It is kaphaja Aushada sadya vyadhi, in which a hard painless nodule resembling the water bubble and shines like the bronze (kamsya) originates in shukla mandala (Sushrutha)
According to videha it is due to vitiation of kapha and vata dosha

**Treatment :-**
1) Ashastra krutha (Surgery is contra indicated) 2) Shareera shodhana (Vaman virechana etc.) and shiro shodhan (Nasya) 3) Application of the following kshara anjana a) Apakwa yava get bhavana in milk for 7 days get dried and should prepare kshara, then add saindhava lavan, tuttha and gorochana, get pakwam and use as anjan, b) Arjaka, asphotha, kapitta, bilwa nirgundi jathi pushpa - prepare kshara and add saindhava lavana, tuttha and gorochan, use as anjan c) Phaninjakadi kshara anjan.

## EPISCLERITIS (Sirajala - sirapidika)
It is the inflammation of sub conjunctival episclera along with the superficial lamellae of sclera
**Etiology :-** 1) Associate with Rheumatoid arthritis , endogenous toxins allergic reactions like in tuberculosis.
**Symptoms :-** 1) Pain and discomfort in the eyes.
2) No discharge lacrimation and photophobia

**Signs** :- 1) A hard pinkish nodule develops sub conjunctivally, 2 to 3 mm away from the limbus

2) Nodule is tender and deeply fixed, never ulcerates.

3) Hyperaemia of the surrounding conjunctiva.

Complication   -          (1) Scleritis               (2) Uveitis

**Treatment :**
1)      Hydrocortizone acetate 1% drops and sub conjunctival injections
        (once in a week)
2)      Elimination of septic focus.

## DIFFERENTIAL DIAGNOSIS

|               | Episcleritis           | Phlycten          | Inflammed Pinguecula                   |
|---------------|------------------------|-------------------|----------------------------------------|
| 1) Age        | Elderly person         | Young             | Elderly person                         |
| 2) Location   | Away from the Limbus.  | on the Limbus.    | Away from Limbus, in Horizontal meridian |
| 3) Tender ness | Present                | Absent            | Present                                |
| 4) Ulceration | Absent                 | Present           | Absent                                 |
| 5) Appearence | Pinkish Red.           | Pinkish White     | Pinkish white                          |

### SCLERITIS (Sirajala - Sira Pidika)

The inflmmation of the sclera is known as scleritis.

**Etiology :** -1) Toxic & allergic influences(Tubercular - Bacterial, septic focus)
2) Endogenous infections :-    T.B,  Syphilis, leprosy  -  Viral infection etc.
3) Secondary infections from pericular or intra ocular tissues
4) Exogenous infection  ex :- conjunctival lesions.
5) Systemic & metabolic ex :- Rheumatoid arthritis.

**Pathology** :- marked infiltration of scleral Lamellae with lymphocytes and
necrosis of the scleral fibres with ultimate thining of the sclera.

**Symptoms -** 1)Marked pain may radiate to the frontal region.

2) Lacrimation but no discharge.

**Sign :-**1) Pinkish red area with hyperaemia of surrounding conjunctiva.

2) The patch of scleritis is slightly elevated and markedly tender

**Complications : -** 1) Tongue shaped corneal opacity

2) Uveitis  3) Ciliary  staphyloma.

**Treatment : -** Same as episcleritis.

**Pinguecula :-** Pistaka - Balasa graditha

This is a small raised yellowish white nodule occur in the bulbar conjunctiva, in the horizontal meridian, a little distance away from the limbus
either on temporal or nasal sides

It may be due to chronic Exposure to dust and smoke Histologically it
consist of proliferated elastic tissue undergoing degenerative changes

No symptom except slight discomfort

**Treatment : -** Not Required

## Diseases of shukla mandal by Sushrutha

Total diseases       =     11

1)    Aushada sadya    =     4
      (Ashastra kruth)

2)    Shastra sadya     -     7

| S. No. | Name of the disease | Treatment |
|---|---|---|
| 1 | Shuktika | |
| 2 | Arjuna | Aushada Sadyam |
| 3 | Pistaka | (Ashastra Kruth) |
| 4 | Balasa Graditha | |
| 1 | Prasthari arma | |
| 2 | Shukla arma | 1) Lekhan/Chedan |
| 3 | Kshathaja arma | 2) Pratisaran |
| 4 | Adimamsa arma | |
| 5 | Snayu arma | |
| 6 | Sirajala | |
| 7 | Sira Pidika | |

## Diseases of shukla mandal by Vagbhat

Total diseases      =     13

1) Aushada Sadya    =     6

2) Shastra Sadya    =     7

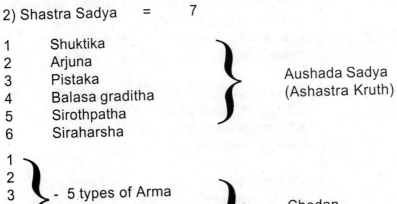

1      Shuktika

2      Arjuna

3      Pistaka                  Aushada Sadya

4      Balasa graditha     (Ashastra Kruth)

5      Sirothpatha

6      Siraharsha

1

2

3    - 5 types of Arma

4                          Chedan

5                          Pratisaran

6      Sira jala

7      Sira Pidika

## Diseases of Shukla madala

| No. | Name of the disease Modern name | Main features | Treatment `Principle |
|-----|--------------------------------|---------------|----------------------|
| 1) | Prasthari arma (pterigium) | It is **sannipataj** Vyadhi in which a thin, spreading reddish blue coloured membrane forms on shuklamandal (Sushrutha) soft, Spreading pain less blackish red membrane form on shukla mandal (vagbhata) | Sadya vyadhi 1) Lekhan Pratisaran if not 2) Chedan pratisaran |
| 2) | Shukla arma (Pterigum) | It is **kaphaj** vyadhi in which A slowly growing, soft, pale white coloured membrane develops on shuklamandal | Sadya vyadhi 1) LekhanPratisaran if not 2) Chedan-prati Saran |
| 3) | Kshataja arma or Shonita arma or Lohita arma (Pterigium) | It is **Raktaja** vyadhi, in which a soft, red coloured membrane resembling the colour of of lotus develops on shukla mandala. | Sadya vyadhi 1) Lekhan, pratisaran 2)Chedan, Pratisaran |
| 4) | Adhimamsa arma (pterigium) | It is **sannipataj** vyadhi in which A soft, thick, widely spreading, chocolate coloured membrana (yakruth varna) develops on shukla Mandala. | sadya vyadhi Chedan, pratisaran |
| 5) | Snayu arma (Pterigium) | It is **sannipataj** vyadhi in which a hard, wide, yellow coloured membrane resembling the snayu develops in shukla mandal | Sadya vyadhi Chedan, Pratisaran |
| 6) | Shuktika (Xerosis) | It is **Pittaja** Vyadhi in which Blackish white patches or dots (like in jala shukti or mirror with dust particles spreads in shukla mandala with pain burning and discomfort. | 1) Ashastra kruth 2) Pittaja abhish yanda chikitsa 3) Sheeta anjanas 4) Sadya vyadhi |

| 7) | Arjuna (Sub conjunctival haemorrhage, Mole, or melanoma) | It is **Raktaja** vyadhi, in which Red coloured dot or patch Originates in Shuklamandal (Red colour as the blood of rabbit) | 1) Sadya Vyadhi 2) Ashastra Kruth 3) Pittaja or Rakta Abhisyandi Chikitsa. |
|---|---|---|---|
| 8) | Pistaka (Pinguecula) | It is Kaphaj vyadhi in which shukla mandala is spread with white, round, fresh papules (Whitish like rice flour, fresh like water) | 1) Sadya vyadhi 2) Ashastra kruth 3) Kaphaja abhishyanda Chikista |
| 9) | Sirajala (Haemangioma of sclera or scleral staphyloma) | It is **Raktaja** vyadhi in which a A hard, big, red coloured capillary net seen in Shukla mandala. | 1) Sadya vyadhi 2) Like Arma 3) Chedan, Pratisaran |
| 10) | Sira pitica (episcleritis) | It is **Sannipataj** vyadhi in which a white nodule encircled with capillary net is seen in shukla Mandala. | 1) Sadya vyadhi 2) Like Arma 3) Chedan, Pratisaran |
| 11) | Balasa graditha (Pinguecula) | It is **Kaphaja** vyadhi in which a hard, painless nodule, resembling the water bubble, shining like bronze originates in shukla mandala. | 1) Sadya vyadhi 2) Ashastra Kruta 3) Application of kshara Anjanas. |

# कृष्णागत रोग

## सव्रणशुक्ल

निमग्नरूपं हि भवेतु कृष्णे सूच्येव विद्धं प्रतिभाति यदैव ।
स्रावं स्त्रवेदुष्णमतीव रुक् च तत् सव्रणशुक्लमुदाहरन्ति ॥

(सु॰ उ॰ 5/4 म॰ अ॰)

## सव्रणशुक्ल की साध्यासाध्यता

दृष्टे: समीपे न भवेतु यस्य न चावगाढं न च संस्रवेद्धि ।
अवेदनावन्न च युग्मशुक्रं तत् सिद्धिमाप्नोति कदाचिदेव ॥
विच्छिन्नमध्यं पिशितावृतं वा चलंसिरासक्तमदृष्टिकृच्च ।
द्वित्वग्गतं लोहितमन्ततश्च चिरोत्थितं चापि विवर्जनीयम् ॥
उष्णाश्रुपात: पिडका च कृष्णे तस्मिन् मुद्गनिभंच शुक्रम् ।
तदप्यसाध्यं प्रवदन्ति केचिद् अन्यच्च यत्तित्तिरिपक्षतुल्यम् ॥

(सु॰ उ॰ 5/5,6,7)

पितं कृष्णेथवादृष्टौ शुक्रंतोदाश्रुरागवत् ।
छित्त्वा त्वचं जनयति तेन स्यात् कृष्णमण्डलम् ।
पक्वजम्बुनिभं किंचित् निम्नं च क्षतशुक्रकम् ॥
तत् कृच्छ्रसाध्यं याप्यं तु द्वितीयपटलव्यधात् ।
तत्र तोदादि बाहुल्यं सूचीविद्धाभकृष्णता ॥
तृतीयपटलच्छेदादसाध्यं निचितं व्रणै: ॥

(अ:हृ:उ:१०अ:)

## अव्रणशुक्र

सितं यदा भात्यसितप्रदेशे स्यन्दात्मकं नातिरुग्श्रुयुक्तम् ।
विहायसीवाच्छघनानुकारि तद्व्रणं साध्यतमं वदन्ति ॥
गम्भीरजातं बहलं च शुक्रं चिरोत्थितं चापि वदन्ति कृच्छ्रम् ॥

(सु॰ उ॰ 4/8 अ॰)

शङ्खुशुक्लं कफात् साध्यं नातिरुक् शुद्धशुक्रकम् ।

(अ:हृ:उ:१०अ:)

120

## अक्षिपाकात्यय

संच्छाद्यते श्वेतनिभेन सर्वं दोषेण यस्या सितमण्डलं तु॥
तमक्षिपाकात्ययमक्षिकोपसमुत्थितं तीव्ररुजं वदन्ति॥

(सु० उ० 1/9 अ०)

दोषै: सास्त्रौ: सदृक् कृष्णं नीयते शुक्लरुपताम् ॥
धवलाम्रोपलिप्ताभं निष्पावार्धदलाकृति ॥
अतितीव्ररुजारागदाहश्वयथुपीडितम्
पाकात्ययेन तच्छुक्रं वर्जयेत्तीव्रवेदनम् ॥

(अ:ह:उ:१०अ:)

## अजकाजात

अजापुरीषप्रतिमो रुजावान् सलोहितो लोहितपिच्छिलाश्रु:
विदार्य कृष्णं प्रचयोभ्युपैति तं चाजकाजातमिति व्यवस्येत्॥

(सु० उ० 1/10 अ०)

आताम्रपिच्छिलास्रस्रुदाता म्रपिटिकातिरुक्।
अजाविट् सदृशोच्छायकृष्णया वज्यसिसृजाजका ॥

(अ:ह:उ:१०अ:)

# DISEASES OF KRISHNA MANDALA
## (Diseases of cornea and iris )

A) According to Sushruth                )(          B) According to Vagbhata
4 Diseases                              )(          5 Diseases

1) Savrana shukla (Shukra)              )(          1) Kshatha Shukla
2) Avrana Shukla (Shukra)               )(          2) Shuddha Shukla
3) AjakaaJatha                          )(          3) Ajaka
4) Akshi Pakathyaya                     )(          4) Pakathyaya Shukra
                                                    5) Sira Shukra.

1, 2, 3, 4, of Sushrutha and vagbhata are same but wording difference, The 5th disease of Vagbhata is the part of savrana shukla of Sushrutha . So the both classifications are merely same.

## 1) SAVRANA SHUKRA (SUSHRUTHA) (KSHATA SHUKRA (VAGBHATA) (ULCER CORNEA OR ULCERATIVE KERATITIS)

It is Rakthaja Asadhya Vyadhi (Sushrutha),
Pittaja Kasta sadhya vyadhi (Vagbhata)

**Note : -** (When doshas vitiate 3 rd patala of krishna mandal it becomes Asadhya) (Vagbhata)

**Description : -** The krishna mandala is vitiated (injured) form a small, round ulcer, with severe pain (as pierced by needle ) and hot lacrimation.

1) The word Succhyeva Viddham is not only applicable to the nature of the pain (Suchividdha vath Shoola), But also to the shape of the ulcer (small, rounded pin pointed as pricked by the needle)

2) The Word **nimaghna rupam** donotes the inflammatory condition of krishna mandala in which it appears as dipped, or sunken

3) **Ushnashrutha :-** Discharges more hot lacrimation

4) **Ateeva ruk :-** With severe untolerable pain Vascularisation of cornea

5) **Raktha rajinibham:-** as a complication (Videha).

6) Because of inflammatory process, krishna mandala appears in red colour like pravala (videha), pakwa jambhuphala (Vagbhata)

7) The stages of the disease explained as

I) a) Utthana (simple superficial lesion) (b) Avagadha deep lesion) by sushrutha

II)     a) Vitiation of      Pradhama patala    -    Kasta Sadhyam
        b)     "    "        Dwitheeya patala   -    Yapyam.
        c)     "    "        Truteeya patala    -    Asadhyam

by " Vagbhata "

8)   According to vaghata the severity of the disease increases by the progression of disease from Ist to IIIrd patala and become more complicated.

## Sadhya Asadhyatwa of Savrana Shukla (Prognosis)

| Sadhyam | Asadhyam |
|---|---|
| 1) Vranam which is not nearer to drusti (not nearer to central cornea in which refractive media is not obsructed). | 1) Vranam near to drusti (Central corneal opacity, refractive media will be obstructed) |
| 2) Na avagadham (Uthana). not deeply spreaded or if pradhama patala (epithelial layer) only affected | 2) Avagadham (deeply spreaded ulcer, if affects 2nd and 3rd patala i.e., stroma and endothelium) |
| 3) Ashru srava rahitham ( no Lacrimation) | 3) Ashru srava Sahitham (with lacrimation) |
| 4) Avedna (No pain) | 4) Ativedanam (more pain) |
| 5) Single ulcer | 5) Multiple ulcers |
| 6) Cornea if not perforated | 6) cornea if perforated |
| 7) No Iris prolapse | 7) with Iris prolapse |
| 8) Non Spreading ulcer | 8) Spreading or serpiginous ulcer. |
| 9) Sira rahitham (Avascular) | 9) Sira yuktham (Vascularised) |
| 10) Prakrutha Varnam(Transparent) | 10) Vikrutha Varnam (Opacities) |
| 11) Pitikaa rahitham (No extra growth) | 11) Pitica yuktam (phlyctenular kerato conjunctivitis.) |
| 12) Shotha rahit (Non inflammed) | 12) Shotha yuktham (inflammed) |

## SIRA SHUKLA  (A.H.)

It is explained by vagbhata as 5th disease of krishna mandala (4 common according to Sushrutha & Vagbhata). The symptoms of this disease are explained by Susrutha in savrana Sukra only.

It is due to the vitiation of 4 doshas (Tri doshas + Raktha), in which the Krishna mandalam is vascularised (Sira yuktha Shukram), signs and symptoms are toda (Pricking pain),Daha (Burning), sirajala (formation of cillary net on cornea) discharge of sheetha or ushna, swaccha or gadha ashru (tears), without specific cause

**Treatment** :-If the vision is not obstructed treatment should be given like Savrana shukara.

**Vishista anjana :-** Should prepare with pundareeka yastimadu Kakoli, simhee, loha, Haridra, rasanjan. The drugs should grinded with goat milk and has to fumigate with yava or Aamalaki patra by dipping in ghritha, should prepare for Anjana.

## 2) AVRANA SHUKLA or SHUDDHA SHUKLA
### (Non ulcerated Keratitis, Corneal Opacities)

The word Avrana Shukra used by Sushrutha and shuddha shukra by vagbhata.

    Rakthaja Sadhya vyadhi.    (Sushrutha)

    Kaphaja Sadhya vyadhi.    (Vagbhata)

Avrana shukla is discribed as secondary to Abhishyanda vyadhi (Syandaathmakam), in which a part of Krishna mandala become white (a) like the thin fresh clouds in the sky (SU), b) like shankha, c) like shankha chandra kunda pushpa and thin fresh clouds (Madhava Kara).

Patient have negligible pain and Lacrimation (Burning sensation also present Madhavakara).

It is sadhya vyadhi But may Become Krichra sadhya when the disease is deeply spreaded (Gambheera), widely spreaded (Bahala) and long standing (Chirotthita).

## 3) AJAKAJATHA OR AJAKA
### (Anterior staphyloma or Iris prolapse)

    Ajakajatha    -    (Sushrutha)

    Ajaka    -    (Vagbhata)

It is Rakthaja Asadhya vyadhi. (Kaphaja Asadhya vyadhi by Dalhana) A red painful growth ( or pitica - vagbhata) resembling the dried pellet of excreta of a goat (Aja pureesha vath pitica) comes out by penetrating the Krishna Mandala, slowly growing in the nature, originates due to the vitiation of Raktha dosha and netra patalas (pradhama - Dwiteeya and Truteeya patalas).

The signs & symptoms are 1) severe pain 2) red sticky discharge 3) perforation of Krishna mandala and 4) Prolapse of a red pitica resembling Aja pureesha, and finally causes 5) blindness.

Generally it arises as a complication of savrana shukla and netra Abhighatha. (Anterior staphyloma is the Ist Stage and Iris prolapse is the next)

Though it is explained as Asadhya vyadhi, treatment can be tried like savrana shukla.

**Treatment Principle of AjakaJatha:-**
      1) Snehan  (2) Anjana (3) Nasya
      (4) Raktha mokshana (5) Agni karma (6) Shastra karma.
A) Triphala ghritha - oral and for nasyam
B) Shukra uthseda Anjana - useful as Analgesic and for correcting  the abnormal pigmentation of krishna mandala.

**ANJANA -** dravyas.
      Narikelaasti, Bhallataka beeja, Harithala, vamshankura- According to Kshara vidhi kshara has to prepare with above  drugs and has  to do mardana and Bhavana with Hasti asti churna, and has to use as Anjana, after anjana vidhi eyes should be washed with Triphala Kashaya.

**Agni karma :-** If the disease does not respond to medical treatment, Agni karma has to do, in this process the prolapsed part has to burnt with swarna shalaka.

**Shastra Karma:-** The prolapsed or bulged part is cleaned well and the selected lateral part is pricked with a needle to  irrigate the infected fluid, Go mamsa churnam+ Ghritha is filled, in the gap and bandaged. Bandage  has to continue for 7 days.  After 7 days if any raised part remains that should be scraped out - for shamana chikitsa, Ksheerisarpi is advised for nasya. ·
      Treatment according to **Yogaratnaker :**

1)     Sira mokshana 2) Rechana with Trivruth churnam (3) Vata hara ghritas for seka Aashchyotan Tarpana etc. (4) Netra Pooranam : Collect the periosteum of cow bones + lukewarm water in a kamsya patra, grind well and use for poorana (5) Shambooka mamsa rasa ( get pakwa in on  smoke less fire) + Karpoora Ashchyotan or Anjana (6) Shashakadi ghritha Panam.

## 4) AKSHI PAKATHYAYA  OR PAKATHYAYA SHUKLA
      (Serpiginous ulcer, complicated ulcerative keratitis,
      hypopyon ulcer - keratomalacia  - panophthalmitis.)

Akshi pakathyaya    -     Sushrutha
Pakathyaya Shukla   -     Vagbhata.

      It is tridoshaja asadhya krishna mandala vyadhi, it arises as a complication of  abhishyanda (abhishyanadath uthpannam), in which the entire Krishna mandala becomes white by the vitiation of Tridoshas. The associated symptoms are severe pain, and drusti nasham. (Loss of vision)

      " It should be rejected for the treatment. "

## SUSHRUTHA AND VAGBHATA'S COMPARATIVE DESCRIPTION :

| | Sushrutha | Vagbhata |
|---|---|---|
| 1) | It is called as Akshi Pakathyaya | Pakathyaya shukla |
| 2) | Vitiating doshes are Tridoshas | Vitiating doshas Tridoshas + Raktha. |
| 3) | The infection (white discolouration) spreads only in Krishna Mandala. | Infection spreads not only in Krishna mandala but also in drusti mandala. |
| 4) | Symptoms are<br>1) Pain<br>2) Drustinasha (Loss of vision) | Symptoms are<br>1. Pain<br>2. Drustinasha(Loss of vision)<br>3. Raga (Hyperaemia)<br>4. daha (Burning)<br>5. shotha (Oedema)<br>6. Pakam (Suppuration) |

If the patient is strengthy, without complications, treatment can be tried like shukra vyadhi.

## SHUKRA VYADHI CHIKITSA
### (Savrana and Avrana shukra)

1) Lekhana or Gharshana with Anjanas is the main treatment procedure explained for shukra vyadhi.

**The treatment prininciple is**

a) Snehan b) Swedana    c) Shodhana  1) Sthanika
                                     2) Sarvadehika
          (a, b, c. for body purification)
d) Lekhana or gharshan

**Sthanika shodhana** With seka, Aashchyotan, tarpana putapaka etc.
**Sarvadehika shodhana** With Rakthamokshana, shirovirechana, virechana.

1) **Oral administation of :-** Triphala choorna or kalka or kashaya with or without ghritha,or Triphala ghritha, or Tikthaka ghritha or ghritha got pakwam in Nishotha Kashaya should give for virechan, tarpan etc then rakta mokshana or jalauka mokshana is advised at temporal region.

2) Then sekam with the medicated milk or decoction prepared with -kamala pushapa, ksheera kakoli, Draksha, yastimadhu, vidari kanda, sugar + goat's milk or water.

3) If pain redness, watering of eye reduces then Lekhana anjana has to use

126

4)      If the affected part is rough and unveven Gharshana is advised. (Rubbing of affected area with medicated powders)

Ex.- 1) Fine powder of Shirisha beeja, Maricha, pippali, saindhava lavana-should use for gharshana.

2) Saindhava lavana got bhavana in triphala kashaya - also used for gharshana.

5)      **Lekhana Anjanas**:-1) Metalic powders (Swarna, rajatha, Tamra etc. ), Rasa Aushada (Gyrika manashila etc.), Lavana, Ratna, Dantha, Shrunga and drugs of Avasadana varga - mix in equal quality, grind well and the fine powders has to use as anjana.
2) Kukkutanda twak bhasma, Lashuna, Trikatu, Karanja and Ela - mix equally, grind well and the fine powder has to use as anjana.

**3) Tamraadi Choornaanjan.:-**Tamra bhasma 16 parts, shanka bhasma 8 parts, manashila 4 parts, maricha 2 parts, saindhava lavana 1 part - powdered together and has to use for anjana.

**4) Shankhaadyan :-** Jan Shankha, kola asti, Nirmali beeja, Draksha, Yastimadhu, madhu (equal parts), grinded together and the fine powder has to use as Anjana.

**5) Kshaudraadhyanjan -**Madhu, samudraphena shirisha pushpa, godantha (equal parts) grinded together and the fine powder has to use as anjan.

**6) Mudgaadyanjan :-** Fried mudga (without seed coat), shanka, cheeni, madhu (equal parts) as anjan.

(7) Shankha, shukthi, Yastimadhu, draksha, Nirmali phala, madhu grinded together and the fine powder has to use as Anjan.

8) Yasti madhusara (the essense of Yastimadhu)+ madhu is used as Anjana.

9) The essense of vibheethaki majja + madhu is used as Anjana.

**10) Maha neela gutika :-** Bruhathi moola, yastimadhu, Tamra bhasma, saindhava lavan, shunti.Grind with Aamalaki kashaya, pasted to the Tamra patra (copper vessel), fumigate with yava. ghritha and Aamalaki patra, has to prepare vati with water or honey and has to use for Anjana.

11) Vamshankura, purified Bhallathaki beeja, Taala, Narikela The drugs are burnt with Tila nala - Prepare kshodaka, add Hasti asthi choorna to the kshar odakam, grind well and has to use as anjana. (This anjana brings the normal pigmentation to cornea)

12) Buds of jathi, laaksha, gyrika, chandana grind with water and has to use as varthi anjana.

**13 Dantha varthi:-** The teeth of - Gaja - Varaha, Ostra, Go, Ashwa, Aja, khara + Shankha, muktha, samudra phena - equally- add (1/4 weight) maricha grind well and has to use as anjana.

**14) Tamaala Patraadi varthi.:-**
Tamaala patra, Go dantha, shankha, samudra phena Kharaasti, Tamra bhasma, grind with go mootra and has to use as varthi **anjana**

15) Rathna, dantha, shrunga, dhathu, Trikatu, Ela, Karanja, beeja Lashuna, swarna ksheeri, grind well and use as Anjan.

16) Vydoorya spatika Shankha, Muktha, pravala, Roupya, Loha, Traphu, Tamra, Naga, Aala, Manahshila, Kukutanda twak bhasma, Samudra phena, Rasanjan, Saindhava lavana - grind with Aja ksheera and has to use as Anjan.

17) Sura, Go dantha, Samudra phena, shirisha pushpa - grind well and has to use for Gharshana - Lekhana anjana.

18) Laangali kshara has to do bhavana either in Aamalaki Kashaya or vana Tulasi Kashaya and has to use as choorna anjan.

**19) Go, khara Aswa, Osthra** Dantha ; + Shankha, samudra Phena, get bhavana and mardana in Arjuna Kashaya - and has to use as varthi anjan.

**20) Chandrodaya varthi:-** Hareethaki, Vibheetaki, Pippali, maricha vacha kusta Shankha nabhi, manahshila, grind with Aja ksheera and has to use as varthi Anjan.

**21) Chandraprabha varthi:-** Rasanjana, swetha maricha, pippali, yastimadhu, Vibheethakaashthi, Shankha nabi, manahshila - grind with Aja ksheera and has to use as varthi anjan.

22) Samudra phena choorna - grind with Lemon juice and has to use as Anjan.

**23) LamajjaKaadyanjan:-** Lamajjaka (Truna Vishesha), Neela Kamala, sugar, sariba, Chandana, **each 1 karsha** sariba kashaya 1 prastam, get it pakwam and has to use as Anjan.

**24) Chanda naadi varthi:-** Chandana, gyrica, Laaksha, Maalathi pushpa - grind well and has to use as varthi anjan.

**25) Danthaadyanjan -** Teeth of Go- khara, oshthra + Shankha, samudra-phena + powdered well and has to use as choorna anjan.
26) Swarna Makshika bhasma + madhu as Anjan.

27) Karanja beeja + phalasha pushpa swarasa - grindwell and use as varthi anjan.

28) Karpoora choorna + vata ksheera as varthi anjan.

29) Vydeha varthi :- Rasanjan, Shiileya, kumkuma, manahshilla, Shankha, swetha maricha, sugar as varthi anjan.

30) Nishotha moola kwatham + madhu as Anjan.

**Nasya :-** 1) Krishnadya taila nasya:- pippali vidanaga yastimadhu, saindhava lavana shunthi - prepare kalka, add aja ksheera, tila taila - has to prepare taila according to taila paka vidhi- and this taila is advised for Nasya.

**Ashchyotanam:-**1)Yastimadhu, Rasanjan, Kamala, Laaksha prapaundareeka, usheera, sariba - kashaya has to prepare + stanyam Aashchyotanam
2) Jathi patra, yastimadhu - get fry in ghritham - add cool water and has to use for eye wash.
3) Haridra yastimadhu, Krishna sariba, swetha lodhra - kashaya has to prepare for sekam.

**Internal yogas**
1) Shadanaga guggulu 2) Lohadi guggulu 3) Patoladi ghritam 4) Krishnasariba Kwath + madhu - Orally.

## CORNEAL ULCER OR ULCERATIVE KERATITIS)
### (Savrana Shukla)

**Classification - I**

**A) Purulent ulcer or Suppurative keratitis**
1) Ordinary pyogenic corneal ulcer.
2) Hypopyon ulcer or serpiginous ulcer.
3) Mycotic ulcer.   4) Marginal ulcer.

**B) Non purulent corneal ulcer**
1) Ulcer in association with trachoma.        2) Dendritic ulcer.
3) Lagophthalmic ulcer   4) Ulcer due to vitamin A deficiency
5) Neurotrophic ulcer.

**C) Allergic corneal ulcer :**
1) Phlyctenular ulcer.

**d) Degenerative ulcer:**
1) Atheromatous ulcer 2) Moorens ulcer.

**Classification - II**
A) Superficial keratitis, (a) Purulent b) Non Purulent
B) Deep Keratitis

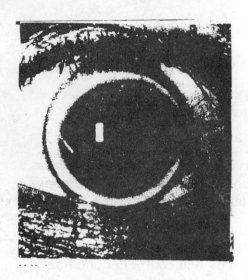

Arcus Senilis

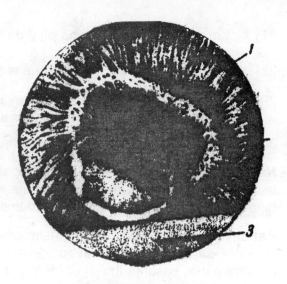

Creeping Ulcer of the cornea:
1. Posteriror synechia; 2.Growing edge of
the Ulcer 3.Hypopyon.

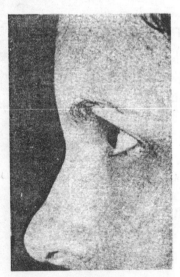

Keratoconus

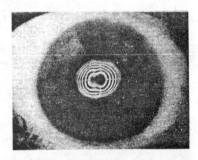

Keratoscopic appearance of the
corneal reflex in an advanced case of
keratoconus

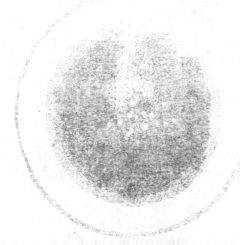

Superficial Punctate Keratitis

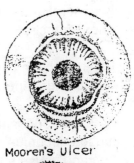

Mooren's Ulcer

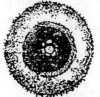

Mycotic Ulcer of cornea

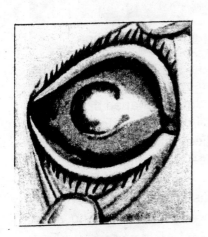

Panophthalmitis

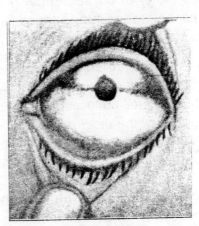

Phthisis bulbi

# MODE OF INFECTION

1) In general ulcers occuring in central cornea are usually due to Exog enous infection whether bacterial, viral or micotic.

2) Ulcers occuring in periphery of cornea are often toxic or **allergic** or due to endogenous infection.

3) From ocular tissue :- owing to the anatomical continuity, the inflam mation of conjunctiva sclera or Uveal tract, may spread to the cornea and cause the disease

## Definition of corneal ulcer
Loss of corneal substance as a result of infection or trauma and formation of a raw excavated area, is known as corneal ulcer.

## Causes of corneal ulceration
1) Corneal epithelium can't be penetrated by most of the organisms, except Diphtheria bacillus and gonococcus.
2) Trauma to cornea by penetrating injuries, misdirected eye lashes, foreignbodies and conjunctival concreations.
3) Unhealthy condition of the corneal epithelium like in glaucoma, corneal oedema and keratomalacia etc.

## Pathology of corneal ulcer :-
It canbe divided into 3 stages.
1) progressive stage 2) stage of regression 3) Stage of cicatrization.

**1) Progressive stage :-** (disease increases in this stage) surrounding the ulcer there is marked infiltration of cornea with puscells, necrosis sloughing off the epithelium occurs. ulcer crater is formed ( Saucer shaped defect) the margins of the ulcer projects above the surface of cornea due to imbibition of fluids, other complications are - ciliary congestion, Iritis Hypopyon forma- tion, vascularisation of peripheral cornea, opacities in the vitreous etc.

**2) Stage of regression :-** Infiltrations start to disappear. polymorphs are replaced by large mononuclear cells, leucocytes in the surrounding zone and digests the necrotic tissue.

**3) Stage of cicatrization :-** Healing of the defect occurs by the formation of granulation tissue from the margins of the ulcer, the newly formed layer is non transparent.

## Pathology of perforating types of corneal ulcer :-

Ulcerative process spreads into deeper corneal tissue and perforation follows, the commonest causes are sudden exertion on the part due to cough sneezing and spasm of the orbicularis muscle.The complications are
1)      Drainage of aqueous and abolition of anterior chamber.
2)      Anterior synechia - anterior staphyloma and Iris prolapse.
3)      Adherent leucoma.
4)      Sub luxation of lens - Anterior polar cataract.
5)      Intra ocular haemorrhages due to sudden lowering of intra ocular pressure.
6)      Panophthalmitis.

## Pathology of sloughing corneal ulcer :-

If the infecting agent is highly virulent or the body resistent power is very low, the whole or a part of cornea may slough out leaving a very big gap in the cornea, pseudo cornea is formed, the associated complications are, Iris prolapse, occluded pupil, dislocated lens, intra ocular haemorrhages, secondary glaucoma, panophthalmitis.

## Signs - symptoms of corneal ulcer :-

**Symptoms :-** Pain or discomfort or burning sensation in the eye, Lacrimation photophobia, head ache, blurring of vision, Blepharo spasm.

**Signs :-** 1) Congestion of conjunctiva & cornea. 2) hazy Cornea.
3) Ulcer crater with over hanged margins and the floor filled with necrotic tissue material.
4) The ulcer area gives green staining with 2% fluorescein drops.
5) No window reflex in cornea.
6) ciliary congestion and conjunctival hyperaemia.
7) Iritis with Hypopyon formation (if virulently infected).
8) Peripheral or total corneal vascularisation.

## General treatment principle
1)      Local & systemic Broad spectrum antibiotics.
2)      1% Atropin ointment application
3)      Ointments should apply at nights to prevent adhesion.
4)      Dark glasses has to use (no bandeging)
5)      In progressive nature of ulcer, the margin should be cauterised to prevent the spreading nature of the ulcer.
6)      Treating the peipheral infective focus.

## 1) Dendritic corneal ulcer:-

It is a type of corneal ulcer with a branched apearence caused by Herpes simplex virus.

## Predisposing causes :-
Febrile conditions like influenza malaria or pneumonia etc.

**Signs :-** 1) Vesicles appear at the termination of the corneal nerves, which soon rupture and produce ulcers in star shape or as branched figure.
2) Loss of corneal sensation. (3) Ciliary Congestion. 4) Lacrimation.

## 2) Lagophthalmic Ulcer:-
**Causes :** 1) Coma vigil (2) Orbicularis oculi muscle function failure ( paralysis of facial nerve.) 3) Proptosis (4) ectropion.
Because of above causes a person cannot able to close his eyes properly leads to exposure Keratitis, the ulcer is usually located at the lower part of the cornea, near the Limbus.

## 3) Neurotrophic ulcer :- It occurs as a result of defect in the sensory nerve supply of the cornea, due to
1) Injection of alcohol in to gasserian ganglian to treat trigeminal neuralgia.
2) Neoplasms pressing on the Gasserian ganglion.

**Signs :-** 1) Oedema of corneal epithelium which exfoliates and become ulcer. (2) ciliary congestion (3) Loss of corneal sensation (4) Pain (5) No Lacrimation(6) Defective vision.

## 4) Phlyctenular Keratitis and ulcer:-
It is an allergic reaction of cornea to some endogenous toxins, bacterial in origin, (usually tuberculous.) Localised lymphocytic infiltrations of cornea occurs and break down to form ulcers.

**Signs :-** Whitish nodules formation at limbus (2) ciliary congestion 3) lacrimation (4) Blepharo spasm. 5) Ulceration of cornea.

## Stages

1)     Phlyctenular keratitis (nodules formation)
2)     Phlyctenular ulcer (Nodules break down and ulcer forms)
3)     Fascicular ulcer (ulcers from periphery, spreads to centre)
4)     Phlyctenular pannus (corneal ulcers, blood supply spreads from all angles)

**5) Hypopyon ulcer or Ulcus serpens:-**

It commonly occur in the old, the debilitated, and in the alcoholics, the infecting organism is pneumo cocus and the source is the chronic dacryocystitis.

**Signs :** (1) Greyish white disc shaped ulceration seen near the centre of cornea (2) The ulcer spreads at one sector with a crescentic edge, stops and again spreads in the another sector (serpiginous character) 3) Iritis with Hypopyon (4) ciliary congestion (5) Oedema of eye lids (6) early perforation of cornea (7) secondary glaucoma.

**Symptoms :-** same as ordinary corneal ulcer but more marked.

**6) Mycotic ulcer :-** (Due to fungus infection)

Causative agents : - Fungus aspergillus fumigatus, candida albicans, streptothrix actinomycosis.

**Signs :-** 1) Dry circular yellowish white ulcers on cornea surrounded by yellowish gutter of demarcation 2) hypopyon formation (3) ciliary congestion. 4) Material scraped from the ulcer shows the presence of fungus.

**7) Marginal corneal ulcer ;-** It is usually seen in the old, debilitated people, gout patients, and as a complication of acute mucopurulent conjunctivitis.

**Causative organisms are :-**

Koch - weeks bacillus, - morax - Axenfeld diplobacillus

**Signs :-** 1) Peripheral corneal ulceration (near timbus ) with surrounding corneal infiltration.

    2) Vascularisation of cornea.

    3) Ulcer may heal rapidly but reccurance is common.

| Primary marginal ulcer | Secondary marginal ulcers |
|---|---|
| 1) a) catarrhal ulcers (gout), | 1) Phlyctenular Keratitis |
| 2) b) Septic focus from ear | 2) Trachomatous keratitis |
| nose throat c) moorens | 3) Purulent conjunctivitis |
| ulcers. | 4) Rosacea Keratitis. |

**8) Atheromatous ulcer :-** It is an ulcer devlops in an old leucoma due to degenerative changes (poor nourishment, low resistence power) the epithelium of leucoma easily get infected and an ulcer develops. The ulcer is very resistent to treatment

**9)     Mooren's ulcer :-** It is a superficial ulcer starts at the margin of cornea and spreads gradually in the entire cornea. Base of the ulcer soon becomes vascularised, the deeper structures of cornea are normal, and the cornea never perforates.

The Patient have severe neuralgic pain, lacrimation and photophobia. The ulceration is probably due to metabolic disorders and malnutrition.

**10)     Superficial keratitis:-** Inflammation of corneal tissue is known as keratitis in which **Ulcer may or may not**  form
It is of two types.
(1) Superficial Keratitis and  2) Deep keratitis,
Punctate erosions inthe superficial layers of cornea is known as **superficial** punctate keratitis.

**Etiology :-** (1) Virus infection by
a) Herpes simplex - virus (b) herpes zoster virus (c) Herpes Febrils (d) TRIC virus (e) Adeono virus (f) Virus of measles. vaccinia and mumps. (g) acne roscea (h) variola.
2) Inflammatory conditions of eye lids.
3) Kerato conjunctivitis sicca
4) Expossure to ultra voilet rays.

**Viral keratitis**
**a) Herpes simplex keratitis :-** (Superficial Keratitis)
Multiple superficial epithelial erosions spread like dendritic ulcer - corneal sensation reduces, and the inflammation extends even into the stroma (diffuse deep keratitis)

**b) Herpes zoster ophthalmicus :-** The gasserian ganglian is affected, virus spread along the Ist branch of V Cranial nerve - and causes superficial punctate keratitis, By the secondary infection it may also cause keratitis profunda. (corneal sensation completely lost).

**c) Herpes Febrills :-** Minute opacities, fissures, vesicles form on the cornea and associated with malaria, influenza etc.
**d)  TRIC virus keratitis**  : - Punctate keratitis seen in as the complication of Trachoma
**e)     Adeno virus - type 8 virus - keratitis :-** (Superficial punctate keratitis) Follicular hypertrophy of conjunctiva, multiple sub epithelial infiltrations in cornea, with a preauricular lymphadenopathy, it is very contageous and recover spontaneously within 3 to 6 weeks.

**f) Measles viral Keratitis :-** Catarrhal conjunctivitis with superficial keratitis develops.

**g) Vaccinia viral keratitis :-** Superficial punctate keratitis and also disciform type of keratitis develops.

**h) Mumps :-** May cause superficial punctate keratitis.

**i) Acne Rosacea Keratitis :-** Marginal sub epithelial infiltrations spreads to the centre of cornea, and cornea soon vascularises.

**j) Variola :-** Nodules formation in conjunctiva and cornea, later nodules ulcerates and causes grave danger to cornea.

**11) Deep keratitis :-**
Inflammation of the deep layers of cornea - stroma etc.

**1) Interstitial keratitis**
cellular infiltrations of deeper layers of cornea followed by vascularisation.

**Causes** Syphilis - Tuberculosis and leprosy etc.
**a) Syphilitic interstitial keratitis**
Hazy-dull- lustreless cornea (Ground glass cornea with), vascularisation radial brush like vessels appear on cornea (Salmon patches) and the general symptoms of syphilis also exist.
**b) Tubercular Interstitial Keratitis :-**Lesions are similar as syphilitic but the lesions limited to one sector of cornea only.

**c) Interstitial keratitis due to leprosy**
Infiltration of deeper layers of cornea, with the dense opacites which spread from periphery to centre of cornea, and does not clear up easily.

**2) Disciform keratitis.** Causativa agent is herpes simplex virus, greish white disc shaped opacities appears in the deeper layers of central cornea, oedema of corneal stroma causes Thickened cornea, fall of vision, diminished corneal sensation, and the opacities may not disappear completely.
**3) Keratitis profunda**
It is a type of deep keratitis associated with uveitis and the exact cause is not known.

**4) Intra corneal Abscess.**
It is due to purulent inflammation of corneal tissue usually as a result of penetrating injury.
**5) Sclerosing keratitis**
It occurs as a complication of scleritis, There is deep infiltration of cornea adjacent to the area of scleritis.

## 12) other affections of the cornea;-

1) Arcus senilis :- greyish white circular line in the cornea concentric with limbus - seen in the aged due to lipoid degeration.

2) Arcus juvenilis :- same as above but comes in children congenitally.

3) Kerato conus :- cone shaped cornea due to congenital weakness of cornea.

4) kerato globus (megalo cornea) Diameter of cornea (Normal 12 to 13 mm), it becomes bigger than normal (about 16 mm)

5) Keratectasia - protrusion of cornea without involvement of Iris, following inflammation, without perforation.

6) Argyrosis Dark brown colour of the cornea due to prolonged use of silver preparations.

7) Siderosis :-        Iron foreign bodies embedded in the cornea.

8) Chalcosis :-        copper foreign bodies embedded in the cornea.

9) Blood staining of cornea, it is seen in severe hyphaema due the absorption of blood by cornea.

10) Staphyloma of cornea - protrusion of cornea along with inflamed Iris , it may follow ulceration and perforation.

11) deposition of melanin pigment in posterior surface of cornea due to high myopia and diabetes.

**12) Mustard gas keratitis:-** It is a degenerative condition of cornea which results from the effect of mustard gas vapour onthe cornea.

**13) Kerato Conjunctivitis:-** Deficient secretion of Lacrimal glands and conjunctival glands causes conjunctival congestion, superficial punctate keratitis etc.

**14) Keratomalacia:-** It is due to vitamin A deficiency associated with dry ness of conjunctiva hazy cornea and bitots spots at near limbal conjunctiva infurthur stages cornea may ulcerate and perforate.

**15) Micro Cornea :-** It is congenital abnormality in which cornea is smaller is size.

**16) Megalo cornea :-** It is also congenital abnormality with bigger size of cornea.

# CORNEAL OPACITIES

(Avrana shukla )

Opacities of cornea according to the density are as following .

1) Nebula (Slight discolouration) only superficial layer of cornea is affected

2) Macula     (Brown opacity) Corneal lesion is some what deeper

3) Leucoma -   (White opacity) - Deepest and the thickest lesion.

**Note :-**

In long standing leucoma degenerative corneal ulcer known as Atheromatous ulcer may develop. and Adhesion of Iris to the leucoma is known as adherent Leucoma.


## CAUSES OF CORNEAL OPACITIES

1)     Healed corneal ulcer.

2)     Healed Keratitis

3)     Healed Penetrating injury to cornea.

4)     Healed Operative injury to cornea.

5)     Foreign body Abrasions

6)     Degenerative changes of cornea.


**Symptoms :**

If the opacity is inthe pupillary area it causes visual disturbances.

(Central opacity of cornea obstructs vision and very
Peripheral opacities doesn't obstruct the vision.)

# Diseaes of Krishna Mandala

| S.No. | name<br>Modern name | Clinicial features | Treatment Principle |
|-------|---------------------|--------------------|--------------------|
| 1) | Savrana shukla (ulcerative Keratitis) | Small round painful ulcers, develop in krishna mandala with Hot lacrimation by the vitiation of rakta dosha | Asadya But can try like Avrana Shukla |
| 2) | Avrana shukla (Non ulcerative Keratitis) | Krishna mandala is spread with white opacities like shankha chandra and fresh clouds by the vitiation of Rakta (sushrutha), kapha (Vagbhata) | 1) Shodhan therapy 2) Anjana Applications |
| 3) | Ajaka jatha (Iris prolapse) | A red painful growth comes out by penetrating the krishna mandala and appears like the driedpellet of excreta of goat, by the vitiation of Raktha dosha shukra | 1) Asadya 2) Shastra karma 3) Agni karma 4) Like Avrana |
| 4) | Akshi Pakatyaya (Panophthalmitis) | Krishna mandala completely become white by the vitiation of tridosha | Asadya |

## Diseases of Krishna mandal (Sushrutha)

|   | Total diseases |   |   | = | 4 |   |   |
|---|---|---|---|---|---|---|---|
| 1) | Avrana shukla | = | Ashastra kruth |   |   | = | 1 |
| 2) | Savrana Shukla | ⎤ |   |   |   |   |   |
| 3) | Ajakajatha |   | Asadya |   |   | = | 3 |
| 4) | Akshipakatyay | ⎦ |   |   |   |   |   |

## Diseases of Krishna mandal by vagbhata

| 1) | Shuddha Shukla | = | Ashastra kruth | = 1 |
|---|---|---|---|---|
| 2) | Kshatha shukla | ⎤ |   |   |
| 3) | Ajaka |   |   |   |
| 4) | Pakathyaya shukla |   | Asadya | = 4 |
| 5) | Sira shukla | ⎦ |   |   |

Note : -

Though most of the diseases (except avrana or shuddha shukla) are explained as asadya, treatment principles and yogas are explained for the all.

## सर्वगत रोग

स्यन्दास्तु चत्वार इहोपदिष्टास्तावन्त एवेह तथाधिमन्था
शोफान्विते शोफयुतश्च पाकावित्येवमेते दश सम्प्रदिष्टा
हताधि मन्थोनिलपर्ययश्च शुष्काक्षि पाकोन्यत एव वाते:
दृष्टि स्तथाम्लाध्युषिता सिराणामुत्पात हर्षवपि सर्वभागा:

## संक्रामक व्याधियों

प्रसङ्गाद् गात्रसंस्पर्शान्नि:श्वासात् सह भोजनात् ।
एकशय्यासनाच्चैव वस्त्रमाल्यानुलेपनात् ॥
कुष्ठं ज्वरश्च शोषश्च नेत्राभिष्यन्द एव च ।
औपसर्गिकरोगाश्च संक्रामन्ति नरान्नरम् ॥

(सु॰ नि॰ २ अ॰)

## अभिष्यन्द् का सर्वरोगकारणत्व

प्रायेण सर्वे नयनामयास्तु भवन्त्यभिष्यन्दनि मित्त मूला: ।
तस्माद भिष्यन्दमुदीर्य माणमुपाचरेदाशुहिताय धीमान् ॥

(सु॰ उ॰ 6/5)

## 1. वातज अभिष्यन्द

निस्तोदनं स्तम्भनरोमहर्षसंघर्षपारुष्य शिरोभितापा:
विशुष्कभाव : शिशिराश्रुता च वाताभिपन्ने नयने भवन्ति ॥

(सु॰ उ॰ 6/6)

वातेन नेत्रेभिष्यण्णे नासानाहोल्पशोफता ।
राङ्खाक्षिभ्रूललाटस्य तोदस्फूरणभेदनम् ॥
शुष्काल्पा दूषिका शीतमच्छँचाश्रु चला रुज:
निमेषोन्मेषणं कृच्र्छाजन्तुनामिब सर्पणम् ॥
अक्ष्याध्मातमिवाभाति सूक्ष्मै: शल्यैरिवाचितम् ।
स्निग्धोष्णैश्चोपशमनं सोभिष्यन्द: .... ॥

(अ:हृ:उ:15)

142

## 2. पैतिक अभिष्यन्द

दाहप्रपाकी शिशिराभिनन्दा धूमायनं बाष्पसमुच्छ्रयश्च ।

उष्णाश्रुता पीतकनेत्रता च पित्ताभिपन्ने नयने भवन्ति ॥

(सु॰ उ॰ 6/7)

दाहो धूमायनं शोफ: श्यावता वर्त्मनो वहि: ।

अन्त:क्लेदोश्रु पीतोष्णं राग: पीताभदर्शनम् ॥

क्षारोक्षितक्षताक्षित्वं पित्ताभिष्यन्दलक्षणम् ।

(अ:हृ:उ:15 अ॰)

## 3. कफज अभिष्यन्द

उष्णाभिनन्दा गुरुताक्षिशोफ: कण्डूपदेहौ सिततातिशैत्यम् ।

स्रावो मुहु: पिच्छिल एव चापि कफाभिपन्ने नयने भवन्ति ॥

(सु॰ उ॰ 6/8 अ॰)

स्यन्दे तु कफ़ सम्भवे

जाड्यं शोफो महान् कण्डूर्निद्रान्नानभिनन्दनम ॥

सान्द्रस्निग्धबहुश्वेतपिच्छावत् दूषिकाश्रुता ।

(अ:हृ:उ:15 अ॰)

## 4. रक्तज अभिष्यन्द

ताम्राश्रुता लोहितनेत्रता च राज्य: समन्तादतिलोहिताश्च ।

पित्तस्य लिङ्गानि च यानि तानि रक्ताभिपन्ने नयने भवन्ति ॥

(सु॰ उ॰ 6/9 अ॰)

रक्ताश्रुराजीदूषीकारक्तमण्डलदर्शनम् ॥

रक्तस्यन्देन नयनं सपित्तस्यन्दलक्षणम् ।

(अ:हृ:उ:१२अ:)

## अधिमन्थ

वृद्दैरेतैरभिष्यन्दैर्नराणामक्रियावताम् ।

तावन्तस्त्वधिमन्था: स्युर्नयने तीव्रवेदना: ॥

(सु॰ उ॰ 6/10 अ॰)

## अधिमन्थ के सामान्य लक्षण

उत्पाट्यत इवात्यर्थ नेत्रं निर्मथ्यते तथा ।
शिरसोर्धं च तंविद्यादधिमन्थं स्वलक्षणै: ॥

(सु॰ उ॰ 6/11 अ॰)

## 5. वातिक अधिमन्थ

नेत्रमुत्पाट्यत इव मथ्यतेरणिवच्च यत् ॥
संघर्षतोदनिर्भेदमांससंरब्धमाविलम् ॥
कुंचनास्फोटनाध्मानवेपथुव्यथनैर्युतम् ॥
शिरसोर्धंच येन स्यादधिमन्थ: स सारुतात् ॥

(सु॰ उ॰ 6/12,13 अ॰)

.................... उपेक्षित:
अधिमन्थो भवेत्तत्र कर्णयोर्नदनं भ्रम: ।
अरण्येव च मथ्यन्ते ललाट्क्षिभ्रुवादय: ॥

(अ:हृ:अ15)

## 6. पित्तज अधिमन्थ

रक्तराजीचितं स्रावि वह्निनेवावदह्यते ।
यकृत्पिण्डोपमं दाहि क्षारेणाक्तमिव क्षतम् ॥
प्रपक्वोच्छूनवर्त्मन्तं सस्वेदं पीतदर्शनम् ।
मूर्च्छाशिरोदाहयुतं पित्तेनाक्ष्यधिमन्थितम् ॥

(सु॰ उ॰ 6/14,15)

ज्वलदङ्गारकीर्णाभं यकृत्पिंडसमप्रभम् ॥
अधिम न्थेभवेन्नेत्रम् ।

(अं॰ हृ॰ उ॰15अ॰)

## 7. कफज अधिमन्थ

शोफवन्नातिसंरब्धं स्रावकण्डूसमन्वितम् ॥
शैत्यगौरवपैच्छिल्य दूषिकाहर्षणान्वितम् ॥
रूपं पश्यति दु:खेन पांशुवर्णमिवाविलम् ॥
नासाध्मान शिरोदु:खयुतं श्लेष्माधिमन्थितम् ॥

(सु॰ उ॰ 6/16,17 अ॰)

अधिमन्थे नतं कृष्णमुन्नतं शुक्लमण्डलम् ॥
प्रसेको नासिकाध्मानं पांशुवर्णमिवेक्षणम् ।

(अं॰ हृ॰ 15 अ॰)

## 8. रक्तज अधिमन्थ

बन्धुजीवप्रतीकाशं ताम्यति स्पर्शनाक्षमम् ।
रक्तास्रावं सनिस्तोदं पश्यत्यग्निनिभा दिश: ॥
रक्तमग्नारिष्टवच्च कृष्णभागश्च लक्ष्यते ।
यद्दीप्तं रक्तपर्यन्तं तद्रक्तेनाधिमन्थितम् ॥

(सु॰ उ॰ 6/18,19 अ॰)

मन्थेक्षि ताम्रपर्यन्तमुत्पाटनसमानरुक् ॥
रागेण बन्धूकनिभं ताम्यति स्पर्शनाक्षमम् ।
असृङ् निमग्नारिष्टाभं कृष्णमग्न्याभदर्शनम् ॥
अधिमन्था यथास्वं च सर्वे स्यंदाधिकव्यथा: ।
शङ्खदन्तकपोलेषु कपाले चातिरुक्करा: ॥

(अं॰ हृ॰ उ॰ 15 अ॰)

हन्याद् दृष्टिं सप्तरात्रात् कफोत्थोधीमन्थोसृक्सम्भव: पंचरात्रात् ।
षड्रात्राद् वै मारुतोत्थो निहन्यान्मिथ्याचारात् पैत्तिक: सद्य एव ॥

(सु॰ उ॰ 6/20 अ॰)

## 9. सशोफ अक्षिपाक

कण्डूपदेहाश्रुयुत: पक्वोदुम्बरसन्निभ: ॥
दाहसंहर्ष ताम्रत्वशोफनिस्तोदगौरवै: ॥
जुष्टो मुहु: स्रवेच्चास्रमुष्णशीताम्बु पिच्छिलम् ॥
संरम्भी पच्यते यश्च नेत्रपाक: सशोफज: ॥

(सु॰ उ॰ 6/21,22)

सशोफ: स्यात्त्रिभिर्मलै:
सरक्तैस्तत्र शोफोतिरुग्दाहष्ठीवनादिमान् ।
पक्वोदुम्बरसङ्काशं जायते शुक्लमण्डलम् ॥
अश्रूष्णशीतविशद पिच्छिलाच्छघनं मुहु: ॥

(अं॰ हृ॰ उ॰ 15 अ॰)

## 10. अशोफ अक्षिपाक

शोफहीनानि लिङ्गानि नेत्रपाकेत्वशोफजे ॥

(सु॰ उ॰ 6/23 अ॰)

अल्पशोफेल्पशोफस्तु पाकोन्यलक्षणैस्तथा।

वाग्भट ने अशोफ अक्षिपाक को अल्पशोफ अक्षिपाक कहा।

(अं॰ ह॰ 15 अ॰)

## 11. हताधिमन्थ

उपेक्षणादक्षि यदाधिमन्थो वातात्मक: सादयति प्रसह्य।

रुजाभिरुग्राभिरसाध्य एष हताधिमन्थ: खलु नाम रोग: ॥

(सु॰ उ॰ 6/23 अ॰)

हताधिमन्थ: सोपि स्यात् प्रमादात्तेन वेदना: ।

अनेकरूपा जायन्ते व्रणो दृष्टै च दृष्टिहा॥

(अं॰ ह॰ 15 अ॰)

## दूसरा हताधिमन्थ:

अन्त:सिराणां श्वसन: स्थितो दृष्टि प्रतिक्षिपन्॥

हताधिमन्थं जनयेत्तमसाध्यं विदुर्बुधा:

(सु॰ उ॰ 6/24 अ॰)

अन्तर्गत: सिराणां तु यदा तिष्टति मारुत: ।

स तदा नयनं शीघ्रं दृष्टि निरस्यति॥

तस्यां निरस्यमानायां निर्मथ्त्रन्निव मारुत: !

नयनं निर्वमत्याशु शूलतोदादिमन्थनै: ॥

अथवा शोषयेदक्षि क्षीणतेजोबलानलम्।

उत्पन्नमिव संशुष्कमवसीदति लोचनम्।

हताधिमन्थं तं विद्यादसाध्यं वातकोपत:

-डल्हण (सु. उ. 6 अ.)

## 12. वातपर्याय

पक्ष्मद्वयाक्षिभ्रुवमाश्रितस्तु यत्रानिल: संचरति प्रदुष्ट: ।

पर्यायश्चापि रुज: करोति तं वातपर्यायमुदाहरंति ॥

(सु॰ उ॰ 6/25 अ॰)

तद्वर्जिंत्यं भवेन्नेत्रमूनं वा वातपर्ययी ॥

(अ. ह्र. उ. 15 अ.)

## 13. अन्यतोवात

यस्यावटुकर्ण शिरोहनुस्थो मन्यागतो वाप्यानिलोन्यतो वा ॥
कुर्याद्रुजोति भ्रुवि लोचने वा तमन्यतोवातमुदाहरन्ति ॥

(सु॰ उ॰ 6/26 अ॰)

मन्याक्षिशंखतो वायुरन्यतो वा प्रवर्त्तयन् ।
व्यथां तीव्रामपैच्छिल्यरागशोफं विलोचनम् ॥
सङ्कोचयति पर्यश्रु सोन्यतोवातसंज्ञित: ॥

(अ. ह्र. उ. 15 अ.)

## 14. शुष्काक्षिपाक

यत् कूणितं दारुणरुक्षवर्त्म विलोकने चाविलदर्शनं च यत् ।
सुदारुणं यत् प्रतिबोधने च शुष्काक्षिपाकोपहतं तदक्षि ॥

(सु॰ उ॰ 6/27 अ॰)

वातपित्तातुरं घर्षतोद्भेदोपदेहवत् ।
रुक्ष दारुणवर्त्माक्षि कृच्छ्रोन्मीलनिमीलनम् ॥
विकूणननविशुष्कत्वशीतेच्छा शुलपाकवत् ।
उत्क: शुष्काक्षिपाकोयम्

(अ. ह्र. उ. 15 अ.)

## 15. अम्लाध्युषित

अम्लेन भुक्तेन विदाहिना च संछाद्यते सर्वत एव नेत्रम् ।
शोफान्वितं लौहितकै: सनीलैरेतादृगम्लाध्युषितं वदन्ति ॥

(सु॰ उ॰ 6/28 अ॰)

अन्नसारोम्लतां नीत: पित्तरक्तोल्वणैर्मलै:
शिराभिर्नेत्रमारूढ: करोति श्यावलोहितम् ।
सशोफदाहपाकाश्रु भृशं चाविलदर्शनम् ॥
अम्लोषितोयम्

(अ. ह्र. उ. 15 अ.)

## 16. सिरोत्पात

अवेदना वापि सवेदना वा यस्याक्षिराज्यो हि भवन्ति ताम्रा: ।
मुहुर्विरज्यन्ति च ता: समन्ताद् व्याधि: सिरोत्पात इति प्रदिष्ट: ॥

(सु. उ. 6/29 अ.)

रक्त राजीततं शुक्लमुष्यते यत्सवेदनम
अशोफाश्रूपदेहंच सिरोत्पात: सशोणितम

(अ. हृ. उ. 15 अ.)

## 17. सिराप्रहर्ष वा सिराहर्ष

मोहात् सिरोत्पात उपेक्षितस्तु जायेत रोगस्तु सिराप्रहर्ष: ॥
ताम्राच्छमसरं स्रवति प्रगाढं तथा न शक्नोत्यभिवीक्षितुं य ॥

(सु॰ उ॰ 6/30 अ॰)

उपेक्षित: सिरोत्पातो राजीस्ता: एव वर्धयन
कुर्यात्सास्र सिराहर्ष तेनाक्ष्यु व्दीक्षणाक्षामम्

(अ. हृ. उ. 15 अ.)

148

# SARVA GATHA ROGAS

The diseases which are explained under this group arises by spreading in all parts (Pakshma varthma - Swetha and Krishna Mandala). so only named as sarva gath roga.

**According to Sushrutha** - 17 diseases, they are :
### 4 types of abhishyanda
1) Vataja Abhishyanda      2) Pittaja Abhishyanda
2) Kaphaja Abhishyanda      4) Rakthaja Abhishyanda
### 4 types of adhimantha
5) Vataja adhimantha      6) Pittaja adhimantha
7) Kaphaja adhimantha      8) Raktaja adhimantha.
### 3 types of Akshi pakas)
9) Sa shopha Akshipaka      10) Ashopha Akshipaka
11) Sushkaakshi paka

12) Hathaadhi manda      13) Anila Paryaaya
14) Anyatho vatha      15) Sirothpaatha
16) Siraaharsha      17) Amladyushitha

**According to vagbhata Sarvaakshi rogas 16 they are :**
17 disease of Sushrutha - 2 diseases = 15 (Sirothpatha, siraharsha not explained why because these two he explained in shukla gatha rogas) and added Akshi pakatyaya, so totally 16 diseases According to vagbhata

# ABHISHYANDA

(Abhi = from four sides (all angles) - (syanda = Discharge.)
It is a contagious disease (Sankramika vyadhi) and becomes the cause for the most of the eye diseases In this disease watery or sticky eye discharge comes from the all angles of the eye.
It is of 4 types. 1) Vataja 2) Pittaja 3) Kaphaj 4) Rakthaja Abhshyand

### 1) VATAJ ABHISHYANDA
### (Sub acute Catarrhal conjunctivitis)
It is vataja sadhya vyadhi
**Signs & symptoms :-** As per sushruth
Nistodana = Suchi viddhavath shoola (Pricking pain in the eye.)
2) Stambana = Stiffness ; 3) Romaharasha = horripilation
4) Sangharsha = Foreign body sensation 5) Parushya = kaathinya (roughness)
6) Shirobhitapa = head ache 7) Vishushkabhava = dryness
8) Shishirashrutha = cool lacrimation (SU)

**Description of sushrutha :-** In vataja Abhishyanda patient feels headache, stiff, hard, dried eyes with, foreign body sensation, cool Lacrimation and with Pricking pain inthe eyes.

149

**Vagbhata :-** 1) Shankha, Akshi, Bhru, lalata - Toda, spurana, and bhedana
(pricking, cutting type of pain inthe Shankha, Akshi, bhru, and lalata );

2) Chala ruja - Radiating type of pain in above places
3) Shuska alpa dushika = dried and little eye discharge
4) Sheetha ashru  =  Cool Lacrimation
5) Nimeshonmeshana Kruchram  = difficulty in opening and closing the eye lids.
6) Janthunaamva sarpana  = Patient feels that Krimi is spreading in the eyes (foregin body sensation)
7) Nasanaaha  = Nasal obstruction
8) Alpa shopha = Oedema of eye
9) Snigda ushnaashcha upashamana feels happy with oily and hot treatments.

**Discription Vagbhata :-** In vataj abhishyanda the Patient feels radiating, pricking cutting pain in the Shankha, Akshi, bhru ,and lalata; cool Lacrimation, dried less eye discharge, difficulty in opening and closing the eyes, Nasal obstruction, oedema, foreign body sensation in the eyes and the patient feels happy with oily and hot treatments.

## 2) PITTAJA ABHISHYANDA
### (Acute Catarrhal conjunctivitis)

It is pittaja vyadhan Sadhya vyadhi, The disease inwhich the patient feels daha (burning sensation inthe eye), paka (suppuration), dhooma - bhashpa samucchaya (smoky sensation), ushna ashru (hot Lacrimation), Peetha netra (yelloish eyes), Shishirabhinanda (Feels happy with cool touch or cool medications, is described as pittaja abhishyanda.

**Vagbhata extra points :-**
1) Varthma shopha and shyava varthma = oedema and black discolouration of eye lids.
2) Antah kleda = exudation in the eyes.
3) Feels severe burning sensation like in Agnidagdha vrana.

## 3) KAPHAJA ABHISHYANDA
### (Acute muco purulent conjunctivitis)

It is kaphaja vyadan vyadhi.
The disease, in which the patient feels gurutwa (heavyness), shopha (oedema), Kandu (itching sensation), upadeha (Sticking of lids together) Pischila srava (Sticky Discharge), ushnabhinanda (patient feels happy with hot treatments), is explained as kaphaja Abhishyanda.

**Extra points of vagbhata :-**Nidra =(Sleeping mood), and  Aruchi (Anorexia).

## 4) RAKTHAJA ABHISHYANDA
### (Acute muco Purulent conjunctivitis)

It is rakthaja vyadhan sadhya vyadhi

The Signs & symptoms are merely equiavlent to pittaja Abhisyanda The special symptoms are (1) Lohitha netra (red eyes),
2) Tamrashru (Red Lacrimation)(3)Raktha raaji (red capillary net appearence)

## VATAJA ABHISHYANDA CHIKITSA

1) a) Nidana Parivarjanam (Treating of the cause), b) Rest c) Sheetho pachar (1 to 4 days) d) ushnopachar (in niram stage)

2) In saama dosha 4 days langhana etc., pathyas has todo (sweda pralepa, Tiktanna, dhooma, Pachan drugs and Langhana are advisable)

3) Ghritha, Kashayarasa, Guru ahaar, anjana and snana are not to do in saama stage.

**4) Treatment Principle :-** (after Ama Pachana) (a) Sneha panam (ghritha pana) (b) mrudu sweda (c) Raktha mokshana (at upanasika, lalata and apanga) (d) sneha virechana (e) sneha - Niruha vasti (f) sneha tarpana (g) sneha Putapaka (h) Sneha dhooma (i) sneha nasya (j) Aschyotan (k) sneha Pariseka (l) Shiro Vasti (m) Pradeha (n) Abhyanga (o) Sneha anjana.

**5) Snehana:-**
(a)  In take of ghee after meals
(b)  In take of medicated milk and ghee prepared with triphala
(c)  In take of medicated milk and ghee prepared with Vidarigandhadi drugs.
(d)  In take of medicated milk and ghee prepared with the dashamoola

After the above medication mrudu sweda is adviced.

**6) Mrudu sweda :** (Seka) with any of the folowing :-
1) Vata hara bhadradarvadi kashaya (2) Anupa mamsa
3) Amla dravas like kanji (4) Sukoshna chatursneha
5) Sukoshna dugda + saindhava lavana (6) Vasavara (7) payasa (8) Upanaha
9) Snigda dravyas + mamsa + Dadima phala rasa + Amalaki phala rasa.
10) Salvana sweda. 11) Haridra Rasanjan + milk + sindhava lavan
12) Erenda moola - patra + twacha siddha dugda - useful in seka **nasya, putapaka** etc.

13) Kantakari moola sukoshna dugda for - seka.

14) The decoction of Saindhava lavana, musta, yastimadhu, pippali, + milk Sechana

## 7) Aashchyotan yogas (eye drops)

a) With the decoction of Bilwadi panchamool, Bruhati, Erenda and shigru,
b) with the decoction of Nimba patra and Lodra

c) **Netra Bindu:-** Used for eye drops
(Gulab jala 1,2 botlles, Karpoora 6 masha, Ahiphena 2 tola, Rasanjan 8 tola)

d) **Phullika drava :-** Used for eye drops
(Gulabjala 2 kg, Mishri 4 tola, saindhava lavana 4 tola ,spatica 4 tola)

e) **Rasanjan drava :-** Used for eye drops
(Rasanjan 12 grams, spatica 24 grams, Honey or mishri 24 grams, Gulabjal 8 ounce)

f) Tankan or spatika eye drops
g) The medicated milk prepared from
   (Erenda moola, patra, twacha )
h) The medicated milk prepared from Kantakri moola

## 8) Pindika:-
Hot pindika ( Poultice) is prepared with erenda patra moola and twacha

## 9) Anjana :- with the following remedies.
a) Yastimadu, Haridra, Hareetaki, and Devadaru should mix equally and grind with Aja Ksheera
b) Swarna gyrika 1, pippali 4 parts, shunti 8 parts should grind with Aja Ksheera to Prepare vati
c) The rasakriyanjan prepared with, Shunti + Saindhava lavana+ ghrithamanda is used as **anjan**
d) Madhu, saindhava lavana, swarna gyrica, grinded well and has to use as anjan.

## 10) Bidalaka :-
a) Lodhra, fry in ghritha and has to paste to the eye lids
b) Hareetaki, fry in ghritha and has to apply to the eye lids
c) Rasanjan 50g, spatica 24g, Ahiphena 10g, Nimapatra 3, Ksheera 500g, gyrica 24g and has to paste to eye lids.
d) **Bhmyamalak** + saindhava lavana and Kanji, should mix in a **copper vessel** to paste to the eye lids.
e) **Saindhavalavan,** Daru haridra, Gyrica, hareetaki, and rasanjan has **to paste** to the eye lids.

## 2) Pittaja Abhisyanda Chikitsa

A)    1) Langhana ( for aama Pachanam)
2) sneha pana (3) Raktha Mokshana
4) Virechana (1to 4 for systemic treatment.)
5) Local treatment seka Aashchyotan Anjan Nasya Alepa Tarpana Putapak etc. has to do.
6) Pittaja visarpa or Pitta hara chikitsa should give.   '

B) 1) Common yoga for seka, Aashchyotan and for nasya:- Medicated ghee prepared from Gundra (truna visesha), shali, Doorva, Paashana bhedha, Daru haridra, Haridra, Ela, Uthphala, Lodhra, swetha kamala, Neela kamala, sharkara Kusha, Ikshu, vetha, Padmaka, Draksha, madhu, Raktha chandana, Yastimadhu, stanya, sariba.

c) **Seka yogas** :- Chandan, Nimba patra. yastimadhu, Rasanjan, Saindhava lavan, grind with water and should use as seka with honey .

D) **Aashchyotana yogas :**
1) Nimba patra kalka has to paste to the Lodhra and heated :- The powder + stanya, after filtration should use for Aashchyotan.

2) Medicated milk prepared from Draksha, yastimadhu, manjista, jeevaneeya dravya .

3) The fine powder of yastimadhu, Lodhra, Draksha, sharkara, and kamal should prepare a potali and dipped in the stanya - this stanya is filtered used for Aashchyotana.

4) Yastimadhu, patha Lodhra - powdered and kept in a potali and is dipped in ghrita, this ghrita is filtered and used for Aashchyotana 5) Gambari twak, or Aamalaki phala, or Hareetaki phala or Katphala can be used by dipping the potali in water like above.

e) **Pindi**  (1) Amalaki  Or (2) mahanimba patra pindi can be used.

f) **Bidalaka :-** Chandana, sariba, Manjista, padmaka, yastimadu jatamamsi, Tagara, lodhra, jathipushpa - gyrica - can be applied to the eye lids.

**G) Anjana -** 1) Phalsha pushpa or moola swarasa or shallaki swarasa + madhu + sharkara - as Anjana.

2) Trivruth or Yastimadhu + Madhu+ Sharkara as- Rasakriya anjan.

3) Musta, Samudra phena, Kamala Vidanga, ela, Aamalaki, beejasar as Rasa kriyanjan

4) Talisa patra, Ela , gyrika, musta, shankha + stanya or cow milk as choorna anjan.

5) Gyrika + stanya (6) Phalasha pushpa + madhu (7) Samudra Phena + madhu or stanya (8) yastimadu, draksha, Lodra vacha  Sharkara, Kamala + stanya. 9) Yastimadu lodra, Draksha, sharkara kamal + stanya. 10) Swarna bhasma stanya or cow milk 11) Amalaki Rasakriyanjan with stanya or cow milk 12) Netrabala chandan, udumber twak + stanya

## KAPHAJ ABHISHYANDA CHIKITSA

**1) Treatment principle :-** General Principles and sira vyadana then sweda, Avapeedan, nasya, Anjan, Dhoomapan seka, pralepa, Kavalagrah, Ruksha Ashchyotan, Ruksha putapaka, Apatarpan - Tiktha ghritha, (kaphahara) Aahara and vihara (Sushrutha)

**2)** Langhana, swedana nasya, Tikthabhojan Teekshna Pradamana nasya, Teekshna upanaha, Ruksha and Teekshna virechan. ( yogaratnakar)

**3) Pindi**  1) Shighru patra Kalka (lukewarm pindi is used)

2) Nimba patra + shunti + saindhava Lavana, luke warm pindi is used

**4) Aashchyotan :-**   Saindhava lavana and Lodhra has to fry in ghritha + sauveeranjan, grind with water and, the extracted swarasa is used for Ashchyotana.

**5) Bidalaka :** 1) Rasanjan or 2) Shunti, hareetaki or 3) Vacha, Haridra Shunti or 4) Gyrika, shunti is used as varthma lepam (Bidalaka)

**6) Anjan** 1) Saindhava lavana, Hingu, Triphala, Yastimadhu, Anjan, Tutha,Tamra and prapaundareeka, grinded with water, varthi  is prepared for Anjan.

2) Hareetaki , Haridra, yastimadu as varthi anjan.

3) Trikatu, Triphala, Haridra, Vidanga sara in equal parts + Tagara, kusta,Devadaru, shankha, patha, vyosha, manashila. As varthi anjan .

4) jathi pushpa, karanja Pushpa, shigru beeja + or pushpa water, as varthi anjan.

5) Puthi Karanja,Phalasha pushpa, shigru Pushpa, Bruhathi dwayam (phala and pushpa) Rasanjan, Saindhava lavana, Draksha, chandan, manashila harital, lashuna + water as varthi anjan.

6) Ksharanjan also used.

# RAKTHAJA ABHISHYANDA CHIKITSA

A) Antah Shodhana
　　1) Snehana with Kaumba ghritha (100 yrs old ghritha)
　　2) Mamsa rasa bhojana 3) Sira Mokshana 4) virechan 5) shiro virechan

**B) Sthanika upachara :-** (Local Treatments)
　　1) Pradeha (2) Parisheka (3) nasya (4) Dhooma (5) Aashchyotan (6) Abhyanga (7) Tarpana (8) Snigda puta Paka (9) anjana (Prasadana)
(Mrudu sweda, jalaukavacharana, Ghritha pana has to do when severe pain is associated )

I) **Seka :-** Triphala Lodhra, yastimadu, sugar, musta should grind with cool-water, and used for .

II) **Pralepa :-** Neelothphala, usheera, Daruharidra, Kaleeyaka (Agaru) yastimadu, musta, Lodra should grind with shathadautha ghritha to paste around the eyes.

III)　　**Aashcyotan** (putting of eye drops with the following medicines)
1)　　Sthanya (Breast milk)
2)　　Dugda or ghritha (milk & ghee)
3)　　The ghee got bhavana with Lodhra
4)　　The medicated water has to use prepared with
　　Triphala + Sharkara + water
5)　　shigru patra swarasa + madhu =
6)　　Bhumyamalaki swarasa 7) Amalaki phala swarasa

IV) **Anjan :-** With the following medicines
1) Shriparni, padhala (patha), Arjuna, Dhathaki, Aamalaki, Bilva, Bruhathi, Bimbi Lodhra, manjista, grinded with madhu or ikshu rasa for anjan.
2) Chandan, kumuda, Teja pathra, shilajithu, kesara, Loha,
Tamra, Tuttha, Nimba Niryasa, Rasanjan, Trapu, Kamsyamala grinded with madu prepare varthi for Anjan.
3) kulutthaadyanjan (Kuluttha got bhavana in aja ksheera, saindhavalavan, Haridra, Rasanjan , as Anjan.

**V) Bidalaka :**
1) Neelkamal, musta, Daruharidra, kaleeyaka yastimadu, muktha Lodhra padmaka, grinded with shatadautha grhitha and is used as varthma lepam.

**Note :** ( Rakthaja abhishyanda, rakthaja adimanda, Siraharsha, sirothpatha are having similar treatment principles.)

# CONJUNCTIVITIS

Inflammation of conjunctiva characterised by redness of the eye and conjunctival discharge is known as conjunctivitis.

## Causes:-

1) Exogenous :- Causative agents entered in to conjuctival sac from outside (May be micro organisms - foreign bodies, chemicals)

2) Endogenous :- Blood borne infection, allergic response or due to metabolic defects.

3) Infection spreading from surrounding structures. i.e.- skin. lacrimal apparatus,cornea, sclera, orbit, and uveal tract.

## CLASSIFICATION OF CONJUNCTIVITIS

(a) Infective Conjunctivitis
- 1) Bacterial
- 2) Viral
- 3) Bedsonia group
- 4) Special infection

## 1) Due to Bacterial infection:-

a) Acute Catarrhal or muco purulent conjunctivitis
   - I. Acute
   - II. Subacute
   - III. Chronic

b) Purulent conjunctivitis

c) Membranous Conjunctivitis

d) Pseudo membranous conjunctivitis

e) Angular conjunctivitis

## 2) Due to Viral infection:-

a) Acute haemorrhagic conjunctivitis

b) Follicular conjunctivitis
   - I. Acute
   - II. Chronic

c)c. in measles

d) c. in varicella or chicken pox

e)c. in herpes zoster ophthalmicus

f) c. in vaccinia

g)c. in mumps

h).c. in infuenza

i)c. in yellow fever and dengue fever.

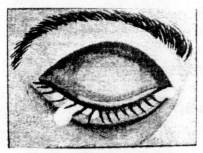

Acute purulent conjunctivitis

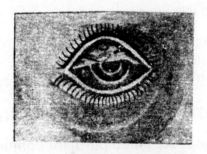

Membranous conjunctivitis

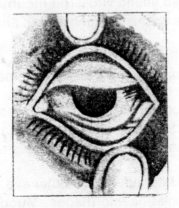

Pseudo Membranous Conjunctivitis

3) Conjuctivitis due to bedsonia group of organisms
    a) Swimming - bath conjunctivitis
    b) Trachoma
    c) Inclusion blennorrhoea of the new born.

4) Conjunctivitis due to specific infection.
    a) tuberculous conjunctivitis
    b) Syphilitic       "
    c) Tularensis     "
    d) C. in Leprosy  "
    e) Parinaud's     "

B) Allergic conjunctivitis
    a) simple allergic Conjunctivitis
    b) phlyctenular C.
    c) Vernal conjunctivitis or spring catarrh

(C) Conjunctivitis following injury
(D) Conjunctivitis associated withskin diseases
(E) Due to B. complex defficiency (pyridoxine defficiency)

## CONJUNCTIVITIS DUE TO BACTERIAL INFECTION

**A/I/a). Acute catarrhal or acute muco purulent conjunctivitis**
It is the commonest cause for " red eye".

**Causative organisms :-**
    Koch - week bacillus, staphylococcus, pneumococcus, strepto coccus, influenza bacilli and also adeno virus.The **Incubation period** is 3 to 4 days. It occurs to the people dosha with unhygienic and dirty habbits.

**Conjunctival discharge** :- It contains tears, mucous, epithelial cells, bacteria, Leucocytes, fibrin and may be R.B.C. (blood stained discharge)

**Symptoms :-** Discomfort (foreign body sensation), photophobia, watering of eye, blurring of vision (due to conjunctival discharge covering on cornea ), sticking together of eye lids at nights, rainbow haloes around thelight etc.

**Signs :-** It starts in one eye later affects the other eye. conjunctival congestion, oedema of lids. petechial haemorrhages. **Mucopurulent discharge** Accumulates at inner canthus - outer canthus - lower fornix, roots of cilia, and causing matting of eye lashes .

**Complications :-** 1) passes into chronic stage 2) marginal corneal ulcer 3) Blepharitis 4) chronic dacryocystitis.

**Treatment :-** (a) Prophylactic b) curative
a) Taking care from spreading of infection to the other eye, sleeping on infected side, personal belongings should kept separate.

**b) Curative :-**
1)   Conjunctival sac should be washed with hot normal saline
2)   Sulfacetamide drops 3 to 4 times a day.
3)   Broad spectrum antibiotic drops or ointment.(Ointment should use at night to prevent sticking of eye lids).
4)   No Bandaging but shoud use dark glassess.
5)   Steroids are contra indicated
6)   culture of the discharge for the isolation of infecting organism and to find its sensitivity to antibiotic for proper treatment.
7)   If cornea is involved 1% atropin sulphate ointment should use.

**A)1/a/ II) Sub acute muco purulent Conjunctivitis**
　　Etiology  -  Clinical picture and pathology same as above
　　but signs and symptoms are less severe than
　　Acute catarhal conjunctivitis

**A/1/a/ III) Chronic catarrhal conjunctivitis**
　　It is a chronic catarrhal inflammation of conjunctiva.

**Causes** 1) for not treating the Acute catarrhal conjunctivitis in time.
2) Continuous irritation of conjunctiva due to smoke, dust, abuse of alcohol and refractive error. 3) Misplaced eye lashes, 4) chronic dacryocystitis and 5) chronic rhinitis

**Symptoms :-** Burning sensation in the eyes, sense of grittyness and photophobia.

**Signs :-** Congestion of palpebral conjunctiva and fornix, thin sticky discharge.

**Complications :-** Blepharitis, corneal ulcers and opacities.

**Treatment** 1) General- Avoiding the irritant causes, ex. correction of refractive error etc.
2) Local  :- Culture of conjunctival swab and if infection present proper antibiotic should use.3) Drops of zinc sulphate + Acid boric.
4) In more severe cases conjunctival sac has to be painted with 1% silver nitrate soultion..

## A/1/b) Acute purulent conjunctivitis

It is acute conjunctivitis with purulent discharge (frank pus from conjunctival sac of eye ball)

## Occurs in two forms
a) Gonococcal conjunctivitis  - in adults
b) Ophthalmia neonatarum    - in new born.

## a) Gonococcal Conjunctivitis :-

The causative agent is Neisseria gonorrhoeae, it is due to direct contact of gonorrhoea from genitalia, incubation period - few hours to 3 days. gonococci forms clusters on the surface of conjunctiva due to inflammatory reactions, epithelium degenerates and infection spreads into deeper layers, lead to oedema of sub conjunctival tissue due to accumulation of inflammatory cells and exudates. if the infection is not controlled it spreads into the cornea and causes corneal ulcers, finally healing occurs without scaring

**Signs** :- Divided into 3 stages

## Ist stage :- stage of Infiltration  ( 1 to 5 days)
pain and tender eye ball, bright red coloured conjunctiva, chemosis of conjunctiva, watery discharge, pseudomembrane formation, swelling of eye lids,and with enlarged preauricular lymphglands.

## 2nd state  - stage of blenorrhoea  (5 day to several weeks)
Frank pus discharges down to the cheeks, oedema of lids and conjunctiva reduced.

## 3rd stage  -  Stage of slow healing
Pain and odema reduces, papillary formation on tarsal conjunctiva, hyperaemic bulbar conjunctiva, reduced discharge- resolution is complete and chronic stage is never attained.

**Complications**  1) Oedema - ulceration of cornea
2) perforation of cornea 3) Uveitis with hypopyon

**Treatment:-** a) prophylactic b) curative

**Phyphylactic** :- Patients belongings should be kept separate, used dressings should be destroyed, sleeping on the side of infection, and the healthy eye should be protected from spreading of infection.

**Curative :-**

1) eye wash with normal saline - as far as possible.
2) Pencilline eye drops, frequently (10000 units/l - CC of distilled water,) systemic pencilline injections and Broad spectrum antibiotic ointment at nights. to prevent adhesions.
3) If corneal ulcer present 1% atropin sulphate ointment should apply.

## B) OPHTHALMIA NEONATARUM

It is a bilateral purulent conjunctivitis occuring in the new born within first three weeks of life.

**Causative organisms :-** Gonococcus - some times by B. coli, pneumococcus, staphylococcus aureus, streptococcus haemolyticus, virus (inclusion blenorrheoa of new born)

**Mode of infection** :- During the birth, in the face presentation, the infection spreads from infected vagina by gonococcus.

Clinical picture :- Absence of tears for a month, conjunctival and corneal epithelium become very thin and the remaining Symptoms are like in the adult.

**Complications -** 1) corneal ulcer -corneal, opacity - maldevelopment of macula and nystagmus.2) Adherent leucoma 3) Anterior staphyloma.

**Treatment** 1) Prophylactic :- Immediately after bith1% silver nitrate drops or pencilline drops has to put 2) perfect antinatal check up.

**II) Curative - like in the adults.**

**A/1/c ) Membranous conjunctivitis:-** It is rare, and is characterised by conjunctivitis with membrane formation on the conjunctiva.

**Etiology** a) ill health following eruptive fevers and unhygienic living condition. (b) Causative agent in majority of cases is coryne bacterium Diphtheriae (klebs - Loeffler Bacilli) which are usually associated with staphylo cocci, and pneumococci - (some times streptococus haemoly ticus).

**Pathology -** 1) Inflammation of conjunctiva 2) Fibrinous exudate is deposited not only on the surface but also within the conjunctiva 3) Exudate forms a membrane on conjunctiva of palpebral and bleeds when removed, necrosis of conjunctiva, ultimately the membrane sloughs off and heals by granulation tissue, during the healing it causes symblepharan (Adhesion between palpebral and bulbar conjunctiva), Ankylo blepharon (Adhesion between lidmargins), Entropion, trichiasis, and corneal ulcer.

**Clinical course of MILD CASE :-**
1) Oedema of lids 2) Conjunctival congestion 3) muco purulent discharge,
4) Yellowish white membrane on palpebral conjunctiva.

**Severe case :-** Divided into 3 stages.
1) Stage of infiltration :- It lasts for 5 to 10 days, red, hot, hard, swollen pain ful eye lids with scanty discharge. Due to stiffness of lid it is impossible to evert, on separating the lids with retracter greyish yellow membrane can be seen with marked hyperaemia, and the Pre auricular lymph glands also enlarges.

**2nd stage - stage of suppuration**
Pain is less, soft lids, copious discharge and membrane the sloughed off leaving red raw granulating surface.

**3rd stage -** stage of cicatrization
Healing takes place by granulating tissue and causes complications like symblepharon. Ankyloblepharon, Trichiasis and corneal ulcer.

**Treatment** 1) Isolation of the patient

2)      Culture and sensitivity of conjunctival swab.
3)      Crystalline pencilline drops frequently
4)      Instillation of Anti diphtheric serum every one hour into eye.
5)      1% atropine sulphate ointment if cornea is involved.
6)      Broad spectrum antibiotic ointment at nights.
7)      After the membrane has sloughed off eye should be covered with
        soft contact glasses to prevent adhesion.
8)      Anti diphtheric serum 50000 units I.M. twice a day.
9)      Crystalline pencilline 5 lack units, I.M. - twice a day.

**A/I/d) Pseudo membranous conjunctivitis**
1) Formation of false membrane on Tarsal conjunctiva and fornix.
2) Develops only on surface of conjunctiva not within its substance
3) Easily can be removed without bleeding points
4) Signs of Acute catarrhal conjunctivitis present
5) Etiology, clinical picture is same as above but not severe (mild, low virulent).

**Treatment :-** Like acute muco purulent conjunctivitis

**A/I/e) Angular Conjunctivitis**
It is commonly associated with nasal discharge, The infecting agent is morax Axenfeld diplobacillus, highly contageous disease, incubation period is 4 days.

**Symptoms :-** Irritation, itching sensation inthe eyes.

**Signs** :-1) hyperaemia and Excoriation of epithelium of inter marginal strip of conjunctiva of lid margin, inner canthus and outer canthus.
2) Congestion of bulbar conjunctiva at inner and outer angle.
3) Scanty muco purulent discharge.
4) Excoriation of the skin of surroundings.

**Complication** :- Marginal corneal infiltration or ulcers

**Treatment :-** 1) 1% zinc sulphate  + 2 % Boric acid drops  3 times a day
2) Tetra cycline eye ointment at bed time.

## A/2    Viral conjunctivitis
Several number of viruses can cause conjunctivitis, the conjunctival reactions to viral infection may be variable, chiefly they are as follows:
1) Inflammation of conjunctiva with follicles formation.
2) Oedema of conjunctiva with sub conjunctiva haemorrhages.
3) Simple hyperaemia
4) Ulcers or membrane formation.
5) Some virus cause punctate opacities in the superficial layers or in the deep layers, some disappears and some remains permanently in the cornea.

## (A/2) Follicular Conjunctivitis
"Conjunctivitis with follicles formation"
(Follicle = Localised aggregation of lymphocytes in the sub epithelial adenoid layer of the conjunctiva, apearing as tiny round translucent swelling).

Follicles are formed in the following conditions.
a) Folliculosis        b) Follicular conjunctivitis
c) Trachoma           d) Drug allergy to atropin eserine and pilocarpin

## Acute Follicular conjunctivitis :-
Follicle formation with signs of acute catarrhal conjunctivitis, causative agent is virus.
a) Acute herpetic follicular conjunctivitis :-

Causative agent is herpes simplex virus, conjunctival follicles are large, vesicles appear in the cornea  (vesicles merge and causes dendritic corneal ulcer)

## b) Epidemic kerato conjunctivitis :-

Causative agent is, type 8 adeno virus, Acute follicular Conjunctivitis with marked inflammation of conjunctiva (in the cornea superficial punctate keratitis develops).

c) Pharyngo conjunctival fever

Causative agent is type 8 adeno virus, here acute follicular conjunctivitis is associated with viral pharyngitis and fever .

d) chronic follicular conjunctivitis :- Slight congestion of conjunctiva, scanty discharge, follicles formation at upper tarsal and lower fornix conjunctiva.

## A/2/B) Folliculosis

Discrete follicles in the lower fornix, No sign of inflammation or discharge follicles are arranged in parallel rows, conjunctiva in between follicle is clear, it may be due to unhygienic condition and due to refractive error (hyper metropia) it is associated with enlarged tonsils and adenoids.

## c) Trachoma  (Explained in varthma rogas)

## A/2/C) Conjunctivitis in measles :-  Inflammed conjunctiva with muco puru-lent discharge, Kopliks spots may appear on conjunctiva, in virulent cases superficial punctate keratitis develops.

## Conjunctivitis in varicella  (Chicken pox):-

Phlycten like lesion appears in lidmargin conjunctiva, and at the limbus it may undergo resolution or may ulcerate, marginal corneal infiltration and kerato malacia proceeds.

## Conjunctivitis in herpes zoster Ophthalmicus :-

Causative agent is herpes zoster virus, conjunctival congestion with petechial haemorrhages seen, rarely follicle develops, if lst branch of 5th nerve is involved pustules may form.

## Conjunctivitis due to vaccination :-

 Causative agent is pox virus, it is due to contamination after contact with vaccination vesicle of another perosn. The clinical features are Oedema, rednes of eye lids purulent Conjunctival discharge, and cornneal complications.

## Conjunctivitis inmumps :-

Causative agent is myxo virus, a mild conjunctivitis without marked discharge is seen , interstitial keratitis may also develop

## Conjunctivitis in infuenza :-

Causative agent is the ARBOR  virus, sub conjunctival haemorrhages with marked congestion of  Bulbar conunctiva is seen.

## A/3)  Conjunctivitis due to bedsonia group of organisms

These group of organisms are not true virus, occupy the middle place between small bacteria and virus.

1) Inclusion blennorrhoea of new born (Inclusion conjunctivitis)
The Causative agent is called TRIC agent
TR = Trachoma ; IC=inclusion conjunctivitis, the causative organism is similar to the trachoma agent which is derived from mother's genital tract.
**The Clinical Features are :-** Papillary hyertrophy of conjunctiva of the lower fornix, later on follicles formation, signs of acute conjunctivitis with purulent discharge present

**2) Swimming bath conjunctivitis :-**
It is also known as inclusion blennorheoa of adult, infection spreads in the swimming pool from the genital tract, features of acute conjunctivitis with follicle formation present.
3) Trachoma - explained.

## A/4) Conjunctivitis due to specific - infections
### 1) Tuberculous conjunctivitis
The Infecting agent is tubercular bacillus, types
a) one or more ulcers in conjunctiva (Palpebral and bulbar)
b) Small nodules appear in the conjunctiva.
(c) Hyper trophic type - Hypertrohied granulation tissue at fornix or tarsal conjunctiva.
Definite diagnonis is possible only by histological examination of conjunctival lesion

2) **Syphilitic conjunctivitis:-** The Conjunctiva may be affected in all stages of syphilis.

**Ist stage :-** Extra genital chancre in conjunctiva, with swelling of the eye lid.
**2nd stage -** A simple conjunctivitis is associated
**3rd Stage -** Gummata may develop in the conjunctiva, it breaks down and produce indolent ulcers.

### 3) Conjunctivitis in leprosy
In nerve type of leprosy, due to affect of sensory nerves, conjunctiva may be exposed and cause hyperaemia of conjunctiva with catarrhal conjunctivitis and  In lepromatous leprosy lepromata may develop in the conjunctiva.

**4) Tularensis conjunctivitis :-** The Causative agent is brucella tularens, small necrotic ulcers develop in conjunctiva with oedema of eye lids and with regional Lymphnodes enlargement

**(5) Parinaud's conjunctivitis:-** Granuloma formation in the conjunctiva with enlargement of regional lymph glands.

## B)     Allergic conjunctivitis.

Inflammation of conjunctiva due to allergic reactions, It may occur in three forms.
1) Simple allergic conjunctivitis
2) Phlyctenular conjunctivitis
3) Vernal conjunctivitis or spring catarrh

### 1) Simple allergic conjunctivitis:-
It occurs due to exogenic and endogenic allergens.

**Exogenous allergens :-** Pollens, vegetable and animal dust and drugs like atropin, eserin, pilocarpin

**Endogenous Allergens :-** Bacterial products from a septic focus particularly due to staphylococcus.

**Symptoms :-** (1) irritation and itching of the eyes 2) photo phobia and 3) watering.

**Signs :** 1) Marked Hyperaemia of conjunctiva 2) Chemosis of conjunctiva 3) scanty watery discharge 4) Eosinophils in conjunctival smear 5) Oedema of lids.

**Treatment :-** 1) Allergen has to be removed
2) Hydrocortisone acetate 1% ointment at bed time.

## 2) Phlyctenular conjunctivitis

It is an allergic inflammatory reaction of the conjunctiva to some endogenous toxin which is bacterial in origin.

**Exciting factor :-** Unhygienic condition, tuberculo toxin, and staphylo coccus.

**Symtoms** Discomfort in the eye, irritation, reflex lacrimation (Photophobia if cornea involves)

**Signs :-** 1) One or multiple phlyctens formation on conjunctiva at limbal area 2) Pinkish white nodule, 1 to 4 mm in size originates a little distance from limbus, the bulbar conjunctiva surrounded by phlycten is congested and rest of the conjunctiva is clear.3) lacrimation present but no discharge.4) In the presence of secondary infection total conjunctiva becomes congested. 5) It associated with enlarged tonsils and cervical glands.

**Pathology** :- The phlycten is the compact mass of lymphocytes and poly morphs, underneath the epithelium, phlycten ulcerates and heals by granulation (Very little scar formation), ulcerates in to cornea causing phlyctenular Keratitis.

**Treatment : -** If no secondary infection.
1) Hydro cortisone acetate 1% drops frequently,
2) If secondary infection present - treatment should be given like acute muco purulent conjunctivitis.
3) if cornea is involved 1% atropine sulphate ointment has to apply.
4) Treatment of Tuberculosis or any other septic focus
5) Vitamins and proper nourishment.

**3) Spring cattarh or vernal conjunctivitis**
It is hypersensitive reaction of conjunctiva to exogenous allergens. (Prevale in summer and subsides in winter).
**Symptoms :-** Itching, burning, photophobia, Lacrimation
**Signs :-** Palpebral type & bulbar type (2 types)

**Palpebral type :-** Hard, flat, bluish white papillae separated by furrows, giving a coble stone appeerence, white ropy conjuntival discharge with eosinophils.

**Bulbar type :-** it is less common there is gelatinous thickned to accumulation of tissue around the limbus
**Treatment :** Cold water eye wash, disodium cromo glycate drops reduce itching, and Dexamethosone drops for best relief.

## 5) ADHIMANTHA (GLAUCOMA)

Severe pain inthe eye is the prime symptom of Adhimantha, it is described as the complication of abhishyanda vyadhi.
1)  Vataja Abhishyanda causes vataj adhimantha main symptoms is pricking pain in the eyes.
2)  Pittaj Abhishyanda cuases pittaja Adhimantha, main symptom is burning pain in the eye
3)  Kaphaja Abhishyanda causes kaphaj adhimantha, main symptom is heavy ness and itching sensation in the eye
4)  Rakthaja Abhishyanda causes Raktaja Adhimantha, main symptom is Raktha prakopa vedana.

**Samanya Lakshanas :-**
1) Severe pain in the eyes like scooping it from the orbit, 2) Crushing type of pain or churning type of pain (Manthana vatha shoola)

3) Half headache ( Arthava bhedak)  4) Vataj complications

**Types of adhimantha**
1)    Vatika Adhimantha
2)    Piithika Adhimantha
3)    Kaphaja Adhimantha
4)    Rakthaja Adhimantha.

## 1) VATIKA ADHIMANTHA
### (Acute congestive glaucoma)

It is a disease in which the patient have scooping type or breaking type or spastic type or pricking type or cutting type of pain in the eyes, exudations, foreign body sensation, extra growths, dirty appearance with  Aadmana (increased tension in the eye ball), Kampana (Shivering) and half headache.

**Vagbhata added** the points like karna nada (Tinnitus), churning type of pain in head eye and root of the nose, and  with giddiness

**Chikitsa:-**  Like vataja abhishyanda, (sneha sweda siramokshana, (Lalata sira vyadana) virechana and vasti; seka Ashchyotan Anjana Tarpana, putapaka dhooma, Nasya, shiovasti etc. has to do.)If the disease is not controlled with above treatment principles, vagbhata suggested " Daha karma" at and  above the " Bhru".

**Varthi Anjana**
1) vataja :- Rajatha patra should be painted with go dadhi, it should become bluish and get it dried and grind with masthu, prepare varthi for Anjana.

## 2) PITTAJA ADHIMANTHA
### Acute congestive glaucoma

It is sarvagatha sadhya vyadhi, The signs & symptoms are
1) eye spread with red capillary net (Raktha raajeechitham) 2) watering of eyes. (Netra srava) 3) severe Burning sensation (Burning pain like burning with fire or chemical or kshara) 4) Hyperaemia of eyes like yakruth (chachlate colour)5) Oedema of eye lids (Varthma shopha) 6) Perspiration (Swedana) 7) Burning sensation of the head (Shirodaha) 8) Murcha (unconscious state) 9) Visualises the things in yellow colour.

**Chikitsa ;-** Like pittaja Abishyanda

**Anjana  for pitta and Raktha adhimantha :-** Buds of jathi pushpa, Shankhanaabhi, Triphala, Yastimadu, Bala moola twak, should grind with Aakashodaka (Rain water) varthi is  prepared for Anjan.

# 3) KAPHAJA ADHIMANTHA
## (Simple chronic glaucoma or chronic congestive glaucoma)

It is sarvagatha sadhya vyadhi, signs & symptoms are.
1) Netra shotha (oedema) 2) srava (Lacrimation) 3) Kandu (itching) 4) cool, heavy sticky discharge comes 5) Harshana (hypersensitvity) 6) shiro ruja (headacha)  7) Visualise the things as smoky, dirty and imperfect (Nose apears as oedematous) 8) difficulty in visualisation and opening of eye lids 9) Oedema of nose.  **Vagbhata** added a peculiar sign, that is " **Natham Krishnam - unnatham shukla mandhalam** "Sunken cornea and bulged sclera.

**Chikitsa**  - Like kaphaja Abhishyanda

**Anjana -** Saindhava lavana, Triphala, Trikatu, shankha nabhi samudra phena, shyleyaka sarjarasa, should grind with water, and varthi is  prepared for Anjana.

# RAKTHAJ ADHIMANTHA
## (Congestive glaucoma or secondary glaucoma)

It is Sarva gatha sadya vyadhi, the signs & symptoms are.

1) Sparshanaakshama (Tenderness - unbearable pain)
2) Eyes becomes red and discharges red secretion
3) Visualises the objects in Red colour (Agnivath)
4) Krishna mandala appears as dipped in the blood like reeta phala (Arista phala).
5) Severe pricking pain & burning sensation in the eyes and head.

**Vagbhata :-** The pain is experienced at Shankha, dantha, kapola, lalata,
**Chikitsa :-** Like rakthaja Abhishyanda

## Adhimantha Sadhya Asadhyatha
If it is not treated in time causes blindness within the following duration

| as per Sushrutha | Vataja, 6 days | Pittaj-1 day | Kaphaj,7 days | Rakthaj, -5 days |
|---|---|---|---|---|
| as per Vagbhata | 5 days | 1 day | 7 days | 3 days |

# GLAUCOMA

Increased intra ocular pressure which is created by solid, liquid contents of eye and the elasticity of its coats, is known as Glaucoma.

Normal intra ocular pressure is 16 to 23 mm Hg. by schiotz tonometer, the solid and semi solid contens which are responsible for the maintenance of intra ocular pressure are, Lens, vitreous, Uveal tract and retina and the Liquid contents which are responsible for the maintenance of intra ocular pressure are blood and aqueous humour.

Changes in the volume of above may lead to raised intra ocular pressure (Glaucoma) "Normal pressure is required for the maintenance of the optical properties of refracting surfaces".

## Physiological variations of I.O.P pesent in 24 hours :-
The difference should not be more than 5 mm Hg.

1) Early morning pressure is maximum.2) sharp fall soon after sun rise.
3) Gradually decreases upto evening4) First 6 hours of night gradually raises
5) Increases in the mid night and becomes maximum upto early morning.

## Factors resposible for rise of Intra ocular presure
1)    Increased aqueous production
2)    Decreased aqueous out flow due to obstruction of its drianage
3)    Increased blood volume or decreased venous out flow.
5)    External pressures on the eye. ball.

## Classification of Glaucoma

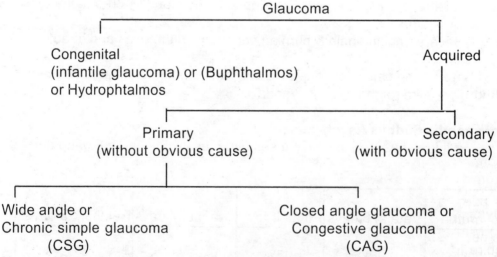

**Note :-** When sense of perception and projection of light is lost, commonly in the final stage of Glaucoma is termed as absolute glaucoma.

# I. INFANTILE GLAUCOMA (CONGENITAL)
## (Buphthalmos - Hydrophthalmos)

**Causative mechanism :-**
Congenital abnormality at the angle of anterior chamber, absence of canal of schlemm, causes Aqueous obctruction in the eye ball, and leads to increased intra ocular pressure.

**Symptos :** 1) Photo phobia                    2) Defective vision.

**Signs :** 1) epiphora 2) Blepharospasm 3) intolerance to light 4) hazy cornea 5) oedemaof cornea 6) elongated (oval) eye ball (resembles the eye of an ox, so only termed as buphthlmos) progressive enlargement of cornea (becomes 12 to 14 mm diameter instead of 10.5 mm) and sclera (becomes thin)
7) Anterior chamber is deep
8) Lens become flat and may be subluxated
9) Iris becomes tremulous
10) Cupping of optic disc
11) Error of myopia due to elongated eye ball
12) Raised intra ocular pressure.

**Treatment :-** Surgical correction of Aqueous passage.

# 2) PRIMARY WIDE ANGLE GLAUCOMA
# OR
# CHRONIC SIMPLE GLAUCOMA
# (CSG)

No obvious cause can be explained for the rise of pressure 2) The angle of anterior chamber remains wide .

**Causative mechanism :-**
Actual cause is not known but the rise of pressure may be due to some changes in the trabeculae, schlemm's canal or in the Exist channels from schlemm's

**Symptoms :**
1) Mild headacha 2) eye ache 3) Changes in the lens accommodation (require frequent change of presbyopic glasses) 4) defect in field of vision 5) gradual dimness of central vision 7) Night blindness in the later stages.

**Signs :-** (No early signs)1) Hazy cornea 2) Sluggished pupil reaction 3) Rise of Intra ocular pressure 4) cupping of optic disc 5) Defect in the field of vision 6) In the later stages central vision also affected and eye becomes complete blind 7) Angle is wide

**Treatment :-** 1) Pilocarpine nitrate (miotic) 2% drops. 2) Diamox 250 mg caps Bid. or Tid.

**Operations :-** 1) Trabeculectomy b) Iridencleisis c) Elliots sclero corneal trephine.

# PRIMARY CLOSED ANGLE GLAUCOMA
## (Acute congestive Glaucoma)

Intra ocular pressure is raised as a result of obstruction in the out flow of the aqueous humour due to narrowing of the angle of Anterior chamber. Probabilities for the occurence :-
1)      Small eye (hyper metropic eye)
2)      Shallow anterior chamber
3)      Bigger ciliary body & lens
4)      Forward displacement of Iris
5)      Cloudy day (rainy season) pupillary dilatation causes obstruction of angle due to dim light.

**Clinical course:-**
a) Prodromal stage.
b) Phase of constant instability
c) Acute congestive attack
d) Chronic congestive attack
e) Stage of absolute glaucoma

**a) Prodromal stage :-**
Symptoms :- Blurring of vision with haloes around the light and mild headache.
**Signs :-** 1)Sudden rise of I.O.P. for a short period, no congestion, slight corneal oedema, pressure increases due to stress, strain and in the dark illumination.
**(b) phase of constant instability:-**
**signs and symptoms:-** The features described above become more and regular, seviority appears more at evenings, and quickly comes to normal by rest or sleep.

## c) Acute Congestive attack :-

**Symptoms :-** Severe eye ache, headache, marked vision loss, (presence of only perception and projection of light) photophobia, and Lacrimation.

**Signs :-** 1) Oedema of eye lids 2) Ciliary & conjunctival congestion 3) hazy and insensitive cornea 4) shallow anterior chamber 5) moderately dilated pupil 6) Iris is discoloured 7) Marked rise of intra ocular pressure 8) eye ball is tender 9) Ophthalmoscipic examination is not possible due to corneal oedema.(Optic disc is congested, no cupping) 10) Vision is markedly reduced, only perception and projection of light present.11) The associated systemic disturbances are 1) Vomiting 2) Fever 3) irregular pulse etc.

## d) Chronic congestive stage : -

**Signs :-** 1) eye remains congested and irritable.
2) Tension remains permanently elevated
3) Field defects like previous.
4) Cupping of the optic disc
5) Vision remains deppressed.
**Note :-** If the treatment not given evena at this stage, it passes into absolute glaucoma.

## E) Stage of absolute glaucoma

**Signs :-**
1) The eye completely become blind, (no perception of light)
2) Irregular venous anastomosis around the limbus (Medusa head)
3) Cornea is hazy and insensitive
4) Anterior chamber is very Shallow
5) Iris atrophy
6) Pupil is dilated, no reaction to light
7) Optic disc is deeply cupped
8) Tension is very high and eye becomes stony hard.
9) The Other changes are :- Ulceration of cornea, glaucomatous pannus, equatorial staphyloma, panophthalmitis, phithisis bulbi.

**Treatment :-** In lst and 2nd stages (1) Miotics (pilocarpine drops 2%, (2) Peripheral iridectomy operation.

**in 3rd stage :** 1) Miotics 2) Diamox 250 mg Tid, 3) Treatment for pain & congestion 4) peripheral irridectomy

**4rth Stage :-**    Trabeculectomy or iridencleisis
**5th Stage :**    Enucleation of eyeball.

# SECONDARY GLAUCOMA

Secondary glaucoma arises because of pre existing disease

**Causes** 1) Due to inflammation :-
Corneal ulcer, uveitis, acute scleritis, endophthalmitis, oribital cellutlitis etc.

The angle of anterior chamber is blocked because of inflammatory exudates and causes glaucoma.

2) **Post inflammatory :-**
a) Intumescent cataract - causes shallow anterior chamber and causes glaucoma
b) Burst morgagnian cataract causes closer of angle, so causes glaucoma
c) Sublauation of Lens of flocculent Lens matter, causes glaucoma. (Iris being pushed forwards)
4) Due to intra ocular haemorrhage
5) glaucoma due to intra ocular tumours
6) Post operative glaucoma ex :in Aphakia.

**Treatment :-** 1) Treat the cause
2) Paracentesis
3) If intra ocular tumours present, enucleation has to do.

## 9) SASHOPHA AKSHI PAKA
### (Cellulitis of eye ball or uveitis or Panophthalmitis )

It is sarva gatha, sannipathaja, vyadana sadhya vyadhi .

**Signs & Symptoms :-**
Eye becomes coppery red colour (Pakwa Udumbara sannibham) and assoicate with kandu (itching), Ashru srava (Lacrimation), daha (Buring sensation), upadeha (Stickyness), Harshana (Sensitivity), Toda (Pricking pain) gurutwa (Heavyness), Red oedema with frequent Sticky hot or sticky cool discharge.

**As per Vagbhata - It is due to " Tridoshas + Raktha vitiation"**
**Note :-** Sa shopha Akshi paka is sadhya vyadhi but panophthalmitis is asadhya vyadhi so it can be compared to Uveitis (Inflammation of second layer of eye ball) Cellulitis of eye ball.

# 10) ASHOPHA AKSHI PAKA

**It is Tridoshaja, sarvagatha, Vyadana sadhya vyadhi**

Except shotha all the symptoms of sashopha Akshi paka are present in this disease. (Vagbhata called it as " Alpa shopha akshi paka")

**Treatment of Sashopha and  Ashopha akshi paka :-**
" Treatment is like Rakthaj abhishyand (Sira vyadnasadhya vyadhi) "

**Treatment principle :-** 1) Snehan 2) Swedan 3) Sira vyada (at Apangasta or upanasika sira)

**Sthanika upacharas Local treatments :-**
Parisheka Aashchyotan, Nasya, putapaka, anjana, etc.

**Anjana yoga :-** 1) Ghritha + Saindhava lavan which is kept in a copper vessel, has to use as Anjan.

2) Sura or Aasava + Saindhava lavan which iskept in a copper vessel for a month, has to use as Anjan.

3) Dadhi which is kept in a copper vessel for a month has to use as Anjan.

4) Raktha mokshana, then apply kamsya malam + ghritam

6) Madhuka sar + gyrika + madhu, as Anjan.

7) Jathi Pushpanjan :- (Jathi pushpa, saindhavalavan, Aardrak, pippali, vidanga + Honey.)

**Aashchyotan yoga :-** 1) Shunti + stanya, add saindhava lavana or Ghritha,kept for a month, then use as Aashchyotan

2) Daruharidra + prapundareeka kwatha as Aashchyotan.

**Treatment principle as per vagbhata (Astanga Hrudya ):-** 1) Sneha - Sweda - Raktha mokshana then again snehan and rechana with Nishotha Kwatha + Draksha + Hareetaki + Ghritha.

2) Swetha lodhra fry in Ghritha, pack in a cloth dip in the lukewarm water, use the lekewarm water parisheka, for the reduction of pain.

**Sandhava yogas especially explained to get relief from redness,pain , and foreign body  sensation.**

1)      Take the essence of Tamra in Gomutra, Should keep in a Iron vessel, fumigate with ghritha and use as anjana.

2)      Go dadhi (masthu), collect in the copper vessel, add pippali, saindhava lavana, mix well and use as anjana.

3)      Take shankha and stanya in a copper vessel, fumigate with shami patra or yava which is dipped in the ghritha, and use as anjana, it reduces foreign body sensation and pain in the eye.

4)      Udumbhara phalam  + stanyam, collect in Iron vesel, fumigate with shami patra which is dipped in the ghritha, and use as anjan, it reduces pain burning and lacrimation.

5) Shigru pallava swarasa, collect in copper vessel, fumigate with ghritha and use as Anjana.

6) Mruth kapala collect in the Kamsya vessel, do bhavana in Tilakwatha, fumigate with Nimba patra which are dipped in ghritha and used as anjan

7) Talisadi Gutikanjan with stanyam.

8) Vyaghradi Kalka Anjana.

**Note :-** After the above anjana applications, aschyotana should do with stanya

## 11) HATHADHIMANTHA
### (Atrophic bulbi or Phthisis bulbi due to acute congestive glaucoma)

It is a sarva gatha, vataja, asadya vyadhi, arises by neglecting the vataja adhimantha.

Netra sosha (atrophy of eye ball) & Teevra vedana (severe pain) are the main features of the disease

**As per Vagbhata : -** An ulcer forms in the eye that causes loss of vision and severe pain in the eye ball, it occurs by neglecting vataj adhimantha

**It is of two types**
1) Vitiated vata by filling the blood vessels, pushes the eye ball forward andproduces severe pain (Pricking, crushing) in the eye (inter calary staphy loma due to increased intra occular pressure)
2) Vitiated vata suppress the Teja bala and agni of the eye ball by that the eye ball shrinks like the lotus.( Atrophic bulbi or phthisis bulbi)

It is Asadhya vyadhi but can be treated like vataj adhishyanda vyadhi.

## 12) ANILA PARYAYA (VATA PARYAYA)
### (occular pain due to chronic glaucoma or Trigeminal neuralgia)

It is sarvagatha vataj, vyadana sadhya vyadhi,

The Vitiated vata causes severe pain, some times in the Pakshma, some times in Bhru and some times in the eye ball, is known as vataparyaya or anila paryaya (Shifting pain).

**Vagbhata's Additional points :-** Eye ball becomes smaller (microphthalmas) Treatment is like vataj Abhishyanda and anyathovata.

176

# 13 ANYATHO VATA
## (Reffered pain in the eye or Spenoidal sinusitis )

It is sarvagatha, vataja ,vyadana sadhya vyadhi,

The Vitiated vata causes severe pain in the eyes or in the bhru (Root of by the nose ) by spreading from peripheral parts like karna (ears), Shira (head), manya (Sides of neck) greeva (neck), hanu (jaws) etc. (Referred pain in the eye from other parts)

**Chikitsa :-** 1) Anila paryaya and Anyathovatha should be treated like vataja Abhishyanda.

2) Sneha, sweda, Raktha mokshana,vasti, sneha Rechan, Tarpan, putapaka Bhojan poorva ghrithapana), and milk with meals .

3) Oral intake of ghee, prepared from veeratarvadi Ksheera

4) Oral intake of ghee, prepared from Mesha shrungi.

# 14) SHUSHKAAKSHI PAKA
## (Xerophthalmia)

It is sarvagatha, vataja, Aushada (Ashastra Krutha) sadhya vyadhi.

Eye lids are closed (dropped) and are opened with difficulty, lids become hard rough, and eye looks dirty lustreless

**Vagbhata :-** Vata + Pitta vitiates, eye lids become hard rough and causes difficulty in opening and closing the lids, it associate with foreign body sensation, pricking pain, cutting pain, exudation, suppuration and the patient likes cool applications.

**Treatment :-**1) Ghrithapanam (oral administration of Ghee), 2) Jeevaneeya ghritha Tarpan, 3) Brumhana taila or Anutaila nasyam, 4) Saindhava lavana +Lukewarm milk for eye wash (pariseka), 5) Bidala with fried lodha+ghritha ,

**6) Anjana : -** 1) Anjana with Shunti + Stanya + Ghritha

2) Anjana with Anupa vasa(Animal fat) + Shunti or saindhava, Lavan

3) Saindhava Lavan + Deva daru + Shunti + mathu lunga swarasa + ghritha Raskriya anjana - with stanya.

4) Anjana with haridra Devadaru, saindhava, lavana ghritha and madhu

5) Anjana with Kesha masi (Hairs ) + Ghritha (Masi is prepared in mallaka samputa).

6) Shunti + Saindhava lavana, Rasa kriyanjan with ghritha

7) Anjana with Madhu, saindava lavan and gyrica.

## 15) AMLADYUSHITHA (Allergic chemosis)

It is sarvagatha pittaja aushada sadhya vyadhi,(Ashastra Krutha)

Eye becomes inflammed, oedema of eye ball occur with bluish red lines due to in take of Amla Katu, lavana tredominent diet is known as Amla dyushitha.

In Astanga hrudaya it is termed as " Amloshitha ",Vagbhata added the points like shotha (oedema) Raga (hyperaemia ), srava (Exudation), paka (suppuration, jwalana (Burning), Ashrusrava (Lacrimation) and lustre less eye.

**Treatment :-** like pittaj Abhishyanda but Raktha mokshana is contra indicated. (Triphala ghritha Tilwaka ghitha purana ghritha roral administration for virechan, then application of sheetha anjanas are advised).

## 16) SIROTHPATHA
### (Allergic Conjunctivitis, angio neurotic Oedema or episcleritis.)

It is sarvagatha rakthaja vyadan Sadhya vyadhi, eye suddenly becomes red and spread with capillary net, may or may not contain the pain and the disease subsides naturally .

" The occurence the resolution of the the disease is natural ",

**Chikitsa** 1) Raktaja Abhishyanda Chikitsa. 2) Raktha mokshana. 3) Anjana with Madhu + Ghritha. 4) Anjana with Saindhava lavan + Kaseesa + Stanya. 5) Anjanan with Swarna gyrica + madhu. 6) Anjana with Shankha nabhi, manashila, Tuttha Daruharidra, saindhava lavana + madhu. 7) Anjana with Sura swetha maricha makshika and sireesha pushpa.

## 17)SIRA HARSHA
### (Allergic hyperaemia Acute orbital cellulitis)

It is sarvagatha, Rakthaja, vyadan, sadya vyadhi, it occurs due to neglecting the sirothpatha in which red sticky discharge comes from the eyes and patient cannot able to see the objects.

**Treatment :-**
1) Rakthaja Abhishyanda Chikitsa. 2) Anjana with Phanitha + Madhu. 3) Anjana with Rasanjan + madhu. 4) Anjana with Kaseesa, Saindhava lavan. + Madhu. 5)Anjana with Vetramla + Stanya + Phanitha+ Saindhava lavan

**Note :-** Sirothpatha and sira harsha are the symptoms observed in somany lesions of conjunctiva, either inflammatory or allergic or traumatic (episcleritis- scleritis).

# Sarvagatha rogas (Susrutha)

Total 17 diseases

I)      1 Disease  Asadya (Hathadhimanda)

II)     2 Diseases - Ashastra kruth,  they are,

a) Shuskakshi paka

b) Amldyushitha

III)    14  Diseases  - Vyadana sadya vyadhies, They are

4 Abhishyanda

4 Adhi manda

2 Akshi paka (Sashopha - Ashopha)

Anyatho vatha

Anila paryaya

Siroth patha

Sira harsha

Sarva gatha roga according to vagbhata :-

Total -1 6

1)      2 Diseases are Asadya

a)  Hathadhimanda

b)  Akshi Pakatyaya

II)     14 diseases  sadyam ( rest of the diseases)

# SARVAGATHA ROGA

| S.No. | Name of the disease Modern Name | Vitiated Dosha Prognosis | Clinical features | Treatment Principle |
|---|---|---|---|---|
| 1. | Vataj abhishyanda (sub acute catarrhal Conjunctivitis) | Vataj | Patient feels head ache, Pricking pain in the eyes, foreign body sensation, cool lacrimation and desires hot therapy. | 1) Vyadan Sadya 2) Aashchyotan Anjan etc. |
| 2. | Pittaja Abhishyanda (Acute catarrhal Conjunctivitis) | Pittaja Sadya | Patient feels burning pain Supuration in the eyes, eyes appear in yellow colour with hot lacrimation and desires cool therapy. | 1) Vyadan Sadya 2) Pittahara Aashchotan, anjana etc. |
| 3. | Kaphaj Abhishyanda (Acute mucopurulent conjunctivits | Kaphaj Sadya | Patient feels heavyness oedema itching, stickyness, coolness, the eyes appears in white colour and desires hot therapy. | Vyadan sadya 2) Kaphara Ashchyotan, anjana etc. |
| 4. | Raktaj Abhishyanda (Acute mucopurlent Conjunctivits) | Raktaj Sadya | Features like pittaja Abhishyanda in addition to those, red eyes red lacrimation with capillary net appearance | 1) Vyadan Sadya. 2) Rakta hara Aashchyotan, Anjan etc. |
| 5. | Vataj Adhimantha (Acute congestive glaucoma) | Vataj Sadya | Head ache, Pricking crushing Scooping and breaking type of pain in the eye ball, foregn body sensation, Lacrimation, admana Kampanan. It occur by neglecting vataj abhishyanda. | 1) Vyadan Sadya 2) Vataja abhishyanda treatment 3) Daha at above bhru. |
| 6) | Pittaj Adhimantha (Acute congestive glaucoma) | Pittaj Sadya | It occurs by neglecting Pittaj Abhishyanda, capillary net, buring, hyperamia, oedema of eye lids, purspiration and unconscious ness the patient visualises the things in yellow colour. | 1) Vyadan sadya |
| 7) | Kaphaj Adhimantha (chronic simple glaucoma) | Kaphaj Sadya | It occurs by neglecting the kaphja abhishyanda, oedema, Lacrimation, Itching sensation coolness, heavness, stickyness, sensitivity in the eye ball, Headache and visualises the things in white colour. | 1) Vyadan Sadya |

| 8) | Raktaj Adhimantha | Rakthaj | It occurs by neglecting rakthaja abhishyanda, tenderness, unberable pain, redness, redexdation, and visualises the objects in red colour. | 1) Vyadan Sadya |
| 9) | Sashopha Akshipaka (Uveitis, cellulits of eye ball, pain ophthalmitis) | Tridosh (Rakth-aj), (Sadya) | Red oedema like pakwajambu Phala, assoiciated with pain, itiching, exudation, stickyness in the eye ball. | 1) Vyadan Sadya |
| 10) | Ashopha Akshipaka | Tridosh | Except shopha all the symptoms are similar to above. | Vyadan Sadya |
| 11) | Halthadhimantha (Atrophic bubi , Phthisis bulbi, acute congestive glaucoma) | Vataj Asdaya | Pain, atrophy of eye ball, forward protrusion of eye ball, shrinkage of eye ball. | Asadya |
| 12) | Anila paryaya (Ocular shifitng pain, trigemenal neuralgia) | Vataj Sadya | Severe shifting pain in the pakshma, bhru, eye ball. | Vyadan Sadya |
| 13) | Anyatho vata (referred pain in the eye ball) | Vataj Sadya | Pain referred to bhru eye from ear, head neck & jaw. | Vyadan sadya |
| 14) | Shushkakshi paka | Vataj Sadya | The closed eyes are opened by diffucult, hard rogh, lustreless, dirty eye ball. | Aushada sadya |
| 15) | Amladyushutha (Allergic chemosis ) | Pittaja Sadya | Inflammation of eye ball due to in take of amla, lavan, katu, ahara | Aushada Sadya |
| 16) | Sirothpath (Allergic conjunctivitis ) | Rakthaj Sadya | Eye suddenly becomes red with capillary net, subside naturally | Vyadan Sadya |
| 17) | Siraharsha (Allergic hyperaemia) | Rakthaj Sadya | Photophobia, red sticky exudation occurs by neglecting sirothpath. | Vyadan Sadya |

# दृष्टिगत रोग

## दृष्टि का प्रमाण

कृष्णात् सप्तममिच्छन्ति दृष्टिदृष्टिविशारदा: ॥

(सु॰ उ॰ 1/13)

नवमस्तारकांशो दृष्टि: ॥

(सु॰ उ॰ 35/12)

मसूरदलमात्रां तु पंचभूतप्रसादजाम् ॥
खद्योतविस्फुलिङ्गाभामिद्दां तेजोभिरव्ययै: ॥
आवृतां पटलेनाक्ष्णोर्बाह्येन विवराकृतिम् ॥
शीतसात्म्यां नृणां दृष्टिमाहुर्नयनचिन्तका: ॥

(सु॰ उ॰ 7/3)

## नेत्र पटल

द्वे वर्त्मपटले विद्याच्चत्वार्यन्यानि चाक्षिणि ॥
जायते तिमिरं येषु व्याधि: परमदारुण: ॥

(सु. उ. 1/17)

तेजोजलाश्रितं वाह्यं तेष्वन्यत् पिशिताश्रितम् ॥
मेदस्तृतीयं पटलमाश्रितं त्वस्थि चापरम् ॥
पंचमांशसमं दृष्टेस्तेषां बाहुल्यमिष्यते ॥

(सु॰ उ॰ 1/18)

## प्रथम पटलगत तिमिर

सिराभिरभिसंप्राप्य विगुणोभ्यन्तरे भृशम् ॥
प्रथमे पटले दोषो यस्य दृष्टौ व्यवस्थित: ॥
अव्यक्तानि स रूपाणि सर्वाण्येव प्रपश्यति ॥

(सु॰ उ॰ 7/6)

सिरानुसारिणि मले प्रथमं पटलं श्रिते ।
अव्यक्तमीक्षते रूपं व्यक्तमप्यनिमित्ततः ॥

(अ. ह. उ. १२ अ.)

## द्वितीय पटलगत तिमिर

दृष्टिभृशं विह्वलति द्विवतीयं पटलं गते ॥
मक्षिकामशकान् केशांजालकानि च पश्यति ॥
मण्डलानि पताकांश्च मरीचिः कुण्डलानिच
परिप्लवांश्च विविधान् वर्षमभ्रं तमांसि च ॥
दूरस्थानिच रूपाणि मन्यतै च समीपतः
समीपस्थानि दूरे च दृष्टेर्गोचरविभ्रमात् ॥
यत्नवानपि चात्यर्थ सूचीपाशं न पश्यति ॥

(सु॰ उ॰ 7/7,8,9,10 अ॰)

प्राप्ते द्विवतीयं पटलमभूतमपि पश्यति ॥
भूतं तु यत्नादासन्नं दूरे सूक्ष्मं च नेक्षते ॥
दूरान्तिकस्थं रूपं च विपर्यासेन मन्यते ॥
दोषे मण्डलसंस्थाने मण्डलानीव पश्यति ॥
द्विवधैकं दृष्टिमध्यस्थे बहुधा बहुधास्थिते ॥
दृष्टेरभ्यन्तरगते ह्रस्ववृद्दविपर्ययम् ॥
नान्तिकस्थमधःसंस्थे दूरगं नोपरिस्थिते ॥
पार्श्वे पश्येन्न पार्श्वस्थे तिमिराख्योयमामयः ॥

(अ. ह्. उ. १२ अ.)

## तृतीय पटलगत तिमिर

ऊर्ध्वं पश्यति नाधस्तात्तृतीयं पटलं गते ॥
महान्त्यपि च रूपाणिच्छादितानीव वाससा ॥
कर्णनासाक्षि युक्तानि विपरीतानि वीक्षते ॥
यथादोषं च रज्येत दृष्टदर्षे वलीयसी ॥
अधः स्थिते समीपस्थं दूरस्थं चोपरिस्थिते ॥
पार्श्वस्थिते तथा दोषे पार्श्वस्थानि न पश्यति ॥
समन्ततः स्थिते दोषे संकुलानीव पश्यति ॥
दृष्टिमध्यगते दोषे स एकं मन्यते द्विवधा ॥
द्विवधास्थिते त्रिधा पश्येद् बहुधा चानवस्थिते ॥
तिमिराख्यः स वै दोषः

(सु. उ. अ. 7/11,12,13,14 )

183

प्राप्नोति काचतां दोषे तृतीयपटलाश्रिते ॥
तेनोर्ध्वमीक्षते नाधस्तनुचैलावृतोपमम् ॥
यथावर्णं च रज्येत दृष्टिर्हीयेत च क्रमात् ॥

(अ. हृ. उ. १२ अ.)

## चतुर्थ पटलगत तिमिर

सर्वै दोषः चतुर्थं पटलं गतः ॥
रुणद्धि सर्वतो दृष्टिं लिङ्गनाशः स उच्यते ॥
तस्मिन्नपि तमोभूते नातिरूढे महागदे ॥
चन्द्रादित्यै सनक्षत्रावन्तरीक्षे च विद्युतः ॥
निर्मलानि च तेजांसि भ्राजिष्णुनि च पश्यति ॥

(सु. उ. 7/15,16,17)

तथाप्युपेक्षणमाणस्य चतुर्थं पटलं गतः ॥
लिङ्गनाशं मलः कुर्वन् छादयेद् दृष्टिमण्डलम् ॥

(अ. हृ. उ. १२ अ.)

## विभिन्न तिमिर लक्षण

तत्र **वातेन** रूपाणि भ्रमन्तीव स पश्यति ॥
आविलान्यरुणाभानि व्याविद्धानि च मानवः ॥
**पित्तेना**दित्यखद्योतशक्रचापतडिद्गुणान् ॥
शिखिबर्हविचित्राणि नीलकृष्णानि पश्यति ॥
**कफेन** पश्येद्रूपाणि स्निग्धानि च सितानि च ॥
गोरचामरगौराणि श्वेताभ्रप्रतिमानि च ॥
पश्येदसूक्ष्माण्यत्यर्थं व्यभ्रे चैवाभ्रसंप्लवम् ॥
सलिलप्लावितानीव परिजाड्यानि मानवः ॥
तथा **रक्तेन** रक्तानि तमांसि विविधानि च ॥
हरितश्यावकृष्णानि धूमधूम्राणि चेक्षते ॥

(सु. उ. 7/18 से 22 )

## 1. वातज तिमिर

तत्र वातेन तिमिरे व्याविद्धामिव पश्यति ॥
चलाविलारुणाभासं प्रसन्नं चेक्षते मुहुः ।

जालानि केशान् मशकान् रश्मींश्चोपेक्षितेत्र च ॥
काचीभूते दृगरुणा पश्यत्यास्यमनासिकम् ॥
चन्द्रदीपात्यनेकत्वं वक्रमृज्ज्वपि मन्यते ॥
वृद्ध: काच:दृशं कुर्याद्रजोधूमावृतामिव ॥
स्पष्टारुणाभां विस्तीर्णां सूक्ष्मां वा हतदर्शनाम् ॥
स लिङ्गनाश:

(अ. ह. उ. १२ अ.)

## 2. पित्तज तिमिर

पित्तजे तिमिरे विद्युत्खद्योतदीपितम् ।
शिखितित्तिरिपत्राभं प्रायो नीलं च पश्यति ॥
काचे दृक् काचनीलाभा तादृगेव च पश्यति ।
अर्केन्दुपरिवेषाग्निमरीचीन्द्रधनूंषि च ॥
भृङ्गनीला निरालोका दृक् स्निग्धा लिङ्गनाशत: ।
दृष्टि: पित्तेन हृस्वाख्या सा हृस्वदर्शिनी ॥
भवेत् पित्तविदग्धाख्या पीता पीताभदर्शना ।

अ. ह. उ. 12 अ

## 3. कफज तिमिर

कफेन तिमिरेप्राय: स्निग्धं श्वेतं च पश्यति ॥
शङ्खेन्दुकुन्दकुसुमै: कुमुदैरिव चाचितम् ।
काचे तु निष्प्रभेन्द्वर्कप्रदीपाद्यैरिवाचितम् ॥
सिताभा च सा दृष्टि: स्याल्लिङ्गनाशे तु लक्ष्यते ।
मूर्त कफो दृष्टिगत: स्निग्धो दर्शननाशन: ॥
बिन्दुजलस्येव चल: पद्मिनीपुटसंस्थित ।
उष्ण संकोचमायाति छायायां परिसर्पति ॥
शंखकुन्देन्दुकुमुदस्फटिकोपमशुक्लिमा ।

(अ. ह. उ. १२ अ.)

## 4. रक्तज तिमिर

रक्तेन तिमिरं रक्तं तमोभुतं च पश्यति ॥
काचेन रक्ता कृष्णा वा दृष्टिस्तादृक् च पश्यति ।

185

लिङ्गनाशोपि तादृक् दृङ् निष्प्रभा हतदर्शना ॥

(अ. ह. उ. १२ अ.)

## 5. सान्निपातिक तिमिर

सन्निपातेन चित्राणि विप्लुतानि च पश्यति ॥
बहुधा वा द्विधा वापि सर्वाण्येव समन्ततः ॥
हीनाधिकाङ्गान्यथवा ज्योतींष्यपि च पश्यति ॥

(सु. उ. 7/23,24 अ.)

## संसर्गज व त्रिदोषज लिङ्गनाश

संसर्गसन्निपातेषु विद्यात् संकीर्णलक्षणान् ।
तिमिरादीनकास्माच्च तैः स्याद् व्यक्ताकुलेक्षणः ॥
तिमिरे, शेषयोर्दृष्टौ चित्रो रागः प्रजायते ॥

(अ. ह. उ. १२ अ.)

तिमिरं काचतां याति काचोप्यान्ध्यमुपेक्षया ।
नेत्ररोगेष्वतो घोरं तिमिरं साधयेद् ध्रुवम् ॥

(अ. ह. उ. १३ अ.)

## 6. परिम्लायि रोग

पित्तं कुयात् परिम्लायि मूर्च्छितं रक्ततेजसा ।
पीता दिशस्तथोद्यन्तमादित्यमिव पश्यति ॥
विकीर्यमाणान् खद्योतै वृक्षांस्तेजोभिरेव च ॥

(सु. उ. 7/25)

रक्तजं मण्डलं दृष्टौ स्थूलकाचानलप्रभम् ।
परिम्लायिनि रोगे स्यान्म्लाथ्यानीलं च मण्डलम् ॥
दोषक्षयात् कदाचित् स्यात् स्वयं तत्र च दर्शनम् ॥

(सु. उ. 7/26,27 अ.)

रागोरुणो मारुतजः प्रदिष्टः पित्तात् परिम्लाथ्यथवापि नीलः ॥
कफात् सितः शोणितजस्तु रक्तः समस्तदोषोथ विचित्ररूपः ॥

(सु. उ. 7/28)

अरुणं मण्डलं वाताच्चंचलं परुषं तथा ॥
पित्तान् मण्डलमानीलं कांस्याभं पीतमेव वा ॥

श्लेष्मणा वहलं स्निग्धं शङ्कुकुन्देन्दुपाण्डुरम् ॥
चलत्पद्मपलाशस्थः शुक्लो बिन्दुरिवाम्भसः ॥
संकुचव्यातपेत्यर्थं छायायां विस्तृतो भवेत् ॥
मृद्यमाने च नयने मण्डलं तद् विसर्पति ॥
प्रवालपद्मपत्राभं मण्डलं शोणितात्मकम् ॥
दृष्टिरागो भवेच्चित्रो लिङ्गनाशे त्रिदोषजे ॥
यथास्वं दोषलिङ्गानि सर्वेष्येव भवन्ति हि ॥

(सु. उ. 7/29 से 33)

## 7. पित्तविदग्धदृष्टि

पित्तेन दुष्टेन गतेन दृष्टि पीता भवेद् यस्य नरस्य दृष्टिः ॥
पीतानि रूपाणि च मन्यते यः स मानवः पित्तविदग्ध दृष्टिः ।
प्राप्ते तृतीयं पटलं तु दोषे दिवा न पश्येन्निशि वीक्षते च ॥
(रात्रौ स शीतानुगृहीतदृष्टिः पित्ताल्पभावादपि तानि पश्येत् ॥)

(सु. उ. 7/35,36)

## 8. श्लेष्मविदग्धदृष्टि

तथा नरः श्लेष्मविदग्धदृष्टिस्तान्येव शुक्लानि हि मन्यते तु ॥
त्रिषु स्थितः पटलेषु दोषो नक्तान्ध्यमापादयति प्रसह्य ॥
दिवा स सूर्यानुगृहीतचक्षुरीक्षेत रूपाणि कफाल्पभावात् ॥

(सु. उ. 7/37,38)

## उष्णविदग्धदृष्टि

उष्णतप्तस्य सहसा शीतवारिनिमज्जनात् ॥
त्रिदोषरक्तसंपृक्ते यात्यूष्मोर्ध्वं ततोक्षिणि ।
दाहोषे मलिनं शुक्लमहन्याविलदर्शनम् ॥
रात्रावान्ध्यं च जायेत विदग्धोष्णेन सा स्मृता ॥

(अ. हृ. १२ अ.)

## 9. धूमदर्शी

शोकज्वरायासशिरोभितापैरम्याहता यस्य नरस्य दृष्टिः ॥
स धूमकान् पश्यति सर्वभावांस्तं धूमदर्शीति वदन्ति रोगम्

(सु. उ. 7/39)

## 10. ह्रस्वजाड्य

स ह्रस्वजड्यो दिवसेषु कृच्छ्राद्ध्रस्वानि रूपाणि च येन पश्येत्॥

(सु. उ. 7/40 अ.)

यो बासरे पश्यति कष्टतोथ रूपं महाच्चापि निरीक्षतेल्पम्॥
रात्रौ पुनर्यः प्रकृतानि पश्येत् स ह्रस्वजाड्यो मुनिभिः प्रदिष्टः।

योग रत्नाकर

दृष्टिमध्यस्थिते दोषे महद्घ्रस्वं ना पश्यति।
रात्री पित्ताल्पभावाच्च तानि रूपाणि पश्यति॥

## 11. नकुलान्ध्य

विद्योतते येन नरस्य दृष्टिर्दोषाभिपन्ना नकुलस्य यद्वत्॥
चित्राणि रूपाणि दिवा स पश्येत् स वै विकारो नकुलान्ध्यसंज्ञः॥

(सु. उ. 7/40)

द्योतते तकुलम्येव यस्य दृङ् निचिता मलैः॥
नकुलान्धः स तत्राह्नि चित्रं पश्यति नो निशि।

(अ. ह. उ. १२ अ.)

# दोषान्ध

अर्केस्तमस्तकन्यस्तगभस्तौ स्तम्भमागताः॥
स्थगयन्ति भृशं दोषा दोषान्धः स गदोपरः।
दिवाकरकरस्पृष्टा भ्रष्टा दृष्टिपथान्मलाः॥
विलीनलीना यच्छन्ति व्यक्त मत्राह्नि दर्शनम्॥

(अ. ह. उ. १२ अ.)

## 12. गम्भीरिका

दृष्टिर्विरूपा श्वसनोपसृष्टा संकुच्यतेद्भ्यन्तरतश्च याति॥
रुजावगाढा च तमक्षिरोगं गम्भीरिकेति प्रवदन्ति तज्ज्ञाः॥

(सु. उ. 7/41)

# आगान्तुक लिंगनाश

बाह्यौ पुनर्द्राविह सम्प्रदिष्टौ निमित्ततश्चाप्यनि मित्ततश्च॥
निमित्ततस्तत्र शिरोभितापाज्झेयस्त्वभिष्यन्दनिदर्शनैश्च॥

(सु. उ. 7/42)

## अनिमित्त लिंगनाश

सुरर्षिगन्धर्वमहोरगाणां सन्दर्शनेनापि च भास्वराणाम्॥

हन्येत दृष्टिर्मनुजस्य यस्य स लिङ्गनाशस्त्वनिमित्तसंज्ञ:॥

तत्राक्षि विस्पष्टमिवाभाति वैदूर्यवर्णा विमला च दृष्टि:॥

(सु. उ. 7/43,44)

## अभिघातहता दृष्टि:

विदीर्यते सीदति हीयते वा नृणामभीघातहता तु दृष्टि: ॥

(सु. उ. 7 अ.)

## अम्लविदग्धदृष्टि

भुशमम्लाशनाद् दोष: सास्त्रैर्वा दृष्टिराचिता॥

सक्लेदकण्डुकलुषा विदग्धाम्लेन सा स्मृता॥

(अ. हृ. १२ अ.)

## धूमर

शोकज्वराशिरोरोगसतप्तस्यानिलादय: ।

धूमाविलां धूमदृशं कुर्यु: स धूमर: ॥

(अ. हृ.उ. १२ अ.)

## औपसर्गिक लिङ्गनाश

सहसैवाल्पसत्वस्य पश्यतो रूपमद्भुतम्॥

भास्वरं भास्करादि वा वाताद्या नयनाश्रिता:॥

कुर्वन्ति तेज: संशोष्य दृष्टि मुषितदर्शनाम्॥

वैदूर्यवर्णा स्तिमितां प्रकृतिस्थामिवाव्यथाम्।

औपसर्गिक इत्येष लिङ्गनाश:

(अ. हृ. उ. १२ अ.)

## वाग्भट का मत से दृष्टिरोग

विना कफाल्लिङ्गनाशान् गम्भीरां ह्रस्वजामपि।

षट् काचा नकुलान्धश्च याप्या:, शेषांस्तु साधयेत्॥

द्वादशेति गदा दृष्टौ निर्दिष्टा: सप्तविंशति:॥

(अ. हृ. १२ अ.)

# DISEASES OF DRUSTI MANDAL

1) Diseases of Drusti mandal are 12 according to sushrutha

II) " 27 according to vagbhata

I) Sushruta's classification of " Drustimandal diseases ".

12 Diseases , they are as follows

Note:- 1) Vataj linganash (Timira - kacha - Lingaanash are the progressive stages of the disease)

2) Pittaja Linganash "

3) Kaphaja Linganash ..

4) Raktaj Linganash "

5) Sannipathaja Linganash

6) Parimlayi "

7) Pitta vidagdha drusti 8) Kapha vidagdha drusti 9) Dhooma darshi 10) Hraswa jadya 11)Nakulandya 12) Gambheerika

## II) Vagbhata's Classification of Drustimandal diseases
### 27 Diseases , they are as follows

He counted Timira Kacha Linganasha as separate diseases, so

1 to 6 - 6 types of Timira
7 to 12 6 types of Kacha
13 to 18 6 types of Linganash

19) Pitta vidagdha drusti     20) Amla vidagdha drusti
21) Ushna Vidagdha drusti     22) Doshandha or Nakthandhya
23) Dhooma darshi     24) Hraswajadya
25) Nakulandya     26) Gambheerika
27) Aupa sargika Linganash.

## Sadya - Asadyatha
### I) According to Sushrutha - A) Sadya (curative diseases)
6 types of Timira, Kaphaj Linganash (shastra sadya), Dhooma darshi, pitta vidagdha drusti and kapha vidagdha drusti are **Sadya**

**B) Yapyam :-** 6 types of Kacha:- **c) Asadya** (incurable), 5 types of Linganash (6 types - Kaphaj Linganash), Gambheerica, Hraswajadya and Nakulandya.

## II) According to Vagbhata:
**A) Sadya (Curable diseases)** 12 they are:- 6 types of Timira, Kaphaj Linganash, pitta vidagdha drusti, ushna vidagdha drusti, Naktandya
**B) Yapya - 7 diseases :-** 6 types of kacha and Nakulandya
**c) Asadya 8 diseases:-** 5 types of linganash, Gambheerica Hrawajadya, Aupasargic Linganash.

# * TIMIRA, KACHA, LINGANASH *

Timira Kacha and Linganash are the progressive stages of a disease, occur by the vitiation of Netra patalas and explained as a terrific disease that obstructs the vision

**Timira** = Partial obstruction of the vision

**Kacha** = Pigmentation of the drusti in which Vision moderately obstructed

**Linganash** = Vision completely obstructed

**Timira -** occurs by the vitiation of I, II, III, patalas (sushrutha), I, II patala (Vagbhata)

**Kacha -** occurs By the vitiation of III patala in which drusti is pigmented (Vagbhata).

If drusti is pigmented in III patala it is called kacha if not Timira (Sushrutha)

**Linganash** - By the vitiation of IV patala Drusti is completely obstructed and called Linganash (sushrutha - Vagbhata)

**Timiraakhyah Timira Sangya**

" **Raga praapthasya cha Timirasya Kacha ithi sangya**

**Runaddhi sarvatho drusti Linganasha Ucchyathe.**"

# Symptoms of Timira Based on Patalas
## (By Vagbhata)

| | | |
|---|---|---|
| 1) | I Patala | 1) Avyakta rupa darshan (indistinct vision) But some times get normal vision without obvious cause |
| 2) | II Patala | 1) Non existing things are visualised<br>2) Nearer objects are seen with difficult<br>3) Smaller objects of distance are not seen<br>4) Distant objects are seen as nearer<br>5) Near objects are seen as distant |

| Site of the dosha in drusti — Symptoms | |
|---|---|
| **If the lesion are** | **Objects oppear** |
| a) Circularly Present | - Circular |
| b) in middle of drusti | Diplopia (Double vision) |
| c) in many places | Polyopia (Multi vision) |
| d) In the interior of drusti | - Big objects seen as small and small objects are seen big |
| e) at Lower part of drusti | - Nearer objects are not seen. |
| f) The upper part of dusti | - Distant objects are not seen. |
| g) Sides of drusti | - on the same side objects are not seen |

(Timira)

| | |
|---|---|
| 3) III patala | When doshas reach this patala it is termed as kacha |
| (Kacha ) | 1) patient have upper vision but not lower vision<br>2) Objects are visualised as covered by cloth<br>3) Gradually pigmentation agravates and vision reduces. |
| 4) IV patala (Linganasha) | 1) Dusti completly obstructed but can identify only the bright light . |

**Note :-**

**In the lesions of the diseases of Drusti mandal**

If treatment is not given intime, the doshas spread from Ist patala to 4th patala and cause total blindness

Ist patala symptoms can be corelated to refractive errors, immature cataract

2nd patala symptoms - Can be corelated to immature cataract, vitreous opacities, Aqueous precipitants (Blood - pus, Foreign bodies) Refractive errors etc.

3rd patala symptoms can be corelated to Lental opacities and Retinal abnormalities

4th Patala symptoms can be coreleted to mature cataract.

## Symptoms of Timira based on patalas
### (By sushrutha)

| S.No. | Patala Sankhya | Symptoms |
|-------|----------------|----------|
| 1) | I Patala (KalaKaasti Aashritam) | 1) Avyakta rupa darshan (Indistinct vision) but some time get normal vision without obvious cause |
| 2 | II Patal (Medo aashritam) | 1) Dusti Vibhrama (Improper vision) a) Midya padartha darshan (Nonexisting things are visualised) ex flies, mosquitoes hair cobweb, rings, flags, rays, stars, rain, Darkness etc seen in their absence. b) Indriartha vibhrama (Existing things are improperly Visualised) **ex** Distant objects are seen as nearer. Near objects are seen as distant and cannot able to recognise the hole of a needle |
| 3) | III patal (mamsa aashritam) (Timira) (kacha) | 1) Patient have upper vision (urdwa drusti) but not the lower vision (Na adho drusti) 2) Bigger objects are visualised as covered by cloth 3) ear Nose eye etc Indrias are visualised in opposite. 4) If doshic vitiation is severe, the drusti is pigmented and called Kacha 5) According to the Site of the dosha, symptoms are explained, those are as follows. |

194

| Dosha Sthanam (Site of the dosham) | | Symptoms |
|---|---|---|
| **If the lesion is at** | | |
| a) Upper part of drusti | = | Distant objects are not seen |
| b) Lower Part of Drusti | = | Nearer objects are not seen |
| Sides of drusti | = | on the same side objects are not seen |
| d) on four sides | = | objects are seen as mixed |
| e) middle of Dusti | = | Diplopia (Double vision) |
| f) in two places of Drusti | = | Triplopia (Triple vision) |
| g) in many places of drusti | = | Polyopia (Multivision) |

4) IV Patala:- Drusti completely obstructed but can identify the
(Linganash):- bright light (Perception and projection of light)
Tejo jala
Aashritam

# Symptoms of Timira Kacha Linganash Based on doshas
## By Sushrutha

| Vitiated Dosha | Timira | Kacha | Linganasha |
|---|---|---|---|
| 1) Vataj | objects appear as moving dirty, irregular and in Red colour ( Aruna Varna) | Drusti appears in Aruna (red) or Shyava aruna (Blackish Red) | Drusti appears in Aruna varna (Red colour) rough and Floating |
| 2) Pittaja | Objects appear as khadyotha (sparkling creature), Aditya (sun) Vidyul latha (sparks) and in blue, black or in yellow colour | Drusti apears in blue or,yellow or dirty colour | Drusti apeears in blue, whitish yellow (Kasmsyabham) |
| 3) Kaphaj | Objects appear as oily, whitish, Like floating in the water, smaller objects appear as stout, rigid and moveing clouds also seen in its absence | Drusti appears in white colour | Drusti appears oily stout and whitish like shankha chandra etc, it appears as a water drop on lotus petal, get constricted in bright light dilated in shade and spreads by pressure. |
| 4) Raktaj | objects appeear in Red colour, dark (tamas), somky (dhoomavath) (Haritha, syava peetha and in Krishna varna) | Drusti appears in red colour | Drusti appears in Red colour like lotus and Pravala. |
| 5) Sanni pathaj | Objects appear in multi or mixed colours (chitra varna), wide spreaded, Diplopia, polypia mixedvision improper vision (Non existing things are visualised and existing things are improperly visualised. | Drusti appears in many colours (Chitra varna) | Drusti appears in many colours colour (Chitra varm) |
| 6) Parimlay | All the sides appear in yellow colour like risingsun, the trees appear as covered by bright things and sparkling small creatures (khadyotha) | Drusti appers in in peetha Neelam (Bluish yellow) | Drusti appears in peetha neela (Bluish yellow) |

## Symptoms of Timira Kacha Linganasha based on Doshas

(By Vagbhata)

1) Vataj  The objects appear as moving, drity, irregular and in red colour, Non existing things are visualised and some times objects appear normal, If treatment is not given in this stage (Timira) it turns in to **Aruna Kacha** in which the drusti appears in red colour, non exist ing things are visualised, and existing things are improp erly. visualised, one thing appears as many, straight things appear as curved, regular as irregular and vice versa, If the disease agravates it turns into **Linganash** in which drusti appears in dirty red colour and cannot able to see the objects.

2) Pittaja  In Timira the objects appear in Blue colour, as bright as vidruth, Khadyotha and shikhi pincha, if treatment is not given it turns into **Neela Kacha** in which the drusti appears blue and can visualise only the bright things like sun moon light rays etc. If treatment is not given it turns into **pittaja Linganash** in which drusti appears oily bright less, bluish and constricted (Hraswa drusti) and the objects are seen smaller

3) Kaphaj  In Timira objects appear oily, in white colour, like shanka chandra etc. in Kacha Drusti appears white and objects are seen as dim or dark and in **Linganasha** drusti appears white as shankha and chandra drusti becomes hard, get constricted in brightness and dilated in the shade, fluctuant like a water drop on the petal of lotus flower and the vision is completely obliterated.

| | |
|---|---|
| 4) Raktaj | In Timira objects appear in red **(Aruna Varna)** colour and dark (Andhaakara) in Kacha and Linganasha drusti appears Bright, less red, black and the vision is completely obliterated. |
| 5) Samsargaj | |
| 6) Sannipataja | Mixed symptoms of the above are observed. |
| **Note :** | I) In Timira due to partial impairment of vision sushrutha or vagbhata given the desciption of the objects which are properly or improperly visualised. |
| | 2) In Kacha drusti mandal is mostly vitiated by vatadi doshas and attain the colour accordingly vision is mostly impaired so only sushrutha and vagbhata described the vision as dark or smoky and explained only the colour of the drusti mandal but not the description of the objects. |
| | 3) In Linganasha sushrutha and vagbhata described only the colour of drusti mandala according to the vitation of doshas and explained that vision is com pletely obstructed but can identify the brightness. |

## TREATMENT PRINCIPLE OF TIMIRA- KACHA - LINGNASH

A)   Sadya vyadhies ( Curable diseases) :-
      6 types of Timira (Aushada sadya), Kaphaj Linganasha,
      (Shastra Sadya).

B)   6 types of Kacha are Yapya (Should be maintained)

C)   5 types of Linganash are Asadya ( in curable)
      (6 types - Kaphaj Linga nash)

**Note :-** Timira is complex disease, can be corelated to the syndrome of the diseases of refractive media .

      The refractive errors, cataract, Opacities of vitreous aqueous and Retinal diseases, The Signs and symptoms are grouped under the description of Netra patalas ( I to IV) and doshas.

# THE COMMON TREATMENT PRINCIPLES OF TIMIRA

**Pathya : -** (Beneficial for the eye)

Triphala ( Hareetaki vibheetaki Amalaki ), Trikatu (pippali maricha - shunthi), Yasti madhu, Anjan (Rasanjan Sauveeranjan Etc.) Haridra, Daru haridra, shigru Shatavari, Ashwagandha, Bala, sariba, manjista, Nimba, Vidanga, Sumudrphene, Tankan Guduchi Bhumyamalaki Nirmaleephala (Kataka beeja) Karpoora, chandana Kasthuri Lavanga Pundareeka usheera musta Tulasi Padmaka Neelothphala Devadaru Nirgundi Rasna Goghritha Aja gritha goksheera Aja Ksheera Go mutra Ajamutra, saindhava lavan, sita, madhu, stanya, jaangala mamsa, multon of carnivorous birds (chala janthu, mamsa ) Punarnava, Brungaraj, Kumari, Karanja, taila, Sarshapa taila, godhuma tail, swarna bhasma, Rajatha bhasma, Tamra bhasma, Nagabhasma, vanga bhasma, Loha bhasma, makshika bhasma, gyrika bhasma, kaseesa bhasma, Abraka bhasma, spatika bhasma, muktha bhasma, praval bhasma, Heeraka bhasma, shalidharya, shastika dhanya, kodrava, Godhuma yava, vana kulutha, mudga, kushmanda, patola, karkotaka, karavellaka, varthaka, Tarkari, kareera shighru, jeevanthi, Sunishannaka, Tanduleeyaka, vastuka, moolaka, Draksha, Dadima Aakashodaka, **Shodhan karmas** (Vaman virehan Nasya Vasti Raktha mokshan). **Local Treatments:-** (Seka Aashchyotan, Pindi Bidalaka Tarpan, putapaka, Anjan etc. Prasanna manas wearing chappals (pada pooja ) and umbrella and shirovestana to save the uttamangam (Head).Shathavari  Ksheera or payasa, Aamalaki Ksheera or Payasa, Triphala Ksheera or payasa, eating of yava odana (Food) shirasnana with cool water Reguler pratice of shiro Abhyanga and avoiding of excessive Katu Amla lavana Vidaha Kshara guru Abhishyandi food

**Apathya**  (Not to do for health of eyes)
1)      All the points those explained in Netra roga Nidana
2)      Suppressing natural urges (vegavarodha)
3)      Paada Peedan or Paada gharshan (giving pain to foot)
4)      Shiro Abhyanga dwesha (Rejecting head massage)
5)      Not wearing umbrella or shiro vestana
6)      Observing the bright, dim, very distant, very nearer, smallest, biggest and moving objects
7)      Using polluted outdated anjanas.

8)	Chronic exposure to dust smoke heat and cold
9)	Improper cleaning or washing of eyes and face.
10)	Tobacco and alcohol habit
11)	Not treating the chronic specific systemic infections in time.
12)	Immediate opposite exposures like hot cold, bright -dim, distant vision - near vision, etc.
13)	Krodha klesha shoka Bhaya Ativyayama eye strain shirobhighatha Tensions emotions anxiety etc Mano dosha
14)	Resting the head upwards or down wards while sleeping.
15)	Ati sweda
16)	Not protecting the eye from foreignbodies (Labour working in stone crushing or cement or other chemical factories etc.)


1) Systemic Purification by virechan, Rakthamokshan etc shodan Karma
2) Local therap by Anjan Tarpan Nasya etc netra kriyakalpas.


**1) a) Jeevanthyadi ghrita** -oral administration :- Jeevanthi 100 phala, water 1 drone. decoction should prepare with 1/4 residue (Padaava sesha) then added I prastha ghee, 2 prasta cow milk, each 1 karsha of kalka dravyas like prapoundareeka ,kakoli ,pippali Lodra, saindhavalavana ,sadapa ,yastimadu, Draksha, sugar ,Devadaru ,Triphala etc ghee has to prepare according to ghrithapaka vidhi and orally given in Timira.


b) Jeevanthi decoction 1 Prastha
1 prasta cowmilk ,kalka dravyas each 1 Karsha - they are ksheer kakoli, jeevaka, sharkara, shatavari, meda, pundrahya, yastimadu ,neelothphala - Ghee has to prepare according to ghritha paka vidhi and given orally in Timira


**2) Patoladya ghritha** -  Oral administration:- Patola, Nimba, katuki, Daruharidra ,usheera ,Triphala, vasa, Dhanvayasa ,Trayanthi ,parpataka - Each 1pala, Amalaki 1 prasta, water 1 drona, decoction should prepare and should reduce to 1/4 (Aadaka), Kalka drvyas are musta Kiratha tiktha yastimadhu, Kutaja, chandana, kuru veru (udeeccha) pippali - each 1/2 phala, 1prasta cow ghee- ghee prepared according to ghritha paka vidhi and should use in Timira nasa karna and charma rogas.

**3) a ) Triphala ghritha :-** ( Vagbhat) Triphala 8 phala, water 1 Aadaka decoction should reduce to 1/4,
cow milk is taken equal to decoction, triphala kalka 1Phala, ghee 1/2 prasta ghee shoould prepare according to ghritha paka vidhi - sugar or Honey added and given Orally in Timira.

b) Triphala kalka, Triphala kwatha, cowmilk, cow ghee (quantity and preparation according to gritha paka vidhi) it is used in Timira (Vagbhat)

c) Maha Triphala ghrita - (Vagbhat) Aja Ksheera 1Prastha, Triphala Kashaya 1 prastha, Vasa swarasa 1 prastha, go ghritha 1 prastha,
**Kalka drugs** each 1 phala they are yastimadu, kakoli, ksheerkakoli, vyaghree, pipali, guduchi, Neelothphala, sugar, draksha, ghee should prepare according to ghritha paka vidhi and is used orally in Timira.

d) Triphala ghritadi yoga in Timira (Vagbhat) Triphala ghritha, Triphala yastimadu and Honey, mixed well and kept for a month, later on daily at night it is used for vision improvement

e) Maha Triphaladya ghritha (Chakradatta) Triphala quatham 1prastha, vasa swarasa 1 prasta Aamalaki swarasa 1 prastha, Brungaraj swarasa 1 prastha Aja Ksheera 1 prastha amrutha swarasa 1 prastha, Kalka drugs are pippali sugar draksha Triphala Neelothphala yastimadu ksheerkakoli mudgaparni Nidagdhika (1/4th weight of ghee)
ghee should prepare acording to ghrithapaka vidhi and is given " Before middle and after meals" for vision improvement.

f) Anya Triphala ghritha (Chakradatta) or Triphala ghritha :-
        Triphala, Trikatu, Draksha, yastimadhu, Katuki, prapoundareeka, sukshma, Ela vidanga, Naga kesar, Neelothphala, Sariba Bala chandana dwayam, Haridradwayam, each 1 karsha, ghee 1 Prastha, cow milk 1 prastha, Triphala quath 3 prastha. Ghee should prepare according to ghrithapaka vidhi and given in Timira.

g) Dwitheeya Triphala ghrita (Bhava mishra):- Hareetaki 100, vibheetaki 200. Aamalaki 400, 4 times water is added and 1/4th decoction should prepare, **Kalka drugs** are yastimadu, sugar, draksha, nidigdhika, madhooka, kakoli, ksheerakakoli, Aamalaki, Haridra, vibheetaki, Nagkesar, pippali, chandana, methi, Uthphala, 1 tula vasa swarasa, 1 tula brungaraj swarasa, 1 Prastha Goghritha - Gritha has to prepare according to gritha paka vidhi and given orally for the improvement of vision.

h) Triphala choorna + ghee - in Timira

i) Triphala kashaya + ghee - in Timira

**4) Maha Vasadi Quatham:-**
Vasa, musta, nimbatwak, Patola patra, Kakuki, guduchi, Raktha chandan, Kutaja, Indrayava, Daruharidra, Chithramoola, shunthi, kiratatiktha, Triphala yava - 16 times water is added and reduced to half - This decoction is orally used in Netra rogas.

5)     a) Triphala choora or Kashaya with Tailam is given in vataja Timira
        b) Triphala choora or Kashaya with ghee is given in Pittaja Timira
        c) Triphala choorna or Kashaya with madhu is given is kaphaja Timira

6) Makshika bhasma, Loha bhasma, swarna bhasma, Yastimadu, Sita, (Sugar) Purana ghritha, madhu and Triphala - orally administered in Timira
7) Makshika, Lohabhasma, swarna bhasma, yastimadu Sita, Purana Ghritha, (Sugar) Madhu and Triphala - Orally administered in Timira
8) Triphala can be used daily with food items (Sweets Tiffins ) for improvement of vision.
9) Draksha or Triphala with sugar and Honey oral administration for the improvement of vision.
10) Daily face wash or eye wash with Triphala Kashaya controls the eye diseases.
11) Triphala churna yastimadu, lohabhasma + ghritha or Honey - oral administration.

## ANJANAS
1) Timira roga hara Choornanjan :- Sauveeranjan (Srotonjan) 64 parts, tamra loha rajatha and swarna bhasma each 1 part, these bhasma are melted and dipped in th decoctions of madhuradi gana drugs separately for 7 times, added vydoorya bhasma, muktha bhasma and shankha bhasm - perfectly grinded and preserved for Anjana in timira.

2) Jata mamsi Trijathaka Loha bhasma Kumkuma Neelothphala Hareetaki tutha swetha Kaca shankha samudra phena maricha sauveer raanjan pippali yastimadhu - The medicines are equally taken perfectly grinded and should use as anjana when chandra enters into Ashwini Nakshatra - it is useful in Timira

**3) Drusti prasadan Anjan :-** Sauveeranjan is melted and dipped in the following liquids 7 times each Draksha swarasa Kamala mrunata swarasa Go ksheera, madhyam vasa swarasa varshodaka etc. The Anjana is powdered and preserved in shankha and is used for the clarity of vision

**4) Bhaskara choorna :-** Tuttham is heated with Badara sticks and dipped in Ajaksheera go ghritha and honey separtely each item. The purified tultam 2 phala makshika maricha srotonjana Katuki Tagora saindhavalavana lodra manah shila Hareetaki pippali Ela Sauveeranjan samudra phena each 1 karsha, Yastimadu ' phala, all the items are fried in a moosha and powdered, it is useful in Timira arma shukra.

**5) Timirantakanjan :-**
    Naga bhasma 30 parts, ganda pashana 5 parts Tamra bhasma 2 parts, Talaka 2 parts, vanga bhasma 1 part, sauveeranjan 3 parts all the drugs are melted powdered and used as anjana in Timira

**6) Tuttanjan :-**
    Tuttham is heated and dipped in gomutra gomaya rasa Kanji stanya Ghritha madhu and Vatsanabhi 7 times in each item after wards tuttham is powdered and used for anjana in Timira.

7) Lead is melted and dipped in triphala Kashaya Brangaraj swarasa Vatsanabhi, Kashaya, Ghritha, Aja Ksheera, Yastimadu Kashaya 7 times in each liquid, then it moulded as anjana shalaka and is used with or without anjana

**8) Drusti shakthikara anjan**
    Parad naga each 1 part, sauveeranjan 2 parts, 1/16 Karpoora - Grinded and used as anjana in Timira.

**9) Drusti Shakthikara anjan**
    Ghridra mukha bhasma + ghritha + Sauveeranjan used as anjana

10) Sauveeranjan and ghritha, kept in the mouth of Krishna sarpa later drug is collected bhasma is prepared and added Jatamamsi Choorna, given as anjana in corneal tear.

**11) Kukkuta vistanjan:-**
    Cow milk is taken in a pot, dead Krishna sarpa and scorpions are added and kept for 21 days, Later on the milk is chilled and cheese removed,that is given to the hen and after wards the Hen faecal material is collected for giving anjana

**12) Drusti shakthikara rasakriya:**
    Krishna sarpa, vasa, shankha, Kataka Sauveeranjan - Rasakriyanjan

**13 Aprathisaranjan :-**
Maricha 10, Makshika 1/2 Karsha, Tuttha 1 phala, yastimadu 1 Karsha, mix with cow milk - make it bhasma and use as anjan in Timira

**14) Aksha beejadi gutica**
    Tala beeja (Aksha beeja) maricha Amalaki tuttha Yastimadu - should grind with water and used as varthi anjan in Timira

**15) Shanmakshik yoga anjan in timira :**
Maricha 1 part, Aamalki 2 parts, swetha kamal 3 parts, tuttha 4 parts sauveeranjan 5 parts, makshika 6 parts - Grinded and given Anjana in Timira.

## 16 Ratnadi Choornajan -

Ratna, rajatha, spatica, swarna, sauveeranjan, Tamara, Loha, shankha, chandana, kumkuma, Gyrica, choornanjan is given in Timira

## 17) Vyaghra vasyanjan

Vyaghra vasa or varaha vasa or Grudhra vasa or kukkata vasa or sarpa vasa + Yastimadu choorna given as anjan in Timira.

18) Sauveeranjan is heated and dipped in mamsa rasa ksheera ghritha separately and choornanjan is given in Timira

## 19) Vimala varthi anjan

Shankha priyang manahshila, Trikatu triphala grinded and varthi anjan is given

## 20) Kokila varthi - Loha raja, trikatu, Saindhava lavan Triphala sauveeranjan - grinded and varthi anjan given .

## 21) Sukhavathi varthi :- kataka, shankha, bhasma, trikatu, saindhavalavan, sugar, samudra phen, rasanjan, vidang, manahshila, kukkutanda twak,- grind with water and varthi anjan is given with madhu

## 22) Chandrodaya varthi - Hareetaki, Vibheetaki, pippali, maricha, Vacha, Kusta, shankhanabhi, manahshila, the powder is grinded with Ajaksheera for varthi anjan.

## 23) Hareetakyadi anjan -

Hareetaki 1 part, haridra 1 part, pippali 1part, saindhava lavan 1/4 part grinded and varthi anjan prepared.

Usheera kashaya + pippali saindhava lavana goghritha madhu as anjan.

## 24) Muktaadi Mahanjan -

Mukttha, karpoora, kachalavana, agaru, maricha, pippali, lavana, sailavala, shunthi, Kankola, kamsya, Haridra,Trapu, manahshila, shankhanabhi, Abhraka, Tuttha, kukkatandatwak, Hareetaki, vibheetaki, Kumkuma, yastimadu, Rajavartha, Tulasi, navapushpa, karanja, Nimbatwak, Arjuna, musta, Tamra, aswagandha, methi - each 1 masha, the fine powder with madhu is given as anjan in Netra rogas.

# NASYA YOGAS

## 1) Jeevanthi Tailam
jeevanthi 100 phala - water 1droni decoction should reduce to 1/8 - Tila taila, and go ksheera 1 prasta each one pala Balatraya shathavari and jeevanth, Yastimadu 4 phala - Tailam is prepared and preserved in Iron vessel Later on used as Nasya in most of shalakya diseases.

## 2) Erendadi Tailam
Erenda, simheephala, Devadaru, vacha, Tagara, ghoshaya Bilvamoola, tila Tailam - cow milk (equallly ) Oil  is prepared according to taila paka vidhi for nasya

## 3) Tila tailam          Aksha tailam
Brungaraj swarasa Asana kashaya equally taken and oil prepared in an iron vessel for nasya
4) Brungarajadya taila
5) Nrupavallabha taila          For nasya
6) Abhijith taila

**Tarpan yogas :-**
1) with ksheeri sarpi (Ghee prepared from milk
2) Cowmilk + kukkuta or varaaha or mayura or Tittiri etc birds vasa perfectly heated together and ghee is extracted, the ghee +Yastimadu usheera chandana and heated according to ghritha paka vidhis. This medicated ghee is used for Tarpana in Timira.
3) Medicated ghee prepared according to the vitiation of doshes is used for Tarpanam.
Vasti or Rakthamokshana also advised according to the condition of the patient.

# VATAJA TIMIRA CHIKITSA

1) **Rakta mokshana**  (Contra indicated in kacha)
2) **Virechan** :- by the oral administration of
a) Medicated ghee prepared from Dasha moola kashaya cow ghee cow milk and Triphala kalka.
b) Triphaia Kashaya or pancha moola kashaya or Dasha moola kasha + cowmilk + erenda tail. etc.
c) Dashamoola ghritha + Trivruth churna etc.
3) **Shaman** Chikitsa by the oral administration of

| | |
|---|---|
| a) mesha shrungi ghritha | b) Triphala ghritha |
| c) Patolodya ghritha | d) purana ghritha |
| e) Ksheerisarpi | f) Kakolyadi or vidarigandadi |

ghrita

## 4) Nasya :-
    a)      Jeevantyadi taila    b) Gomaya tailam

    c)      Anu tailam    d) Kakolyadi or vidari gandhadi taila or ghritha

    e)   -  sahadi taila or ghritha

(Taila or ghritha, saha (mudga parni), Ashwa gandha, Ati bala and shatavari)

    f) Jalodbhavadi ghritha (matsya, Kacchapa mamsa, milk - ghee should prepare according to ghritha paka vidhi .

    g) Erenda mooladi ghritha or taila h) Trivrutadi tail nasya

    i) Ksheera sarpi (ghee prepared from milk)

5)      **Vasti** with vatara taila or ghritha

6) a)    **Tarpan** and snehan putapaka, with medicated ghee prepared from shatahwa kusta jatamamsi, Kakoli, Ksheer kakoli, Yastimadu, sarala, kusta, Devadaru, ghee and milk.

    **b) Tarpan** With ghritha manda or Ksheeri sarpi .

    c) Tarpan with the medicated ghee prepared form- cow milk and vasa of animals, ghee should preopared and yasti madu usheera, chandan are added, pakwa ghritha, is used for tarpan.

## 7) Puta Paka & Anjan
with Ghridra, Harina mamsa, Saindhava, Lavang, ghee and Honey .

## 8) Anjan :
    a) Ghridra Krishna sarpa, Kukkuta vasa + Yastimadhu churna

    b)Srotonjan or sauveranjan should in heat and dip in Triphala kashya, in mamsa rasa, ghritha and ksheera - after that the anjan head and dip should be powdered and preserved for usage

    c) Anjan with vyaghra varaha vas.

9)      a) Triphala churna with taila or ghee should take orally, daily for improvement of vision

    b) Triphala Kashaya with Taila or ghee should take orally, daily for the improvement of vision

    c) Triphala ghritha + Lukewarm milk

    d) Aamalaki phala Kashaya

    e) Triphala ghritha + yastimadu churna + Honey

    f) Triphala churna + Yastimadu + Loha bhasma + Ghritha + Madhu

    g) Regular oral usage of go ghritha after meals.

h) Oral usage of madicated ghee prepared from Rasna, Triphala quath Dasha moola quath, Jeevaneeya Kalka ghritha.

I) The medicated ghee prepared with Dashamoola quath + Triphal Kalka + milk + Ghee

J)Oral administration of Triphala makshika loha bhasma swarna bhasma Yastimadu sugar and Ghee,

## Vataj Kacha Chikistsa

1) Raktha mokshan is contra indicated
2) Srotonjan should kept in the mouth of krishna sarpa for amonth then it is collected and add saindhava lavan and Jathi pushpa swarasa for the usage.
3) Above srotonjan should do bhavan in milk for 3 days then if can be used for anjana

## PITTAJA TIMIRA CHIKITSA

1) **Sneha Karma -** Oral administration of
   a) Triphala ghritha
   b) Mesha shrungi ghrita
   c) Purana ghritha
   d) Ksheeri sarpi
   e) Kakolyadi ghritha
   f) Vidari gandhadi ghritha
   (oleation and shodhan with one of the above)
2) Raktha mokshan (sira vyadana)
3) Rechana -
   a) Sharkara, Ela, Trivruth churna + Madhu
   b) Triphala Churna + Ghee (cow ghee)

4) Cool applications to eye lid and eye drops (Shirolepa, mukha lepa and varthma lepa)

5) **Anjan :-**
a) Sariba, padmaka, usheera, mukta, lodra, chandana-as varthi anjana
b) Tejpatra, kamala, Anjan, Nagkesar, karpoor, yastimadu, swarna gyrika - as choornanajan.
c) Rasanjan, cheeni, manahshila, madhu, Yastimadu-as Rasa krianjan
d) Rasanjan or Sauveeranjan + Equally tutta as pratyanjan
e) Sauveeranjan 5 parts + Tuttam 5 parts + Karkatak Shrungi 3parts + Aamalaki 3 parts + Spatika 1 part + Karpoor 1 Part used as anjan

6) Nasya And for oral administation :-
   a) Ksheeri sarpi or ghritha manda
   b) Kakolyadi ghritha  c) Vidharigandhadi ghritha
   d) Jeevaneeya drugs + Sheeta veeya drugs + sharkara + Cow milk + cowghee The pakwa ghritha is used for nasya

**7) Putapaka :-** With Jangala mamsa + Ksheeri sarpi + Madhuradi gana drugs (Like Kakolyadi drugs) are used

**8) Oral adminstration of**
   a) Triphala churna + Ghritha
   b) Triphala Kashaya + Ghritha
   c) Triphala Yastimadu, Loha bhasma, Ghritha and Madhu
   d) The medicated ghee prepared from, Bala, shatavari, kakoli Mishri syreyaka, Triphala and ghee is used for oral administration

**Pittaja Kacha Chikitsa**
1) Raktha mokshana contraindicated
2) meshashrunga, Sauveranjan, Rasanjan; srotoaanjan are useful
3) Phalasha pushpa , Rohitha pushpa , Madhukapushpa + madira + madhu as  Rasa Krianjan

## KAPHAJ TIMIRA CHIKITSA

1) Ghritha prepared with Giloya kwatha, Triphala - pippali Kalka ghritha and given for oral administration
2) Rakthamokshan
3) a) Rechan with the decoction prepared with poogiphal, Haretaki, Shunthi, pippali, Trivruth, Danthee beeja - Given for oral administration.
b) Trivruth  ghritam oral administration for virechan.

**4) Nasyam with:-**
   a) Tailam prepared with usheera Lodra Triphala priyangu, taila,
   b) Gomaya taila
   c) Tailam prepared from Hreebera, Devadaru, Haridra, Daru haridra (Kalka), Milk dashamoola Kwatha and Tila taila.
   d) Maricha yastimadu Vidanga Devadaru .

**5) Anjana**
   a) Manahshila Trikatu shankha bhasma madhu saindhava lavan Kaseesa Rasanjan + Water, as Rasa Kriyanjan
   b) Kaseesa Rasanjan Shunthi Guda as Kasakrianjan.
   **c) Vimala Varthi Anjan :-**
   Shankha priyang manashila trikatu triphala  Lohabhasma, Trikatu, saindhaval avan, Triphala Rasanjan
   d) Kokila varthi anjan:- Maricha saindhava Lavana, pippali, samdraphena, sauveeranjan.
   **f) Hareetakyadi Varthi:-**
   Haretaki 1 part, Haridra 1part, pippali 1part, saindhava lavan 1/4

**g) Sukhavathi varthi** :
Nirmali phala shankha bhasm, Trikata, Saindhava lavan cheeni, samudra phena Rasanjan vidanga manashila Kukkutanda twak + water and Honey
h) Chandrodaya Varthi - Hareetaki, vacha, Kusta, pippali, Maricha, vibheetaki, shanka nabhi, Manshila + Aja Ksheera

**6) Dhoom** - With vidanga, patha, Apamarga, usheera, Ingudee

**7) Tarpan** :- With the medicated ghee prepared from Ksheeri vruksha Kashaya 4 parts, Haridra and usheera kashaya 1/4 part, ghritha 1part.

**8) Putapaka:-** With jangalamamsa, pippali, madhu, saindhava lavana, etc. medicines

**Kaphaj Kacha chikitsa** : - Rasakriyanjan :- Guda, samudra phena, sauveeranjan, pippali, maricha, Kumkama, madhu

**Sannipathaj Timira Chikitsa**
1) All the treatments explained previously should used according to the necessity
2) **Anjan** :-  The medicated ghee prepared from usheer kwatha + pippali saindhava lavan + Ghrita + Honey .
3) **Nasya** :- lastimadu kadi taila (yastimadu vidanga maricha devadaru taila cow milk)

**Sarvaj Kacha chikitsa**
**Anjan**  :- Sauveeranjan shouuld heat immers in Asta mutra and triphala Kashya 7 to 21 times - prepare the fine powder and should fill it in long bone of (in marrow space ) Nisha char animals by perfect packing and should kept it in water for a month after that the powder should be collected and grind with Mesha shruga pushpsa swarasa or Yastimadu churnag for anjana.

## PARIMLAYI TIMIRA CHIKITSA AND RAKTAJ TIMIRA CHIKITSA

1)      Like pittaja Timira chikitsa
2)      a) Drakshadi varthi anjan (Draksha, usheera, Lodra, Yastamadu, Shankha, Tamra, padmaka, chandana, Aja Ksheera)
b) Karpora Samudraphena swetha Kanchana and Chandana.

3)    Nasya with
a)    Anutaila
b)    Vidarigandhadi Ghritha
c)    Kakolyadi ghritha
d)    Ksheri sarpi

**Note :** - In Kacha all the treatments of Timira can be given except Raktha mokshana, if Raktha mokshana is compulsary Jalaukamokshana can be advised

## KAPHAJ LINGANASHA SHASTRA CHIKITSA

**Indications of kaphaj Linganash shastra Chikitsa :-**

1)    Completely formed or pakwa drusti (Mature cataract)
2)    Hard (Solid state, not semi solid)
3)    with Complete loss of vision
4)    only kaphaj linganash
5) Drusti should not contain following 6 abnormalities.
       a) Aavarthaki - Chala drusti with black and red colour.
       b) Sharkara - Vere hard drusti like arka ksheera
       c) Rajeemathee - Thin elongated drusti with lines like shali shooka (Rice grains with capsule)
       d) Chinnamshuka - Irregular drusti with cutting pain and burning sensation.
       e) Chandrakee - drusti is bright as Bronze and multi pigmented like pea cock feathers.
       f) chathrakee - Drusti is multi pigmented and resembling umbrella
                                                          (Vagbhata)
7) Drusti Should not Contain the following features.
       a) Semi lunar shape b) like sweat drop c) like a pearl d) fixed (Sthira)
       e) Vishama (irregular) (These symptoms are seen when associated
       with Iritis, Synechia and immature cataract) f) Thin at central part g)
with vessels h) Bright (Partial opacification) i) Painful (If associated with glaucoma) j) Blood collections (Uveitis with hypaema) (sushrutha)

8) The Apakwa linganash (immature cataract) is contra indicated because the drusti is imperfectly formed, irregular, thin like cheese on curd, spreads upwards during surgery, causes pain etc. complications and drusti revitiates even after surgery so only apakwa linganash is contra indicated for surgery.

9) The common contra indications of siravyadan are also applicable here

10) Only kaphaj Linganash without other doshic vitiations is indicated for the surgery.

# PROCEDURE OF
# KAPHAJ LINGANASH
# SHASTRA CHIKTSA

In a normal season , after sneha sweda karma. the patient is asked to sit down on a stool comfortably, asked to see towards nasal side, and should give co operation while the operation, The head and Limbs should be properly holded by the assistants not to move during the operation. The eyes are properly opened to expose the middle part of eye perfectly. " Vyadana Karma has to do with Right - hand in left eye operation and with left hand in Right eye operation". The instrument used for yadana Karma is "YAVA VAKRA shalaka, The puncturing area is known as " DIIVA KRUTHA CHIDRA" where blood vessels are absent and so doesn't cause bleeding complications.

### Selection of the Site of vyadana karma:-

1) 2 Part sof Shukla mandala towards apanga should leave for puncturing (Sushrutha)

2) 1/2 angula from Krishna mandala and 1/4 angula from apanga should leave for puncturing (Vagbhata)

While puncturing proper care should be taken if not, cause so many complications

### Signs of adequate vyadana karma :-
1) No Pain     2) Some specific sound comes during puncturing
3) Water bubble like dosha comes out through punctured area
4) Drusti prapthi (Visualisatiion)

### Signs of in adequate vyadana Karma :-
1) Pain 2) Bleeding 3) Lacrimation 4) Oedema 5) Hyperaemia 5) Head ache
7) Improper visualisation obstructed vision (vyadan karma is not get succeded again sneha sweda vyadan should perform)

### Post vyadana regimen:-
1)      Stanya pariseka
2)      Vata Kapha hara mrudu sweda (Kara sweda).
3)      Gentle pressure on eye ball with blunt end of shalaka to expel the Kapha perfectly.

4) Blowing out the nose by closing the opposite nostril (ucchinghan) to expel out the residual kapha.

5) After perfect elimination of doshas

If vision is normal Ghritha drops instillation or ghritha pichu should put at the site and Netra bandana( eye bandage) is applied.

6) Patient is advised to lie down on opposite side or in supine position

7) for every 3 days Bandage should be removed for Cleaning, mrudu sweda and for observation- up to 10 days.

8) Langhana or post oleatiion regimen should follow

9) Bed rest 10) following pathya vidhi up to 10 days

11) Application of Drusti prasadan anjanas

**Apathya :-** Contra indications for the maintenance of health
1) Sneezing 2) Coughing 3) Blechings 4) spittings 5) Bending the head 6) Drinking more liquids 7) Bathing 8) Brushing of teeth 9) Eating hard or solid items. 10) Body movements etc are rejected for 10 days ofter operation

## TREATMENTS FOR THE COMPLICATIONS:

1) in red eye or haemorrhagic lesions due to vyadana karma in improper place - is treated with Yastimadu - ghritha + stanya pariseka.

2) If vyadana Karma did more nearer to Apanga, causes pain oedema exudation etc lesions in that condition Bhru madya mrudu sweda and lukewarm ghritha pariseka advised.

3) If vyadana karma didi more nearer to krishna mandal, causes inflammation, at that condition virechan, Jalaukamokshan, Luk ewarm ghritha Aashcyo tan advised

4) In Atiyoga of vyadana karma, sneha sweha Anuvasan Vasti are advised.

In apakwa Linganash extraction Luke warm madhura ghritha Aashchyotan and shiro vasti should do

**5) In pain burning sensation oedema and in Hyperaemia:-**

  a) sariva gyrica Doorva yava + Ghritha (Pakwa ghritha) mukha or varthma lepa

  b) Fried Tila and swetha sarshapa, should grind with Mathulunga swarasa for mukha or varthma lepa

  c) Draksha yastimadu Kusta saindhava, lavana grinded with Aja ksheera for mukha or varthma lepa.

  d) Ksheera Kakoli sariva Teja patra manjista yastimadu grinded with Aja ksheera for mukha or varthma lepa.

e)   Devadara, Daru haridra padmaka shunthi grinded with Ajaksheera for mukha lepa or varthma lepa.

6) Pariseka or Aashchyotan yogas
   a) Lodra saindhava lavan Yastimadu Draksha kwatha + Aja Ksheera as eye drops
   b) Yasti madu, Nelothphala, Kusta, Draksha, Laksha, sharkara, saindhavalavana, Kwatha+ Aja Ksheera as eye drops
   c) Shathavari, prushni parni, musta, Aamalaki, padmaka (Kalka), Aja ksheera ghritha (Pakwa ghritha) used as eye drops.
   d) Bhadradarvadi Kakolyadi ghritha  - Lepa seka Anjan.

7) If pain is not relieved with above treatment (lalata, Apanga, upanasika). Dhaha karma is adviced .

8) Drusti prasadan Anjanas
   a) Mesha shrunga pushpa shireesha pushpa dhava pushpa jathee pushpa Muktha pisti Vydoorya - Grindred in Aja Ksheera Pasted and kept in a copper vessel for a week - varthi is prepared and Anjana is given with Rose water.
   b) Srotonjan Pravala samudra phena manashila maricha grinded with Aja Ksheera - Varthi Prepared and Anjan is given with Rose water.

## 7) PITTA VIDAGDHA DRUSTI
### (Day blindness)

The vitiated pitta dosha deranges the drusti produces yellow pigmentation to the drusti and visualises the objects in Yellow colour if doshas spread into 3rd patala causes day blindness (can not see the objects at day time)Due to pitta prakopa but can see the objects at night due to pitta shaman.

It is pittaja aushada sadya vyadhi (Ashastra Krutha)

It can be corelated to central opacity of Lens and cornea macular lesions central retinal lesions, retinitis pigmentosa, Amblyopia etc.

## 8) KAPHA VIDAGDHA DRUSTI
### (Naktandya)  (Night blindness - nyctalopia)

The vitiated kapha dosha deranges the drusti, prouced white pigmentation to the drusti and visualise the objects in white colour. if dosheas spread in to 3rd patala causes night Blindness (Cannot see the objects at night) due to kapha prakopa but ue to Kapha shaman or Kapha vilayan can see the objects at day time.

It is kaphaja Aushada sadya (Ashastra kruth) vyadhi. It can be corelated to Night blindness due to vitamin A deficiency and peripheral retinopathy.

213

# TREATMENT PRINCIPLES OF PITTA VIDAGDHA DRUSTI AND KAPHA VIDAGDHA DRUSTI

## A) In Pitta Vidagdha Drusti

1) Ashastra Krutha (Aushada Sadya.)
2) Pitta Dosha hara chikitsa should give .
3) Pittaja Abhishyanda chikitsa should give .
4) Oral administration of Triphala ghritha or Tilwaka ghrith for Oleation.
5) Vaman etc shodhan Karma should do for body purification
6) Local Treatments like seka, Aashcyotan,Tarpan, Putapaka, Anjan, Nasya etc. should give.
7) Oral administradtion of Chakshushya drugs.

## B) In Kapha Vidagdha drusti

1) Ashastra Krutha (Aushada sadya )
2) Kapha dosha hara  Chikitsa should give
3) Kaphaja Abhishyanda Chikitsa should give
4) oral administration of Trivruth ghritha or Tilwaka ghritha or purana ghritha for Oleation.
5) Vamana etc shodhan Karma should do for body purification.
6) Local Treatment like seka, Aashchyolan, Tarpan, putapaka, Anjan, nasya etc. should give.
7) Oral administration of Chakshushya drugs.

## COMMON ANJANA YOGAS FOR PITTA VIDAYGDHA DRUSTI AND KAPHAVIDAGDHA DRUSTI

1) Gyrica, Saindhava lavan, pippali Godantha masi (Equal parts).
2) Gomamsa choorna, maricha, shireshabeeja, manahshila (equal parts)
3) Kapittha vruntha + madhu - as anjan
4) Swayam guptha beeja + madhu-as anjana
5) Kubjak, ashok chal, Amra, priyang, padmaka, Neelothphala, Renuka, pippali,Hareetaki, Aamalaki + Madhu or ghee, The medicine should preserve in vamshi naala (tube of the bamboosa stick) as Anjan.
6) Arma jambu pushpa rasa, Renaka + madhu ghritha as anjan
7) Rakta padmaka or kamala Neelothphala kesar gyrica should grind with Gomayaras and used as gutikanjan.

# ANJANAS IN PITTA VIDAGDHA DRUSTI

**1) Rasanjanaadyanjan :-** Rasanjan Jathi patra ras (Or ghee or Aamalaki ) madhu Taleesa Patra, swarna gyrica , should grind with Gomaya rasa and used as choornanjan.

**2) Kashmaryaadyanjan :-** Kasmari pushpa Yastimadu Daru haridra, Lodhra, Rasanjan, fine powder prepared and given as anjana with madhu.

**3) Saindhavadyanjan :-** Saindhavalavan, mudga, Trikatu, Sauvereranjan, manahshila. Haridra, Daruharidra, Goyakruth, Swetha Chandan, used either as choornanjan or Gutikanjan.

4) Swarna bhasma + gheee or Honey - as anjan

5) Gomayarasa + go ksheera + Goghritha (pakwa) as Rasakriyaanjan.

6) Swarna gyrica + Talisa Patra choorna as Rasakriyaanjan

7) karpooraadyanjan :- Karpoora Sauveranjan, Should grind with mamsarasa, Koorma or Rohit matsya pitta and used as Ananjana.

## Anjanas in Kaphavidagdha drusti or Nakthandya

1) Srotonjan, saindhavalavan Pippali Renuka should grind with Aja mutra for varthi anjan

2) Renuka pippali (Vitusha beeja) Sukshma ela, should grind with Gomaya ras or yakruthrasa for anjana.

3) Pippali of yakruth pippali yoga + madhu as anjan.

4) Fried (In ghee or taila) Yakruth or pleeha, grinded with sarshapa taila - used as anjan.

5) Maricha rubbed in curd, the essence is used as anjana.

6) Shaphari matsya Kshara as anjan

7) Hingula or Tankana or Karnamala + madhu, as anjan.

8) Ghritha + Gomaya rasa + madhu - as Rasa Kriyanjan.

9) Gyrica + Talisa patra as Rasakriyanjan

10) Tagar Trikatu Triphala Haritala manahshila samudra phena, grinded with Ajaksheera and used as varthi anjan.

11) Karanja Neelothphala swarna gyrika, kamalkesar, grinded with gomaya ras and used as varthi anjan

12) Pure vatsanabhi choorna manhshila grinded with mathulunga swarasa for anjana (R.R.S.)

13)  Trikatu Keep in Aja yakruth and allow to dry later on Trikatu should be collected and anjana given with chiri Bilwa rasa (R.R.S) .

14)  Maricha grinded with the blood of bed bug, used for anjana (R.R.S).

15)  Rasanjan Haridra, Daru haridra jathipallava Nimba pallava, grinded with Gomaya rasa for anjana

16)  Triphala grinded with yakruthras - as anjan.

17)  Tagarqqdyanjan:- Tagara pippail shunthi Yastimadu Talis patra Haridra darau haridra musta etc are grinded with yakrath rasa fro anjana

18)  Renuka, pippali aja asti- majja Ela Aja yakrth - Grinded well and given as Anjana .

19)  Manashila Hareetaki Trikatu Bala Tagara Samudrapena - Grinded with goat's milk for anjana.

20)  Go mutra, go or Aja pitta madyam Yakruth Aamalaki Swarasa - Grinded and used as Anjana .

21)  Gomootra Gogritha samudraphena pippali Katphala saindhava lavan and madhu Rasakriya is prepared and preserved in the Vamshi Nala (Cavity of bomboosa Stick)

22)  Aja vasa yakruth and ghee pippali saindhavalvan madhu Aamalaki swar as  Rasakriyanjan

23)  Srotoanjan grinded in Yakruthras as anjan


**Nasya** 1)  Brungarajadya tail

2)  Nrupavallabha taila

3)  Abhijith taila

4)  Medicated ghee prepared with medha Lodhra guduchi manjista daruharidra Yastimadu tila taila and go ghritha.

**Tarpana**  With Ksheeri sarpi :-

**Oral Remedies :-**  1) Triphala ghritha 2) maha Triphala ghritha 3) Nrupa vallabha ghritha 4) Maha Triphaladya ghritha 5) jeevanthyadi ghritha 6) Patoladya gritha 7) Ksheeri sarpi or purana ghritha (daily usase with meaals).8) Triphala choorna or Kashaya, with ghee 9) Mahavasadi quath 10) Yakruth Pippali voga (Puta Paka) 11) Yakruth or pleeha of a cow and goat which is fried in taila or ghritha is gred in Taila or ghritha 12) Tamboola Yaktam khadyotam (the small sparkling creature with betal leaf)13) Rohitha matsya eggs + brunga ras. 14) Oral intake of Jeevanthi Atimuktha (Madhaveelatha) Erenda shephalee Shatavaree etc. Leaves which are fried in ghee 15) Sapthaa mruta loha.

### 9) DHOOMADARSHI
(Smoky Vision or Hazyvision)

It is pittaja sadya vyadhi in which drusti is vitated due to headache fever exertion and crying etc causes and visualise the things as smoky or hazy

It is a symptom appears commonly in the errrors of refractive media (Precipitations in aqueous and vitreous, Retinal lesions inflammation of cornea(Keratites) refractive errors like myopia hyper metrpia etc. corneal oederna immature cataract uveitis Glaucoma etc.) The transparent media be comes hazy so only visualises the things as hazy.

### USHNA VIDAGDHA DRUSTI
(By vagbhat)

It is a disease of drusti occurs due to ushnabhitapthasya jala praveshaath etc causes (Exposure to cold immediately after exposure to heat) Because of immediate opposite exposures The tridoshas and Raktha vitiates, the vit'ation reaches the head, eyes, and so the person visualises the things imperfectly at day time and cannot visualise at night.

### AMLA VIDAGDHA DRUSTI
(By Vaghbhata)

It is a lesion of drusti, occurs due to excess usage of sour (Amla ) things, the Tridoshaas and Rakatha vitiate the drustimandala and causes collection of exudation and dirt in drusti mandal, itching sensation and visual errors.

**Note : - Amla vidagdha drusti, Ushna vidhgdha drusti, Dhooma darshi and pittavidagdha drusti are having similar treatment principles**

### 10) HRASWA JADYA

It is pittaja asadya vyadhi in which drusti mandal is vitiated, causes difficult and imperfect vision at day time and bigger objects are seen as smaller.

**Commentry -** 1) Vision is very poor at day time it self so at night the patient cannot see any thing .
2) Poor vision at day time may get vision at night due to pitta shaman it can becorelated to Retinitis pigmentosa etc,diseases.

### 11) NAKULANDHYA
( A type of night blindness )

It is Tridoshaja Asadya Vyadhi in which drusti mandal is vitiated causes shining of the drusti as like mangoose, visualises the things in multi colours and so cannot see the things at night

**12 Gambheerika** (Phthisis bulbi - Endophthalmitis) It is vataja Asadya vyadhi in which drusti mandal is vitiated and causes shrinkage of the eye ball with irregular size and shape. It associates with severe pain.

## DOSHANDHA OR NAKTHANDHYA
### (By Vagbhata)

The vitiated doshas cause the drusti inactive and covered at night so cannot visualise the things- But at day time doshas are activated or dissolved from drusti so only can visualise at day time (It is a type of Night blindness)

## AUPASARGIKA LINGANASHA
### (By Vagbhat)

The Vatadi doshas vitiate the drusti and causes painless blindness due to the eye exposing to bright things (Sun etc) or observing the wonders or super natural things etc. (Structural abnormality is not present but only functional derangement present)

**Note :**
Dhoomadarshi - Amla vidagdha drusti, ushna vidagdha drusti and pitta vidagdha drusti are having similar treatment procedures (Pittahara chikitsa)
1) Pitta dosha chikitsa
2) sheeta veerya applications and anjana
3) Virechana
4) Go shakruthrasa - Goksheera go ghritha (Pakwa ghritha) Anjana
5) Rasa kriyanjan prepared with Gyrica, Talisa patra
6) Ksheeri sarpi Nasyam - Tarpana Aashchyotan .
7) Nasya with medicated ghee prepared with meda Lodra guduchi manjista daruharidra yastimadu - Goghritha tila taila go ksheera etc.
8) Sira vyadana

## BAHYA NETRA ROGA OR BAHYA LINGANASHA

2 diseases, they are

1) Sanimittaja Linganasha
2) Animittaja Linganasha        - Asadyam (Incurable)

**1) Sanimittaja Linganasha :-**
The Aetiopathology for the disease can be explained, ex: Shirobhighata shiro abhitapa, poisonous touches to eyes etc. The signs Symptoms are exhibited like in abhishyanda (Structural abnormality causes loss of vision. But the causative factors are other than doshas).

## 2) Animittaja Linganasha :-

Aetiopathology of the disease is obscure, the blindness occurs without structural deformity (eye appears bright like vydoorya but visual perception is absent)
It occurs due to observing the super natural things, exposing to bright things, curse of the deva, gandarva, Rushi and maha sarpa etc.
Sanimittaja and Animittaja Linganash are Asadya

## Abhighataja Linganash :-

Due to injuries if dursti is injured and destructed, is known as Abhighataj Linganasha

## NAYANAABHIGHATHA (INJURIES OF EYE BALL)

Injuries to the eye ball may occur two types 1) Moortha (visible or direct injuries) 2) Amoortha (invisible or indirect injuries) .

The injuries to the eye ball occur due to following causes.
1) Penetrating injuries, contusion injuries, crushing injuries etc. 2) insect bite, 3) Sunstroke 4) Sun rays 5) Burns 6) Tikshna anjanas 7) effect of sun, moon, stars, grahas, super natural things etc. 8) Exposure to dust, smoke, foreign bodies chemicals, vapour Bright light and polluted water 9) Regular habit of tobacco alcohol 10) eye straining factors 11) Crying fear anxiety etc emotional factors 12) Langhana 13) Sleepless ness, night arousal day sleeping etc. 14) Ati sweda 15) Vascular and nervous dis orders etc.

## Clinical features :-

1) Severe pain 2) Oedema 3) Hyperaemia 4) Congestion of vessels 5) Sub conjunctival haemorrhages 6) Photophobia 7) Lacrimation or exudation or Haemorrhage 8) head ache 9) Inflammation 10) Foreign body sensation 11) Reflex blepharo spasm 120 Dim vision or hazy vision or loss of vision occurs depending upon the seviority of the injury. 13) Distruction of eye ball 14) Sunken eye ball 15) proptosed eye ball

## Sadya - Asadyaatwa:
If Ist patala only injured - Sukha sadya .
If 2nd patala also injured kasta sadya
If 3rd patala also injured Asadya and rejected for the treatment
Pishchita netra, shithila netra, Hata druk and anthahpravista netra- are **Yapyam**

**Treatment principles :-**

1) Nasya, Lepa, pariseka, Tarpan, snehan, Sheeta upachar (Cool therapy), Vranaharaupachar (wound healing therapy), pittaja and Rakthaja Abhishyanda chikista etc should give - If the injury is within 7 days duration, If not vataja Abhishyanda chikitsa (Sneha - Sweda (Bhaspa sweda) Should give .

2) In sunken or antah Pravista netra eyes should be tried to push out by prana yama sneezing vomiting and restricting. deglutition etc. .

3) In Proptosed eye - Deep inspiration cool water shiro seka etc. should do

4) Sadya vrana chikitsa should do, if vision is not Disturbed.

5) Gritha for Tarpan, Nasya and for oral the Ghee is prepared with Aja Ghritha 1. Prasta, Aja Ksheera 1 Aadak, madhu 2 phala, Neelothphal 2 phala, jeevak 2 phala, Rushabhak 2 phala etc.

# DRUSTIGATHA ROGA

12 diseases According to Sushrutha
1 to 6 Timira - Explained in table form

| S.No. | Name modern name | Dosha prognosis | Clinical Features | Treatment principle |
|---|---|---|---|---|
| 7. | Pitta Vidagdha drusti (Day blindness) | Pittaj Sadya | Drusti is vitiated and visualise the things in yellow colour, if pitta dosha enters 3rd patala causes day blindness. | Ashastra kruth |
| 8. | Kapha Vidagdha drusti (Night blindness) | Kaphaj Sadya | Drusti is vitiated and visualise the things in white colour, if doshas enters into 3rd patala causes night blindness. | Ashastra kruth |
| 9. | Dhooma Darshi (Smoky vision) | Pittaj Sadya | Drusti is vitiated due to head-ache, fever exertion etc and visualise the things as smoky | Pittaja Abhishanda chikitsa |
| 10. | Hrawajadya (Retinitis • pigmentosa) | Pittaj Asadya | Drusti is vitiated and causes difficulty in vision at day time (bigger objects are seen smaller) | Asadya |
| 11. | Nakulandya ( A type of night blindness) | Tridoshaj Asadya | Drusti is vitiatied and shines like the drusti of mangoose, objects are seen in multi colours and can't see at Nights. | Asadya |
| 12. | Gambheerika (Phthisis bubli endophthalmity) | Vataj Asadya | Drusti is vitiated and eye ball is shrinkan and become irregular with severe pain. | Asadya. |

## BAHYA NETRA ROGA.

| | | | |
|---|---|---|---|
| 1) | Sanimittaja Linganasha | Aetiopathology is obvious, Shirobhi tapa, shirobhi, ghatha inhalation of poisonous flowers strucutral abnormality causes lose of vision. | Asadya. |
| 2) | Animittaj Linganasha | Aetiopathology is obscure blind ness occurs without structural deformity . | Asadya. |

221

# CATARACT
(Timira    Kacha    Linganasha)

**Defination:-** Opacification of (formation of opacities) lens or its capsule is known as cataract .

**Description:-** Lens is the Biconvex transparent structure placed behind the Iris by the support of zonule or suspensory Ligament , it converges the light rays to form image on retina. It contains capsule, subcapsular epithelium cortex and nucleus. The fibres from foetal life are concentrically arranged in the lens like the scales of an onion. The most interior fibres are the oldest fibres (fibres of foetal life).So many factors cause the lental opacities (Denaturation of lens) and affect the vision, it is known as cataract.

## Aetiology and pathology of cataract:

1. Lens is a Avascular structure so inflammatory changes cannot occur mostly Degenerative changes occur.

2. Lens fibres from foetal life are concentrically placed in the lens like the scales of an onion, so by age the central fibres of lens (Nucleus)are crushed and leads to Lental sclerosis (Degeniration) with increased refractive index of lens.So physiologically threre are chances for senile cataract.

3.Senile biochemical changes in Lens
a) Gradual increase of Lental degeneration.
b) Diminished Lens metabolism (Impaired auto oxidative system of Lens).
c) Decreased essential amino acids, Glutathione nucleotides, Ascorbic acid enzymes vitamines and minerals
d) Altered calcium and phosphates ratio in Lens and extra Lenticular fluids.
e) Altered Sodium and potassium ratio in Lens and extra lenticular fluids.
f) Increased osmotic pressure in Lens and decreased osmotic pressure in extra Lenticular fluids - So causes imbibition of fluids into Lens and causes opacification.
g) Increased cholesterol and disappearance of inter cellular fat membrane
h) Reduction of soluble proteins and aggravation of insoluble proteins .
i) Increased acidity and proteolysis causes digestion of soluble proteins (into white milky fluid) and coagulation of insolubleproteins in which the nucleas appears as floating.

**1.**

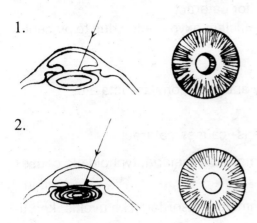

**2.**

1. Iris shadow in immature cataract

2. No Iris shadow in mature catarct

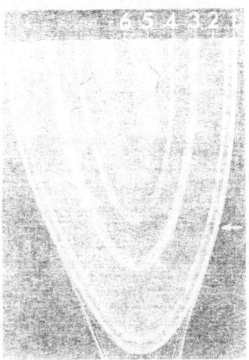

The structure of the lens in an adult of 40 years, as shown in the optical beam of the slit-lamp; 1, anterior capsule; 2, cortex; 3, adult nucleus; 4, infantile nucleus; 5, foetal nucleus; 6, embryonic nucleus

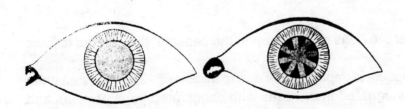

Lental sclerosis

Incipient cataract
(Peripheral type)

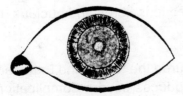

Incipient cataract
(Central type)

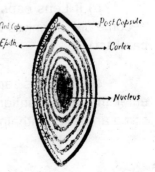

Ant Cap.
Epith.
Post Capsule
Cortex
Nucleus

223

4) Congenital or developmental causes for cataract.
**ex:-** maternal malnutrition, infections, defficient oxygenation due to placental haemorrhage etc.

5)Traumatic causes for cataract
**ex:-** penetrating, injury, contusion Injury and radiational trauma etc.

6)Increased osmotic pressure in the Lens- causes cataract.

7) Systemic infections like diphtheria, small pox, malaria, typhoid etc causes cataract.

8) As a complication of peripheral inflammatory disorders like uveitis, keratitis
glaucoma etc causes cataract

9) Metabolic disorders
**ex Diabetes** - Hypo thyroidism etc causes cataract

10) Defficiency of Amino acids vitamines and minerals - causes cataract

11) Usage of toxic drugs
**ex** Naphthalene, Thalium, cobalt, selinium, steroids etc, causes catarct

12) Physical influences on capsule and sub capsular epithelium - causes cataract.

13 Cataract in association with multiple syndromes, skin lesions Bone lesions etc.

14) Ultimate state of the Lens depends upon the capsule, they are as follows

a) If Lens capsule is impermeable due to thickness - The digeste Lends fibres (Milky fluid) stagnated in the Lens with coagulated Lens proteins and with the floating nucleus (morgagnian cataract)

b) If Lens capsule is permeable lens matter diffused out - and lens become flat, shrinked with undigested lens fibres and nucleus (hyper mature cataract)

c) If the lens capsule get ruptured the toxins and Extra lenticular fluids enter the lens disintigrate it and produces severe complications like Glaucoma and endophthalmitis.

**Classification of cataract :-**

I)      a) Congenital or developmental cataract  b) Acquired cataract

II)     A) Immature b) mature c) Hyper mature cataract

III)    a) capsular cataract b) cortical cataract c) Nuclear cataract.

IV)    Clinical types of cataract

1)      Congenital or developmental cataract    2) Senile cataract

          3) Metabolic cataract    4)   Osmotic cataract

5)      Cataract in Osseous diseases

6)      Cataract in skin diseases (syndermatotic

7)      Cataract with multiple syndromes

8)      Traumatic cataract  9) Toxic cataract    10)   Complicated cataract

11)    Cataract due to systemic infections

12)    Defficiency or malnutrition of cataract

13)    Occupational cataract.

## SENILE CATARACT

Senile cataract - generally starts after the age of 50 yrs. and occur equally in men and women. It is usually bilateral but starts in one eye then in the other

**Clinical features:-**

It can be divided into 2 large groups, they are.

1) 20 to 25 % - nuclear cataract

2) 75 to 80 %  cortical cataract

**1) Nuclear cataract or Hard cataract:-** The nucleus of the lens becomes diffusely cloudy due to physiological Lental sclerosis, while the cortical fibres remain transparent. The nucleus may become brown red and even black.

**Clinical features -** 1) Visual disturbance (Progressive myopia due to increased refractive index of Lens.) 2) Obstruction of vision (Hypermature stage does not occur ) 3) 0/E = with Ophthalmoscope by pupil dilatation, fundus appears little hazy and nucleus appears black against the red reflex.

4) If maturity (Sclerosis) reaches up to capsule, vision completely obstructed and ophthalmoscopy is not possible.

## 2) CORTICAL CATARACT

The clinical features can be explained in 4 stages

( cortical cataract means denaturation or opacification of cortex of Lens.

1)  Incipient stage    2) Intumescent stage
3)  mature stage    4) Hyper mature stage

**1) Incipient stage :-**
Few opacities develop either in the periphery or at the centre and are arranged like the spokes of a wheel. The subjective symptoms are polyopia rainbow haloes, and impairment of vision. If the opacity is in the centre part of Lens the patient complains of defective vision more in day time and if the opacity is in the peripheral part of Lens, defective vision is more at night.

**Signs :-** 1) On ophthalmoscopic examination the opacities appear as black spots against red reflex of funds 2) In oblique illumination the pupils appear greyish (In lental sclerosis also) the pupil appears greyish But confirmation only by above ophthalmoscopic examination in which black opacities are not seen against red reflex in Lental sclerosis.

**2) Intumescent stage :- Symptoms** are same as above but in addition myopia develops due to alteration in Lental Curvature.

**Signs :-** opacities become more diffuse and irregular, Lens is swollen, pushes the iris forwards, Anterior chamber become shallow and leads to secondary glaucoma (Iris shadow present)

**3) Mature stage :-** whole Lens become opaque, its Anterior surface shows mother of pearl appearance, vision mostly reduced, can recognise only hand movements no fundal glow at pupillary area, Loss of 3rd purkinje's image and Iris shoadow is absent.

**4) Hyper mature stage** :- Mature cataract if delayed without proper treatment leads to hypermature catarct .
1) Soluble Lens proteins digested and become milky fluid insoluble proteins coagulates, due to the permeability of Lens capsule the fluid of Lens get lost, Lens become flat and shrunken, Iris become tremulous, Anterior chamber become deep, degeneration of suspensary ligament, sub luxation of Lens and secondary glaucoma follows.
2) Lens fibres of cortex digested and become milky, nucleus sinks to the bottom of thickend capsule, such cataract is known as morgagnian cataract.

**Dangers of hyper maturity :-**
1)  Sub luxation of Lens    2)  Secondary glaucoma
3)  irido cyclitis    4)  endophthalmitis

**Treatment :-**
1) No drug has significant effect in causing disappearance of opacities
2) Surgical interference in mature stage is un avoidable.

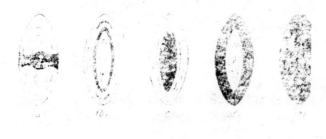

Schematic representation of the clinical types of Cataract
a. Spindle; b. Lamellar; c. Nuclear; d. cortical e. complete

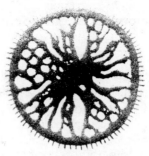

Coronary Cataract

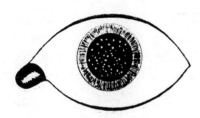

Punctate Cataract

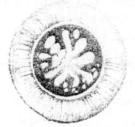

Coralli form cataract

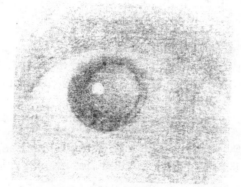

Morgagnian cataract showing the lenticular
nucleus

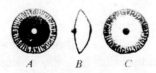

ANTERIOR POLAR CATARACT.

*A*, seen with oblique illumination; *B*, section of lens; *C*, seen with the
ophthalmoscope.

227

## II) Congenital or developmental cataract:-

The child is born with Lental opacities or it develops soon after birth. The exact cause is not known and the opacities are mostly stationary in nature. The following are some of the causes

1) Hereditory tendency. 2) maternal malnutrition 3) maternal infection by German measles etc. 4) defficient oxygenation due to placental haemorrhage etc.

## Types :-

1) Punctate cataract or blue dot cataract :- Small multiple opqaue dots are scattered all over the Lens, they appear as tiny blue dots on oblique illumination with slit lamp (These cannot obstruct the vision)

## 2) Fusiform or spindle shaped or coralli form or disciod Cataract

Spindle shaped or coral shaped small opacities develops in Lens, those does not cause visual obstruction.

## 3) Embryonal nuclear cataract :-
Some of the the central nuclear fibres remains opaque due to early developmental anomaly, other fibres are normal (Rubella infection in first trimester of pregnancy causes nuclear cataract which is progressive in nature) in general it does'nt cause visual obstruction

## 4) Coronary cataract :-
Non progressive club shaped opacities develop in deeper cortex and peripheral nucleus (peripheral cortex and depper nucleus is normal) vision cannot obstructs.

## 5) Lamellar or zonular cataract :-
Grey disc shaped opacities (Spokes of a wheel) develops in some layers due to nutritional defficiency, the other layers are normal, it is a bilateral heriditory tendency.

## 6) Anterior capsular cataract :-
it is congenital due to delayed formation of anterior chamber, Acquired due to contact of ulcerated cornea to the anterior Lens capsule. Anterior Lens capsule and some times subcapsular cortical fibres also involves.

## 7) Posterior capsular cataract ;-
It is due to persistance of posterior part of vascular sheath of Lens, incase of persistent hyaloid artery.

## III) Traumatic Cataract :-
It is due to injury to Lens or its capsule

1) Penetrating injury such as needle or a thorn causes cloudiness or opacity at the site of injury with in few hours due to entry of aqueous humour and toxins, within few days the entire Lens may become opaque with complications like glaucoma, endophthalmitis, etc.

2) Contusion injury causes rupture of Lens and causes complete cataract.

3)　　　Radiational trauma due to exposure of
　　a)　　　Infra red rays, ex - glass workers, furnace workers
　　b)　　　Ultra voilet rays, Prolonged exposure to sunlight
　　c)　　　irradiation - exposure to x rays frequently.
　　d)　　　Due to electric, shock etc, causes cataract formation.

## IV Osmotic cataract :-

Changes in the Osmotic pressures in Aqueos (Body fluids) and Lens causes cataract formation.

a) precipitation of sodium calcium etc in Lens than aqueous b) reduction of phosphates potassium etc in Lens than aqueous, cause increased osmotic pressure in lens that aggrevates the imbibition of water, aqueous, extra lenticular fluids and toxins in to the Lens, causes proteolysis and cataract formation.

## V) Cataract due to systemic disorders :-
1)　　　Infective Fevers like diphtheria malaria, typhoid, typhus, cholera, small pox, scarlotine fever, etc may cause cataract.
2　　　Severe toxic states Extreme cachexia, nephritis, pernicious anaemia etc.
3)　　　Massive blood loss
4)　　　Less authentic types Tuberculosis, ornithosis, cooley's anaemia, profound anaemia, ankylostomiasis etc.

## VI) Complicated Cataract :-
It is due to complications of peripheral Lesions like
Ulcerative keratitis, irido cyclitis, choroiditis, syphilis, Rubella, Toxo plasmosis, High myopia, Glaucoma, intra ocular neoplasm, vitreo-retinal dystrophies, Retinal detachment etc. causs cataract as a complication.

## VII) Toxic cataract :-
It is due to usage and exposure of toxic drugs like
1)　　　Hydro carbons　　　　　　ex naphthalene
　　　　　　　　　　　　　　　　　　　Dinitro phenol
2)　　　Salts - Thalium cobalt selinium, etc,
3)　　　Anti mitotic agents ( 1-4, Dimethane sulfanoxy butane)
4)　　　Enzyme inhibitors ( Iodo acetic acid)
5)　　　Prolonged administration of miotics
6)　　　Prolonged usage of cortico sterioids
7)　　　Prolonged usage of synthetic antihistamines
8)　　　Prolonged usage of concentrated sulfanamides
9)　　　Prolonged usage of morphine group drugs.

All these drugs produce Lenticular opacities very quickly with other systemic lesions, like increased or altered metabolism, spleenic hepatic lesions, degenerative changes (Local -systemic), neurological lesions and vascular lesions etc.

**VIII) Metabolic Cataract :-**

It occurs due to impairment of Lens and body metabolism

**1) Diabetic cataract ;-** Diabetic people get the cataract earlier than others, among the lesions, 70% Anterior cortical cataract , 21% nuclear cataract, 7% posterior cortical cataract and 2% subcapsular cataract. punctate flasky white opacities appear with plenty of vacuoles - Gradually due to hydration complete lens becomes opaque.

**2) Galactocaemic cataract:-** develops in infants due to inability to metabolise galactose in to glycogen owing to absence of enzymes (Galactose I phosphate urivdyl transferase)

**3) Hypo calcaemic cataract :-** Hypo calcaemia (and more calcium in Lens) Produces osmotic pressure differences between aqueous (Less osmotic pressure ) and Lens (more Osmotic pressure), causes imbibition of fluids in to Lens leads to opacification.

**4) Hypothyroidism Cataract :-** Small flasky opacities develop in superficial cortex of Lens and does not obstruct the vision.

**5) Myotonic cataract :-** Lenticular changes occur due to intence contraction and Less relaxation of muscles, the punctate opacities develops and after long time total Lens may become opaque.

**6) Defficiency cataract :-** Reduction of Amino acids, soluble proteins, Gluta thione, Ascorbic, acid Riboflavine, Nicotinic acid, vitamin A and D etc. and changes in sodium potassium ratio and calcium phosphate ratio causes the formation of cataract.

**7) Amino aciduria or organic aciduria** :-
        Essential amino acids are eliminated out due to metabolic deffects and other causes, leads to cataract formation.

**IX) Syndermatotic Cataract:**

Cataract formation is due to skin lesions like 1) Atopic dermatitis (Eczema); sub capsular plaque radiating to anterior and posterior cortex develops (It is a heriditory tendency - constitutional allergic basis)
2) Rothmund syndrome - Cataract and skin lesions are associated
3) Warner syndrome - Subcapsular and posterior cortical opacities (Striae) develops and soon become intumescent and mature.

# X) Cataract with multiple syndromes

**1) Vander hoever's syndrome :-** syndrome of Brittle bones, Blue sclera and deafness with zonular or corical cataract.

**2) Conradi's syndrome:-**
widespread skin lesions, mental retardation and Total cataract

**3) Mandibulo oculo facial dyscephaly (Bird face) :-**
along with Microphthalmos micro cornea, congenital Bilateral partial or total cataract are associated.

**4) Marfan's syndrome :-**
Spherophakia, dislocated Lens and with localised Lenticular opacities

**5) Turners syndrome :-**
Development of cataract due to long standing retinal detachment

**6) Mayriac's syndrome:-**
development of typical diabetic cataract

**7) Torsten sjogren Syndrome :-**
Zonular or total or Anterior polar or posterior cortical cataract develops.

**8) Mongolism :-**
Punctate arcuate sutural Lenticular opacities develop

9) In certain anomalies of Brain also Lenticular opacities develops

## CATARACT SURGERY

1) Discission or Needling
2) Needling and aspiration    These methods are in complete and complicated, so not practicing
3) Extraction of Lens
   a) Intra capsular Lens extraction
   b) Extra capsular Lens extraction
4) Intra Ocular Lens implantation (I.O.L)

**Investigations before operation :-**

1) Patient should have pupillary reaction to light
2) Perception of light, 3) Projection of Light, 4) good macular function
5) Catract should be in mature stage, (should identify only hand movements no fundal glow at pupillary region lens should appears as white pearl through pupil, No Iris shdow and 3 rd purkinje's image)
6) Patient should not have infection of conjunctiva Lacrimal sac, eye lids, eye margins, uveal tract sclera and cornea etc.
7) Intra ocular pressure should be normal, if not should be controlled
8) urine for sugar and albumin should investigate, if positive should be controlled.
9) Bloodpressure, Bleeeding clotting time, should be estimated and controlled
10) Other routine invoestigatons should also do to control the complication for the success of operation.

**Intra capsular Lens extraction:-**

Removal of Lens with its capsule, is known as intra capsular lens extraction (Vitreous loss is the major complication after some period)

**Preparation of the patient :-**

1) One day before, the patient should be admitted inthe hospital, in the morning laxatives and at night sedatives should give to controle the tensions of the patient.

2) On the day of operation, light breakfast should give, eye lashes should cut-from their bases, and clean property.

3) Half an hour before the operation 2% G. homatropine drops (Pupil dilator) should put 3 to 4 times with 10 minutes interval

**4) Anaesthesia :-**

    a) 4% Cocaine drops with adrenaline (1:1000) should put in Conjunctival sac 4 to 5 times with 5 minutes interval

    b) Facial nerve should be blocked with 2% Novacaine solution, 1-2 cc, should inject at temparo mandibular joint, to paralise orbicularis oculi muscle.

    c) Retro bulbar ciliary block, with 2% Novocaine solution, 1/2 to ICC, should inject at the junction of medial 2/3 and Lateral 1/3 of Lower orbital margin, needle should pass backwards medial and slight upwards, to paralise the iris, to reduce intra ocular pressure and to dilate the pupil .

**Stepes of Operation :-**

1) Eyelids should be sterilized with spirit, conjunctival sac should be washed with normal salina face mask is put and eye lids are separated with universal eye speculum.

2) Conjunctiva episcleral tissue is hold at timbus in 6$^0$ clock position with fixation forceps, conjunctival flap should be separated at the site of incision.

3) Cataract knife with its sharp edge, to wads the sugeon is introduced from the temporal side ( 9$^0$ clock position in right eye, 3$^0$ clock position in left eye) after passing through the anterior chamber, counter puncture is made at the opposite limbal area and by sawing movements the upper segment of sclero corneal junction is cut.

4) Sutures are given widely to keep the cornea in position, the incised corneal flap is bended down wards to face the anterior chamber and Iris.

5) With Iris forceps - Iris scissors Iridectomy should perform at pupillary area for easy lens extraction and to prevent glaucoma

6) Lens with capsule should be extracted by separating it from suspensary ligament with intra capsular forceps by the gentle pressure and rotatory movements from the periphery of anterior lens capsule at 6$^0$ clock position and lens is removed. 7) Iris is reposited with a repositor .

8) Suturing should complete and air is inserted into anterior chamber with syrenge to form anterior chamber without adhesions

9) Conjunctival flap is resposited, G. pilo carpine drops are inserted (to con strict the pupill) and bandaged.

10) Patient should lie flat on his back for 24 hours.

11) Next day bandage should be removed and observed for any conjunctival discharges oedema, condition of anterior chamber, pupil Iris and aqueus whether they are normal or abnormal and also asked about perception of vision (counting the fingers etc)

12) G. pilcarpine drops should continue for 5 days, later G. atropine drops should continue for 5 weeks

13) Operated eye should cover with a pad for a month, later proper powered spectacles are given

The aphakia 9) Absence of Lens) is corrected by -
for **Distant vision** 10.00.D. spherical lens
If astigmatism associated + 2 or 3. D. 180 Cylindrical lens should be added
for **near vision** - 13.00 D spherical, + 2 or 3.D. 180°Cylindrical lens, should used

|  | Spherical | Cylindrical lens | Axis |
|---|---|---|---|
| Distant vision+ 10.00 D | | + 2 or 3. D | 180° |
| Near vision | + 13.00 D | + 2 or 3. D | 180° |

# EXTRA CAPSULAR LENS EXTRACTION

Extraction of Lens matter by leaving the capsule inside (Chances of after cataract which may need second operation in future - Vitreous prolapse is not present)

**Method :-** a) Preparation b) Anaesthesia c) Corneal incission
d) iridectomy are same as intra capsular extraction)

Anterior Lens capsule is incised with a cystitome or with cataract knife with, the tip of lens expressor lens matter is removed from the lower part by firm counter pressure on sclera at 12 0 clock position Or after incission of capsule the Lens matter can be removed by cryo's apparatus.

**Note :-** Post operative care is as like intra capsuler or extraction.

## INTRA OCULAR LENS IMPLANTATION (I.O.L)

Operative technique is like extra capsular extraction but after extraction of Lens matter, artificial Lens is introduced into capsule instead of spectacle.

1) **Aphakia** - Absence of the crystalline lens in the eye.

**Causes :-** 1) Operative removal of the Lens due to cataract formation 2) Dislocation of lens into vitreous humour 3) spontaneous absorption of the Lens after discission.

**Clinical features :-** 1) Dim vision (high Hyper metropia) 2) Jet black pupil 3) deep anterior chmaber 4) Tremulousness of Iris (Irido donesis) 5) Absence of 2nd, 3rd purkinje's images 6) absence of accommodation 7) Linear scar at upper Limbus if aphakia is due to cataract operation.

## TREATMENT :-PRESCRIBING CONVEX SPECTACLE

Distant vision = + 10.00 D sperical and
+ 2 or 3 $180^0$ cylindrical Lens

Near vision = + 13.00 D sperical and
+ 2 or 3. $180^0$ cylindrical Lens.

2) Microphakia - Smaller Lens (It is a congenital abnormality)

3) Spherophakia = Presence of spherical Lens

4) Lenti conus = Presence of conical shaped Lens

5) Cataract = opacification of Lens

6) Ectopia Lentis = Due to weakness of zonule the Lens is dragged to the opposite side.

7) Sublaxatin of Lens = Partial dislocation of Lens.

8) Luxation of Lens =
Dislocation of Lens either into Anterior chamber or posterior chamber

9) Coloboma of Lens = Improper formation of Lens

10) Immature cataract = Partial opacification of Lens

11) mature cataract = Total opacification of Lens

12) Lental sclerosis = Degeneration of fibres of Lens (nucleus) by age.

13) After cataract -
These are the opaque Lens residues when the Nucleus and cortex are removed by an extra capsular extraction operaton.

# DISEASES OF UVEAL TRACT (VASCULAR LAYER OF EYE BALL)
## TERMINOLOGY OF UVEAL TRACT LESIONS:

1)  Uveal tract    = Iris ciliary body and choroid
2)  Anterior Uvea = Iris and ciliary body
3)  Posterior Uvea = Choroid
4)  Uveitis = inflammation of Uveal tract
5)  Iritis = inflammation of Iris
6)  Cyclitis = inflammation of choroid
7)  Choroiditis = Inflammation of Choroid
8)  Irido cyclitis = Inflammation of Iris and ciliary body
9)  Anterior Synechia - Adhesion of Iris with cornea
10) Posterior synechia - Adhesion of Iris with Lens.

11) Iris bombi - due to seclusio pupillae Iris bulged forwards due to pressure of aqueous humour, known as Iris bombi

12) Irido donesis - Moving of iris along with head movement
due to Aphakia or subluxation of Lens.

13. Irido dialysis - separation of Iris from ciliary body
14. Rubeosis iridis - formation of new vessels on Iris due to diabetes etc causes.

15) Iridencleisis - A piece of Iris is included in a scleral wound at  limbus as filtering wick through which Aqueous flows out into sub conjunctival  space and intra ocular pressure is reduced, it is done especially in peripheral anterior synechia
16) Irotomy - This operation is carried out to lower the intra ocular pressure in cases of Iris bombe and secondary glaucoma in which 4 punctures are made in the Iris for proper aqueous circulation.

17) Iridectomy dialysis - Taking a part of iris from its ciliary attachment to open the angle of anterior chamber.
18) Peripheral iridectomy ;- making a small button hole in the peripheral part of Iris for free circulation of aqueous humour.

19) Enucleation - Removing of eye ball in absolute glaucoma, malignant intra ocular tumours, phthisis bulbi and sympathetic ophthalmia.

20) Evisceration:- In panophthalmitis etc lesions the suppurative infective material of eye ball is scooped out after removal of cornea by leaving only scleral cup.

# CONGENITAL ABNORMALITIES OF UVEAL TRACT

**1) Persistent pupillary membrane:-** The pupil in the foetus is closed by a thin membrane that disappears in the 7th month of foetal life, But some times a few shreds of this membrane remain and called persistent pupillary membrane, it causes visual obstruction.

**2) Congenital Aniridia:-** Failure of the development of Iris ( A rudimentary Iris present - smaller and hidden behind the sclero corneal margin)

**3) Congenital coloboma of Iris and choroid:-**
Imperfect development of Iris and choroid with gaping.

**4) Coloboma of Macula:-**
Defect in the choroid at the region of macula.

**5) Albinism :-** Deficiency of pigment in the Uveal tract gives rise to photophobia defective vision and nystagmos.

**6) Hetero chromia Iridis -** The 2 Irides may be in different colour or one sector of the Iris has a different colour from the rest of the Iris tissue.

**7) Choroideremia:-** Entire or partial absence of the choroid.

# IRITIS

**IRITIS** :-
It is the inflammation of the Iris, often associated with inflammation of ciliary body hence called Irido cyclitis (Anterior uveitis)

**Causes ;-**a) Exogenous inflection (perforated corneal ulcer, penetrating injury to the eye ball)
b) Secondary infection (From interstitial keratitis, scleritis)
c) Endogenous infection (Via blood stream such, as syphilis Tuberculosis, Leprosy, Gonorrhoea, Brucellosis, toxoplasmosis)
d) Allergic reaction (Bacterial toxin, Lens protein, symphathetic ophthalmia)
e) Metabolic disorders (Diabetes, gout, Rheumatism)

**Pathology:-**
Inflammation of iris causes 1) exudation of albuminous fluid with lecucocytes and fibrin into stroma and anterior chamber 2) collection of unusual exudates in the stroma causes oedema of iris 3) Aqueous becomes turbid with hypopyon and hyphaema 4) Irritation to sensary nerve endings causes pain 5) changes in the pupillary reaction 6) Formation of posterior synechia (Adhesion between Iris and Lens) 7) Occlusio pupillae (collection of exudates in the pupil 8) seclusio pupillae (Adhesion of whole pupillary margin to the Lens capsule) 9) Development of degenerative patches on Iris due to chronic inflammatory changes.

**Symptoms:-**
1)      Pain in the eye that radiates to forhead cheek and teeth
2)      Lacrimation and photophobia due to reflex irritation.
3)      Dim vision due to turbidity of aqueous, collection of exudates in pupil, and due to posterior synechia.

**Signs:-**
1)      Circum corneal congestion (due to Anterior ciliary vessels)
2)      Some extent of Conjunctival congestion
3)      Anterior chamber is hazy deep with hypopyon or hyphaema.
4)      Iris is muddy in colour due to collection of exudates
5)      Pupil small irregular and sluggish in reaction to light
6)      ciliary tenderness when associated with cyclitis

**Complications**
1) Posterior synechia
2) Occlusio pupillae          } cause secondary glaucoma
3) Seclusio pupillae
4) Complicated cataract
5) Corneal opacities

**Treatment** 1) Improvement of general health
2) Analgesics - Antibiotics
3) Sub conjunctival hydro cortisone injections
4) Atropin eye ointment
5) Cause should be treated 6) using of dark goggles
7) Surgical interference

## Specific varieties of Iritis

**1) Syphilitic Iritis:-**
a) in severe congenital syphilis, pseudoglioma may develop with interstitial keratitis
b) In late secondary or tertiary stage, yellowish vascularised nodules (Gummatus iritis) appear at pupillary margin and at ciliary borders of iris
c) Plastic exudation that may cause broad posterior synechia
d) Nodules heal leaving depigmented patches
e) Washer mann and kahn reaction positive

**2) Gonorrhoeal iritis:-** Greenish gelatinous fibrinous exudates in anterior chamber and with Extensive posterior Synechia.
**3) Tuberculous iritis:-** Mutton fat keratic precipitates, Koeppe's nodules at pupillary margin, hypopyon with caseating material and thesclero corneal junction is eroded ultimately.
**4) Diabetes Iritis:-** Formation of new vessels on iris (Rubeosis iridis), definite hopopyon and secondary glaucoma
**5) Allergic Iritis:** Lens protein allergy in Extra capsuler lens extraction followed by second operation (needling for cataract).
**6) Reiter's Uveitis:-** Uveitis associate with spondylosis, sacroiliitis with the history of urethral discharge. The clinical features are ocular pain ,congestion, fibrinous exudation in anterior chamber and with posterior synechia.
**7) Stills disease :-** Juvenil rheumatoid arthritis with chronic Uveitis (Band degeneration of cornea, complicated cataract and Blindness)
**8) Sarcoid Uveitis:-** This type of anterior Uveitis associated with the presence of Iris nodule at ciliary Junction, Large pale K.P may be present ,it associate with sarcoidosis in bones, skin, viscera, Lymph glands and lungs (sarcoidosis is a mild or attenuated Tuberculosis)
**9) Leprosy Uveitis:-** Iris nodules develops which contain leucocytes and Leprosy bacillus. K.P. and other common signs of Uveitiis are also present.
**10) Herpes simplex Uveits :-** It is a sequel to herpetic keratitis
**11) Herpes zoster Uveitis:-** It associates with herpes zoster ophthalmicus.
**12) Hetero Chromic Uveitis :-** Associate with atrophic and discoloured Iris.

# CYCLITIS

It is an inflammation of ciliary body. It always associate with some degree of Iritis, so usually termed as Irido cyclitis or anterior uveitis.

## A) Acute cyclitis:-

Aetiology    -    Same as Iritis
Pathology    -    2 types, as follows

### a) Serous type :-

The inflammatory exudate poured into anterior chamber is albuminous and toxic, causes impairment of corneal endothelial nutrition and the inflammatory cells sticks to the lower triangle of cornea, called Keratic precipitates.

### b) Plastic type:- The fibrinous exudate which poured into posterior chamber organises and causes total posterior synechia

The exudate which has extended into anterior vitreous produces cyclitic membrane behind the lens, The fibrinous exudate of vitrious may cause retinal detachment, the exudate that organised in the medial surface of ciliary body causes destruction of ciliary Process that results reduced aqueous secretion and producing hypotony (phthisis bulbi) of eye ball.

II) Signs and symptoms of Acute cyclitis:

## A) Serous type :-
1) Pain and redness of eye ball
2) Moving spots before the eye
3) Dim or hazy vision
4) Circum corneal congestion
5) Ciliary tenderness
6) Grey spots on the posterior suface of cornea (Keratic precipitates -K.P)
7) Deep anterior chamber
8) Cloudy aqueons
9) Oedema of eye lids.
10) Raised intra ocular pressure at first, later intra ocular pressure reduces.

## B) Plastic type :-
1) Extensive posterior synechia
2) Deep anterior chamber
3) Formation of cyclitic membrane behind the lens
4) Hypotony of eye ball
5) phthisis bulbi results.

**Treatment :-** As like Iritis

## II Chronic Cyclitis :-

Chronic inflammation of ciliary body.

**Diagnostic Points :-**

1) Keratic precipitates on back of cornea,
2) Dust like opacities in the anterior vitreous
3) Atrophic changes (Heterochromia of Iris)
4) Considerable reduction of vision.
5) Other common symptoms of cyclitis

## III) Purulent irido cyclitis :-

(Panophthalmitis)

It is a suppurative inflammation of anterior Uvea, vitreous and Retina, If the irido cyclitis is not controlled properly or if the infection is virulent, the purulent infection gradually extends to the posterior segment and causes panophthalmitis

**Clinical features**

Fever, headache, pain, redness in the eye ball, marked reduction of vision, swelling of eye lids, ciliary and conjunctival congestion, cloudy cornea, Hypopyon purulent vitreous (Yellow reflex at pupil on oblique illumination) constricted pupil with sluggished reaction, inflammed Tenons capsule, Finally ends with phthisisbulbi. Evisceration operation should do in time.

## IV) Sympathetic ophthalmitis:-

It is a serious condition characterised by plastic inflammation of Uveal tract in one eye due to the effect of a similar inflammation in the other, following a penetrating injury.

## CHOROIDITIS - (POSTERIOR UVEITIS)

The inflammation of the choroid is known as choroiditis. in most cases retina affects secondarily and the anterior part of the Uveal tract may be concomitantly affected.

**Signs & Symptoms ;-**

a) Visual disturbances (Floating specks may appear, defective visual acuity, distortion of objects (meta-morphopsia) objects may appear smaller (Micropsia), objects may appear bigger (macropsia), Flashes, sparks, bright circles may appear due to stimulation of sensory cells of retina (photopsia), defective field of vision and central vision)

b) On ophtholmoscopic examination retina shows patches of inflammatory exudates derived from choroid.

c) Vitireous opacities appear due to collection of inflammatory exudates. Destruction of nerve cells of retina in various parts depending upon the type of infection and vurulence of the organism.

**Complications**
1)    Complicated cataract
2)    Optic neuritis & atrophy
3)    Degeneration of visual field.

**Types of Choroiditis :-**
1) Suppurative choroiditis - The whole choroid and retina are inflammed and ultimately leading to panophthalmitis.

2)Non suppurative Choroiditis - Isolated foci of inflammation scattered over the fundus.

3) Disseminated choroiditis - Inflammatory patches in the fundus with healthy area in between.

4) Anterior choroiditis - Anterior part of choroid afftects, it commonly associate with interstitial Keratitis.

5) Central choroiditis - Central part of choroid affects.

6) Juxta papillary choroiditis - Choroid nearer to optic disc affects with defect in the field of vision

7) Diffuse choroiditis - Greater part of fundus is affected by gradual spread.

8) Toxoplasmosis uveitis - Caused by Toxoplasma gondii, transfered from mother to child in utero - the characteristic uveal lesion is a Circum scribed inflammation of choroid at Posterior pole

9) Toxocara canis uveitis - It is caused by the larvae of a nematode called Toxocara canis which Lives in cats and dogs. it causes white granulomatos lesion in choroid.

10) Tuberculous Posterior Uveitis- produces tubercles in the choroid near posterior pole.

11) Syphilitic posterior Uveitis, occur in congenital or acquired syphilis.

12) Sympathetic ophthalmitis- is a plastic inflammation of the Uveal tract in one eye following a similar inflammation in the other

13) Panophthalmitis - It is an intense purulent inflammation of the entire Uveal tract(Polymorpho nuclear leucocytosis) which fills the eye ball with pus and ends in complete destruction of eye ball. Commonly associate with penetrating injury to cornea and removal of eye is invariably indicated.

**14) Behcets syndrome:-**Recurrent iritis with hypopyon and Ulcerative lesions of mouth and genitalia optic atrophy is common and prognosis is bad.

**15) Stevens Johnson Syndrome:-** It is characterised by skin rash, stomatitis, conjunctivitis, keratitis, corneal ulcer, Uveitis and panophthalmitis.

**16) Vogt- Koyanagi syndrome -** Uveitis associated with alopecia, vitiligo poliosis and hyperacousis

**17) Harada's syndrome:-** Uveitis with Retinal detachment

**18) Heerfordt's disease:-** Uveitis with enlargement of parotid glands and facial paralysis

**19) Endophthalmitis :-**Generalised inflammatory condition of Uveal tract with lymphocyes and the other tissue are secondarily affected. Retinal detachment and phthisis bulbi commonly follows.

20) Degenerative changes of choroid like choroidal sclerosis and senile macular degeneration etc also causes choroidal lesions

**Common treatment principles of choriditis**

1)      Protection of eye from light with goggles
2)      Atropine drops or ointment TID or QID
3)      Sub conjunctival or Retrobulbar hydrocortisone injections
4)      Systemic antibiotics
5)      Antihistamine drugs
6)      Systemic cortisones or hydrocortisones.
7)      Control of specific infections
8)      Rest
9)      Analgesics and Anti inflammatories if needed
10)     Surgical procedures if needed
11)     For most of the chronic wide spreaded infections of choroid prognosis is very bad.

# THE PUPILS

Pupil is the central perforation of Iris, it regulates the amount of light admitted to the interior of the eye. The average diameter is about 3 mm. it is controlled by sphincter pupillae (For constriction of pupil) and dilator pupillae (for the dilatation of pupil.)Examination of the size (3mm), shape (Circular), position (central), margins (regular) and pupillary reaction is very important for the diagnosis of the diseases.

**A) Size of the pupil :-**
Average size of pupil is between 2 to 5 mm in diameter and vary in size due to following factors
    1) Infants and old - small pupil  2) Adolescents - Bigger pupil
    3) Brown eyes smaller pupil than blue eyes.
    4) During sleep first dilated then constricted
    5) In Hypermetropia pupil is smaller than in myopia.

B) Shape of the pupil is normally circular But is lesions of central nervous system it may become oval or D shaped.

**C) Position of Pupil -** In normal it is central But may become eccentric in Flat sarcoma of Iris, synechia, cerebral diseases (neurosyphilis), and in congenital abnormalities.

**d) Margins of Pupil -** Normally pupillary margins are regular but may be irregular due to synechia, uveitis and neuro syphilis.

The following conditions may cause abnormality in the size shape and position of the pupils.
1) Congenital anisocoria (unequal size of pupils)
2) " coloboma of Iris (Gaping in Iris)
3) Artificial coloboma of Iris due to sugery for cataract, glaucoma and Iris
    prolapse.                              4) Traumatic lesions.
5) Inflammatory lesions like uveitis synechia and due to corneal perforation etc.
6) Eccentric pupil due to flat sarcoma of Iris.
7) Iris atrophy due to increased intra ocualar pressure.
**E) Pupillary reactions-** 1) Reactions of the pupil to light
**a) Direct light reflex -** light should be focussed into one eye from the side by covering the other and pupillary constriction should be noted.
**b) Consensual light reflex -** Light should be focussed on one eye and pupil constriction should be noted in the other eye.
**2) Reaction of the pupil to shade :-**
Pupil will be dilated in the shade or dimillumination.
**3) Convergence and divergence Reaction : -** Pupil constricts when a person gazes at a near object and dilates when gazes at a distant object.
**4) The Pupil reaction to painful stimuli (cilio spinal reflex):-**
    By Pricking the skin of neck or head the pupils dilate for a while.

**F) Unilateral constriction of the Pupil :-** Irritation of the parasympathetic nerve fibres of the 3rd cranial nerve which supplies the sphincter pupillae is the causative fator.

**Ex.** 1) unilateral cerebral irritation or.

2) Intra cranial lesion irritating 3rd cranial nerve at base of skull

3) Local use of miotics **ex** - pilocarpine, eserine drops.

4) Paralysis of sympathetic fibres which supply the dilator pupillae.

**G) Unilateral dilatation of Pupil :-** Stimulation of the sympathetic nerve fibres which supply the dilator pupillae

**Ex.** 1) Irritative lesion of ocular sympathetic 2) Due to cocaine.3) Paralysis of parasympathetic fibres of 3rd cranial nerve 4) Lesion of ciliary ganglion or peripheral nerve endings. **ex** - mydriatics .

**H) Bilateral constriction of Pupil :-** Effect of the drugs acting on pupillo constrictor centre of the brain. Ex. 1) opium, morphine, chloral hydrate. 2) pineal tumour 3) neuro syphilis.

**I) Bilateral dilatation of Pupil :-** it is due to peripheral neuritis

**Ex**: - 1) Dugs taken internally like, Belladonna, Hyoscine, strammonium

2) Complication of diphtheria 3) Anaemia 4) Thyrotoxicosis 5) Botulism 6) coma.

**Mydriasis -** Causing dilatation of pupil

**Mydriatics -** The medicines those cause pupil dilatation, these are used for examination of posterior compartment of eye ball, in the treatmet of Iritis Irido, cyclitis and corneal ulcer to prevent, synechia.

**Ex.** 1) Atropine solution or ointment 2) Scopolamine 3) Homatropine 4) Platyphy 5) Phenamine etc .

**Note :-** Mydriatics are contra indicated in glaucoma.

**Miosis : - causing constriction of pupil**

**Miotics -** The medicines those cause pupil constriction. These are used for the management of Glaucoma

**ex** 1) Pilocarpine solution or ointment 2) Eserine 3) furamon 4) Phosphacol

**Corectopia -** It is a congenital abnormality in which the pupil present not in the centre of Iris.

**Anisocoria -** Inequal size of pupils

**Polycoria -** Multiple pupils in Iris myotonic pupil or Adies pupil- Slow constriction and dilatation of pupil.

**Occlusio Pupillae:-** Pupillary area is filled with Organised exudates and causes difficulty in refraction and aqueous circulation.

**Seclusio pupillae :-** Adhesion of entire pupillary margin to the Lens capsule Above 2 conditions causes glaucoma and Iris bombi due to obstructed aqueous circulation.

# RETINA

## A) Congenital and developmental defects of Retina

1) Coloboma of choroid and retina:- ophthalmoscopically a white area of exposed sclera can be detected as a congenital defect.

2) **Opaque nerve fibres** (or medullated nerve fibres):- As a developmental defect some times myelinated nerve fibres are also found. Ophthalmoscopically it appears as opaque white patches with a feathered edge at the margin of disc.

3) **Albinism -** Defective development of retinal choriodal pigments - causes photo phobia, nystagmus and defective vision etc.

4) **Aplasia -** Hypoplasia of macula may occur congenitally and cause blindness.

5) **Congenital pigmentation of the retina :** small oval grey spots or groups of poly gonal black spots may present in retina due to the accumulation of retinal pigment epithelium, it doesn't cause any serious problems.

6) **Colour blindness :-** Total colour blindness - is rare, it is due to defective development of cones and some defects in higher cerebral centres.
Partial colour blindness - is relatively common and exact cause is obscure.

7) **Retro lental fibroplasia (Retinopathy of prematurity)**
It appears in the premature infants with the birth wight less than 1.5 kg.

The clinical features are 1) Grey appearance of peripheral retina 2) formation of Vasularised retro lental membrane 3) Retinal separation 4) shallow anterior chamber 5) peripheral anterior synechia 6) secondary glaucoma 7) Atrophic changes in the eye ball.

## B) INJURIES OF THE RETINA

The injuries to the eye ball causes the following lesions .

1) **Contusion of Retina** Is caused by a severe blow on the eye ball, causes oedema of the retina at the posterior pole, with or without haemorrhages, the fluid exudes from capillaries and collect predominantly in the outer reticular layer of henle and in the rod and cone layer. The dimness of vision depends upon the intensity of lesion.

2) **Retinal rupture -** It occur in association with rupture of choroid.

3) Retinal haemorrhages occur with or without oedema .

4) **Retinal separation -** Due to injury, haemorrhage, exudates collection, give rise to separation of retina.

5) **Solar Retinopathy:-** Injury to retina due to Bright light exposure (eclipse blindness) causes blindness is known as solar retinopathy.

## C) Retinitis :-

Inflammation of the retina is known as retinitis it usually associate with choroid (choroido retinitis) or optic nerve (neuro retinitis).

**Pathological changes :-** Congestion, Oedema, exudation of plasma and leucocytes, extravasation of blood in to the retina, choroido retinal atrophy and blindness.

**Common Clinical features.**
If macular region is involved causes.
1) Distortion of the shape of objects ex:- straight lines appear as wavy ( meta morphopsia)
2) Objects appear smaller than normal (micropsia)
3) Objects appear bigger than normal (macropsia)
4) Impaired visual acuity 5) photo phobia.
6) if lesion present very peripheral, only blurring of vision present.
7) On ophthalmoscopic examination fundus shows slightly hazy retina, haemorrhagic points, spots, exudations, pigmentary changes, blurred disc margins etc .are found

**1) Purulent retinitis  Or septic  retinitis : -**
Retina is infected with virulent pyogenic Organisms, the infection spreads from choroid, finally it may cause panophthalmitis or endophthamitis.

**2)Cyto megalic inclusion disease.**
Human cyto megalo virus infection is characterised by distended tissue in which nuclei contrain large acidophilic inclusion bodies. It causes macular lesion or exudative chorio retinitis.

**3) Syphilitic** Retinitis arises in association with Uveitis, in which diffuse retinitis, attenuated vessels depigmented retina and optic atrophy are present.

**4) Massive exudative** retinitis - Coats disease, It is a rare disease of the young which presents a large raised yellowish white area as the result of haemorrhage and exudate collections between the outer layers of retina. Vision get lost due to retinal separation and glaucoma

**5) Sub acute infective  Retinitis** ( Septic retinitis of Roth)
The characteristic feature is the presence of round or oval white spots (Roths spots) in the posterior part of fundus, commonly arises due to Bacterial endo carditis and puerperal septicaemia, vision mostly impaired and also causes death.

**6) Vasculitis retinae**
Exudations are seen around the vessels. inflammation of veins is knwon as Phlebitis in which veins become thickened congested and tortuous
Inflammation of the arteries is known as Arteritis.

**7) Eales disease  Or periphlebitis retinae :** Profuse recurring haemorrhages into the vitreous

**8) Retinitis proliferans :-** The retinal haemorrhages organise and cause vitreal and Retinal bands or membranes  that cause atrophic changes in retina.

**9) Photo retinitis -** Inflammation of retina due to bright light exposure.

**10) Sarcoidosis** ( epitheloid granuloma)  Clinical features - candle wax spots, whitish areas, Oedema of optic disc, optic atrophy, choreo retinitis, periphlebitis, etc. the disease occurs in association with posterior Uveitis.

**11) Toxo plasmosis :-** It is protozoan infection from cats,it causes chorio retinitis.

12) Toxo cara canis, toxocara cati and Ascaris lymbricoides etc round worms produce retinal lesions.

## D)  RetinoPathies:-

Retinopathies occur in association with some general diseases like hypertension diabetes nephritis toxaemias of pregnancy, arterio sclerosis etc. The retinal changes are probably caused by increased capillary permeability and degenerative changes in the retinal tissue from anoxaemia.

**1) Hypertensive retinopathy:-** It may occur in 4 types.

a) In simple hypertension without sclerosis seen in the young, the retinal signs are constriction of the arteries which appear to be pale with acult angled branching, while haemorrhages may occur but not exudates.

b) Hypertension with involutionary sclerosis, occuring in older patients, the picture of arterio sclerotic Retinopathy appears, vascular constricutions, dilatations, sheathing of vessels, deposition of hard exudates, haemorrhages without any oedema.

c) Arterio sclerosis in the young (Diffuse hyperplastic sclerosis) Hyper tension with glomerulo nephritis produces the ophthalmoscopic picture as, narrow and tortuous veins with nicking at arterio venous crossings, multiple haemorrhages, oedema cotton wool patches, hard  exudates collection which scattered diffusely and produce macular star, vision is seriously impaired and causes death from uraemia.

d) malignant hypertension extreme attenuation of vessels, Entire retina may be clouded, generalised oedema, papilloedema, cotton wool patches, macular star and vision is gravely affected.

## 2) Retinopathy in toxaemias of pregnancy

It occurs in late months of pregnancy, it has many of the characteristics of hypertensive retinopathy, The features are narrowing of vessels, angiospasm, oedema, haemorrhages, profuse exudations and generalised to cause retinal detachment if Angiospasm weight gain present that indicates systemic retention of fluid, that may cause blindness and harm for the mother and child, hence termination of pregnancy is advised.

## 3) Lupus erythematosis retinopathy

If occurs in 10% patients, of Lupus erythematosis, in which cotton wool spots in posterior retina, flame shaped haemorrhages, and minor papilloedema, other symptoms are part of sjogren's syndrome (Kerato conjunctivitis, scleritis epi scleritis, Uveitis and butterfly skin eruptions)

## 4) Diabetic retinopathy

It usually occur in elderly persons with other features of diabetes, presence of dot (Punctate haemorrhages) or blot (larger haemorrhages) cr clusters of grapes like haemorrhages, development of micro aneurysms due to degeneration of vessel wall, hard white yellow waxy exudative patches at posterior pole, Oedema is not marked, Arterio sclerosis hypertension and renal disease are often superimposed upon the diabetic fundus, finally it causes retinitis proliferans, retinal detachment and blindness.

## 5) Proliferative or Neovascular Retinopathy

Progressive obliteration of the pre capillary arterioles results in focal areas of retinal anoxia followed by a neo vascularisation These new formed vessels originally within the retina but break in to vitreous where they are responsible for recurrent vitreous haemorrhages, finally Organisation of vitreous and retinal separation occurs.

## 6) Renal retinopathy

It is found commonly in chronic glomerulo nephritis with hypertension. signs of advanced arterio sclerosis are found in retinal arteries, other signs are oedematous fundus, blurred disc margins, flame shaped haemorrhages, soft cotton wool patches of exudates, macula star and hyaline, lipoid exudative deposits appear in later stages, It occurs Bilaterally and causes blindness.

## 7) Arterio Sclerotic retinopathy

Sclerosis of the retinal arteries is due to high blood pressare and usually seen in elderly persons.

## Changes in the vessels of retina-

1) Tortuosity of the small arteries especially at macula
2) alterations in the size breadth of the areterial lumen.
3) The vein is concealed at the crossing by the sclerosed artery.
4) The vein is compressed at the crossing by the sclerosed artery so that the peripheral portion of the vein is dilated while the central portion remain normal

5) Copper wire arteries - owing to the thickening of the arterial wall by the sclerosis , light is reflected back from its wall giving a coppery appearance

6) In more advanced sclerosis, light is reflected back from arterial wall giving a silvery appearance (Silver wire arteries)

7) minute miliary aneurisms are some times seen.

8) Flame shaped haemorrhages along the vesels 9) White solid exudates usually found in the posterior part of fundus.

10) No Oedema of retina or disc.

## Complications:-
a)     Amaurosis fugax - blurring of vision due to retinal arterial spasm
b)     If arterio sclerosis is neglected, leads to retino pathy (with haemorrhagic exudates)
c)     Thrombosis of retinal vein
d)     Optic atrophy.

## E) Neoplasm of Retina

### 1) Primary Neoplasms :-
Retino blastoma or Glioma of the retina or neuro epithelioma of retina :-

This is a malignant growth, congenital in origin occurs in children under 5 years of age. The tumour is composed of small round densely packed cells with largenuclei arranged around the vessels. It rapidly spreads in the eye ball and cauces retinal detachment, vitreal degeneration enlargement of eye ball and the infection also spread in to cranial cavity along the optic nerve.

**Symptoms :-** Yellowish white reflex at pupil, pain in later stages, dimvision, secondary squint, enlargement of eye ball etc.

### Signs - Ist stage
Yellowish white plaques either covered by retina or vitreous or blood vessels or haemorrhagic exudates are seen with ophthamoscopic examination. (Amaurotic cats eye)

**2nd stage :-** wide spread of tumour in the eye ball and development of glaucoma is seen.

**3rd stage : -** extra ocular stage or stage of metastasis, eye ball is enlarged, pushed forwards and retro ocular extention of the infection through optic nerve (Involves all the tissue which it comes in contact

**Treatment : -** Enucleation of the eye ball should be undler taken as quick as possible, if not it causes death.

### 2) Secondary Neoplasms :-
Secondary neoplasms of retina occurs by the invasion of primary and secondary choroidal neoplasms

## 3) Retinoschisis

Splitting of the retina at the level of outer plexiform layer (smooth sharply demarcated detachment) due to retinal cysts.

# F) VASCULAR DISORDERS OF RETINA

**1) Retinal arterial hyperaemia -** is caused by inflammatory lesions of the retina choroid, characterised by fullness and tortuosity of the arteries.

**2) Retinal venous hyperaemia :** - It is caused by congenital heart disease heart failure, increased intra orbital pressure, increased intra cranial pressure thrombosis of central retinal vein etc. The venous hyperaemia is characterised by dilatation and tortuosity of the veins.

**3) Anaemia of Retina :-** If is due to Thrombos is of central retinal artery, spasm of the retinal arteries, compression due to sudden rise of intra ocular pressure , cardiacfailure, profuse loss of blood, and in quinine amblyopia.

**Clinical features:-** are pallor disc, narrowing of retinal arteries, loss of vision etc.

**4) Retinal haemorrhages :-** The causes are a) Injuries b) lesions of retinal and choroidal vessles c) diseased blood vessels (Atheroma) commonly associate with heart and kedney diseases and in the old people. d) Circulatory problems, e) changes in the composition of vessel wall and blood f) Valvular heart disease and cardiac hypertrophy g) Loss of blood etc.

**Signs symptoms :-**
1) pre retinal haemorrhages (Sub hyloid haemorrhages) - the bleeding occupies between internal limiting membrane and vitreous, the haemorrhage occupies a circular shape but later spreads horizontally, occur at macular region.

2) Intra retinal haemorrhage
      a) Superficial type (it occur in nerve fibre layers.)
      b) deep type (it occur in nuclear layers)

The interference with vision depends upon the size and location of the haemorrhage. Minute haemorrhages are absorbed without any traces, bigger haemorrhages causes lesions and visual disturbances.

**5) Oedéma of retina :-** This may be diffuse or localised, the retina appears pale cloudy instead of bright red appearance. Oedema tends to throw the retina into radiating folds. (Star shaped folds)

**6) Macular Oedema : -**
Extra cellular fluid may accumulate in the foveal region by leakage from the local capillaries. it is of 2 types.
a) Cystoid oedema (simple, without foveal structural alteration)
b) Non cystoid or amorphous Oedema, when the normal capillary architecture at the macula has become destorted.

**7) Central serous retinopathy -** Circular dark raised swelling of macula, caused by exudation from the para foveal or choroded capillaries, impairs the central vision upto some extent.

**8)** Exudative retinopathy of coats (explained in Retinitis)

**9)** Proliferative retinopathy (or reinitis proliferans) explained in Retinitis

**10)** Retro lental fibroplasia (Explained in congenital developmental abnormalities.)

## G) RETINAL CHANGES IN THE DISEASES OF BLOOD

Retinal haemorrhages occur in blood diseases due to capillary permeability because of deficient oxygenation.

**1) Anaemia :-** In severe anaemias the veins are frequently engorged and in the posterior half of retina haemorrhages appear which are in flameshape, occationally are associated with soft exudates and fundus appears pale

**2)** Sickle cell haemoglobin peripheral arterioler occlusion are common in the retina and retinitis proliferans develop.

**3) Plycythaemia :-** In more severe cases marked venous engorgement, cyanosis of veins, Oedema of the disc and retinal haemorrhages occur.

**4) Leucaemia : -** Engorged and tortuous veins, round and flame shaped haemorrhages, soft exudates, fundus is pale or orenge coloured, oedema of retina and optic disc etc occurs due to capillary anoxia.

5) Occlusion of central retinal artery. The site of obstruction is just behind the lamina cribrosa where there is normally narrow vessel. The obstruction commonly occur due to thrombus embolus and arterio spasm of peripheral vessels.

**Clinical features :-**
　　　1) Sudden complete loss of vision
　　　2) Pupil widely dilated and no reaction to light .
　　　3) Retina be comes miiky white
　　　4) Macula pink (cherry red spot)
　　　5) Vessels are thin attenuated.
　　　6) Thrombosis of Retinal vein,:- It usually occur in elderly arterio sclerosis person and involves either central retinal vein or one of its tributaries. If central vein Obstructs that is just behind lamina cribrosa and tributaries obstruct at arterio venous crossings.

Thrombosis causes venous engorgement with dilated and tortuous veins, fundus is scattered with haemorrhages. vision greately reduces if macular area affected and within few weeks causes atrophic retinae with fine pigmentary chonges.

# H. DEGENERATIVE CONDITIONS OF RETINA

1) Senile macular degeneration (Hereditory) It occurs in the aged persons.

**2) Circinate retinopathy .**
It is due to chronic oedema involving a considerable area of the retina at and around the macula, as a part of hypertensive or diabetic retinopathy .

3) Benign peripheral retinal degeneration.

There are a number of retinal degenerations which do not-threaten the retina, even seen in many normal eyes

Ex.     1) Snow flakes (dotted white appearance at ora serrata)
        2) Paving stone degeneration (Due to chorio retinal atrophy)
        3) Reticular pigmentary degeneration
        4) Equatorial drysen, commonly found in elders with peripheral cystoid degeneration.

**4) Angioid streaks:-**
Dark browny pigmented streaks which anastomose with each other and may be mistaken for blood vessels, situated near the optic disc at a deeper level than the retinal vessels, these are due to changes in the elastic tissue of Bruch's membrane, paget's disease of bone, Ehlers Danlos syndrome and sickle cell disease may be associated with angioid streaks.

**5) Pigmentary retinal dystrophy (Retinitis pigmentosa)**
It is a congenital and familial disease characterised by night blindness and ultimately causing total blindness. the exact aetiology is obscure.

a) Small jet black pigments start in the equatorial region then gradually spreads centrally and peripherally and resembles bone corpusles b) Attenuation of retinal vessels c) degeneration of rods. d) field of vision show concentric contraction e) Ring scotoma is found in corresponding with the degenerated zone of retina. f) As the case progresses the field becomes smaller and at last reduced to restricted area around the fixation point, eventhough the central vision retained for a long time. g) Disc atrophies and appears in waxy yellow colour, Optic atrophy sets in and gradually increases h) In the later stages cataract develops i) Ultimately it causes total blindness.

# I) DETACHMENT OF RETINA OR RETINAL SEPARATION.

Retina is separated from underlying choroid eithr by fluids or solids. Retina mostly depends on choroid for its nutrition, if it is separated from choroid it may under go degenerative changes.

1) Primary detachment of retina, the cause is not obvious, usually associated with a tear or hole in the retina, This is commonly found in a) old persons with peripheral choroideo retinitis b) High myopia c) Contusion injury to the eye ball

2) Secondary datachment of retina the cause is obvious, they are a)Intra ocular tumours b) Exudative choroiditis c) Fibrous tissue formation in vitreous d) Haemorrhage between choroid and retina.

**Clinical features :-**
1) Vision gradually reduces and may become blind 2) Appearance of shades in visual fields when gazing in a fixed direction and retinal tear can be identified in ophthalmoscopic examination.

**Treatment** 1) Cause should be treated 2) Surgical correction (Diathermy coagulation to drain the sub retinal fluids to produce adhesion between choroid and Retina.

# DISEASES OF THE OPTIC NERVE

The optic nerve is the second cranial nerve meant for visual perception. it is a tract formed by the ganglian cells of retina. it comes out from eye ball by piercing the sclera at Lamina cribrosa a little distance to the posterior pole of eye ball. it enters the cranial cavity through optic foramina and ends at Lateral geniculate body, from here optic radiations reaches the visual cortex of occipital lobe of cerebrum for visual perception and discrimination.

**Optic nerve may be divided into,**
1) Intra ocular portion (in eye ball)
2) Orbital portion (eye ball to optic canal)
3) Intra canalicular portion ( in optic canal)
4) Intra cranial portion ( in cranial cavity)

The optic disc is known as head of the optic nerve present a little inside to the posterior pole where all the ganglian cells are united to form optic nerve. there is a funnel shaped central small depression known as physiological cup. Optic disc is cirular but some times oval, light pink in colour and much lighter than the rest of fundus. The margins often present 2 rings an inner scleral and outer choroidal, the central artery and vein of the optic nerve pass along the inner wall of the disc.

# A) Congenital Abnormalities of optic disc
1) Coloboma of optic disc (partial formation of the optic disc

## B) Inflammatory conditions :- 1) Inflammation of optic nerve is known as optic neuritis 2) inflammation of optic nerve head is knownas papillitis 3) Inflammation of orbital part ofoptic nerve is knwon as retro bulbar optic neuritis

| I) Papillitis (Intra ocular optic neuritis ) | II) Papilloedema (Plerocephalic oedema or chocked disc) |
|---|---|
| 1) Inflammation of the optic nerve head, The cause is obscure, But may arise due to general debility septic focus etc. | 1) Non inflammatory oedema of optic disc, commonly due to raised intra cranial pressure, orbital tumour, abscess, Hypertention, nephritis and leukaemias etc |
| 2) Disc is hyperaemic with blurred margins and the disc swelling rarely more than 2 Dioptres | 2) Disc margins are blurred and the disc swelling is frequently high (6 to 10 Dioptres) |
| 3) Venous engorgement and haemorrhages less marked | 3) Venous congestionand haemorrhages are marked (macular star) |
| 4) Loss of sight is sudden and profound | 4) loss of vision is gradual and negligible |
| 5) usually unilateral | 5) usually bilateral |
| 6) condition is temporary and recovers in 2-3 weeks. If condition is severe disc becomes pallor due to optic atrophy. | 6) Condition is progressive if not treated in time and causes blindness due to optic atrophy |
| 7) Central scotoma for red and green objects. | 7) Gradual concentric contraction of the fields. |
| 8) Treating the aetiology septic focus; B. complex and cortisione therapy may be benificial | 8) Cause should be treated, B Complex therapy cortisone therapy may be benifical. |

## III) Retrobulbar optic neuritis :-

Inflammation of the orbital part of the optic nerve is known as retro bulbar optic neuritis.

**1) Acute stage :-** It is due to disseminated sclerosis, Neuromyelitis optica, infection from sphenoid and ethmoid cells, lead and methyl alcohal poisoning.

**Signs and symptoms :-** Pain with movement of eye ball, especially in upward direction, sudden profound loss of vision, hyperaemia and blurring of disc margin, scotometry shows central or pericentral scotoma - especially for red and green objects.

**2) Chronic stage or Toxic amblyopia :-** It is due to toxic effect of Tobacco, quinine Arsenic ethylalcohol etc. causes Bilateral gradual blurring of vision, vision is normal but misty, fundus is normal and with centro caecal or central scotoma. **Treatment :-** Stoppage of consumption of tobacco alcohol etc and administriation of B12 - B Complex etc.

## IV) Optic atrophy

Atrophy of the optic nerve is called optic atrophy
**1) Consecutive atrophy :-** It occurs in association with certain diseases of retina **eg :-** Diffuse chorio retinitis, retinitis pigmentosa, etc (Here ganglian cells undergo degeneration. )
**2) Secondary atrophy ;-**
It occurs as the complication of the papillitis - papilloedema etc. diseases.

**Signs & symptoms : -**
The colour of the optic disc dull white, margins blurred, physiological cup filled up with glial tissue, and blood vessels show pathological changes like narrowing sheathing etc.

**3) Primary optic atrophy :-** It occurs without obvious lesion of fundus. But observed mostly due to syphilitiic affection, disseminated sclerosis, pressure on the optic nerve, haemorrhage in optic nerve sheath, massive haemorrhagic disorders, Arsenic poisoning, cranial stenosis, Toxic amblyopias, malnutrition etc.

**Signs & Symptoms : -**
The optic disc is bluish white in colour, enlarged physiolgical cup, clear margins and no vessel chunges.

**Treatment** 1) Cause should be treated 2) Stopage of toxic things like Tobacco methyl alchohol etc.3) B1, B6, B12 administration etc.
**Tumours of optic nerve :-** Rare but some times the following malignant tumours arise 1) Glioma it it arises in optic nerve fibres 2) meningioma it arises in the endothelial cells of meningeal sheath of optic nerve. These 2 should be excised)

# AQUEOUS HUMOUR

It is a clear watery fluid occupying the anterior and posterior chambers of the eye ball. it is not a stagnated fluid but continuously secreted by ciliary process of ciliary body and passed over the Lens, through pupil enters into the Anterior chamber and then drained into vascular system

Reaction - AlK aline (PH 7.1 to 7.3) specific gravity - 1.002 to 1.004
Viscosity - 1.029., Refractive index - 1.34

## Composition :-
Water 98. 69 %, Solids 1.3% (It closely resembles cerebrospinal fluid)

## Functions:-
1)     Maintains intraocular pressure ( 18 t0 23 mm Hg in schiotz tonometer)
2)     Gives shape for the eye ball
3)     Act as a refractive media
4)     Supplies nutrition and drains the metabolites from the surrounding structures.

## Aqueous affection
1)     Increased intraocular pressure of eye ball is due to stagnation of aqueous flow or increased aqueous secretion.
2)     Severe aqueous leakage causes lowered intra ocular pressure, causes shrinkage of eye ball (phthisis bulbi)
3)     Aqueous is a transparent water like structure, acts as a refractive media but if it is polluted with inflammatory precipitations, vision is obliterated (Interstitial keratitis, corneal ulcer, corneal perforations, uveitis and due to post operative lesions).
4)     Collection of pus in the anterior chamber (Aqueous) is known as hypopyon
5)     Collection of blood in the anterior chamber is known as hyphaema
6)     collection of macroscopic deposits in the lower part of cornea due to uveitis, the precipitations floats in the aqueous known as keratic precipitates.

## Vitreous humour :-
It is a transparent colourless jelly like substance fills the posterior compartment of eye ball behind the lens. It is separated from Lens by a retrolental space. its outer surface presents a thin condensation of its structure known as hyaloid membrane, vitreous is traversed by a canal from optic disc to posterior capsule of lens known as hyaloid canal, It has no blood supply but receives nourishment from surrounding tissue, It is incapable for inflammatory changes, but degenerative changes only occur .

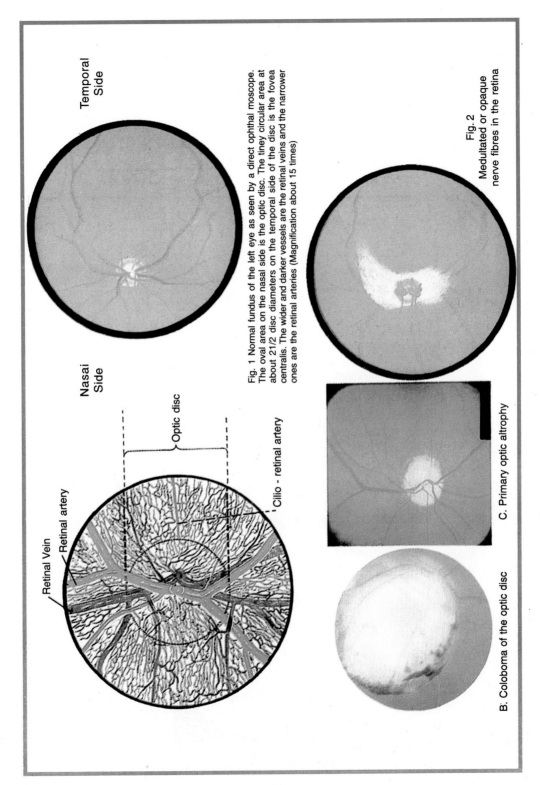

Temporal
Side

Nasai
Side

Retinal Vein

Retinal artery

Optic disc

Cilio - retinal artery

Fig. 1 Normal fundus of the left eye as seen by a direct ophthal moscope. The oval area on the nasal side is the optic disc. The tiney circular area at about 21/2 disc diameters on the temporal side of the disc is the fovea centralis. The wider and darker vessels are the retinal veins and the narrower ones are the retinal arteries (Magnification about 15 times)

Fig. 2
Medulated or opaque
nerve fibres in the retina

C. Primary optic altrophy

B. Coloboma of the optic disc

257

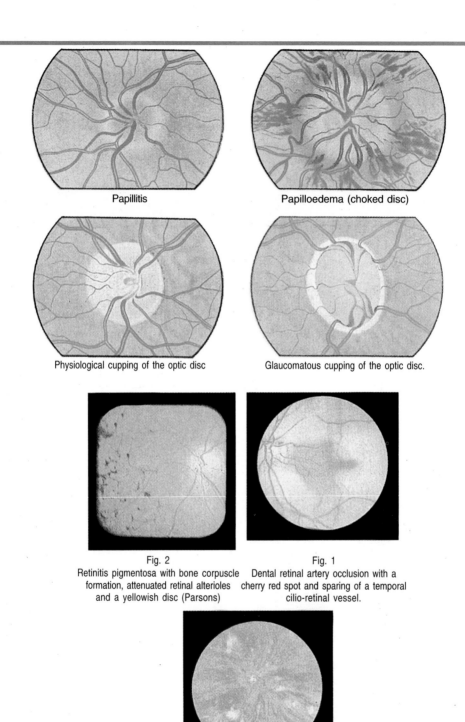

Papillitis

Papilloedema (choked disc)

Physiological cupping of the optic disc

Glaucomatous cupping of the optic disc.

Fig. 2
Retinitis pigmentosa with bone corpuscle formation, attenuated retinal alterioles and a yellowish disc (Parsons)

Fig. 1
Dental retinal artery occlusion with a cherry red spot and sparing of a temporal cilio-retinal vessel.

Fig. 2
Central retinal vein thrombosis (Parsons)

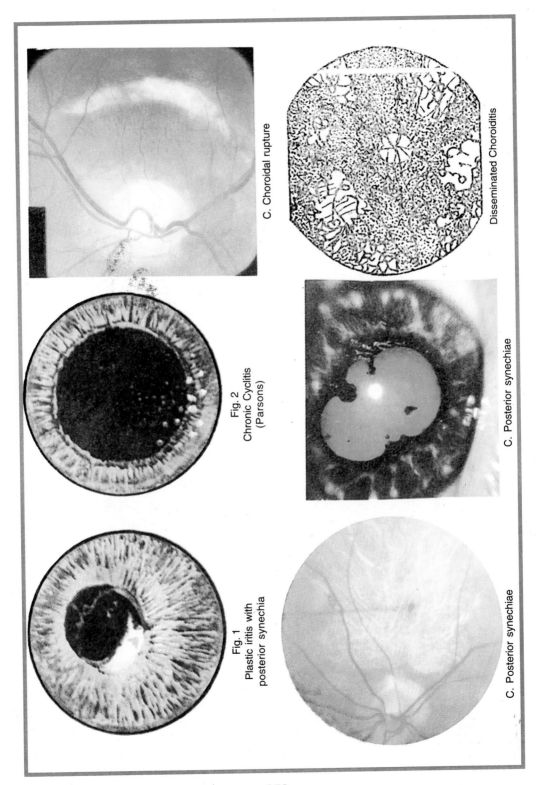

C. Choroidal rupture

Disseminated Choroiditis

Fig. 2
Chronic Cyclitis
(Parsons)

C. Posterior synechiae

Fig. 1
Plastic iritis with
posterior synechia

C. Posterior synechiae

259

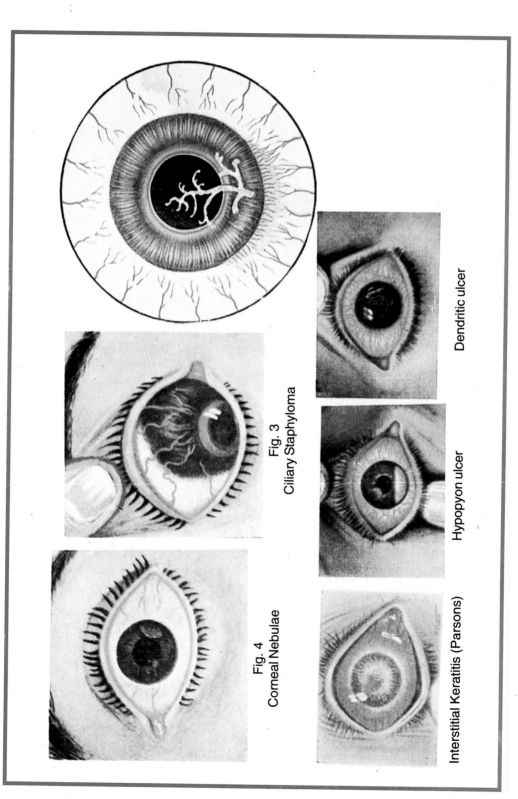

Fig. 3
Ciliary Staphyloma

Dendritic ulcer

Hypopyon ulcer

Fig. 4
Corneal Nebulae

Interstitial Keratitis (Parsons)

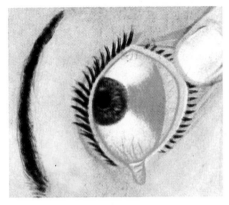

Fig. 4
Subconjunctival Haemorrhage
(May and Worth)

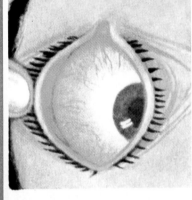

Fig. 2
Scleritis (Parsons)

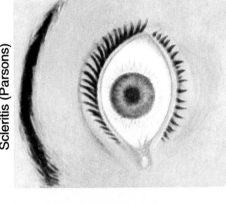

Fig. 2
Circumcorneal or ciliary congestion
(May and Worth)

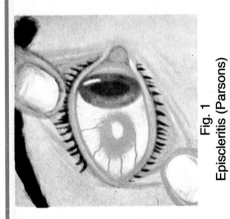

Fig. 1
Episcleritis (Parsons)

Fig. 1
Conjunctival type of congestion
(May and Worth)

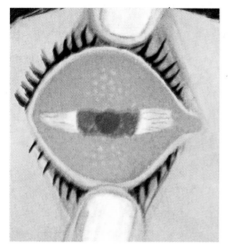

Fig. 2
Trachoma, Follicular Stage
(Parsons)

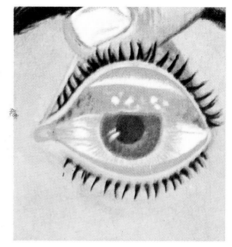

Fig. 3
Trachoma, cicatricial Stage
(Parsons)

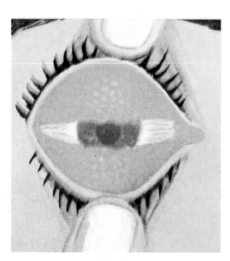

Fig. 1
Trachomatous Pannus
(Parsons)

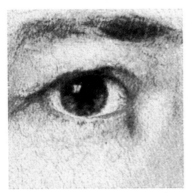

Fig. 1
Chronic Dacryocystitic
with Mucocele of the
lacrimal Sac.

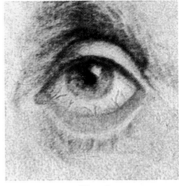

Fig. 4
Ectropion

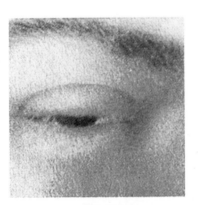

Fig. 2
Acute Dacryoystitis

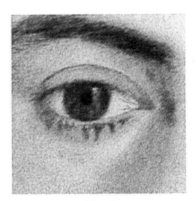

Fig. 3
Blepharitis

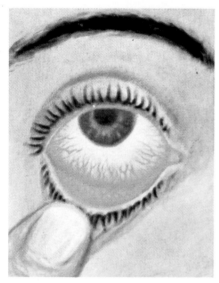

Fig. 1
Acute muco-purulent conjunctivitis
(Parsons)

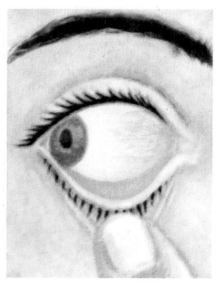

Fig. 2
Angular conjunctivitis
(Parsons)

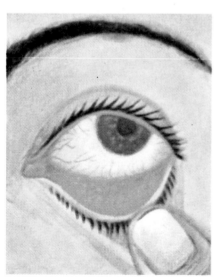

Fig. 3
Folicular conjunctivitis
(Parsons)

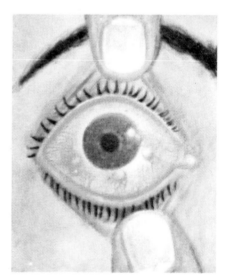

Fig. 4
Phlyctenular conjunctivitis
(Parsons)

**Congenital defects :-** 1) Persistent remains of the hyaloid artery :- usually hyaloid artery disappears before the delivary it self but some times the remnants attached to the posterior pole of lens casule which appears as a small blackish dot when viewed with the ophthalmoscope.

2) Peripheral inflammatory lesions, Neoplasms may produce opacities haemorrhages, degenerative chages in the vitreous that may cause considerable visual defect.

3) Fluidity of vitreous (Synchisis) :- Fluidity of vitreous due to alteration of the consistency of the vitreous due to opacities, high myopia, old age and peripheral inflammatory conditions the patient feels moving spots in the field of vision and finally it may cause retinal separation due to increased pressure.

**4) Shrinkage of Vitreous :-** It occurs due to age (Senile degenerative changes ) vitreous detached posterioly, due to adhesions, retinal separation also occurs. Patient complains of floating spots and flashes of light in visua field.

**5) Muscae Volitantes :-** Thses are fine translucent dots or filaments only seen subjectively especially when they are viewed against a brightly illuminated background. there is no pathological significance but a sensitive myopic patient may fear.
**Treatment :-** No effective treatment is known except correction of the refractive errors.
**6) Opacities of vitreous :-** These occur in the vitreous due to inflammatory changes and haemorrhages of peripheral structures.

    a) Protein coagula of the vitreous:- These dot like opacities visible due to liquefaction of vitreous .
    b) Asteroid hyalitis :- Numerous white particles resembling snow flakes appear in vitreous even in the normal, the disease dosesnot cause any visual defect and the exact cause also obscure.
    c) Synchisis scintillans :- Numerous shining crystalline bodies (cholesterol crystals) are seen in fluid vitreous the crystals churned up with eye ball movement. It is due to long standing Uveitis. It rarely produce symptoms and no effective treatment is known
    d) Degenerative changes of vitreous due to high myopia.
    e) Exudes from Uveitis cause diffuse clouding in vitreous .
    f) Blood from the retinal vessels may invade the vitreous and cause opacities.
    g) Extensive membrane formation, organisation of exudates or haemorrhages(Retinitis proliferans) may cause vitreous opacities.

**Signs - Symptoms ;-** Some degree of visual disturbance discomort from float-ing specks, visual acuity is not greatcly impaired.

**Prognosis -** Mostly opacities are absorbed and residual opacities remain without much problem.

**Treatment**   1) Peripheral lesions should be treated.
2) Supplementation of vitamin C-K P
3) Potassium Iodide by mouth, diaphoretics, cathartics and sub conjunctival saliva injections may benifit to the patient.

**7) Vitreous haemorrhages :-** Blood in Vitreous is always derived from the retinal vessels and vessels of Uveal tract as the vitreous humour has no blood vessels in post natal life.

The causative factors are injuries, Arterio sclerosis, Hypertenisve and dia-betic retino pathy, high myopia, sequela to surgical procedures, Eales disease etc.

If the haemorrhage is minor doesn't Obstruct the vision and it may be absorbed but wide spread haemorrhages cause visual loss and prognosis also bad.

**Treatment -**   1) Cause should be treated
2) It can be tried like vitreous opacities.
3) Not Satisfactory.

**8) Vitreous abscess**  : -
It arises  due to perforation of cornea or penetrating injury to eye ball  or endog-enous infection (endophthalmities) etc.

**Sign:** A yellow reflex at pupil in oblique illumination
**Treatment ;-** Evisceration of the eye ball.

## ERRORS OF REFRACTION

**Refraction :-** The method by which the light rays after travelling through the refractive media falling on retina (fovea centralis) for visual perception is known as refraction

**Refractive media**  : - Cornea, aqueous humour, pupil, Aqeous, Lens, vitreous humour and retina

**Emmetropia -** It is a normal refractive condition of the eye in which the parallel light rays from a distant object are brought to foccus on retina with the accommo-dation at rest.

**Ametropia :-** it is an abnormal refractive condition of the eye in which the parallel rays from a distant object are brought to foccus either before or beyond the retina, is known as Ametropia (Refractive errors)

**1) Myopia** (short sighted) it is a refractive error of the eye in which, with the accommodation at rest, the parallel rays from a distance object are brought to foccus in front of the retina

**2) Hyper metropia** (Long sighted) It is a refractive error of the eye in which, with the accommodation at rest, the parallel rays from a distance object, are brought to focus beyond the retina.

**3) Astigmatism** It is the refractive condition of the eye in which the refraction differs in different meridians of the eye (Ex:- Normal in one meridian and myopic or hypermetropic in another meridian)

**4)Aniso metropia** it is the condition in which there is considerable inequality in the refraction of the two eyes.

**EX:-** 1) Uni ocular trauma (one eye is normal another is affected )
2) Uni ocular Extraction of lens in cataract (3) High myopia etc
4) Congenital causes

**Note :-** If the difference in refraction is more than 2.5-D in the two eyes Causes difficulty for binocular vision Because it produces 5% difference in the size of retinal image.

# MYOPIA (SHORT SIGHTED)

**Defination:-** It is the refractive condition of the eye in which with the accommo-dation at rest, the parallel light rays from a distant object are brought to foccus before the retina in stead of on fovea centralis of macula of retina, is known as myopia or short sighted or Hraswa drusti. In myopia the patient cannot see the distant objects properly (difficulty in distant vision )

**Causes:-** (1) congenital or developmental or Heriditory (2) increased antero pos-terior axis of the eye is the commonest cause which is known as Axial myopia (3) Increased refractive inde of the refractive media will converge the rays so only brought to be focussed before the retina like in lental sclerosis, is known as Index myopia .(4) when the curvature of cornea is greater then normal causes curva-ture myopia (5) The posiuon of the lens moving fowards or increased convexity produces myopia .

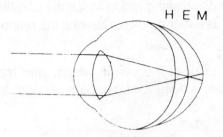

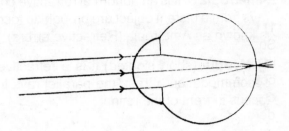

Emmetropia, hypermetropia and myopia. In emmetropia (E), parallel rays of light are focused upon the retina. In hypermetropia (H), the eye is relatively too short; in myopia (M), it is too long

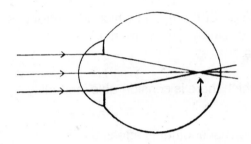

Myopia

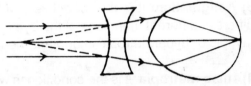

Correction of myopia with concave spherical lens

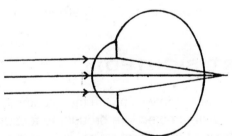

Hyper Metropia

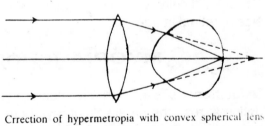

Crrection of hypermetropia with convex spherical lens

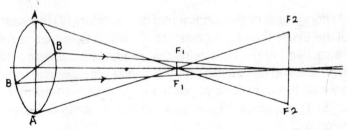

Refraction through an astigmatic surface—Sturm's Conoid

**Clinical types of myopia :-**

**1) Congenital Myopia -**
Some times high Anisometropia (one eye is normal and other eye is high myopia) is seen congenitally and Bilateral congenital myopia commonly associate with convergent squint ingeneral congenital myopia associate with cataract, microphthalmos, Lenticonus, aniridia, megalocornea, retinal separation etc. disorders.

**2) Developmental myopia or simple myopia -**
It is a safe variety without degenerative changes, mypoia may tatain maximum 5 to 6 D. A Child is born as hyper metropic but at the age of 4 yrs it will become emmetropic due to normal development of body But in some conditions the eye maybecome myopic due to accelaration of the maturity (long eye ), It is said to be nonpathological or Non progressive mypoia, commonly observed in school going age group.

**3) Degenerative or progressive or pathological myopia-**
It is a complicated myopia due to degenerative changes in the eye ball, the refractive error may reach even more than 20 D. The associated complications are.
a) Reduction of Vision b) Ectasia of posterior segment of eye with thinning of sclera c) curvature anomalies of Lens and cornea d) Chorio retinal degeneration e) Retinal detachment f) Vitreous degeneration g) Posterior cortical or nuclear cataract h) Retinal haemorrhages i) Large myopic disc with temporal cresc' j) optic atrophy.

**4) Acquired myopia -**
Myopia may also develop due to injuries after glaucoma operation, interstitial kera and due to drugs like steroids sulfonamides etc.

**Signs and symptoms of myopia -**
1) Dimness of vision for distant objects
2) There is no difficulty for near vision unless the defect is too high (Getting head ache while reading writting etc.)
3) In case of High myopia due to affection of near vision the Child holds the book very close to his eyes while reading.
4) If the error is uncorrected the pathological mypoia may cause blind ness.

**Treatment :-**
1) Nutritious food or vitamines supplementation.
2) Prescribing of concave Lens (-) of proper strength or contact Lens.
3) Symptomatic therapy for complications
4) Hygienic measures
5) Eye exercises etc.

## II) Hyper metropia -

**Defination:-** It is the refractive error of the eye in which with the accommodation at rest, the paralel rays from a distant object are brought to foccus beyond the retina, instead of on fovea of macula of retina. In hyper metropia the patient complaints of dim vision for near things.

**Causes -** 1) Shortness of the eye ball in the antero posterior axis, this is the commonest cause due to underdevelopment of eye during child hood., is known as Axial hypermetropia.

2) Refractive index of the refractive media ( mainly lens) may be low, This type is known as Index hypermetropia.

3) If the curvature of the cornea is less than normal (flat), is called curvature hypermetropia.

### Clinical types of Hyper metropia :-
**1) congenital hypermetropia.**This is uncommon and assoicate with other Abnormatlities like microphthalmos.

**2) Developmental hypermetropia:-** Most of normal infants are born with + 4 D hypermetropia, it should be corrected physiologically upto 4 yrs. of age but due to delayed development the hypermetropia continued ,this is known as developmental hypermetropia.

### 3) Acquired hypermetropia
It is due to removal of crystalline Lens on account of cataract surgery (Aphakia), shortening of eye's length following scleral resection operation, partial dislocation of Lens posteriorly can also cause this condition.

### Signs and sympotms:-
1) If there is moderate hypermetropia the Patient complains of dimvision only for near objects.
2) If there is high degree of hypermetropia the patient complains of dim vision for both near and distant objects.
3) If hypermetropia is minimal there are no visual symptoms, as the error is corrected by prolonged contraction of ciliary muscles which causes fatigue of muscles and produces eye strain or asthenopia (eye strain, head ache blurring of vision, pain in the eye, red ness and heaviness of lids)

### Treatment :-
1) hygienic measures 2) eye exercises 3) prescribing of proper power convex Lens (+) 4) Symptomatic treatment of complications.

## III) Astigmatism : -

It is the refractive condition of the eye in which the refraction differs in different meridians of the eye.

**Ex** - In the horizontal meridian the eye is emmetropic but in vertical meridiian It is hyper metropic or mypoic.

**Causes :-** 1) variation in the curvature of cornea - lens or both.
2) Partial dislocation of Lens

**Types :-**
1) Regular astigmatism (simple, compound and mixed) 2) Irregular astigmatism.

**1) Irregular astigmatism :-**. Here the light rays are refracted very irregularly (Different groups of foci in various positions) due to corneal ulcers, keratitis, penetrating injuries, surgical lesions, kerato conus etc.

**Correction :-**
1)      spectacle lenses are not  useful.
2)      Contact lenses are useful upto some extent
3)      Keratoplasty is advisable.

**2) Regular astigmatism :** - Light rays are not focussed at a single point but here the meridians of greatest and least refraction are at right angled to each other (Light rays are not regular totally in all meridians but regular in each meridian that is right angled to each ) It is due to corneal curvature irregularities and subluxation of Lens.
**It is of 3 types**
1) simple astigmatism 2) compound astigmatism. 3) Mixed astigmatism.

**1) Simple regular astigmatism :-**
one meridian is emmetropic and the other either myopic or hypermetropic it is again 2 types a) simple myopic regular astigmatism b) simple hypermetropic regular astigmatism.

**2) Compound regular astigmatism :-** The Both meridians are Ametropic. either myopic or hypermetropic so it is again two types a) Compound myopic regular astigmatism (the two focal lines fall before the retina. b) Compound hypermetropic regular astigmatism ( the two focal lines fall beyond the retina).

3) Mixed regular astigmatism Both the focal lines are ametropic among them one is myopic (focal line fall before the retina) another is hyper metropic (focal line fall beyond the retina).

**Signs and sympotms -** With a small degree of astigmatism there may not be any visual disability but with greater degree distant and near visual disturbances and Asthenopia develops (Red eyes, headache, eye strain and pain while reading etc. ) for especially near works.

**Treatment :-** Regular astigmatism is corrected with cylindrical Lens of proper strength ( in simple astigmatism only with cylindrical Lenses and in compound and mixed astigmatism correction with cylindrical and sperical lenses.)

## IV) Presbyopia :-

This is a physiological phenomenon which affects every eye usually after the ageof 40 yrs, in which the near point of distinct vision receedes beyond the distance at which we are accustomed to read ordinary print (Beyond 28 cm from the eye).

It is physiolgical process in which the crystalline Lens undergo gradual loss of plasticity and weakness of ciliary muscle so only the Lens lost the capacity to accommodate the near point from 28 cm after the age of 40 yrs.

**Symtoms : -**1) Difficulty in doing near works like reading writting sewing composing etc, As the age advances the difficulty increases more and more.

**Treatment : -** 1) age Prescribing the convex Lens of proper strenght
2) Rough calculation of strength of Lens as per age, is as follows.

| S.No | Age | Strength of Lens. |
|------|-----|-------------------|
| 1 | 40 yrs to 45 | + 1. Dioptres |
| 2. | 45 " to 50 | + 1.5.   " |
| 3. | 50 " to 55 | + 2.00 . " |
| 4. | 55 " to 60 | + 2.5    " |
| 5. | 60 " to 70 | + 3.00 |

**Refractive Index :-**
Light rays travels through the air at a speed of about 300000 km/ second

**Refractive index :-** relative measure of transmission of light

Refractive index
of a media

$$= \frac{\text{Light velocity in air}}{\text{Light velocity in 2nd media.}}$$

Refractive index of
human Lens

$$= \frac{\text{Light rays velocity in lens}}{} $$
$$= \frac{300000 \text{ km/ second}}{2,14, 285 \text{ km/second}} = \frac{\text{light rays velocity in air}}{\text{light rays velocity in lens}}$$
$$= 1.4.$$

**Note : -** The refraction depends upon the difference between refractive indices of two media and the affect of the  beam of light traverses the interface between the media.

Refractive index of cornea - 1.38
"          "          Aqueous humour                    1.34
"          "          Crystalline Lens        =        1.4
"          "          Vitreous humour        =        1.34

**Note : -** Refractive index increases in myopia and decreases in Hypermetropia.

# Accommodation of Lens:-

Adjustment of the optical apparatus so as to change the refractive power of the eye, when the image of a near object is brought into foccus on the retina, is described as accommodation.

There is no need of accommodation.For focussing the parallel rays of distant objects, but accommodation is needed to focus the divergent rays of near objects, for that the dioptric power of the Lens should be increased by increasing its curvature, for this mechanism under the influence of nerve impulses there is contraction of ciliary muscle relaxation of suspensory ligament and the fibres attached to the Lens capsule, this results in loosening of capsule and the Lens become more convex in shape owing to its elasticity. After near objects, visualisation to see the distant objects the dioptric power of the Lens should be reduced by flattening of lens (ciliary muscle relaxation, contraction of suspensary ligament and fibres attached to the Lens capsule, causes flattening of Lens). This adaptation takes place continuously for the proper visualisation of the objects at different distances.

If the object is brought closer then a point is reached at which inspite of strong contraction of ciliary muscle the object is not focussed, the rays from that object is so divergent. The nearest point at which the object is clearly focussed with full accommodation is the near point. The distance between the near point and the eyes increases with age due to hardening of Lens and become diffficult appoximately after 40 yrs of age (presbyopia) the far point is at infinity (20feet) and the distance between the far point and near point is called Range of accommodation.

The greater distance between the object and the eye, the lower the degree of accommodation ; and the closer the objects viewed the greater the degree of accommodation.. The accommodation get failure in paralysis, spasm, due to constant near work, after diphtheria, in certain cranial injuries injection of atropine into conjunctival sac, in poisoning with methylalcohol plasmocide, etc.

1) In normal eyes the parallel rays from infinity fall on the principle foccus of the lens.

2) In myopia the rays are convergent and focussed before the retina so only for the correction, divergence sperical Lens( concave) of proper strenght is used for the correction.

3) In hypermetropia the rays are divergent and fall beyond the retina so only for the correction, convergent sperical Lens( + convex) of proper strength is used for the correction.

4) In presbyopia inability to read the small print occurs due to the reduced accommodative capacity of Lens ( the Lens cannot become more convex to focus the more divergent rays of near things) so only sperical convex Lens is used for the correction of this error.

5) In irregular Astigmatism light rays are most irregular in all meridians so spectacle Lendses are not useful only contact Lenses and Keratoplasty are benificial.

6) In simple regular astigmatism cylindrical Lenses correct the error

7) In compound and mixed astigmatism cylindrical + sperical Lenses are needed for the correction of error.

8) Accommodation of Lens required only for Near objects to converge the diverging rays emerging from near things.

9) In hyper metropia or presbyopia correction shold be proper, to give rest for the accomodation of Lens if not causes accommodative asthenopia.

10) The symptoms of accommodative asthenopia are eye strain, head ache, eye pain, redness, heavyness in lids, hazy blurring of vision etc.

11) Simply giving the spectacles cannot control the disease for that cause should be treated, nutritious food, vitamins should be supplemented, patient is advised not to expose to hot, dusty, Bright things.

12) Some children are habitated to handle the books very close to the eyes - that cause visual errors so parents should take care for avoiding those things.

13) Mydriatics (pupil dilator) are used for fundoscopy but it is contra indicated in glaucoma

14) Heavy exercises, intake of toxic things like tobaco alcohal etc. Bright light or dimlight prolonged exposure, chronic exposure to foreign bodies, malnutrition, hypo vitaminosis, injuries, unhygienic conditions, all the common aetiological points causes visual errors, so all those should be avoided.

# VISION

Eye ball is the end organ of optic nerve, it is meant for visual perception. The light rays after travelling through the refractive media has to fall on fovea centralis of macula of the retina.

The white and monochromatic light rays which fall on fovea causes Bio-chemical stimulus in cones and cone fibres, those reach the cerebral cortex through the optic tract and cause photophic vision(Bright and colour vision perception) the rays of low intensity face on the peripheral portions of retina where rods are predominent and causes Bio chemical stimulus in rods and rod fibres, those reach the cerebral cortex through the optic tract and produce scotopic (dim) visual perception. For the normal perception of vision Length of the eye ball ; Normal (position surfaces, refractive Index, functions) refractive media, Normal Intra ocular pressure, Reltina, optic disc, optic tract and visual centre are responsible.

So many factors affects the visual perception, those are .
1) Deviation of visual axis 2) Lesions of appendages of eye ball 3) corneal lesions like flat cornea or Kerato conus, central corneal ulcers or opacities 4) Aqueous precepitations (Hypopyon Hyphaema) 5) Affection of pupillary reflex 6) Accomodatory problems of lens, central lental opacities, cataract 7) Vitreous degeneration, Vitreous haemorrhages 8) Retinal detachment, atrophy, Retinitis impropery production of Rods and cones macular degeneration, macular burn 9) Lesions of optic disc, optic nerve, central connections and visual centre .10) Congenital lesions, traumatic lesions, Idiopathic causes. 11) Malnutrition, Vitamin defficiencies chronic systemic lesions, endocrinal disorders, poisionous thinks regular usage of Tobacco, alcohol (Amblyopias) Above factors causes disturbances in the normal Visual perception.

# BLINDNESS

## Day Blindness (Hemeralopia )

The Vision is poor in Bright light But better in dim light (In dim light the pupil dilates and so the peripheral cornea lens and retina are used for vision).

**Causes :-**
1) Pathological changes in macula.
2) Central opacity of Lens or cornea
3) Congenital abnormality Commonly associate with total colour blindness.

(In Ayurvedic science it is corelated to **pitta vidagdha drusti** in which during the day time due to piita prakopa the person cannot see the things But can see the objects at night due to pitta shaman ).

## COLOUR BLINDNESS

Inability to recognise the colours either partially or in total, is known as colour blindness.

**Causes :-**
    **A) Congenital Causes :-**

        It is bilateral and incurable (either partial or total blindness) No colour is recognised and see the things in grey.

    **B) Acquired Causes :-**
        It is due to diseases of macula, and optic nerve ex: Toxic amblyopias, macular affections in various diseases.

There are 3 Primary colours (Red - green - Blue ) which when mixed together produce rest of the colours of spectrum.

It congenital colour blindness the 3 basic colours are not seen, they are grouped into the following 3 groups.

1)    **Total Colour Blind ness  (Achromics)**
    All the 3 colour factors are not seen

2)    **Mono Chromics :-** Among the 3 only one colour factor is seen .

3)    **Dichromics :-** Among the 3, only 2 colour factors are seen, it is sub divided into
    a) Protanopes    -    Red colour blind
    b) Deuteranopes    -    Green Colour blind.
    c) Tritanopes    -    Blue Colour blind.

## NIGHT BLINDNESS (Nyctalopia)

It is a condition in which the vision is defective at night But good in the day time.

It occurs as a symptom in certain retinal diseases and some times associate with systemic disorders like vitamine " A" deficiency etc.

**Causes :-**

**1) Congenital -Hereditory causes :-**
It associate with other anomalies of retina as in oguchi's disease( usually occurring in Japan.)

**2) Diseases of eye ball like :-**
a) Retinitis pigmentosa b Peripheral chorio- retinitis c) myopic degenerative changes in the peripheral retina. d) Chronic simple glaucoma with marked contraction of visual field . e) Retinal detachment.

**3) Systemic diseases :-**
a) Vitamin A deficiency
b) Pathological changes in liver, like cirrhosis of liver.

**Note :-** It is mainly due to damage of rods or deficient regeneration of visual purple due to vitamine "A" deficiency. that can be measured with adaptometer.

## Amaurosis :-
Amaurosis means complete loss of eye sight.
**Causes :-** 1) Vitreous haemorrhage as in Eale's disease 2) Acute exudative choroiditis 3) Detachment of retina 4) Thrombosis of central vein of retina 5) Acute retrobulbar neuritis 6) Occlusion of central artery of retina 7) Acute congestive glaucoma 8) Injury as by pen knife, arrows or bombs etc. 9) Neuro myelitis optica or Devic's disease 10) Optic neuritis.

## Amblyopia :-
It is a disease in which partial loss of vision occurs not due to any obvious or demonstrable organic lesion ( inherent defect with no demonstrable physical sign ) ex. toxic amblyopia due to Tobacco usage etc.

a) It is due to supression of macular function, Known as amblyopia ex anopsia.It commonly associate with squinting eye in the child .

b) disuse of the macula as in case of uncorrected high myopia or due to opacity of the media (corneal opacity or cataract etc.)

## Hemianopia :-
It is a condition in which one half of the visual field of each eye is affected or damaged .

## Causes :-
Syphilitic meningitis, gumma or tuberculoma at the base of brain,

Tumour or aneurism in the neighbourhood of the optic tract, cerebral haemorrhage ; thrombosis trauma and tumour of the occipital lobe of the brain.

It is produced by a lesion in the optic tract, Lateral geniculate body, optic radiation or calcarian cortex of one side. It is characterised. by sparing of the macular area.

## Diplopia (Double Vision )
When an object appears double it is called diplopia. it is of two types 1) Uniocular diplopia 2) Binocular diplopia .

### 1)    Uniocular diplopia :-
When two images of an object fall on the retina, uniocular diplopia is produced,
**Causes of uniocular diplopia. :-**
a) Sub luxation of lens b) incipient. cataract c) Large irido dialysis d) Kerato conus e) Retinal detachment.

### 2)    Binocular diplopia :-
When the images of an object do not fall on the corresponding points of the retinae, diplopia is produced. Diplopia disappearse by closing one eye. It may be grouped as .

**a) Vertical Binocular Diplopia :-** When one image is situated above or below the other.
**b) Horizontal Binocular diplopia :-** when the images are placed side side, it is called Horizontal Binocular diplopia.
1) Homonymous Binocular diplopia :- The false image present on the same side of the deviated eye .
2) Crossed Binocular diplopia :-   The false image is seen Opposite side of the deviated eye .
**Causes of Binocular diplopia :-**
1) Paralysis of extra ocular muscle.
2) Displacement of eye ball due to space ocupying lesion in orbit.
3) Restriction of the movements of the eye ball due to pterigium or symblepharon etc.

## Phthisis Bulbi :-
It is an atrophic condition of eye ball which becomes soft and shrunken.
**Causes :-**
a) Keratomalacia b) Panophthalmitis. c) Endophthalmitis d) Severe Irido Cyclitis e) Absolute glaucoma.

The solid contents of the eye ball are disintigrated and become pus, Hypotomy follows shrinkage of eye ball.

**Treatment :-** Enucleation of the eye ball.

## Internal Ophthalmoplegia :-

It is a condition in which there is paralysis of intrinsic muscles of eye ball (ciliary muscle, sphincter pupillae of Iris ) Causes loss of accommodation of Lens due to oculomotor nerve palsy.

## External Ophthalmoplegia :-

It is a condition in which there is paralysis of Extra ocular muscles (4 recti, 2 oblique and Levetor palpebrae superioris ) commonly due to syphilis.

## Colour haloes :-

Haloes are seen as coloured ring around artificial lights. The conditions in which colour haloes are seen are as follows.

**1) Acute or sub acute conjunctivitis :-** The flakes of mucous over the cornea give rise to colour haloes owing to their prismatic effect.

**2) Closed angle Glaucoma :-**
The haloes appear in this disease due to Oedema of corneal epithelium and altered refractive index of the corneal lamellae .

**3) Lenticular Haloes :-** Lental changes during early cataract may produce haloes.

**Note :-** Among the above 3 diseases, haloes of acute conjunctivitis can be easily recognised and for the differential diagnois of closed angle glaucoma and early cataract, stenopic slit is passed across the eye if haloes. remains in tact that is glaucoma, and if haloes broken up that is cataract.

## Dimvision :-

It is a symptom, observed in many diseases . It is due to following causes.
1) Central corneal opacity or ulcer.
2) Corneal oedema.
3) Interstitial Keratitis.
4) Keratopic precipitations.
5) Aqueous precipitations (Hypopyon. Hyphaema etc).
5) Occlusio pupillae and seclusio pupillae etc.
6) Lental & Capsular opacities.

7) Glaucoma 8) Vitreous degeneration, haemorrhages etc. 9) Macular degeneration 10) Optic neuritis. 11) Vitamin A deficiency 12) Chronic specific systemic. disorders 13) Toxic amblyopia 14) Hypertensive, Diabetic. retinopathy etc. 15) Lesions of central connections etc. 16) Increased or Decreased Anterio posterior diameter 17) Increased or Decreased refractive index of the media 18) Lesions of Lens accommodation. 19) congenital or developmental or heriditory causes 20) Idiopathic causes.

## BLINDNESS PROFILE AND ITS CONTROL

The Term Blindness implies to loss of perception of light either partially or totally. If the vision is reduced more than 3/60 Those patients can be treated as the blind.

At present Nutritional deficiencies Trachoma ,Glaucoma, cataract, ocular injuries, Retinal lesions, optic nerve lesions and visual centre lesions, are the common diseases that cause blind ness.

As per, I.C.M.R. Survey.

| | | |
|---|---|---|
| 1) Cataract | Blindness | 55% |
| 2) Glaucoma | " | 3 % |
| 3) Nutritional | " | 2% |
| 4) Corneal | " | 20% |
| 5) Posterior segment | " | 20% |

Govt of India has launched National plan for the control of Blindness (NPCB) in 1976, to establish permanent eye care facilities to controle and treat the blindness. The eye care centres are established at different levels of the country. Many primary health centres, Districts hospitals ,medical colleges, and voluntary organisations.etc, are conducting the surgeries for cataract glaucoma etc diseases,and distributing vitamin A, B .Complex, folic acid Iron etc tabs, and educating thepeople to prevent the traumatic eye lesions etc. Like this govt of India is trying maximum to controle the blindness.

# A) KU-POSHANAJANYA NETRA VIKARA
## (Mal- Nutritional and Vitamin deficiency, eye diseases ).

Eye ball the organ of vision is the most important sensory organ among the five (Pancha gyanendria)" Sarvendrianaam Nayanam pradhanam " A blind man though he is having the richest facilities, are merely useless so only it is advised to save the eye from the diseases. There are so many factors responsible for causing the eye diseases, among them nutritional deficiencies and vitamin deficiencies are also causes different types of eye diseases, they are follows.

### 1) Vitamin "A" Deficiency :-
Vitamin A deficiency causes xerosis (Xerophthalmia), Keratomalacia, Night blindness, skin lesions, demyelination, diminished resistence to infections etc. The daily requirement is 4000. I.U. The sources are " Leaf Vegetables, yellow fruits, milk, butter, fish, egg, animal fat, codliver oil, halibut oil carrot, shigru leaves etc.

### Xerosis ;-
The dry lustreless conjunctiva with degenerative changes is known as xerosis (dirty grey coloured patches and Bitodes spots are seen at or near Limbal conjunctiva).

### Keratomalacia :-
Degenerative changes are seen in Conjunctiva (Dirty grey coloured patches, bitods spots and dry lustre less conjunctiva ) and cornea (dull, insensitive, hazy cornea, softening , tissue necrosis and with severe complications.)

### Stages of Keratomalacia :-
1) Night blindness - due to diminished production of visual purple (Rodopsine)
2) Conjunctival degenerative changes.
3) Pre Xerotic changes of cornea (dull hazy cornea with slightly reduced sen sation.
4) Corneal tissue necrosis with epithelial desquamation.
5) Corneal ulceration spreads in total and finally cornea is sloughed out.
6) Complications like Anterior staphyloma, Adherent leucoma, panopthalmitis, Blindness etc arises.

### Treatment :-
1) Oral and systemic vitamine A administration (beneficial in pre xerotic stages).

2) Systemic vitamin "A" 100000 units deep I.M. injection, weekly twice for 4 weeks.
3) Antibioties, Atropin 1 % ointment, lubricant eyedrops etc are given.

## 2)    Vitamin B. Complex :-
Beneficial in Toxic retino neuropathy and Toxic amblyopias

### B1 (Thiamine ) :-
The deficiency causes Beriberi, Toxic retino neuropathy etc.
a) Paraplegic or dry beri beri, causes peri pheral neuritis ptosis and lesions of lateral rectus muscle.
b) Cardiac Beri beri or wet beri beri causes peripheral neuritis and ocular palsies.
c) Cerebral beri beri or Wernicke's encephalopathy causes ophththalmoplegia.

The sources are,
Lean pork, beans, peas, nuts, grains Flour, beaf, Yeast etc.

**Note :-** The daily requirment is 100 mg.

### B2 (Riboflavine ) :-
Sources are same as B1, The deficiency affects Glossitis, cheilosis, Vascularising Keratitis, Burning sensation in the eyes and Photo phobia. The daily requirement is 10 mg .

### Nicotinic acid :-
The deficiency causes pellagra, glossitis and skin lesions, The daily requirement is 150 mg.

### B12 (Cynocobalamine ) :-
The deficiency causes peripheral neuritis, it is useful in Trigeminal neuralgia, Herpes zoster and in Tobacco amblyopia. The daily requirement is 1000 micro grams.
### Vitamin " C" (Ascorbic acid ) :-
The deficiency causes scurey, ocular haemorrhages, chronic inflammation etc. **The daily requirment is 300 to 500**

### Vitamin "D" (Calciferol)
The deficiency causes Rickets, osteo malacia, tetany, altered Calcium metabolism, myopia cataract etc. The daily requirement is 1000 units.

**Vitamin " K" (Dimethylnaphthoquinone) :-**

The deficiency causes intra ocular haemorrhages. **The daily requirement is 20 mg.**

**Vitamin "P" (Flavone ) :-**

The deficiency causes intra ocular haemorrhages. The usual therapeutic dose is 1 gram daily.

The changes in the proteins, fats carbohydrates and minerals of the body tissue also produces visual problems.

1) In senile cataract :- Changes in proteins fats etc causes denaturation of Lens, leads to cataract.

2) Denaturation of scleral coat (Thinning) due to malnutrition may leads to Anterior or posterior staphyloma, myopia etc.

3) Anaemia (Raktha dhathu Kshaya) May produce so many changes in Retina and optic nerve .

4) The changes in the ratio of Calcium and phosphate, sodium and potassium may produce cataract .

5) Iron and Folic acid deficiency (vitamin minarals) also produces visual errors.

# B) EYE DISEASES IN COMMON INFECTIONS

## 1) In Septic Abortions :-
a) endophthalmitis b) Orbital cellulits

## 2) In measles :-
a) Conjunctival hyperaemia, sub conjunctival haemorrhage b) Kopliks spots in Conjunctiva & Xerosis c) acute muco purulent conjunctivitis d) Optic neuritis - dimvision.

## 3) In Diphtheria :-
a) Membranous conjunctivitis b) Paralysis of accommodation c) Paralysis of extra ocular muscles, especially lateral rectas. muscles. especially lateral rectus.

## 4) In Typhoid Fever :-
a) Logophthalmos corneal ulcer b) optic neuritis.

## 5) In Whooping cough :-
a) sub conjunctival haemorrhage, orbital haemorrhage, proptosis.

## 6) In mumps :-
a) Acute dacryo cystitis  b) Uveitis.

## 7) In meninngo coccal meningitis :-
a) Metastatic conjunctivitis b) Loss of pupillary reaction c) paresis of extra ocular muscles d) metastatic endophthalmitis and panophthalmitis e) complete loss of vision due to optic neuritis.

## 8) In Tuberculosis :-
a) Conjunctivitis, Interstitial Keratitis, uveitis, chorio retinitis etc.
b) Tubercular meningitis may lead optic atrophy c) Intra cranial tuber culoma may produce papilloedema .

## 9)     In Syphilis (Acquiried ) :-
In Primary stage chancre of the conjunctiva and conjunctivitis occurs

In Secondary stage :-  Uveitis and nodules develop on the iris.
In tertiary stage :-  Chorio retinitis development of gummata in the orbit.
In congenital syphilis:- Interstitial Keratitis, Uveitis and chorio retinitis develops.

**6)    In Leprosy :-**

Nodules on the skin of the eye lids, falling of the hairs of eye lashes and eye brows, conjunctivitis, Keratitis, pannus formation, leucoma, Lepromatous nodules on Sclera, Granulomatous Uveitis and Dacryocystitis develops.

**C)    Parasitic Infections :-**
**I) In Malaria :-**
   a) Dendritic ulcer of cornea
   b) Embolism of retinal artery develops.

**2) In toxoplasmosis :-**
   Necrotizing chorio retinitis develops particularly in infants.
3    In taenia echino coccuas infection :-
   a)Hydatid cyst in the orbit .
   b) Intra cranial cyst formation may produce papilloedema.

**4)    In Taeniasolium Infection:-**
   a) Cysticercus cyst in retina and vitreous .
   b) Cyst formation the orbit - & Conjunctiva.

**D)    Metabolic diseases.**
1) In gout and Rheumatism
   a) Episcleritis Scleritis and Uveitis develops.
2) In Diabetic mellitas
   a) Changes in refraction.
   (When blood sugar falls causes Hyper metropia, when blood sugar raises cause myopia)
   b) Haemorrhagic iritis and new blood vessels on the Iris.
   c) Diabetic cataract
   d) Diabetic retinopathy
   e) Lipaemia retinitis (Retinal vessels appear as filled with milk.
   f)   extra ocular muscle palsies
   g) Optic neuritis etc develops.

**E) Diseases of Kedney - Nephritis :-**

   1) Passive oedema of eye lids.
   2) Renal retinopathy develops. (Flame shaped retinal haemorrhages and woolly exudates in retina)

**F) Toxaemia of Pregnancy :-**
   1) Loss of vision due to spasm of retinal vessels.
   2) Retinopathy (retinal detachment due to transudation in the sub retial space)

## G) Cardio vascular system :-
1) Hypertensive retinopathy
2) Benign and malignant hyperten.
3) Cardiac regitation from mitralsion Valvular disease causes central retinal artery occlusion.

## H) Blood Diseases :-
1) In Leucaemia
   a) Dilatation of Vessels
   b) Retinal haemorrhages
   c) Sub Conjunctival haemorrhages.

2) In purpura and haemophilia
   a) Sub conjunctival retinal and orbital haemorrhages develop.

3) In pernicious anaemia Retinal haemorrhages are seen with central white spots.

## I) Intra Cranial Lesions :-
   1) Meningitis a) Cerebrospinal meningitis produces unilateral paralysis of 3,4 and 6 cranial nerves, papillitis and endophthalmitis .b) Tubercular meningitis produces papillitis and papilloedema.
2) encephalitis causes 3rd nerve palsy, ptosis, nystagmus and paresis of convergence.
3) In sub dural haematoma papilloedema occurs.

4) In sub arachnoid haemorrhage
   a) Sub hyaloid haemorrhage in retina b) proptosis c) Ocular palsies occur

5) In Intra cranial tumours.
   a) Papilloedema b) Ocular palsies (in pitutory tumour - Bi temporal hemianopia occurs).

6) In head inury .
   a) Contraction of the pupil
   b) Dilatation of pupil without pupillary reflex due to raised intra cranial pressure.
   c) Paralysis of extra ocular muscles if the base of the skull is involved.
   d) Optic atrophy e) Sub conjunctival haemorrhage
   f) Field defects if Visual path way is affected.

7)  In intra cranial aneurisms .
   a) Aneurisms in the vessels of circle of willis causes ocular palsies.
   b) Aneurisms of the internal carotid artery, out isde the cavernous sinus causes optic atrophy.

c) Aneurism of internal carotid artery inside the cavernous sinus causes oculomotor palsies and pulsating exophthalmos.

8) In migraine - central vision defects and hemianopia are produced.

## J)    Demyelinating diseases.

1) In disseminated sclerosis causes Nystagmus, Dim vision, due to retro bulbar neuritis, and extra ocular palsies.

2) In neuro myelitis optica (Devic's disease ) Causes sudden blind ness due to papillitis, and dilatation of pupil due to loss of visual acuity

3) Schlders disease (encephalitis peri-axialis diffusa) causes blindness papilloedema and optic atrophy .

## K)    Diseases of Muscles :-

1) In myasthenia gravis

Causes ptosis and defect in the eye move ments due to weakness of muscles.

## L)    Endo Crine Disorders :

1) In thyrotoxic exophthalmos, or grave's disease (excessive thyroxin secretion).

a) Bilateral Exophthalmos which is reducible on pressure.

b) Retraction of the upper lid .

c) Lid lag on attemp to lookdown .

d) Weakness of convergence

e) Pigmentation of skin of upper lid.

2) In Thyro trophic exophthalmos (Excessive thyrotrophic hormone).

a) Marked proptosis which is irreducible on pressure.

b) Marked chemosis of Conjunctiva and oedema of the lids.

c) Exposure Keratitis

d) External ophthalmoplegia.

e) Optic atrophy

3) Deficient secretion of thyroxin causes cretinism in infants it causes puffy eye lids, posterior cortical cataract and in adults it causes myxoedema it produces solid oedema of eye lids.

4) Parathyroid deficient secretion (Tetany) may cause cortical cataract.

5) Pitutory tumour causes Bitemporal hemianopia (Loss of vision in both temporal sides ) later nasal sides also affects and causes complete blindness.

# INJURIES TO THE EYE LIDS AND EYE BALL

Injuries of the eye lids and eye ball can be grouped under the following categories.
1) Mechanical injuries 2) chemical injuries .
3) Thermal injuries 4) Electrical injuries.
5) Radiational injuries.

I)      **Mechanical injuries :-**
        a) Contusion injuries b) penetrating or perforating injuries c) Retained Foreign bodies.

**a) Contusion injuries caused by blunt instruments :-**
**Clinical Features :-**
**1)      Eye Lids :-**
        Ecchymosis or bruising of eye lids or Haematoma (Black eye) of eye lids occurs. The injury causes swelling of eye lids and surrounding tissue, it may be impossible to separate the eye lids for several days But the blood gradually becomes absorbed and full ocular mobility is restored. Immediate cold compress is needed to stop furthur bleeding.
**2) Conjunctiva :-** Lacerated with sub conjunctival haemorrhages.
**3) Cornea :-** Abrasions, corneal opacities etc. causes dimvision, photophobia discomfort and Lacrimation.
**4) Sclera :-** Get Ruptured with Prolapse of Uveal tissue and even vitreous (if the injury is severe.)
**5) The Anterior chamber :-** Hyphaema, increased intra ocular pressure and reddish brown cornea..
**6) Iris - Pupil :-** Traumatic miosis due to irritiation of nerves, then traumatic mydriasis due to paralysis of pupillo motor fibres, Iridodialysis (detachment of Iris from ciliary body), Antiflexion of Iris, irregular pupil and traumatic aniridia entire iris may torn off from ciliary body and sinks to the bottom of anterior chamber.
**7) Lens :-** Concussion cataract, Sub luxation of Lens, and dislocation of Lens.
**8) Vitreous humour :-** Liquification of vitreous, vitreal haemorrhages, opacities, organisation of opacities (may lead to Retinitis proliferans,)
**9) Retina :-** Retinal oedema, Retinal haemorrhages, and retinal detachment.
**10) Choroid :-** Rupture of choroid and choroidal haemorrhages.
**11) Optic nerves :-** Avulsion of optic nerve which is rare.
**12) Intra ocular pressure :-** Secondary glaucoma or hypotony of eye ball.

**Treatment :-**

**Blackeye :-** Cold compress, bandage,
**Subconjunctival haemorrhage :-** Naturally disappears within 2 or 3 weeks and Local eye drops like argyrol is useful.
**Rupture of Cornea and Sclera :-** Suturing and ulcer therapy.
**Hyphaema and Raised intra Ocular Pressure :-**
Paracentesis to drain the pus.
**Corneal abrasions without glaucoma ;-**
1% Atropin sulphate drops (mydriatics) Hydro cortisone drops and antibiotics are useful
**Irido donesis & Irido dialysis :-** Surgical correction.
**Concussion cataract :-** Cataract surgery.
**Dislocated Lens :-** Lens should be removed.
**Choroidal, Vitreal and retinal Haemorrhages:-** Prognosis is not good, rest and laser therapy etc. are beneficial upto some extent.
**Traumatic Glaucoma :-** (Miotics) diamox caps etc and surgery are useful.
**Any foreign body :-** If lodged in cornea sclera etc.- should be detected and removed.

B)     Penetrating or perforating injuries. by sharp instruments. or small particles travelling at a high speed.

In this lesion apart from actual trauma there is always high risk of introduction of infection into eye ball that cause severe complications.

a) Vertical cut injury of lid may cause cicatrisation and ectropion, a wound on the lid margin produces a notch (traumatic coloboma).
b) Wounds of Conjunctiva (incised or lacerated) associate with sub Conjunctival haemorrhages.
c) A penetrating corneal wound always leaves behind an opacity after healing. there is always a chance of falling of intra ocular pressure immediately following the injury due to leakage of aqueous humour through the perforation.
d) Wounds of the sclera - a penetrating injury of sclera commonly associated with prolapse of uveal tissue and also vitreous. .
e) Wounds of the Lens - cause traumatic cataract and may also cause secondary glaucoma.
f) Infection by spreading through the perforation may cause severe iritis, Iridocyclitis, hypopyon, panophthalmitis etc complications.
g) Risk of sympathetic ophthalmia in the other eye.

**Treatment :-**

i) Injury of lids must be carefully repaired in layers if not causes epiphora ectropion and coloboma of lids.

2) Removal of obvious dirt by normal saline wash very gently.

3) Excision of or separation of entangled intra ocular tissue.

4) Repair of the wound - Anti infective treatment (corneal -scleral tear suturing)

5) Instillation of 1 % atrophin sulphate solution with eye bandage ( contra indicated in glaucoma )

6) Exogenous infection should be controlled by sub conjunctival anti biotics. or cortisones.

7) If lens is affected cataract surgery should be done

8) If secondary glaucoma develops miotic eye drops and diamox 250 mg caps daily twice by month should be given.

9) Corneal opacity should be corrected by Keratoplasty.

10) Anterior synechia is corrected by synecheotomy to prevent secondary glaucoma.

**C) Retained Foreign bodies :-**

These are of two types 1) Extra ocular Foreign bodies and 2) Intra ocular foreign bodies.

**1) Extra ocular foreign bodies :-** particles of coal, dust, iron, husk of paddy, wings of insects etc. lodge in the conjunctiva ( in sub tarsal furrow) or embedded in the corneal epithelium or in the substancea propria. There is immediate discomfort, watering and foreign body sensation ( blepharo spasm and severe discomfort present in corneal foreign bodies). Corneal foreign bodies may produce severe complications like corneal abrasions, opacities and ulcerative keratitis etc.

**Treatment :-**

1) Identification of the location of foreign bodies.

2) Removal of Conjunctival Foreign bodies with a sterile swab stick after application of Local anaestetic drops.

3) Corneal Foreign bodies should be removed with a spud or needle.

4) Application of antibiotic, and atropin ointment.

**2) Intra Ocular Foreign bodies with perforating wound in the eye ball:-**

The foreign bodies which commonly penetrate the eye are, particles of Iron, stone, glass, lead or spicules of wood etc. signs and symptoms depend upon the size and shape of foreign body and the extent of its entry into the eye ball ( The features of perforating or penetrating wound are observed ) it causes spread of infection into the eye and cause gross damage to the eye even end either with endophthalmitis or panophthalmitis.

The metalic particles stimulate Local reaction and fibrosis, Iron particles produces specific degenerative changes known as SIDEROSIS and copper particles produces CHALCOSIS .

**Treatment ;-**
   A Thorough Examination of eye ball is needed to ascertain whether the Foreign body has actually penetrated the eye ball or not.

   1) Clinical examination of each part with corneal loupe, ophthalmoscope, slit lamp and by special radiographic techniques and the location of the Foreign body should be detected.

   2) Either by a hand magnet or forceps the foreign bodies should be removed from the interior of eye ball.

   3) Wound healing therapy.

## CHEMICAL INJURIES OR BURNS

   External contact of chemicals in the form of solid liquid powder or gas, occuring in private houses laboratories or in Industries etc In general chemical burns comprises two main groups a) Alkali burns b) Acid burns.

**a) Alkali burns :-** These are more dangerous than acid burns,usually lime caustic soda, caustic potash, liquid ammonia or ammonium hydroxide etc are responsible agents.

**Changes in the ocular tissue :-**
   The proteins are converted into gel like alkaline proteinates (soap or soft gelatine like ) destruction of cell membrane, Lipoids are digested and become soft, so the chemical agent penetrates deep in to the tissues and causes necrotic changes in the tissues.

**Conjunctiva :-** Marked congestion oedema, necrosis, profuse purulent discharge and symblepharon.

**Cornea :-** Destruction of epithelium, formation of opacities - ulcers and even the cornea may slough out causing anterior staphyloma.

**Uveal Tissue :-** Inflammation and the normal tissue replaced by granulating tissue.

**Lens :-** Become cataractous.

**Eye ball :-** get atrophied.

**Note : -**

At, PH 11. 00 to 11.2 alkalies cause severe damage to the tissue . The severity of the damage increases with the rise of P.H.

## b) Acid Burns or Injuries :-

Inorganic acids like sulphuric acid, Hydrochloric acid, Nitric acid, are the common agents those cause injury to eye ball.

Strong acids causes instant coagulation of all the proteins with the formation of insoluble protinates (coagulative necrosis) this coagulated protein acts as a barrier so that there is no penetration of the chemical in to the deeper tissues and thus the lesion becomes sharply limited.

The ocular lesions are,

**Conjunctiva : -** There is necrosis followed by sloughing of tissues with symblepharon .

**Cornea :-** Sloughout completely and staphyloma forms.

## Treatment of chemical burns.:-

1) Thorough wash of conjunctival sac with plain water or normal saline Immedialtely .

2) Chemical particles if any remained. it must be carefully removed with swab sticks.

3) Necrotic tags of Conjunctiva should be excised .

4) 1 % Atrophine sulphate, Steroids, Antibiotic ointment should be used to subside the inflammation and to create a suitable condition for the repair.

5) Soft contact lens application temporarily to prevent symblepharon.

6) Symptomatic therapy should be given to prevent secondary infection etc.

# III) THERMAL INJURIES TO EYE BALL

These are usually caused by contact with hot bodies like glowing coal or molten metal or hot fluids. The ocular lesions depend upon the size and temparature of the hot body or fluid. it causes severe damage to conjunctiva and cornea. Ex :- at $47^0$ C causes damage of corneal epithelium, at $65^\circ$.C Stroma suffers and at $80^0$ C all the parts affects.

**Treatment :-**

1) Cold therapy 2) Excision of necrotic tags. 3) Instilling 1 % atropine sulphate ointment, steroids and antibiotics to subside the inflammation and burning pain .

4) Severe corneal damage can be corrected by Keratoplasty .
5) Symptomatic treatment.

## IV) Electrical injuries to eye ball :-

High voltage electric current if passess through the head, near the orbit can cause ocular lesions like the follwing .
1) Ciliary and conjunctival congestion .
2) Punctate or diffuse interstitial corneal opacities.
3) Iritis and Irido cyclitis
4) Retinal haemorrhages and optic neuritis.
5) Electrical cataract.

**Treatment :-**

1) Lens extraction in Cataract.
2) Instillation of 1% atropin sulphate, Steroids and antibiotic eye drops.
3) Sub conjunctival cortisones and Antibiotics
4) Symptomatic treatment.

## V Radiational Injury. :-

Any radiation if absorbed by a tissue causes radiational injuries , like the following.

## 1) Thermal Lesions :-

It occurs due to sudden release of a large amount of radiation as in exposure to arc lights or prolonged exposure to arc lights or prolonged exposure to small amount of radiation **ex:-** Development of cataract due to proloned exposure to infra red rays in furnace works and glass workers etc.

**2)    Abiotic lesion :-**

Exposure to ultra voilet rays which occurs in workers engaged in oxy acetylene or arc welding (Photophthalmia)

**3)    Ionizing lesions :-**

the lesions commonly seen in workers who deal with radio active Ionising paints for coating the figures on the dials of clocks, who undergone deep xray therapy or radium therapy to the tumours of lids or eye ball. The Hair follicles eye lashes eye brows and lens (cataract) are affected.

**Treatment :-** 1) Wearing dark glasses to prevent the exposure of infra red or ultra voilet radiation. 2) For photophthalmia cold compress, Atropine, steriods and antibiotics, xylocaine drops, Bandage, relieve the symptoms.

## Burns of Eye lids :-

Fire caustics, ultra voilet light or Beta and gamma radiation may cause great disfigurement, scarring, contraction of tissue, ectropion exposure keratitis and visual disability. Superficial burns affect only a part of the epithelium and are characterised by blistering, they are painful sensitive and rapidly heals without complications. Deep burns involve total destruction of the epithelium, scarring in sensitive surface, slow healing, metabolic disturbances and with complications for the management :-

1) Foreign bodies and necrotic tags should be removed 2) Oily drops instillation to prevent adhesion 3) Blisters are left intact 4) Dusting of antibiotic powders 5) Parenteral administration of antibiotics 6) Anti inflammatory and analgesic drugs 7) Superficial burns heal within 14 days 8) Deep burns which require longer time (More than 30 days) should be treated by skin graft at the earliest oppurtuntiy, this accelerates healing and prevents contracture.

**Burns of Conjunctiva and Cornea :-**

The conjunctiva and cornea may be burnt by caustic alkalis such as caustic soda and lime, by caustic acids such as hydro choric acid salphuric acid Nitric acid etc. Alkalis cause more damage than acids. Burns cause destruction of the conjunctiva and corneal epithelium and induce inflammatory reaction in the subepithelial layer. The common clinical features are congestion and necrosis of conjunctiva, corneal abrasions opacities ulcers Blepharo spasm, photo phobia, Dimvision, symblepharon and may also cause panophthalmitis.

**Treatment :**

1) Irrigating the eye with tapwater or normal saline 2) Causative agent traces should be removed 3) Neutralising the causative agent a) Irrigating with weak acetic acid when injury occurs due to caustic alkalis b) Irrigating with weak sodium bicarbonate when injury occurs due to caustic acids.

4) Instillation of oily eye drops, 1 % atropin sulphate Hydrocortisone drops etc. 5) Putting of soft contact lens to prevent symblepharon 6) Bandaging.

# PARALYSIS OF THE EXTRINSIC OCULAR MUSCLES.

Extrinsic ocular muscles are 6, they are 4 recti muscles and 2 oblique muscles. These perform the following actions.

| S.No. | Name of the muscle | Action | Nerve Supply. |
|---|---|---|---|
| 1. | Superior rectus | elevation and inward rotation. or intorsion | Oculo motor. Nerve(3rd Cranial) |
| 2. | Inferior rectus | Depression, adduction and out ward rotation (Extorsion) | -do- |
| 3. | Medial rectus. | Adduction or inward movement | -do- |
| 4. | Lateral rectus | Abduction or out ward movement. | abduscens nerve (6th cranial) |
| 5. | Superior oblique | Depression, intorsion and abduction. | Trochlear Nerve ( 4th Cranial) |
| 6. | Inferior oblique | Elevation, extorsion and abduction. | Oculomotor nerve (3rd cranial) |

## The Extra ocular muscles and the movement of eye ball :-

1) Adduction or inward movement :- although the medial rectus is the main muscle, The superior and inferior recti also assist.

2) Abduction or outward movement - although lateral rectus is the main muscle, inferior and superior obliques also assists.

3) Direct elevation :- Superior rectus is assisted by inferior oblique

4) Direct depression :- Inferior rectus is assisted by superior obliqe

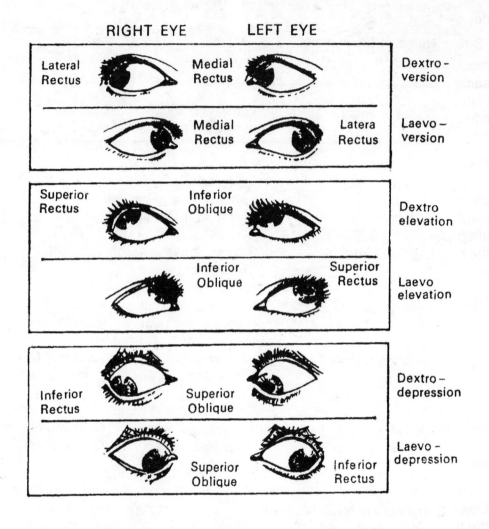

RIGHT EYE        LEFT EYE

Lateral Rectus | Medial Rectus — Dextro-version

Medial Rectus | Latera Rectus — Laevo-version

Superior Rectus | Inferior Oblique — Dextro elevation

Inferior Oblique | Superior Rectus — Laevo elevation

Inferior Rectus | Superior Oblique — Dextro-depression

Superior Oblique | Inferior Rectus — Laevo-depression

Conjugate movements of the eyeball (May and Worth)

5) Wheel rotation inward (intorsion ) :- It is mainly produced by superior oblique and assisted by superior rectus.

6) Wheel rotation outward (Extorsion ) :- It is mainly produced by inferior oblique and assisted by inferior rectus .

The associated movements or conjugate movements of eye balls. are reguulated by the centre in the brain. The conjugate movements occurs in the same direction with the visual axes (parallel,) this conjugate movements are distrubed (convergence or divergence) in the paralysis or paresis of extra ocular muscles either single or more and produces deviated visual axes, that may cause disturbance in the binocular vision.

**Binocular Vision :-**
The both eyes are concerned in the act of vision so the image of an object is focussed on the macula of the both eyes, these two images are involutarily adjusted in the brain for the fusion of two images to form a single image, it is known as Binocular vision, it is possible when the visual axes of the both eyes are parallel and when image fall on macula exactly, if not, it may leads to diplopia and other complications.

**Diplopia :-**   a) Homonymous diplopia
b) Heteronymous diplopia
c) Torsional diplopia
d) Diplopia in palsy of muscles.
e) Diplopia by placing a prism in front of one eye.

**a) Homonymous diplopia :-** In Binocular diplopia if left eye is fixed at an object (normal image form at forea) and right eye  deviates inwards with the image at nasal side, projects the object to the right of its position (Horizontal diplopia)

**b) Heteronymous or Crossed diplopia :-** If left eye is fixed at an Object (normal images  forms at fovea ) & right eye deviates out wards with the image at the right of macula, projects the object to the left of object by crossing. (horizotnal diplopia ) in vertical diplopia the false image may be situated either above or below the true image (False image forms in the position which is opposite to the deviation of eye ball.

**c) Torsional diplopia :-**
If affected eye is intorted the false image leans out wards and if affected eye is extorted the false image leans inwards.

d) Diplopia occurs in ocular palsy and also e) by placing a prism of adequate strength infront of one eye.

# TYPES OF OCULAR DEVIATION

**1) Paralytic ocular deviation :-** In paralysis, defective function of one or more ocular muscles causes occular deviation, it is known as paralytic squint or strabismus.

2) Non paralytic squint or strabismus (Concomitant squint or Strabismus) it is due to anomalies of the power of convergence and divergence, A concomitant deviation is almost always Horizontal one (vertical deviation is rare, if occurs that is paretic origin).

A team of six muscles controles the move ments of eyes, four of them are the recti muscles responsible for rotating the eye ball in four cardinal directions (up, down, out and in ) and the 2 oblique. muscles rotate the eye globe obliquely. The motility of the eye is controlled by voluntary and reflex mechanisms centred in cerebral cortex. **The lesions at the supra nuclear** Pathways produce conjugate deviations or paresis of both eyes equally which does not cause diplopia though themovements and positions are abnormal, due to the maintenance of relative coordination. **The lower neurous** affecting the nuclei, the nerves, the muscles produce diplopia and other paralytic squint features due to disturbed relative coordination. **The Kintetic Squint** is produced due to irritative intracranial lesions, irregular spasmodic contractions, un equal stimulation of nerve centres and due to to over action of certain muscles.

## Aetiology :-

There are various causes for extra ocular muscle palsy, they are

A) Lessions of nerve supplying the muscle.

**Ex :-** encephalitis, neuro syphilis, disseminated sclerosis, neoplasms, Aneurisms, thrombosis haemorrhage or embolism, trauma, peripheral neuritis.

B) Lession of muscle it Self :- Abnormal insertion of a muscle or congenital musculo facial anomalies, trauma, myopathic conditions like myasthenia gravis, thyrotoxic and ocular myopathies.

**Signs and Symptoms :-**

**Symptoms :-**
     1) Diplopia is the chief complaint and may be present in all or in certain directions of gaze.
     2) vertigo nausea uncertain gait are associated if affected eye is kept open. on this account patients frequently keep the affected eye closed or covered.
     3) Loss of binocular vision without diplopia are also observed in certain cases of ocular palsy of congenital origin .
     4) Defective or excessive movement of affected eye in one or more directions.
     5) Compensatory head posture or Tilting of head (ocular torticollis) in one direction, especially found in cases of congenital ocular palsies, it is adopted to prevent diplopia and maintain binocular single vision.

**Signs :-**
     **1) Deviation :-** The angle of squint varies with the direction of gaze. The angle is maximum when the eye attempts to look in the direction of action of the paralysed muscle and there may not be any deviation in opposite direction.
     **a) Primary deviation :-**
     When the good eye fixes an object infront, the deviation recorded in the affected eye is called primary deviation
     **b) Secondary deviation :-**
     When the good eye is covered and the paralysed eye is made to fix an object, the deviation shown in the covered eye is called secondary deviation.
     " The secodary deviation is always greater than the primary deviation in paralytic squint."

**2) Compensatory head posture :-**
     a) In paralysis of the horizontally acting muscles , the head is turned to the direction of action of paralysed muscle.
     b) If a vertically acting muscle in involved, there is tilting of head to one or other side (ocular torticollis ) together with depression or elivation of the chin depending on muscle which is affected (head tilting is more marked in paralysis of the oblique muscles.)
**ex :-** If Right Lateral rectus muscle is paralysed, the right lateral movement of eye ball is restricted so the head turned to the right for the compensation to avoid diplopia etc.

**Note :-** Diplopia Nausea Vomitings etc are counteracted Partially by altering the position of head or by shutting or covering the affected eye.

3) Limitation of movement of affected eye in the direction of action of the paralysed muscle, it is recognised when the patient keeps his head fixed and tries to follow the Examiner's finger which is moved in different direction.

**4) False Projection :-**

The Paralysed eye does not see objects in their correct Location, it is due to increased innervation conveyed to the nerve supplying the paralysed muscle in an efford to force it to act, it can be examined by closing the patient's sound eye and telling him to point out quickly on object infront of him, with paralysed eye.

**Varieties of Ocular Palsies :-**

1) One muscle may be involved or Several muscles may be in volved. Lateral rectus and superior oblique commonly affected Isolately. In complete 3 rd nerve palsy rest of 4 muscles, sphincter pupillae and ciliary muscle etc are totally affected.

a) Single muscle involvement :- Either It is lateral rectus or superior oblique muscles .

b) External ophthalmoplegia:- Involvement of Recti and oblique muscles

c) Internal ophthalmoplegia :-Involvement of ciliary muscles and sphincter muscles.

d) Total or complete ophthalmoplegia :- 4 Recti. muscles, 2 oblique muscles, ciliary muscles ans sphincter muscles are involved.

e) Congenital ocular Palsy - Here diplopia may be absent due to supression of the false image by the brain by adapting compensatory head posture.

**f) Paralysis of the lateral rectus :** -There is limitation of movements out wards, face is tuned towards the paralysed side, Homonymous diplopia occurs on looking towards paralysed side, the images are same level and errect.

**g) Paralysis of Superior Oblique :-** There is limitation of movements down wards and towards sound side, the face is turned down wards and towards sound side, Hornonymous diplopia occurs on looking down, the false image is lower and its upper end is tilted towards the true image.

**h) Paralysis of Oculomotor nerve :-** Most of the muscles are paralysed and ptosis proceeds. on raising the eye lid diplopia with crossed higher tilted image occurs towards paralised side.

**Treatment :-**

1) Indentification of the cause is very important for the assessment of result (No recovery takes place in assoication with head injury) .2) Waiting for some period of time for giving scope for spontaneous recovery.3. If dipopia is trouble some the affected eye should be occluded or using proper prisms.4) Eye exercises 5) Surgical correction.

# CONCOMITANT SQUINT OR
# NON PARALYTIC SQUINT OR STRABISMUS

Concomitant squints are produced by some anomalies of the convergence or divergence mechanism (supra nuclear affection). If is almost always have horizontal deviation (vertical deviation is rare if occurs that is paretic origin. ) The visual axes don't meet at the desired objective point, i.e., one eye is fixed upon a certain object while the fellow eye is turned away, but have full range of movement and achieve the binocular single vision (No problem of diplopia ). It is of two types
> 1) Heterophoria or Latent squint
> 2) Heterotropia or Manifest squint.

## 1) Heterophoria Or Latent Squint :-
It is a condition where there is a tendency of the visual axes to deviate from their normal alignment and which constantly being corrected by the neuro muscular effort prompted by the desire for binocular single vision.

**Orthophoria :-** Normal physiological condition in which the visual axes maintain a perfect parallelism

**HeteroPhoria :-** May be of 5 types depending on the direction of deviation.

| | | |
|---|---|---|
| 1) | Esophoria - | Convergent squint (Nasal side) |
| 2) | Exophoria - | Divergent Squint (Temporal side) |
| 3) | Hyperphoria - | Visual axis of one eye deviates upward in relation to that of the other eye. |
| 4) | Hypophoria - | Visual axis of one eye deviates downward inrelation to the other eye |
| 5) | Cyclophoria - | Wheel rotation of eye ball in ward or out ward (torsional) |

## Etiology :-
Predisposing factors :- ill health,eyestrain worries
anxieties,proffessional prolonged close working (Tailers, proof readers, watch repairers etc). refractive errors anatomical defects (wide or  narrow inter pupillary distane ) Orbital asymmetry etc may cause squint.

## Symptoms :-
If strong neuro muscular power present that compensate the heterophoria and no symptoms are produced.

Symptoms present only in decompensated heterophoria they are,

1) Head ache 2) Aching of the eyes especially after prolonged use of the eyes .3) Difficulty in changing focus from distant to near objects and vice versa 4) Blurring of vision 5) Intermittent diplopia usually under fatigue conditions. 6) Intermittent squint may occur.

**Treatment :-**

1) Cause should be treated.

2) Correction of refractive errors. 3) Eye straining things worries anxieties should be avoided.

4) Improvement of health .

5) Eye exercises

6) Usage of proper power prisms .

7) Surgical correction where heterophoria is due toanatomical defects.

# MANIFEST SQUINT OR HETEROTROPIA

The deviation present all the time, fixation is maintained with one eye but not with both eyes at a time the angle of squint remains constant in all directions. There is no limitation of movements in either eyes. The primary and secondary deviations are equall.

**Types :-**

A)   a) Intermittent - The deviation not presentall the time.

b) Constant - The deviation present all the time.

c) Uniocular - Deviation always manifested by same eye.

d) Alternating - Deviation is manifested and changing in the either eyes at different times.

B)   a) Convergent squint - Visual axes are convergent

b) Divergent Squint - Visual axes are divergent

c) Vertical Squint - Upward or down ward deviation of visual axes.

**Aetiology :-** 1) Congenital defective development of extra ocular muscles 2) Refractive errors 3) Lesions of accommodation 4) Paresis of some extra ocular muscles 5) Heriditory factors 6) Debilitative disorders in child hood.

**Symptoms :-** 1) Physical deformity due to deviation of visual axis. 2) Refractive errors 3) Head ache and eye strain.

**Treatment :-** 1) When the visual axes become parallel binocular single vision is restored. 2) Correction of refractive errors.3) Orthoptic treatment (when angle of squint is small) 4) Surgery (in the presence of big Visual angle.)

# NYSTAGMUS

The Normal fixation of the eyes (Steady fixation) is made possible by the neuro muscular coordination of the extrinsic ocular muscles, the retina, Vestibular apparatuas, proprioceptive end organs of cervical musculature which provide sensary stimuli, motor activity by the effect of oculo motor (3rd Cranial ) nerve, and the muscle tone controle by cerebellum etc. So the lesions of any above may result in " involuntary ocular movements " which is termed as nystagmus.

Nystagmus is defined as a disturbance of ocular posture which consist of involuntary rhythmical oscillatroy rotatory deviations of the eyes, usually affecting the both eyes.

A)      1) Pendular nystagmus (both phases of the movement are of equal speed ) a) Horizontal b) Vertical c) Rotatory d) Oblique

2) Jerking nystagmus (The movement is speed in one phase and slow in another phase )a) To Right b) To left c) to up d) to down e) Right rotatory f) Left rotatory g) oblique up to right h) oblique down to right.

B)      1) Ocular or fixation nystagmus
        a) Physiologically induced nystagmus
        b) Spontaneous nystagmus (Due to blindness, defective central vision etc.

2) Vestibular nystagmus (Due to lesions of vestibular apparatus)
3) Nystagmus of central (Brain ) Origin
4) Congenital idiopathic nystagmus
5) Hysterical nystagmus.

**Clinical Features :-**
        1) These depend upon the type of lesion..
        2) Central vision is poor 3) Giddiness 4) Nausea
        5) Improper fixation of objects (moving)

**Treatment :-**

Cause should be identified and treated.

# DISEASES OF THE ORBIT

The orbit is a quadrilateral bony cavity contains the eye ball with optic nerve extra ocular muscles, Lacrimal gland vessels and nerves. all these structures are supported by Orbital fat. The Periosteum lining the bony walls of orbit is called the periorbita, infront the orbital base is partially closed by a septum extending form the upper and Lower orbital margins to the tarsal plates known as septum orbitale.

## ORBITAL INFLAMMATION

It is of 3 types
1) **Periostitis :-** Inflammation of periorbita
2) **Orbital cellulitis :-** Inflammation of the cellular tissue of orbit .
3) **Tenonitis :-** Inflammation of the Tenans capsule which separate the eye ball from orbital contents.

**1) Periostitis :-**

Inflammation of the periorbita is known as periostitis, it is very rare, peri osteum near the orbital margins is commonly involved. Occasionally deeper periorbita. may be affected.

The pridisposing factors are suppurative processes in paranasal sinuses, Tuberculosis syphilis Trauma etc.

The Clinical features are a tender swelling which is fixed at the orbital margin, redness of the skin, collection of pus at the lession. discharge of pus through newly formed fistula and some times it may burst through orbital roof producing septic meningitis cerebral abscess etc.

**Treatment : -**
1) Treatment should be given for the principal disease (Like Tuberculosis syphilis etc)
2) Broad spectrum antibiotics
3) Evacuationof pus to prevent the spread of infection and to prevent fistula formation.
4) Symptomatic treatment.

**2) Orbital Cellulitis :-**

Inflammationof the cellular tissue of the orbit, usually terminating in suppuration.

**Causes :-** 1) Extension of inflammation from the neighbouring parts (Paranasal sinuses, teeth etc ) 2) Traumatic lesions 3) Facial infection (erysipelus - Furunculosis) 4) Meta static lesions (Pyaemia - septicaemia)

**Clinical Features :-**

1) Swelling of lids with chemois 2) Eyeball is proptosed with reduced movements of the globe 3) Pain and diplopia follows when attempt to move the eye ball 4) Vision rarely affected (Due to retrobulbar neuritis ) 5) Fever headache and discomfort in the body 6) Formation of abscess and spread of infection, if not treated properly and in time.

**Complications :-**

1) Optic neuritis 2) Meningitis - Brain abscess
3) Cavernous sinus thrombosis 4) Pan ophthalmitis.

**Treatment ;-**

1) Cause should be treated 2) Systemic broad spectrum antibiotics 3) Local heat application .4) Pus drainage by giving incision in the skin near the orbital margin .5) Symptomatic treatment.

**3) Tenonitis :-** It is the inflammation of the Tenons capsule of eye ball, It is a rare condition.

**Clinical Features :-** 1) Swelling of lids with chemosis 2) Proptosis 3) Limitation of eye ball movements 4) Painful movements of eye ball 5) Pan ophthalmitis treatment 1) Broad spectrum antibiotics 2) Evacuation of pus if formed 3) Symptomatic treatment.

**Tumours of Orbit :-**

Tumours of orbit are not very common

**1) Benign Tumours :-** Dermoid cyst, Dermo lipoma, osteoma,Angioma, neuro fibroma.

**2) Primary tumours of optic nerve :-** Glioma, Endothelioma, Fibroma

**3) Malignant Tumours :-** Sarcoma, Lympho sarcoma, carcinoma of Lacrimal gland.

**4) Secondary tumours :-** Extension from Naso pharyngial carcinoma, breast carcinoma hyper nephroma and neuroblastoma of adrenal medulla.

**Clinical Features :-**1) Unilateral proptosis, 2) Mobility of globe is impaired 3) Diplopia, 4) Visual loss 5) Palpable growth 6) Papilloedema
7) Optic atrophy.

**Treatment :-** Surgery and Radiation .

# UNI OCULAR PROPTOSIS

It is uni lateral protrusion of eye ball.

**Causes :-**1) Haemorrhage in the orbit .2) Inflammatory lesions of oribt
3) Vascular lesions of orbit4) Neoplasms of orbit.
5) Invasion of some mass into orbit from surrounding structures etc.

## लेख्य रोग

उत्सङ्गिनी बहलकर्दमवर्त्मनी च
श्यावं च यच्च पिठितं त्विह बद्धवर्त्म ॥
क्लिष्टं च पोथकियुतं खलु यच्च वर्त्म
कुम्भीकिनी च सह शर्करया च लेख्या: ॥

(सु. उ. 9/2)

## भेद्य रोग

श्लेष्मोपनाहलगणी च विसं भेद्या ग्रन्थिश्च य: कृमिकृतोंजननामिका च ॥

## छेदन रोग

अर्शोन्वितं भवति वर्त्म तु यत्तथार्श:
शुष्कं तथाबुंदमथो पिडका: सिराजा: ॥
जालं सिराजमपि पंचविधं तथार्म
छेद्या भवन्ति सह पर्वणिकामयेन ॥

(सु. उ. 8/6)

# LEKHANA SADYA ROGA

## Shastra Chikitsa Procedure

**Lekhana sadya rogas are 9 , they are**

1) Utsangini     2) Kumbheeka     3) Pothaki
4) Varthma sharkara     5) Bahala varthma     6) Varthma
bandha
7) Klista Varthma     8) Kardama varthma
9) Shyava Varthma.

**The surgery is explained in 3 Stages :-**

1) poorva karma     (preparation of the Patient)

2) Pradhana Karma (method of operation)

3) Pashchyath Karma (Post operative regimen)

## 1) Poorva Karma (Preparation of the patient for Surgery) ;-

a) Snehan (Oral administration of oleus drugs) b) Vaman c) Virechan d) Patient is asked to lie down (utthana shayan ) on operative table where there is no dust air and heat pollution e) Patient should be controlled or holded by his friends, not to move during Lekhana therapy f) Eye lid should be everted for mrudu Sweda with a soft cloth by dipping in Lukewarm water. g) Everted Eye lid should be firmly gripped to conduct Lekhana therapy successfully.

## 2) Pradhana Karma (Lekhana Therapy ) :-

a) Lekhana procedure commonly associate with pracchana chedana Bhedana etc. Procedures, (according to the condition of the diseases).

b) If eye lid is hard (kapha vata vitiation) Lekhan has to do with shastra

c) If eye lid is soft (Pitta Raktha vitiation) Lekhana has to do with leaves like shephalika etc.

d) In Utsanini Kumbheeka and Varthma Sharkara - **Chedan** and **Lekhana** has to do (in pakwa granthi **bhedan** and Lekhana has to do).

e) In varthmavabandha, klista Varthma, Bahala varthma and Pothaki **pracchana** and **Lekhana** has to do.

f) In shyava varthma and Kardama varthma uniform superficial Lekhana has to do

g) 1)   Chedan pracchana has to do with mandalagra shastra.

   2)   Lekhana with mandalogra shastra or shephalika patra- Gojihwa patra etc.

   3)   Bhedana with Vreehi mukhu shastra,

## 3) PASHCHYATH KARMA (POST LEKHANA REGIMEN)

After the coagulation of beeding or exudations.

1) Mrudu sweda and pratisaran has to do.

With fine powders of manahshila Kaseesa, shunthi, maricha pippali, saindhava lavan rasanjan etc drugs and Honey.

2) After 5 to 10 minutes eye should be cleaned. with Lukewarm water.

3) Then Ghritha seka and Bandhana.

4) Treatment like wound healing therapy

5) 4th day nasya Karma Should do

6) After 5th day onwads Bandage should be removed.

**Note :-**  In pothaki after Lekhana therapy prathisaran is advised with shunthi & saindhava lavan and pariseka with khadhira Aadhakee shigru decoction and Haridra Daruharidra Triphala Yastimadu decoction and madhu ).

## A) Symtoms of Adequate Lekhana therapy :-

1) Bleeding or other discharges should not present.

2) No itching sensation at the lesion.

3) No oedema

4) Relief from the problem ordisease

5) Gaining normal condition.

## B) Symptoms of inadequate Lekhana therapy :-

1) Bleeding 20 Hyperaemai 3) Oedema 4) Abnor mal exudations 5) Dimvision 6) Problem is not relieved 7) Blackish Oedematous rigid eyelids with itching and sticky exudates with itching and sticky exudates 8) Inflammation of eye lids.

## c) Symptoms of Excess Lekhana Therapy :-
1) Pakshma shatha 2) Pain 3) Increased exudations
4) Severe bleeding 5) Agravation of the disease with complications.

**Treatment ;-** 1) Vata hara sneha Sweda Pariseka 2) Lodhra Navaneetha should paste to erenda moola and processed according to puta paka - the extracted swarasa + Aja Ksheera - Aashchyotan has to do 3) Lodhra Navaneetha + Shalidhanya - puta pakwa swarasa + Ajaksheera Aashchyotan has to do swarasa + aja Ksheera Aashchyotan has to do.

# BHEDAN SADYA VYADHIES SURGICAL PROCEDURES :

Bhedan Sadya Vyadhies are 5, they are 1) Anjana namika 2)Lagana 3) Bisa varthma 4) Krimi granthi 5) Sleshmopanaha.

## The Common surgical treatment principles :-
1) Snehan 2) Swedan 3) Shodhan (Virechan etc) 4) Bhedana (giving incision ) with vreehi mukha shastra 5) Pooya nirharan (evacuation of pus) 6) Prakshalan (cleaning the wound) 7) Pratisaran (applicatin of medicine) 8) Bandan (Bandaging) 9) Vrano pachar (Wound healing therapy) 10) Following the pathya vidhi.

1) Poorva Karma (Preparationof the patient) Like in Lekhana therapy
**2) Pradhana karma :-**
a) Giving incision (Bhedana ) with vreehi mukha shastra to evacuate the pus.
b) In pain less bigger sleshmopanaha Lekhana and Bhedana should do .
c) In Bleeding type of upanaha pracchana and bhedan shouuld do.
d) Bigger type of Lagana - Bhedana, Kshara, Agni Karma should do.

**3) Pashchyath Karma :-** Pratisaran and Bandan with the following drugs.
1) In Anjana Namika Pratisaran with - manahshila Ela, Tagara saindhava lavana + Honey or Rasanjan + honey or Deepa shikha masi anjana.

**2) Lagana :-** Prathi saran with - Gorochan yava kshara, Tuttha, pippali and Honey

**3) In Bisa varthma :-** Pratisaran with Saindhava lavan kaseesa, pippali, pushpanjan manahshila Ela and Honey or ghee .

**4) In Krimi grandhi :-** Pratisaran with manahshila ela Tagara saindhava lavan + Honey or Triphala kwatha Tuttha kaseesa saindhava lavan Rasakriya - anjan or Rasanjan + madhu anjan.

**5) Sleshmopanaha :-** Pratisaran with pippali saindhava lavana and Honey.

# CHEDAN SADYA ROGA SHASTRA CHIKITSA PROCEDURES

Chedan sadya rogas are 11, they are
1) to 5) - 5 types of arma
6) Sirajala 7) Sira pidika 8) Parvani 9) Varthma arsha
10) Shushka arsha 11) Vartma arbuda.

**Note :-** Chedan therapy is common for all the diseases

**5 types of Arma chedan Chikitsa :-**
a) Thin smaller membranous arma - only Lekhana therapy suggested.
    Ex. Prastari arma, shukla arma and kshataja arma.
b) Thick wider fibrous membranous arma chedan and Lekhana suggested.
    Ex. Adimamsa arma and snaya arma.

Poorva karma - (preparation of the patient for Excision therapy ).
    1) Sneha and Sweda
    2) Shareer shodhan (Vaman virechana vasti etc.
    3) Shiro shodhan (Nasya)
    4) Oral administration of oleas foods
    5) Lavan Pratisaran to disintigrate the tissue of arma.
    6) Patient should be well prepared, physically and mentally for the
        therapy .
    7) Patient is perfectly holded by his friends during the therapy.

**Pradhana Karma :-** Chedan Karma (Excision therapy )
    1) Patient is asked to see towards apanga (outer canthus ) if the
    arma is towards kaneenika and eye lids are widely opened.
    2) Mrudu sweda at the lesion
    3) Separation of arma from the floor with badisha (hooks ) and thread
    4) Elevation of arma with muchundi (Forceps)
    5) Arma is separated and cut at the krishna mandala, then the flap is
lifted towardsKaneenika Sandhi and 3/4th part of arma is cut with mandalagra
shastra by leaving the 1/4 th part as residue to prevent the complications like
Nadivrana Rakta srava and Drustinasha
    6) The Residual part of arma  should be Scraped out by the applica-
tion of Lekhana anjana afterwards.

**Pashchyath karma :-** Post Excision regimen.
    1) Pratisaran with Yavakshar shunthi, pippali, maricha and lavan.
    2) Mrudhu Swea 3) Ghritha Seka 4) Cheen Bandan 5) After 3 to 5 days
Bandage should be opened to observe the healing process 6) Wound healing
therapy 7) Treatment of the complications if any.

After the excision of arma, if pain is assoicated that should be treated with the following aashchyotan (eye drops)

1) The decoctions should be prepared with Karanja beeja, Amalaki, Yasti madu and milk (should prepare according to Ksheera paka vidhi ) + Honey.

2) Application of Yastimadu, Kamal Kesar, Doorva + Milk + ghee .

3) The residual part of arma should be scraped with the application of Lekhana anjana.

**Symptoms of adequate Excision :-**
1) Getting of normal colour to eyes .
2) Painless movements of eye ball
3) Relief from the problems etc.
4) No bleeding itching and exudation.

## 6) Siajala 7) Sira pidika chedan Chikitsa :-
Similar to arma chikitsa
( 1)Chedan 2) Lekhan 3) Pratisaran)

**8) Parvani Chedan Chikitsa :-** Similar to Arma, 2/3 of Parvani should be cut with mandalagra shastra, and 1/3 should be scraped with Lekhana anjanas.

Pratisaran with saindhava lavan + Honey

**Anjana for the sirajala, Sira pidika and Arma :-**

Shankhadyanjan - Shankha nabhi samudraphena , Matsya Spatika padmaraga pravala Ashmantak Vydoorya pulak, mukta Loha Tamra + equally Srotonjan - Fine powder should prepare for the Anjan therapy.

**9) Varthmarsha 10) Shuskarsha 11) Arbuda Shastra Chiktisa :-**

Same as Arma Chikitsa.
1) chedan 3/4 or 2/3 should be cut withmandalagra shastra.
2) Pratisaran with saindhava lavan kaseesa and pippali choorna.
3) 1/4 or 1/3 Residual part should be burnt with shalaka
4) If any residue is remained that should be scraped by Lekhana or Kshara anjana.

# नेत्र क्रया कल्प

सेकं अश्च्योतनं पिण्डी बिडालक स्तर्पण स्तथा
पुटपाकं अंजनं श्चेति कल्पो नेत्र मुपाचरेत्

## आश्च्योतन और सेक

यथादोषोपयुक्तं तु नातिप्रबलमोजसा।
रोगमाश्च्योतनं हन्ति सेकस्तु बलवत्तरम्॥

(सु. उ. 18 अ.)

## सोक आश्च्योतन विधि

''प्रागेवाक्ष्यामये कार्य त्रिरात्रं लघुभोजनम्।
उपवासस्त्र्यहं वा स्यान्नक्तं वाप्यशनं त्र्यहम्।
ततश्चतुर्थे दिवसे व्याधि संजातलक्षणम्।
समीक्ष्याश्च्योतनै: सेकैर्यथास्वमुपपादयेत्॥
''आश्च्योतनं सर्वाक्षिरोगेष्वाद्य उपक्रम:।
नानाद्रव्यकल्पनया च रागाश्रु घर्षरुग्दाहतोदभेदपाकशोफकण्डुघ्नम्॥

(अ॰ स॰. सू॰ ३२ अ॰)

## सेक आश्च्योतन मात्र

लेखने सप्त चाष्टौ वा विन्दव: स्नैहिके दश॥
आश्च्योतने प्रयौक्तया द्वादशैव तु रोपणे।
सेकस्य द्विगुणो  काल: पुटपाकात् परोमत:
अथबा कार्यनिर्वृत्तेरुपयोगो यथाक्रमम्।

(सु. उ. 18 अ.)

## अंजन प्रयोज्य

व्यक्तरूपेषु दोषेषु शुद्धकायस्य केवले॥
नेत्र एव स्थिते दोषे प्राप्तमंजनमाचरेत्।
लेखनं रोपणं चापि प्रसादनमथापि वा॥

(सु. उ. 18 अ.)

## अंजन प्रमाण

हरेणुमात्रा वर्ति: स्याल्लेखनस्य प्रमाणत:।
प्रसादनस्य चाध्यर्धा द्विगुणा रोपणस्य च॥

रसांजनस्य मात्रा तु यथावर्त्तिमिता मता ।
द्वित्रिचतु:शलाकाश्च चूर्णस्थानुपूर्वश: ॥

(सु. उ. 18 अ.)

## बिडालक

विडालका बहिर्लेपो नेत्रे पक्ष्मविवर्जिते ।
तस्य मात्रा परिज्ञेया मुखलेपविधानवत् ॥

## पिण्डी वा पिंड़िका

पिण्डी कवलिका प्रोक्ता उच्यते वस्त्रपवृकै: ।
नेत्राभिष्यन्दयोग्या सा व्रणेष्वपि निगद्यते ॥

## तर्पण

संशुद्धदेहशिरसो जीर्णान्नस्य शुभेदिने ॥
पूर्वाह्णेवापराह्णेवा कार्यमक्ष्णोस्तु तर्पणम् ॥
वातातपरजोहीने वेश्मन्युत्तानशायिन: ॥
आधारौ माषचूर्णेन क्लिन्नेन परिमण्डलौ ॥
समौ दृढावसम्बाधौ कर्त्तव्यौ नेत्रकोशयो: ॥
पूरयेद् घृतमण्डस्य विलीनस्य सुखोदके ॥
आपक्ष्माग्रात्तत: स्थाप्यं पंच तद् वाक्शतानि तु ॥
स्वस्थे, कफे षट्, पित्तेष्टौ, दश वाते तदुत्तमम् ॥
रोगस्थानविशेषेण केचित् कालं प्रचक्षते ॥
यथाक्रमोपदिष्टेषु त्रीण्येकं पंच सप्त च ॥
दश दृष्टावथाष्टौ च वाक्शतानि विभावयेत् ॥
ततश्चापाङ्गत: स्नेहं स्रावयित्वाक्षिशोधयेत् ॥
स्विन्नेन यवपिष्टेन, स्नेहवीर्येरितं तत: ॥
यथास्वं धूमपानेन कफमस्य विशोधयेत् ॥

(सु. उ. 18 अ.)

## पुटपाक के भेद

तत: प्रशान्तदोषेषु पुटपाकक्षमेषु च ॥
पुटपाक: प्रयोक्तव्यो नेत्रेषु भिषजा भवेत् ।
स्नेहनो लेखनीयश्च रोपणीयश्च स त्रिधा ॥

(सु. उ. 18 अ.)

# NETRA KRIYA KALPAS (TREATMENT PROCEDURES)

In Ayurvedic samhitas, the local treatment procedures of netra are explainled in the name of Netra Kriya kalpa, they are

1.  **Charaka** Mentioned 3 Kriya Kalpa 1) Bidalaka 2) Aashchyotana 3) anjanam (varthi, choorna - rasakriya )

II.  **Sushrutha** mentioned 5 kriya kalpa.
    1) Seka 2) Aashchyotana 3) Anjana 4) Tarpana 5) Putapaka.

III. **Sarangadhara** mentioned 7 kriya kalpa.
    1) Seka 2) Aashchyotana 3) Pindi 4) Tarpana 5) Bidalaka.
    6) Putapaka 7) Anjana.

**" Vagbhata followed sushutha and Bhavanamishra followed sarangadhara in the description of Kriya Kalpa" :-**

**I) Seka :-** It is indicated in acute condition of the diseases. " Medicine is poured on closed eyes (on closed eye lids) continuously, from 4" height, for a specific time, according. to doshas "

**Types :-**

I)   3 types : 1) snehan 2) Ropana 3) Lekhana
II)  2 types : 1) Ushna seka 2) Sheetha seka.

| S.No. | Name of the method | Dosha Predominence | Duration / time. | Nature of medicine |
|-------|--------------------|--------------------|------------------|--------------------|
| 1. | Snehan | In vata disorders | 400 matra kalas (Aparahna) | Luke warm, Oily,madhura Amla Lavana aushada has to use. |
| 2. | Ropana | In Pitta & Raktha disorders | 600 matra Kala (madyahna) | cool, madhura Tiktha Kashaya Aushada has to use |
| 3. | Lekhana | In Kapha disorders | 300 or 200 matra Kala (Poorvahna) | Luke warm, Katu, Tiktha Kashya Aushadas has to use. |

**" In the Acute condition it can be done at any time "**

After the treatment, eyes should be washed or cleaned with Luke warm water, and advised not to see the bright things and not to take Kapha Vrudhikara Aahara and vihara.

**Samyak Seka Lakshanas** 1) Roga Nivruthi ( Relieved from disease) 2) Swabhavika Varna ( getting natural colour) 3) Karya Patutwa, (Perfectness in the functions of the parts) 4) Vedana shanthi (Relief from pain etc)

**Seka Yogas :-**

1) Seka with medicated milk prepared from Erenda twak, patra, moola Ajadugda, is used in vataja Abhishyanda 2) seka with medicated milk prepared from Saindhava Lavana and in Aja dugda is used in vataja Abhishyanda. 3) Seka with medicated milk prepared from Lodhra, Yastimadu, (taken in equal quantity, fry in ghritha,) Ajaksheera is used in Pitta and Raktha abhishyanda.4) Seka with medicated milk prepared from Triphala lodhra Yastimadu manjista Sariba Kamala, grinded with water and can be used in pittaja and Rakthaja Abhishyanda.

## II) AASHCHYOTANA

The medicated drops are put into eyes from 2" height, the doctor has to open the eyes of the patient with his left hand and has to put the drops with his right hand.

In sheetha ruthu And in pitta Raktha disorders cool medicine is used.

In ushna ruthu and in vata and kapha disorder luke warm medicine is used.

The medicine has to Kept in the eyes for 100 matra Kalas, after wards eyes should be cleaned with Luke warm water (Mrudu Sweda), and adivsed not to see the bright things.

**Types :-** 3 types, 1) Lekhana 2) Ropana 3) Snehana

| S.No. | Name of the method | Dosha Pradha natha. | dosage of medicine | Nature of medicine |
|---|---|---|---|---|
| 1) | Lekhana | Kapha Vikaras | 7 to 8 drops | Luke warm, katu Tiktha Kashaya medicine. |
| 2. | Ropana | Pitta & Raktha vikaras | 12 drops | cool, madura tiktha kashaya medicine |
| 3. | Snehan | Vata vikaras | 10 drops | Luke warm, oily madhura amla lavana medicine. |

1) In Kapha vitiation Aashchyotan has to do in Poorvahna (Morning)
2) In Pitta vitiation Aashchyotana has to do in madhyahna (After noon)
3) In Vata vitiation Aashchyotana has to do in Aparahna (evening)

**Note :-** Aashchyotana is contra indicated at night.

# AASHCHYOTANA YOGAS

**1)** Aashchyotana with Triphala kashya is used in all types of Abhishyanda.

**2)** Aashchyotana with Stanya (Breast milk) can be used in vata, pitta and Raktha Abhishyanada

**3)** Aashchyotana with Ksheeri sarpi or ksheeri Navaneetha can be used in vataj pitta and Rakthaj Abhishyanda.

**4)** Aashchyotana with the decoction of Bilwadi panchamoola, Erendamoola, shighru Bruhathi, is used in vataj Abhishyanda.

**5)** Aashchyotana with the medicated milk prepared from Kantakari moola, is used in vataj Abhishyanda .

**6)** Aashchyotana with Aamalaki phala swarasa, can be used in pittaja Abhishyanda.

**7)** Aashchyotana with medicated milk prepared from Draksha Yastimadu, manjista, jeevaneeya dravya and milk

**8)** Saindhava lavana, shunti + ghritha kept for a month, after that with stanya Aashcyotan can be done in Netra paka.

**9)** Aaschyotana with Shigru patra swarasa in Raktaj abhishyanda

**10)** Aaschyotana with  Milk + ghee in Raktaj Abhishyanda.

## III) " PINDI OR KAVALIKA OR PINDIKA "

Medicated paste is kept in a fresh thin cloth and applied on the eyes is named as pindi.
1) In vata diseases - oleus hot medicine has to use .
2) In pitta diseases - Cool medicine has to use.
3) In Kapha diseases Rough hot medicine has to use.

### PINDI YOAGA

1) Pindi with Triphala in all types of Abhishyanda.

2) Pindi with Aamalaki or maha nimba patra in pittaja Abhishyanda.

3) Pindi with Shigru patra, or Nimba patra in Kaphaja Abhishyanda.

4) Pindi with Lodhra which is fried in ghritha, grinded with Kanji is used in pitta and Raktha Abhishyanda.

5) Pindi with Erenda patra, mool in vataj abhishyanda.

6) Pindi with Nimba patra + Shunti + Saindhava lavan - in Kaphaj abhishyanda.

## IV) BIDALAKA (Varthma Lepa)

Application of the medicated paste to the eye lids (externally,) except at the eye lashes (Pakshma).
Types of Bidalaka  According to thickness of the medicated paste,
If the lepam is

| | | |
|---|---|---|
| 1 " thick, | it is Utthama | (The best) |
| 1/3 "    " | Madyama | (Moderate) |
| 1/4"    " | Heena | (Minimal) |

## BIDALAKA YOGA

Application of the mediciated paste to the eye lids with following medicines.

1) Yastimadu, gyrica, saindhava lavana, Daru haridra, Rasanjan+ water in all types of Abhishyanda.

2) Neel Kamal, musta Daruharidra Kaleeyaka Yastimadu Lodra padmaka + Shatadhautha ghritha in Raktaj Abhishyanda.

3) Rasanjana in Kaphaj Abhishyanda

4) Hareetaki + Shunti + Tejapatra in Kaphaj Abhishyanda

5) Kumari + Chitraka patra in Kaphaj Abhisyanda

6) Dadima patra in Pittaj Abhishyanda

7) Vacha + Haridra + Nimba patra used in Kaphaj Abhishyanda

8) Shunti + Gyrica. in Kaphaj Abhishyanda

9) Lodhra get fried in Ghee and used in Vataj Abhishyanda.

10) Chandan + sariva + manjista + padmaka + yastimadu + jatamamsi Tagara + Lodr + jathi pushpa and Gyurica used in pittaj Abhisyanda.

## V) ANJAN

Application of medicine to the internal surface of lid margin from Kaneenika sandhi to apanga sandhi, with anjana shalaka is known as Anjana.

## CLASSIFICATION OF ANJANA ACCORDING TO ACTION OF THE DRUG.

1) Lekhana anjana :- Used in Kapha predominent disorders, drug has to prepare with all except madhura rasa.

i.e. in vata pradhana ; with the predominence of Amla - Lavan rasa

| | | |
|---|---|---|
| Pitta | " | Tikta Kashaya rasa |
| Kapha | " | Katu Tiktha Kashaya |
| Raktha | " | Kashaya  Tiktha |

317

**Note :-** Anjana scrapes and expels the dosha from Netra, varthma, sira, Netra Kosha and Ashru Vaha srotas, through the mouth, Nose and eye.

**2) Ropana Anjanam :-** The drug shoud be oily, with the predominence of tiktha and Kashayarasa, it gives strength and complexion to the eyes.

**3) Prasadan anjan :-** It is Prepared with madhura and sneha predominent medicines

It is used for drusti prasadana (improvement of vision) and to remove the roughness of drusti (Drusti snehana)

**Note :-** In vata rogas at evening, pitta roga at nights and in kapha roga mornings anjana has to do.

II)      **Classification of anjan according to akruthi (nature of the drug)**
1) Gutica 2) Rasakriya 3) Choora

A)      **Gutica or  Varthi:-** Is used in strengthy disorders (mahabala roga) .
B)      **Rasa Kriya :-** Is moderate type of diseases ( in madyama bala roga)
C)      **Choorna:-** Is used in Heenabala roga ( in minimal vitiation)

A) Gutica    a) Lekhana gutica    -       1 Harenu matra (dosage)
             b) Ropana gutica      -       1 1/2 Harenu matra
             c) prasadana gutica,          2 Harenu matra

B) Rasa Kriyaa) Lekhana Rasa Kriya  -   1 Harenu
              b) Ropana Rasa Kriya  -   1 1/2 Harenu
              c) Prasadana Rasa Kriya -  2 Harenu

C) Choorna   a) Lekhana choorna  -    2 Shalaka
             b) Ropana choorna   -    3 shalaka
             c) Prasadan choorna-     4 shalaka

III)    Classification of Anjana according to Karma or Potency of drug
(Dravya veerya )

1) Mrudu anjan                        2) Teekshna Anjan

   a) Snehan
   b) Ropana                          Lekhana
   c) Prasadana

IV)     Classification of Anjanas according to rasa (Drug taste)
1) Madura anjana 2) Amla anjana 3) Lavana Anjana 4) Katu anjana
5) Tiktha anjana 6) Kashaya anjana.

# ANJANA SHALAKA ANJANA PAATRA

| Anjana paatra (Vessel ) | | Rasa of the Anjana drug |
|---|---|---|
| Swarna Paatra | " | madura rasa drug |
| Roupya paatra | " | Amla |
| Mesha shrunga paatra | " | Lavana |
| Tamra or Loha paatra | " | Kashaya |
| Vydoorya paatra | ' | Katu |
| Kamsya paatra | " | Tiktha |

## Anjana Shalaka :-

**Note :-**Shalaka should prepare with the metals as above

**Ex :-** 1) for madura rasa anjana    shalaka should be prepare, with gold;etc
2) for Lekhana Karma,    shalaka should be prepared with Tamra
3) Ropana karma  -  "    "    Loha shalaka
4) Prasadana karma -   "    "    Swarna shalaka

Anjana shalaka should be 10 Angulas length, the two ends. should be blunt (should not sharp ).Like jasmine (flower ) , should be easy for handling, and should not be rough, thin, hard, and breakable.

## when anjana has to apply :-

1) Body should be purified by siravyada virechana Nasya vasti etc.
2) Aamaavasta should be eliminated.
3) The eye should be free from Aama and should exhibit normal doshic symptoms, then only affer Ashchyotan Anjjana has to do.

## ANJANA VIDHI

1) Mangalacharana 2) Devatha prarthana
3) Then patient is asked to sit without fear and tension.
4) Doctor with his left hand, has to open the eyes of the patient, and with his right hand he has to handle Anjana shalaka and has to do Anjana from Kaneenika sandhi to apanga sandhi and from Apanga sandhi to Kaneenika sandhi .
5) Anjan should not be more or less, hard or soft, Teekshna or mrudu, quick or delayed, if so causes injury to eyes
6) After anjana vidhi, by closing the eyes, eye ball should be rotated gently, eye lids should be moved slowly - by this the medicine perfectly spreads in the eyes.
7) The doshas dissolves and comes out in the state of lacrimation,
8) The eyes should be cleaned when discharge stops.
9) If required according to the condition **prathyanjana** has to give.

# ANJAN NISHEDHA
## (Contra indication of Anjana)

Anjan vidhi is not advisable for the following conditions or diseases like shrama, vegavarodha, udavartha, Rodan, madyapan, krodha, Bhaya jwara, shirodosha, Shirasnana, Netra aaghatha, sunstroke, pipasa, vomitting. Jagara, Nasya, rechan, Dhomapan.

If Anjana has given in above states causes Netra raga (Hyperaemia) srava (exudation), shoola (pain), shotha (oedema), Timira (Dimvision), and difficulty in opening and closing the eye lids.

## ANJANA YOGA

**1) Choorananjana yoga :-**
   **a) Sauveer Chooranjan :-**
Heat the sauveeranjan and dip in the Triphala Kashaya, for 6 times then 7th time has to dip in stanya, then the drug should be dried and powdered, this is useful in most of the eye diseases.
   b) Maricha 1/2 part, pippali, samudra phena 1 part, saindhava lavana 1/2 part, sauveeranjan 1 part, togetherly powdered and used as anjan, in Kacha and netra vikaras.
   c) shireesha beeja, maricha, pippali and saindhava lavan, choornajan used in savrana shukla

**2) Rasakriyanjan Yoga :-**
   **a) Krishna sarpa vasa rasakriya anjan:-** Krishna sarpa vasa, Shankha, Nirmali phala, is useful in Andhatwa( Blindness).
   **b) Guduchi rasakriya anjan ;-**Guduchi swarasa 12 grams, madhu 1 gram, saindhava lavana 1 gram mixed and grinded toghether, It is used as anjan, in Arma Timira etc. Netra vikara.
   **c) Babbola patra rasa kriyanjan** Used in Netra srava.
**3) Gutika Or varthi anjana Yoga :-**

**1) Karanja varthi anjan :-**
Karanja beeja choorna Bhavana in palasha pushpa swarasa for many times. and used as the varthi anjana is in Netra pushpa.

**2) Samudraphenadi Varthi anjan :-** Samudra phena, shankha, Kukkutanda twak, shigru beeja,the prepared varthi anjan is used in shukra.

**3) Naktandya nashini varthi anjan :-**
Rasanjan, Haridra, Daruharidra, jathi patra, Nimba Patra - grinded with go maya ras and used as varthi anjan.

**Note :-** Generally Lekhana anjanas will be in powder form.
Ropana and prasadana anjanas will be either in varthi or Rasakriya form.

# VI) AKSHI TARPANA

It is one among 7 Kriyakalpa, it gives nourishment to the eyes and cures the vata pitta vikara (Preventie as well as curative effects).

In this process the unctuous (oily) substance is kept in the eye for a specific time by special arrangements.

Indications 1) Tamyatha 2) Stabdatha 3) Shushkatha 4) Rukshatha 5) Abhighatha 6) Vata pitta vikara 7) Jihwatha 8) Katina varthma 9) Kruchronmeelan 10) Sirothpatha 110 Sira harsha 12) Arjuna 13) Abhishyanda 14) Adhimantha 15) Anyathovatha 16) Vata paryaya 17) Shukra roga 18) Sheerna pakshma.

## Contra indications :-

1) Durdina (cloudy day ), 2) Ati ushna Atisheetha ruthu ( Hot or cold seasons),  3) Chintha (worries ), 4)  Aayasa (un easyness), 5) Bhaya (fear), 6) Shoka (weeping), 7) Shotha (Oedema), 8) raga (Hyperaemia), 9) Vedana (pain), 10) upadrava. (complications),

## Procedure of Tarpana Vidhi
## Poorvakarma :-

Kaya shodhana by vamana, virechan, vasti Rakthamokshan etc and Shiro shodhana with Nasya should do.
It can be given both in the morning and evenings.

## Pradhana Karma :-

In sadharana ruthu (In normal season ) either in themorning or in the evening it should be done.

The place should be Rajo dhooma rahitha. (without dust and smoke), Prakashavan (With bright light). Then the patient is asked to liedwon (utthana shayanam), with the paste of yava or masha, masha pali has to prepare and stick around the eyes in 2 " height, it prevents the medicine not to escape out from eye cavity. The medicine (ghritha manda ) has to melt by putting the vessel in hot water **( Taptha ambu Pravilapitham),** the medicine has to pour into the cavity formed by masha pali while the eyes are closed **(nimeelitha Netram ),** up to the level of eye lashes **(Aapakshmaargrath)** and the patient is advised to open and close his eye lids gradually upto specific time according to vitiation.

| Aushada dharna Kalam<br>Diseased part | Duration of the<br>Procedure |
|---|---|
| 1) In Sandhigatha rogas | 300 matra kalas |
| 2) Varthma " | 100 " |
| 3) Shukla " | 500 " |
| 4) Krishna " | 700 " |
| 5) Drusti " | 800 or 1000 " |
| 6) Sarva " | 1000 " |

--

| | |
|---|---|
| 1) Vataja Vikaras | 1000 " |
| 2) Pittaja " | 800 " |
| 3) Kaphaja " | 600 or 500 " |
| 4) Swasta " | 500 " |

--

| | |
|---|---|
| 1) Vataja 1 day | |
| 2) Pittaja 3 days | Tarpana has to do |
| 3) Kaphaja 5 days | |

--

**as per Jejjata**

| Alpadosha | - | 1 day |
|---|---|---|
| madyama dosha | - | 3 days |
| Ati dosha | - | 5 days Tarpana has to do |

**as per Videha** in healthy condition

| | |
|---|---|
| | with 2 days gap. |
| Vataja | daily |
| Raktha, pitta, dosha 1 day gap (alternatively) | |
| Sanni Pathaj | 2 days gap |
| Kaphaj | 3 days gap |

**Pashchath Karma :-** 1) After specific time of tarpana the micine should be removed by doing a perforation in mashapali at temporal side.

2) The eyes should be cleaned with yava pista.

3) Ushnodaka (Luke warm water) Prakshalana.

4) Shiro virechana & dhooma pana to save the eye from kaphaj disorders

5) Patient is advised not to see Bright - things.

**Samyak Tarpitha Lakshanas :-**
1) Prakasha kshamatha (tolerance to light)
2) Swastyam (health)
3) Vishada netra (fresh eyes)
4) Laghu Lochana (Lightness in the eyes)
5) Swabhavika Nidra (Sound sleep )
6) Swabhavika varna of Netra angas (normal colour and complexion of the parts.
7) Vyadhi nivaranam (health gain)
8) Laghutwam in Nimeshonmeshanam
   (easy in closing & opening the eyes)

## ATI TARPITHA LAKSHANA

1) Gurutwa (heavyness in the eyes)
2) Avilatwa (dirty collections in the eye)
3) Atisnigda (oilyness in the eyes)
4) Ashrusrava (epiphora)
5) Kandu (itching sensation)
6) Upadeha (sticky debris collection in the eye)
7) Kapha complication.

## HEENA TARPITHA LAKSHANA

1) Rukshatha (Roughness)
2) Avilatha (dirtyness)
3) Netra sravas (Lacrimation and discharges)
4) Roga vruddhi (Aggravation of the disease)
5) Rupa darshana avaroda ( indistinct vision)

## VII) PUTA PAKA

Indications and procedure is like Tarpana but the medicine preparation is specific i.e., the medicine is (Swarasa) extracted by puta paka vidhi.
It is of 3 types .
1) Snehana putapaka 2) Ropana putapaka 3) Lekhana putapaka.
**Vagbhata :-** Explained prasadana putapaka instead of Ropana putapaka.

**Ratio of the drugs :-** Flesh 2 phala, dravya 1 phala, liquids 8 phala.

**1) Snehan puta paka :-** Used in Ruksha Netra, vata vikara, the medicine has to kept in the eyes for 200 matra kalas. 2 days can be given.

**The medical combination is** :-

Anupamamsa, vasa majja, kakolyadi varga dravyas, are used. The above medicines are grinded, bolus should be prepared and has to cover with vata hara patra and so on, this should be heated (Puta paka) swarasa should be extracted and used like in Tarpana Vidhi.

**2) Ropana puta paka :-**

Drusti balya. vata pitta Raktha vrana dosha hara. the medicine is kept for 300 matra kala, upto 3 days it should be done.

**Combination of medicine :-**

Jangala mamasa, madhu, ghritha Tiktha dravyas, stanya, the puta paka has to do for the perfect extraction of swarasa.

**3) Lekhana Puta paka :-**

It is used in the vitiation of Kapha dosha (Ati snigda patients). The duration is 100 matra Kala and the period is only oneday.

**Medicine Combination :-**

Jangala mamsa, Yakruth, Lekhana drugs like Kantha loha bhasma, Tamra bhasma, shankha bhasma. Pravala bhasma, saindhava lavana samudraphena, Kaseesa, srotonjan, dadhi, mastu, madhu, shunthi, maricha, pippali etc drugs.

Medicine should be extracted by Puta paka for the therapy.

# " ANJANA YOGA " FROM SUSHRUTH SAMHITHA UTTHARA STANA

**1) Anjana in shukra roga (of the children) :-**
Shankha nabhi and saindhava lavan grined with Godadhi and pasted to Rasanjan, daily 2 times upto 7 1/2 days, Later on the drug should be grinded, varthi is prepared and Anjana is given with water.

**2) Gutikanjan in Kukoonak disease :-**
Trikatu Palandu Yastimadu Saindhavalavan Laksha - equally taken and grinded with water to prepare Gutikaanjan.

**3) Gutikanjan in Kukoonak disease :-**
Nimba patra, Yastimaduka, Daru haridra, Tamra bhasma, Loha bhasma, and srotonjan or Neelanjan equally taken grinded with water to prepare gutikanjan

**4) Kukoonak hara anjan :-**
Manahshila, maricha, shankha nabhi, Rasanjan, Saindhava lavan, Guda, madhu, taken equally and grinded to prepare anjana.

**5) Kukoonak hara anjan :-**
Madhurasa (moorva ), Yastimadu, Aamra twak, ginded with water, to prepare anjana

**6) Kukoonak hara anjan :-**
Krishna loha antardhooma bhasma and ghritha or madhu given as anjan.

**7) Pathyadi varthi :-**
Hareetaki, Tuttha, Yastimadu, each 1 tula; maricha 16 tula, the fine powder of above drugs grinded with water and used as varthi anjan.

**8) Kamsyadi varthi :-** Or Rujapah varthi anjan
Kamsya mala (mase), yastimadu, saindhava lavan, Erendamoola - each 1 Tola; Bruhathi phala and moola 2 tola, grinded with Aja ksheera for 3 days, and pasted to copper vessel, next day again the paste should be grinded with Aja ksheera then pasted to copper vessel like this 7 times should grind and paste to the copper vessel. later on varthi should be prepared and pre-serve in a bottle, the varthi is used as anjana with Rose Water or water. In the pain ful lesions of eye ball.

## 9) Manahshilaadyanjan :-

Manahshila, Devadaru, Haridra, Daru haridra,Triphala, maricha, Laksha, Lashuna, Manjista, saindhava lavana, sukshma ela, swarna makshika bhasma, Lodra, Loharaja, Tamra raja, Tagara, Kukkutanda twak  - equally taken and the fine powder should be grinded with cow milk for 3 days, varthi anjana is prepared and used in Timira, Arma, shukra etc diseases.

## 10) Tagaraadyanjan :-

Tagar, Maricha, Jatamamsi, shaileya, each one part ; manahshila Teja patra 4 parts; srotonjan, Neelanjan 16 parts, Yastimadu 16 parts - powdered and Preserved for anjana to treat the kings.

## 11) Bhadrodaya Anjan :-

Kusta, chandan, Ela, Teja patra, Yastimadu, Anjan, Mesha shrung pushpa, Tagar, Saptha Ratna, Uthphala, Bruhati, Raktha Kamal, Nagakesar, usheer, pippali, Tuttha, Kukkutanda twak, Daraharidra, Hareetaki, Gorochan, maricha, Vibheetak, Gruhagopika - Powdered and preserved the anjana for the treatment of kings.

## 12) Shresta Choornanjan :-

Srotonjan or sauveeranjan 8 parts; Tamra bhasma 1 part; swarna bhasma, 1 part, Rajatha bhasma 1 part,. The medicines or heated and dipped seperately in the following liquids-

Go maya rasa, Gomootra, Dadhi, Goghrith, madhu, tail, Madya, vasa, majja, Eladi gana, Kashaya Draksha rasa, Ikshu rasa, Triphala Kashaya Sarivadi Kashaya etc. 3 times in each above liquids. Then the medicine is packed in a cloth and kept in Rain water for 7 days after wards the medicine is dried and spatica, pravala, Tagar bhasmas are added - The medicine is powdered and preserved to give anjana for the  kings etc.

## 13) Sannipathaj Timira Harnjan :-

Sauveeranjan is heated and dipped 21 times in Astamutra - Triphala kashaya - Then the Anjana is filled in the bone marrow cavity of Nishachar Pakshi and Kept for a month in flowing water after that the anjana is collected and grinded with mesha shrungi pushpa and Yastimadu choorna - and is used for anjan.

## 14) Kaphaja Timira hara anjan :-

Kaseesa Rasanjan Guda shunthi used as Rasa Kriyanjan

## 15) Kaphaj Timira hara anjan :-

Manashila, Trikatu, shankhanabhi, madhu, saindhava lavan, Kaseesa, Rasanjan, grinded with water - and prepared for Rasa kriyanjan.

**16) Kacha roga hara anjan :-**
        Mesha shrunga 1 part, sauveeranjan 1 part, 2 parts shankha nabhi - grinded into fine pwoder for anjana

**17) Kacha roga hara anjan :-**
        Phalasha, Rohitha, madhuk twak choorna, madhu, madhira, added and grinded to prepare the rasakriyanjan

**18) Pittaja Timira hara anjan :-**
        Rasanjan, Madhu, sharkar, manahsila, Yastimadu, grinded with water and used as Rasakriya anjana.

**19) Pittaja Timira hara anjana :-**
        Sauveeranjan, Tuttha, is grinded and fine powder prepared for anjana.

20)     Ghridhra, Sarpa, Kukkuta Vasa and yastimadu, grined and used for anjana in vataja timira

21)     Sroto anjan is grinded with Aja ksheera for 3 days and used for anjan in Kacha.

**22) Gutikanjan in Diwandya :-**
        Saindhava, lavan, shimbhee Trikatu, Sauveeranjan, manahshila, Haridra, Daruharidra. Go yakruth, Rakthachandan - the fine powder is made vati and preserved to use as anjan .

23) Go or Aja Yakruth pleeha fried in sarshapa taila - dried, powdered and used as anjan in Naktandya .

**24) Harenyadyanjan in Naktandya :-**
        Renuka, pippali, Aja asti - majja, Ela, Aja Yakruth - the fine powder is used as anjan.

25) Yakruth rasa + Sroto anjan used as varthi anjan in Naktandya.

**26) Aja medo anjan in naktandya :-**
        Aja meda, Aja Yakruth, Aja ghritha, pippali, saindhava lavan, madhu, Aamalaki, Drakwa, used as Rasa krianjan in Naktandya ( it is preserved in the cavity of Khadhira stick).

**27) Go mutradi Rasa Krianjan in Naktardya:-** Go mutra, go ghritha, samudra phena, pippali, madhu, Katphala, Saindhavlavan, The fine powder should be preserved in the cavity of vamsha stick for anjan.

28) Yakruth rasa - Triphala quath as rasakriya anjan in Naktandya.

**29) Go Mutradi rasakriya In Naktandya:-** Go mutra, go or Aja pitta, madira Yakrutha rasa, Amalaki rasa, should be prepared rasa krianjan for anjana.

**30) Manahshiladyanjan in Naktandya :-**
    Manahshila, Hareetaki, shunthi, maricha, pippali, Bala moola, Tagar, samudraphena, the fine powder should be grineded with Aja ksheera to pre-pare varthi anjan.

**31) Nakthandya Hara anjan ;-**
    Togar, pippali, shunthi, Yastimadu, Talispatra, Haridra, Daruharidra, musta, the fine powder should be grinded with aja Yakruth rasa to prepare varthi in the shape of yava to give anjan in Naktandya.

32) Srotonjan, Saindhava lavan, pippali, Renuka, the fine powder should be grinded with aja mutra to prepare varthi in the shape of yava to give anjana with Rose water in Naktandya.

**33) Kashmaryadi anjan in Diwandya :-** Kashmari pushpa, Yastimadu, Lodra, Daru haridra, Rasanjan, the fine powder should be grinded with Honey to give anjan in pitta vidagdha drusti.

**34) Pittahara sheeta anjan ;-**
    Rasanjan or Karpoora, sauveeranjan should mix with mamsa rasa (of pakshi) and grinded with the pitta of Kacchapa or Rihitha matsya - fine powder is prepared to give anjana in pittaja Abishyanda and pitta vidagdha drusti etc.

**35) Rasanjanadi anjan in pitta vidagdha drusti :-**
    Rasanjan, Amalaki Patra or jathi patra Swarasa, Madhu, Talisa patra, Gyrica, should be grinded with gomaya rasa for anjana.

**36)** Amra and Jambu Pushpa , should be grinded with Renuka Honey and Ghee  to give anjana in Blindness.

**37)** Raktha Kamal, Neel kamal, uthphala, kesari Gyrica, should be grinded with  Gomaya rasa, to prepare vati anjana with Gulabjal in Blindness.

**38) Kubjakadyanjan in blindess :-**
    The flowers of Kubjak, Ashok, shala, Amra, Nalini, priyanga, uthphala, Renuka, pippali, Hareetaki, Amalaki,  the grinded fine powder should be pre-served in the tube of vamshi for anjana.

39) Gyrica ,saindhava lavan, pippali ,Godantha bhasma ,as anjana in Blind-ness.

40) Gomamsa, maricha ,shireesha beeja, manahshila - as Anjana in Blind-ness

41) Kapitta (Patra with patra vruntha) choorna with madhu as anjana in blindess

42) Swayamguptha phala  choorna with madhu as anjana in blindess.

## 43) Shankadyanyanjan :-

Shankha nabhi, samudra phena, mastsya, spatica, padmaraga, praval, Ashmantak mani, vydoorya, muktha, Loha bhasma, Tamra bhasma - (equal parts.) srotonjan (equal, to all in total) the fine powder should be preserved in mesha shrunga vessel for anjana in Arma, sir jala, sira pidika.

## 44) Aklinna Praklinna Varthma hara anjan :-

Samudra phena, Saindhava lavan, shankha bhasma, shimbee, swetha maricha, the fine powder used for choornaonjan .

## 45) Aklinna Praklinna varthma hara anjana :-

Tuuttha, Rasanjan, Anjan, should grind with Rose water in a copper vessel and anjana is given with ghee.

46) Shrotonjan + Madhu given as anjan in praklinna varthma .

47) Amalaki patra phala 5 Tola, 40 tola water should heat up to 1/8 residue, then heated in a copper vessel to prepare rasa Krianjan, in Praklinna varthma.

48) Vamshi Moola Kashaya rasakriya should be prepared in a copper vessel for for anjana, in praklinna varthma roga.

49) Triphala quatha rasa kriya should be prepared in a copper vessel for anjana in praklinna varthma.

50) Phalasha Pushpa quatha rasaKriya should be prepared in a copper ves-sel for anjana in praklinna varthma .

51) Apamarga, quatha rasakriya should be prepared in a coper vessel for anjana in praklinna varthma .

52) Kamsya malam and Karpasa vastra masi and Aja ksheera well grinded for anjana in Praklinna varthma.

53) Kamsya malam and karpasa Vastra masi, maricha choorna, Tamra bhasma is used as anjana with Rose water in praklinna varthma.

**54) Kaseesadi rasa Kriyanjan in puyalasa :-**

Kaseesa, saindhavalavan, Ardraka - and madhu, well grinded and used as anjana.

**55) Rasakriyanjan in Puyalasa :-**

Kaseesa, saindhava lavan, Ardraka, Tamra bhasma, Loha bhasma and madhu well grinded and used as anjana .

**56) Jathipushpanjan in Netrapaka :-**

jathi pushpa, saindhava lavan, Ardraka, pippali, vidanga - the fine powders with madhu used as Rasa Kiryanjan.

57) Saindhava lavan, shunthi and ghritha used as anjana, in Netra paka

58) Dadima, Amlavetas, Ashmanthak, kola, kanji, saindhava lavan - water is added and boiled upto 1/4 residue, then the prepared rasa Kriya is used for anjana in Netra paka.

59) Saindhava lavana and ghee should kept in a copper vessel for a month and anjana is given in Netra paka.

60) Dadhi or dadhi masthu or sura in kept in a copper vessel for a month Later on medicine is collected and anjana given in Netra paka .

61) Ghritha + Kamsya mala, grinded and given anjana in Netra paka.
62) Saindhava lavan + Milk, grinded and given as anjana in netra paka.
63) Yastimadu + Swarna gyrika + madu, as anjan in Netra paka.
64) Saindhavalavan + Ghee + Tamra bhasma + Stanya, as anjana in netra paka.

**65) Shukra vyvarnyahara anjan :-**

Vamshankur, Bhalla tak, Tala, Narikela, should burnt with tilanala, 8 times water added and boiled upto 1/4 the residue, Hasti asti choorna is added to above decoction and grinded for 7 days the dried powdered is preserved for anjana.

66) Saindhava lavan as choornanjan in savrana shukla .

67) Shireesha beeja, maricha, pippali and saindhavalavan as choornanjan in savrana shukla.

68) Tamra bhasma 1 part, Rajatha bhasma 2 parts, shankha nabhi basma 4 parts, manahshila 8 parts, maricha 16 parts and saindhava lavan 32 parts the choornanjan is given in savrana shukla.

69) Shankha nabhi, kolasti, Kataka, Draksha, Yastimadu and madhu, grinded and given as anjana in savrana shukla

70) Madhu, Godantha, Samudraphena and shireesha pushpa as anjan in savrana shukla.

71) Ksharanjan in savrana shukla

72) Mugda bhasma, shankha nabhi choorna, madhu as anjana in savrana shukla .

73) Madhuksar + madhu as anjan in savrana shukla
74) Vibheetaki majja + madhu as anjanin savrana shukla
75) Shankha nabhi, shukthi, madhu, Draksha, Yastimadhu Kataka beeja, as choornanjan in savrana shukla.

76) Ikshu, madhu, sharkara, ksheera, Daruharidra, Yastimadu, saindhava lavana grinded and given as anjana in Arjuna .

77) spatica, praval, shankha nabhi, Yastimadu, madhu grinded and given as anjana in Arjuna.

78) Shankha nabhi, madhu, Sharkara, samudraphena, grinded and given as anjan in Arjuna

79) Saindhava lavan, madhu, Kataka beeja as anjana in Arjuna .

80) Rasanjan and madhu as anjana in Arjuna

81) kaseesa and madhu as anjan in Arjuna

**82) Lekhyanjan in Arjuna shukra :-**
     Dhathu bhasma, Rasa aushada bhasma, Lavan, Ratana, Dantha bhasma, Shrunga bhasma, Trikatu, Karanja beeja, Ela and Avasaadak gana drugs, the fine powder is used as anjana.

83) Phanitha + madhu as anjan in siraharsha.

84) Rasanjan + Madhu = as anjan in siraharsha.

85) Kaeesa, Saindhava lavan and madhu as anjan in siraharsha

86) Amlavetas, stanya, phanitha, saindhava lavan as anjan in sira harsha.

87) Rasanjan, madhu, Ghritha, as anjan in sirothpatha .

87) Saindhava lavan, Kaseesa, Go ksheera, as anjan in sirothpatha

88) Shankhanabhi, manahshila, Tuttha, Daruharidra, Saindhava lavan + Madhu as anjan in siroth patha.

89) Sura, swetha maricha, makshika + Shireesha pashpa swarasa-grinded and given as anjan in sirothpatha.

90) Gyrica + madhu as anjan in Sirothpatha

91) Pata, Arjuna, shreeparni, Dhataki, Amalaki, Bilwam Bruhathi pushpa, Lodra, manjista, the fine powder with madhu or ikshurasa, anjana is given in Rakthaj Abhishyanda.

92) Chandan, Kumuda, Tejapatra, shilajith, kesara, loha bhasma, Tamra bhasma, Tuttha, nimba Niryasa, Trapu kamsyamala, powdered and well grined with madhu, varthi is prepared, for anjana in Rakthaj Abhisyanda.

93) Shunthi, Devadaru, musta, saindhava, lavan jathi pushpa, grinded with sura and Anjana applied in Netra Kanda .

94) Saindhvalavan, mircha , manahshila grinded with matulunga rasa and used as anjan in netra kandu.

95) Kaseesa, Samudraphen, Rasanjan, Jathi pushpa, grinded with madhu for anjana in Praklinna varthma

96) Shunthi, pippali, musta, saindhava lavan, swetha maricha, should be grinded with matulunga rasa - the powder is used as anjana in pistaka.

97) Bruhati or varthak, shigru, Indra varuni, patola, kiratatiktha, Amalaki etc. Riped fruits any of the above is taken, seeds are removed and the cavity is filled with pippali and srotonjan and kept for 7 days, later on medicine should be collected grinded with Honey and used for anjana, in pistaka.

98) Yavaadi ksharanjan in Balasagraditha

99) Poothi Karanja phala or puspa, shigru phala or pushpa, Rasanjan, Saindhava lavan, chandan, manahshila, Haritala, lashun, powdered and grinded with water to prepare varthi for anjana in Kaphaj Abhishyanda .

100) Hareertaki, Haridra, Yasti madu, powdered and grinded with water to prepare varthi, for anjana in Kaphaj Abhishyanda.

101) Saindhava lavan, Hingu, Triphala, Yastimadu, prapaundareeka, Anjan, Tuttha, Tamra Bhasma, grinded with water for Varthi anjan in Kaphaj Abhishyanda.

102) Trikatu, Tiphala, Haridra, vidanga, grinded with water for varthi anjan in Kaphaja abhisyanda

103) Netrabaa, Kusta, Devadaru, shankha, patha, Nakha, Trikatu, manahshila, grinded with water for varthi anjan in Kaphaja Abhishyanda

104) Jathi pushpa, Karanja Pushpa or beeja, shigru beeja or pushpa, Brahati phala or pushpa, Rasanjan, Saindhava lavan, chandan, manahshila, Haritala, Lashuna - grinded with water for varthi anjan inKaphaja abhishyanda.

**105) Vydooryadyanjan in Shuktika :-**
Vydoorya, spatica, pravala, muktha, shankha nabhi, Rajatha bhasma, swarna bhasma, powdered and grinded with sugar and Honey for anjan .

106) Samudra phena, is grinded with stanya or madhu and anjana is given in pittaja abhishyanda.

107) Yastimadu, Lodhra, Draksha, Sharkara, Kamal, grinded with stanya for anjana in pittaja abhishyanda

108) Lodra, Draksha, Sharkara, Kamal , Yastimadu, Vacha, grinded with milk for anjana in pittaja abhishyanda .

109) Amlavetas grineded with milk for anjana in pittaja abhishyanda, .

110) Chandan, udumbar twak, grinded with water for anjana in pittaja abhishyanda

111) Phalasha puspa or moola + Sharkara  + madhu as anjan in pittaja abhishyanda

112) Shallaki Swarasa + Sharkara + madhu  as anjan in pittaja abhisyanda.

113) Nishotha + Sharkara as rasakriyan in pittaja abhishyanda .
114) Yastimadu + sharkara + madhu as Rasakriya anjan in pittaja abhishyanda

115) Mustaadyanjan in pittaja abhishyanda:- musta, samudra phena, kamal, vidanga, Ela, Amalaki, Beejasar as Rasa kriyanjan.

116) Talisa patra, Ela, Gyrica, musta, shankhanabhi, powdered and grinded with cow milk for 3 days, used as anjan in pittaja abhisyanda

117) Aamalaki rasa Kriyanjan with stamya in pitaja abhishyanda

118) swarna bhasma + Stanya as anjan in pittaja abhishyanda.

119) Phalasha pushpa choorna + madhu as anjana in pittaja abhisyanda.

120) Shunthi, saindhava lavan Rasa kriya + Ghritha as anjana in vataj netra roga

121) Aanupa janthu vasa, saindhava lavan, shunthi choorna, as anjan in shuskakshipaka.

122) Saindhava lavan, Daru haridra, shunthi, powdered and grinded with mathulunga rasa, dried, ghee added and preserved, then with milk or water Anjana is given in shuskakshi paka .

123) Haridra, Daru haridradi ghritha (Ghritha prepared according to ghritha paka vidhi) + Saindhava lavan, given as anjan in shuskakshi paka.

124) Shunthi + Stanya or milk as anjana in shuskakshi paka .

125) Swarna gurica 1 part, saindhava lavan 2 parts, pippali 4 parts, shunthi8 parts, grinded with water, varthi is prepared and  Anjana is given with Aja Ksheera in Abhishyanda .

126) Yastimadu, Haridra, Hareetaki, Devadaru, grinded with water, varthi is prepared and anjan is given with aja ksheera in vataj abhishyanda.

127) Madhu, saindhava lavana and Gyrica perfectly grinded and used as anjana in vataj netro roga.

# ANJANA YOGA FROM ASTANGA HRUDAYA

**1) Haritaladi Choornanjan :-**
Haritala, sauveeranjan ( 1:1) and Tamra raja - well powdered and applied as choornanjan in pilla roga and pakshma shatha.

2) Cotton is made varthi and bhavana done in the decoctions of Laksha, Nirgundi, Brunga raj, Daruharidra for 7 times each. The Karpasa varthi is dipped in ghee and burnt, at Last the masi of Karpasa varti should be collected and used for anjana in pilla roga.

3) Saindhava lavan, Triphala, pippali, katuki, Shankha nabhi, Tamra raja, used as varthi anjana in pilla roga.

4) Pushpa kaseesa should be grinded with Tulasi rasa in a copper vessel and is used as anjana in pilla roga .

5) Rasanjan, sarja rasa, pushpanjan, manahshila, samudra phena, saindhava lavana, Gyrica, maricha, should be grinded with Honey, used as anjana in pilla roga.

6) Grandi Tagara should grind with Hareetaki Kashaya Ghee is added and is used as anjana in pilla roga .

7) Devadaru is grinded in Avi mootra, ghee is added and used as anjana in pilla rogs.

8) Karanja beeja, Tulasi, Jathi pushpa, grinded and used as rasa Krianjan in pilla roga.

9) Tutta 1 phala, swetha maricha 20, +30 phala Kanji,grinded in copper vessel and is used for seka or Anjana in pilla roga.

10) Vyaghree twak, Yastimadu, Tamra raja, should be grinded with aja Ksheera and fumigated with the smoke of shami and Amalaki patra which is coated with ghee the medicine is used as Anjana in netra shoola and shotha.

11) Talisadi Vatikanjan with stanya in Netra shoola and shotha.

12)" Sandhava Yoga " Anjanas are explained in Akshi shoola shotha and paka etc.

13) Shunti + stanya and grinded with cow ghee for anjana in shuskakshi paka .

14) Aanupa janthu Vasa + Shunthi + Saindhava Lavana is used as Anjana in Shuskakshi paka .

15) Hairs of human, dipped in the ghee, and burnt in " mallaka samputa " grind with the cow ghee for anjana inshuskakshi paka .

16) Go dadhi is pasted to silver vessel, after drying properly it is collected and grinded with dadhimastu, varthi is prepared, and is used for anjanaa in vataja Abhishyanda .

17) Jathi puspa, shankha, Triphala, Yastimadu, Bala - Grinded with Aakshodak and used as varthi anjana in pittaja Abhisyanda.

18) Saindhavalavana, Triphala, Trikatu, shankha, Samudra phena, shilajith sarja rasa, grinded and used as Varthi anjana in Kaphaj abhisyanda.

19) Go shakruth rasa, Go ksheera, Go ghritha (pakwam) and is used as Rasa Krianjan, in Dhooma darshi.

20) Karanja, Neelothphala swarasa, Gyrica, Kamalkesar, should be grinded with Gomaya ras and used as varthi anaja in Naktandya.

21) Renuka, Pippali, Sauveeranjan, Saindhava, lavan should be grinded with Aja mootra and used as varthi anjan in Naktandya.

22) Triphala, Trikatu, Haritala, Manashila, Samudra phena - should be grinded with Aja ksheera and used as varthi anjan in naktandya.

23) Rasanjan, Gyrica, Talisa patra, Go maya rasa ,madhu ,Go ghritha, grinded and used as rasa Krianjan in Naktandya.

24) Maricha rubbed in dadhi, the essence is used as anjan in Naktandya.

25) Guda, samudra phena, sauveeranjan, pippali, maricha, Kumkuma it is powdered and used as anjana with madhu in kacha.

26) Pippali, saindhava lavana, coocked in usheera kashaya, Go ghritha, Hoeny added, Rasa Kriya is prepared and used for anjana in sannipathaja Timira.

## 27) Rakthaja Timira Roga haranjan :-
Draksha, usheera, Lodra, Yastimadu, shankha, Tamra, chandana, kamala pushpa, padmaka, Neelothphala, grinded with avi ksheera and used as varthi anjana in Raktaj Timira .

28) The teeth and frotal bones of shasha, Go, khara, simha, ostra, and tail of white cow, maricha, shankha, chandana, samudra phena,. grinded with aja ksheera or stanya, used for varthi anjan in timira shukra.

**29) Vimala Varthi :-**
Shankha, priyangu, manahshila, Trikatu, Triphala, grinded and used as varthi anjan for vision improve ment .

**30) Kokila varthi :-**
Krishna loha raja, Trikatu, saindhava lavana, Triphala, sauveeranjan, grinded and used as varthi anjan. for vsion improvement.

**31) Pittaja Timira hara Sauveeradyanjan :-**
Sauveeranjan 5 parts, tuttha 5 parts, karkatak shrangi 3 parts, Amalaki 3 parts, karpura 1 part, powdered and used as choornanjan in pittaja Timira.

**32) Pittaja Timira rogas hara Anjan :-**
Sariba, padmaka, usheera, muktha, Lodra, chandan, used as varthi anjan or choorna anjan in pittaja Timira.

**33) Pittaja Timira Roga hara anjan :-**
Patra, Neelopthphala, sauveeranjan, Nagakesar, Karpoor, yastimadu, Gyrika, powdered and used as choorna anjan in pittaja Timira.

**34)** Vyaghra vasa or Varaha vasa + Yastimadu, powdered and used as choorna anjan in Timira.

**35)** Sauveeranjan should heat and dip in mamsarasa, ksheera, ghritha etc. powdered and used as choorna anjan in Timira .

**36) Ratnadi choorna anjan :-**
Ratna, Rajatha, spatika, swarna, sauveeranjan, Tamra, loha, shankha, chandana, kumkuma, Gyrika, powdered and used as choorna anjan for improovement of vision.

**37) Shanmakshika Yoga :-**
Maricha 1 part, Amalaki 2 parts, jalodbhava 3 parts, Tuttha 4 parts, sauveeranjan 5 parts, swarna makshika 6 parts, powdered and used as choorna anjana in Timira Arma jalasrava.

**38) Akshabeejadi vati :-**
Akshabeeja, maricha, Amalaki, Tuttha, yastimadu, should be grinded with water, used as varthi anjan in Timira.

**39) Prathisaranjan :-**
Maricha 10, Swarna makshika 1/2 karsha, Tuttha 1 phala , Yastimadu 1 karsha, dipped inghee and burnt, the bhasma is used for anjana in Timira.

**40)** Krishna sarpa vasa, shankha, kataka, sauveeranjan grinded and used as - Rasa kriyanjan in Timira .

## 41) Kukkutavistanjan :-

Cow milk is taken in a pot and added dead body of krishna sarpa and 5 scropians kept for 21 days. later on milk is chilled and cheese is collected that should be given to hen to eat after that the pureesha of the hen is collected for anjana in Timira.

## 42) Drusti shakthikaraanjan :-

Parada and Nagabhasma equally, double sauveeranjan, 1/16, karpoora, powdered and given as anjana.

**43)** Ghridhra mukha bhasma + Ghritha + Sauveeranjan powdered and used as choornanjan for vision improvement.

**44)** Ghritha, sauveeranjan, is kept in the mouth of krishna sarpa later collected and burnt perfectly + jata mamsi patra, the fine powder is given as anjana in savrana shukla.

**45)** Nagam (Lead) is melted and dipped 7 times each in Triphala kashaya, Bruangarajras, vatsanabhi Kashaya, Go ghritha, Aja ksheera, Yastimadu Kashaya. The shalaka (naga shalaka) is used as anjan shalka or the naga bhasma is used in the Timira, Arma etc.

**46) Paashupatha Yoga in abhishyanda:-** prapaundareeka, Yastimadu, Daruharidra, each 8 phala; 1 prasta water, boiled and concetrated decoction is prepared, then puspanjan 10 phala, maricha 1 karsha added and heated again - The powder or varthi is used for anjana in Abhishyanda and Drusti vikara.

**47) Tutthanjan:-** Tuttham is heated and dipped 7 times in the following liquids, the Gomutra, Gomaya rasa, kanji, stanya, Goghritha, vatsana, bhi madhu, then tuttam is powderd and used for anjana in Timira.

## 48) Timiranthaka Anjana :-

30 Parts naga bhasma, 5 parts Gandha pashana, Tamra and Talaka each 2 parts, vangam 1part and sauveeranjan 3 parts, mixed and well powdered for anjana in Timira.

## 49) Bhaskara Choorna :-

Tuttham is heated with the fire of badari sticks and dipped in Aja ksheera, Goghritha, madhu - each for 7 times, the purified Tuttam 2 phala, makshika, maricha, srotonjan, Katuki, Tagara, saindhava lavana, Lodra manahshila, Hareetaki pippali, Ela, sauveeranjan, Samudraphena each 1 karsha; Yastimadu 1 phala - burnt in a moosha, well powdered and used for anjana in Timira, Arma, Naktandya.

**50) Drusti Prasadan anjan :-** Sauveeranjan should be heated and dipped in the following decoctions each 7 times, Draksha swarasa ,Kamala mrunala swarsa. Goksheera, madyam, vasa ,Aakashodak. the medicine is powdered preserved and used for anjana inDrusti rogas.

**51) Kaphaja Timira Haranjan :-**
        Maricha saindhavalavana pippali samudraphena each 2 parts, sauveeranjan 9 parts should be collected and powdered in chitta Nakshatra and   used for anjana.

**52) Timira Armadi roga haranjan :-**
        Jatamamsi, Trijathaka, Loha, Kumkuma, Neelothphala, Hareetaki, Tuttha, sita, kacha, shankha, Samudra phena, maricha, sauveerajan, pippali, Yastimmadu, (equally) wellpowdered and used use as anjan when Chandra enters in to Ashwini Nakshatra .

**53) Timira roga hara choornanjan :-**
        Sauveeranjan 64 parts, Tamra, loha, Rajatha, swarna, each 1 part ; There are melted and dipped in madhuradi gana kashaya for each 7 times - These are powdered and added Vydoorya muktha, shankha bhasma, each 1 part well mixed and used as Anjana .

**54) Asadya Shukra dosha haranjan :-**
        Narikelasti, Bhallatak, Tala pallava, Vamshi, burnt and mixed in water, well filtered then ostra asti choorna is added and is used for anjana.

**55) Pundradyanjan in Shukra vyadhi :-** pundra, yastimadu, Kakoli, simhee, Loha, (or Krishna agara) Haridra Rasanjan, should grind with Aja, ksheera, and fumigate with yava or amalatki partra which is  dipped in ghritha, varthi is prepared and used for anjana .

**56) Shukra hara anjan :-**
        The teeth of Go, khara, Ashwa, ostra, shankha, samudra phena, should grind with arjuna kashaya varthi is prepared and used for anjana.

**57) Shukra roga haranjan :-**
        Langali kshara should dip in the amalaki phala swarasa and phaninjaka rasa, the fine powder is used for anjana.

**58) Kathina shukra roga hara anjana :-** Anjana is given with the shanka, kolasti, kataka, Draksha, Yastimadu and madhu .

59) Sura, Hastidantha, samudraphena, shireesha pushpa, the anjana is given in Kathina shukra.

60 ) Pippali, maricha, shireesha beeja, saindhava lavan, is used as choornanjan in Kathina shukra .

61) Saindhava lavan, got bhavan in Triphala Kashaya is used as anjana in Kathina shukra .

**62) Maha neela gutikaanjin in shukra vyadhi :-** (Bruhathi moola, Yastimadu, Tamra raja, saindhava lavana, shunthi, should be grinded with Aamalaki kashaya, pasted to coppervessel, fumigated with yava Aamalaki patra which is diped in ghee, the powder is collected, grinded with madhu and is used for anjana.

**63) Sarva Shukra haranjan :-**
Muktha etc ratnas, Dantha and shrunga of animals, gyrica etc Rasa Aushada, Trikatu, Ela, Karanja beeja, Lashuna, vrana hara Aushada etc are mixed, powdered and used as anjana.

**64) Tamala Patradi Varthi :-** Tamala patra, Go dantha, Shankha, samudra Phena, Gardabhaasti, Tamra etc are grinded with go mutra and Varthi prepared for anjana in shukra vyadhi.

**65) Dantha Varthi : -** The teeth of hasti varaha, ostra, Go, Ashwa Khara etc. Shankha, muktha, samudra phena, 1/4 maricha, varthi is prepared for anjan in shukra vyadhi.

**66) Kshatha Shukrahara Varthi :-**
jathi pushpa, Laksha, Gyrica, chandana, grinded and varthi is prepared for anjana.

**67) Timira roga hara Lekhananjan :-**
One drug of Triphala is burnt and masi prepared, with the Triphala decoctionof the masi is grinded, added saindhavaa lavana, Kachalavana well grinded and used for anjana.

**68) Shuklarmadi rogahara anjan :-** Sita, manahshila, Ela, lavan, shunthi, each 1/2 Karsha; Rasanjan 1/2 phala, should be grinded with madhu and used for anjana.

**69) Kukonaka pthaki roga hara varthi :-** Ela, Rasona, Kataka, shankha, maricha phaninjak, Katphala, should be grinded with sura and used for anjan.

**70)** Haridra, Daruharidra, Lodra, Yastimadu, Katuki, Nimba Pallava, Tamra raja, should be grinded with water and used for varthi anjan in Kukoonaka.

**71)** Loha raja should be heated dipped in ksheera madhu ghritha separately fine powder is prepared for anjana in Kukoonaka.

# ANJANA FORM CHARAKA CHIKITSA

1) Saindava lavana and maricha 1/2 shana, pippali and Samudra phena 2 shana, sauveeranjan 1 shana should be collected and grinded in chitta Nakshatra and used for anjana in kacha, Netra kandu and Kaphaja netra diseases .

2) Bida lavana (Bida churna) should be grinded with Aja mootra (Goats unrine) for 3 days, then choorna anjana is given in Timira, Krimi and pilla roga.

3) Sauveeranjan, Tuttha, swarna makshik, manahshila, vana kuluttha, Yastimadu, loha bhasma, Ratna, pushpanjan, saindhava lavana, vana varaha damstra, kataka, powdered ans used as Choornanjan in Timira etc .

4) Sauveeranjan should kept in the mouth of Krishna sarpa for a month, it is removed dried powdered and added 1/2 quantity of jathi pushpa and saindhava lavana, perfectly grinded and used as choornanjan in Timira etc diseases .

5) Pippali, phalasha pushpa rasa, Krishna sarpa vasa, saindhava lavana, and grinded with old ghee and used for anjana.

6)) Krishna sarpa vasa, Madhu, Amalaki swarasa, grineded and used as Rasakriya anjana in Timira, kacha, Arbuda etc.

7) Amalaki, Rasanjan, Madhu, ghritha, grinded and used as Rasa Kiryanjan in pitta Raktha disroders and Timira .

8) Amalaki Saindhavan lavana pippali maricha and madhu used as Rasa Kriyanjan in timira.

### 9) Sukhavatee varthi.
Kataka, shankha, saindhava lavana, Trikatu, sita, (sugar) samudra phena, Rasanjan, madhu, vidanga, manahsila, kukkutanda twak grinded and used as vati Anjan in Timira etc diseases.

### 10) Drusti prada varthi :-
Triphala, Kukkutanda twak, Kaseesa, Loha bhasma, Neelothphala, vidanga, samudraphena, should be grinded with Aja ksheera in a copper vessel for 2 days and given as vati anjan in Timira.

# ANJANAS FROM RASA RATNA SAMUCCHAYA.

1)      Tamra druthi + madhu or ghritha or stanya used as anjana, in Timira Arma, Abhishyanda .

2) Gandaka druthi + madhu or ghritha or stanya used as anjana.

3) **Shuklari varthi :-** Shambuka, parada, naga, Kamsya Rasanjan bhasma, should be grinded in a copper vessel with chincha patra srarasa-varthi is prepared and anjana given with madhu, in Timira, shuklarma,pilla vyadhi etc

4) **Nava netra dhatree varthi :-**Tamra bhasma 16 parts, Yastimadu choorna 14 parts, kusta choorna 12 parts, vacha choorna 10 parts, Rajatha bhasma 4 parts, swarna bhasma 2 parts, saindhava lavana 8 parts , pippali choorna 6 parts, should be grinded with Aja ksheera for 3 days and collected in copper vessel - it is used as anjana in Abhishyanda, Adhimantha, savrana shukla, Timira etc.

5) **Nayana rogahara Varthi :-** Pippali 1/4 tula, saindhava lavana 1/2 tula, vacha churna 1 tula, Yastimadu 2 tula (Sthalaja) Jalaja Yastimadu 4 tula, tamra bhasma 8 Tula, should be grinded with aja ksheera for 3 days, varthi anjana is given with madhu in most of the eye diseases.

6) Shigru tailam+Karpoora used as Anjana in Timira, Arma and savrana shukla.

7) **Swarnadi Varthi :-**
        Swarna, varata, rasa, should be grinded with putikaranja patra swarasa and varthi anjana is given with navaneeta in Timira and Arma.

8) **Vishaadyanjan :-**
        Vatsanabhi, Shahkhanabhi (1:1) should be grinded with  Amalaki rasa for a day and used as anjana in Timira .

9) **Pushpaharanjan :-**
        shankha, varata, the masi is used as anjan with navaneeta in shukra

10) **Nru Kaphalanjan :-**
        Human skull bhasma is given as anjana with stanya in Timira.

11) **Kacha Andya haranjan :-** Vatsanabhi choorna, manahshila (1:1) grinded with madhiphala rasa and used as anjana at nights in Kacha and Andhatha

12) **Shadanga Varthi :-**
        Karpoora, Rasanjan, Naga bhasma, parada bhasma, pippali churna, loha bhasma, (equally ) grinded with nandyaavartha Pushpa rasa for 3 days, Anjana is given with madhu in Timira arma shukla etc.

## 13) Dwadashanga Varthi ;-

Tamra bhasma, Tuttha, Tankan, Rasanjan, Triphala, Trikatu, Samudra phena, shankha, grinded with lemon juice for 3 days, varthi anjana is used with madhu in Timira, Kacha, Arma, shukra.

## 14) Patala haranjan :-

Sootha bhasma or Rasa sindhura, should be grinded with Laksha and jambeera srarasa, this powder is kept in Kaphardika and cealed with the paste of Tankan + Aja ksheera and preserved in the Dhaanya Rasi for 1 month then the medicine along with Kaphardika is powdered and anjana is given with Honey or ghee in Timira.

## 15) Paradadi Varthi :-

Parada, Naga bhasma, Rasanjan, Loha bhasma, mudga moola choorna , sarjaras (equally) should be grinded with chincha patra swarasa for 7 days, preserved for one day in a copper vessel - Anjana is applied with madhu in Timira, Adimantha, shukra, Arma etc.

## 16) Eeka Trishanga varthi :-

Parada, naga bhasma, Rasanjan, Pravala Kaseesa, Iodra, Tamra bhasma, Renuka, Trikkatu, Gyrika saindhava lavana, Tutta, Samudra phena, Triphala, Mukta bhasma, peetha Rohini Choorna, Babula patra choorna, visnukrantha choorna, putranjeeva choorna, dathura moola churna, chincha, patra choora, shat lavan (Pamshulavana, bidalavan Sauvarch lavan, Kachalavan, Samudra lavan, saindhavlavan,) should be grinded with Nimba patra rasa for 3 days, varthi anjan is given with madhu.

## 17) Garudanjan :-

Kataka, saindhava lavana, Tuttha, Rasanjan, Trikatu, spatica, musta, varata, Trilavan, Tamra bhasma, loha bhasma, Karpoora, Katuki. samudra phena, vacha, Nruka rotika, Naga bhasma, parada, Tankan, Neelanjan, Triphala, Yastimadu, should be grinded with Karanja Twak Kashaya for 7 days - Varthi anjana is given with water in visual problems.

## 18) Timira haranjan :-

Parada 1 part, Naga bhasma 1 part, Neelanjan 2 parts, Karpoora 1/4 part, grinded and applied as anjana in Timira.

## 19) Nagadi Varthi :-

Naga bhasma, parada, Amlaki, Karpoora, Mouktika, Goghritha, pippali, Saindhava lavan, Rasanjan, Jeeraka, Madhu - Should be grinded with Nagavalli Patra swarasa in (Kamsya paatra) Coppper vessel - vati anjan is given with Honey in Abhishyanda, Adhi mantha etc diseases.

343

**20) Tamradi Varthi :**

Tamra bhasma, Nagabhasma, Rajatha Bhasma, Parada, peetha Rohini, Karpoora, pippali, Rasanjan, Saindhava lavan, shankha bhasma, Kamshya bhasma, should be grinded with Hamsa padi moola swarasa- Varti anjan is given in Most of the eye diseases.

**21) Raktanjan :-**

Rakta chandan, choorna collected in a coppervessel - 100 Bhavana and 100 mardana should be given in Bringaraj rasa and anjana is given with madhu.

**22) Timira haranjan :-**

Gandak 1 Part, parada 2 parts, Sauveeranjan 1/8 part, should be grinded with kapittha rasa for anjana in timira.

# CHAKRADATTA - ANJANA YOGA.

**1) Sukhavathi varthi :-**

Kataka, shankha, Trikatu, Lavan, Samudra phena, Rasanjan, Vidanga, manahshila, Kukkutanda twak, should be grinded with water varthi anjana is given with madhu in Timira, kacha, Arma, shukra.

**2) Chandrodaya Varthi :-**

Hareetak, Vibheetak, pippali, maricha, vacha, kusta, Nabhi Manahshila, should be grinded with Aja ksheera and used as varthi anjan in Timira, Kacha, Arma, Naktandya.

**3) Hareetakyadi Varthi :-**

Hareetaki, Haridra each 2 parts ; Pippali 1 part, Lavana 1/4 part, grineded and used As varthi anjan in Timira.

# ANJANA YOGA FROM BASVA RAJEEYA (TELUGU BOOK)

## 1) Trikatukaadyanjan :-

Trikatu, Triphala, jyothishmati, vidanga, Karanja - each 4 part ; prapoundareeka, Yastimadu, Tamra basma, Saindhava lavana, spatika shankah, each 3 parts ; Rasanjan Gyrika, chandana dwayam, Draksha, Haridra, Swetha Lodra - each 2 parts ; Tutta, Daruharidra, Katuki, - each 1 part ; should be grinded with Karanja swarasa, vati should be prepared and is used as anjan with water - in Timira, Adimantha, Arma, shukra and Naktandya.

## 2) Katakaadyanjan :-

Kataka beeja, shankha, saindhava lavana, Trikatu, sharkara, samudra phena, Rasanjan, Madhu, vidanga, manahshila, kukkutanda twak, should be grinded with stanya and used as anjana with lemon juice, it is useful in Timira, varthma roga, Abhishyanda and Arma.

## 3) Garudanjan :-

Ela, Maricha, Tuttha, Saindhava lavan, samudra phena, spatic, Hingula, shankha, chandana, kusta, Laksha, haridra, Kukkudanda twak, skull of the human, manahsila, kataka, karpoora, Devadaru, Rasanjan, Guggulu and should grind spearately with Bringaraj swaras, Aja ksheera, matsyakshi patra swarasa, swetha Kamala swarasa, Neeli swarasa, punarnav swarasa and vati is prepared for anjana with water in Timira, Dhoomadarshi and Andhatwa.

## 4) Maha Garudanjan :-

Kathak, saindhava lavan, Tutta, Trikatu, spatika, shankha, Kaphardhika, Rasanjan, Manahsila, Tamra bhasma, Loha bhasma, Karpoora, katuki, Samudraphena, vacha, skull of human, Naga bhasma, Rasa bhasma Tankan, sauveeranjan, Triphala, Yastimadu, Gorochan, should be grinded with Karanja swarasa and the preared vati is used for anjan with water in Andhatwa Timira.

## 5) Nayanamrutam :-

Karpoora, Sauveeranjan, Tutta, Rasanjan, Daruharidra, katuki, Kaphardika, Saindhavalavana, Trikatu, Samudra phena, Yastimadu, Chandan, Shankha, should be grinded with mathulunga swarara and prepared vati is used for anjan with Honey or in all types of eye diseases.

## 6) Rasa Krianjan :-

Rasa bhasma, praval bhasma, Nagabhasma, kaseesa, Rasanjan, Saindhava lavan, Trikatu, Tamra bhasma, Tutta, Gyrika, Lodra, putranjeevi seeds, manahshila, musta, shireesha beeja, Abhaya, Chinchabeeja, sauveeranjan - should be grinded with Nimba patra swarasa in a copper vessei and anjan is given with Honey. in Timira, Arma, etc diseases.

345

**7) Netranjan :-**

Pippali, Sauveeranjan, Karpoora, Nagabhasma, Rasa bhasma, Loha bhasma, vatsanabhi should be grinded with Nandyaavarth rasa in a Iron vesel for a day and vati anjan is given .

**8) Tamradyanjan :-** Tamra bhasma, Dhanyabhraka, Tuttha, Kaphari each 10 Nishka, the powder should heat in a pan with 30 karsha gandhaka, by closing the pan with same sized pan to prevent the medicated vapours not to escape out. After formation of perfect mixture the medicine should be coolled then it is diluted in 1 prasta of water, the pure solution is kept in the heat of sun to make the liquid concentrate, then 1karsh Tutta and shilajith powder is added vati is prepared for anjan with madhu or ghritha and is used in most of the eye diseases.

**9) Rasanjanadyanjan :-** Ativisha, pippali - grinded in Gomutra, vati is pre-pared for anjana in Timira. Samudra phena, spatica, Hingula, Rasanjan, Kacchapa Prusta Asti, manahsila, Trikatu, ( double to manahshila), saindhava lavan (double to Trikatu,) Loha bhasma (equal to saindheva lavana,) Ati visha (equal to lohe bhasma ) grinded welll and anjana is given with Honey or ghee in Timira and Arma.

**10) Saindhavadyanjan :-** Saindhava lavan, Rasa bhasma Nagabhasma, Amalaki, Rasanjan, Pippali etc should be collected in a copper vessel and grinded with ghee, honey, Nagavalli swarasa and sugar, vati is prepared and used for anjana .

**11) Tarakadya vati Or Taranjan :-** Rajatha bhasma, Tamra bhas, Rasa bhasma, Tuttha, Khapari, Daruharidra, Kakuti, Rasanjan, kamsya bhasma, shankha should be grinded with Hamsapada patra swarasa and vati prepared for anjana.

Gaja kesari :- Manahshila, naga bhasma Tuttha, (Dobule to naga) slight karpoora, should be grinded with dronapushapa ras and vati prepared for anjan.

**12) Chandrakaanjan :-** Tuttha, Tamra bhasma, Loha bhasma, yastimadu, vacha, palatutta, lavanga, saindhava lavan, Shankha, Tritaku, vidanga, Rasa bhasma, Kataka, Daruharidra, Vata, Amalaki, Talaka, Karanja beeja, Neelanjan and Should be grinded with Nimba swarasa, matulunga swarasa to prepare vati for anjana .

13) Spatika, Iodra, Rasanjan, Tagara ,Tuttha ,Naga bhasma, Kaphari, saindhava lavana, Karanja beeja, Yastimmadu, Trikatu, vidanga, Hareetaki, and Should be grinded with Bringaraj rasa - Mathulunga ras to prepare vati for anjan .

14) Kataka, Manhshila, Amalaki, Kshёeratutta ,Hingula, Yastimadu, Iodra, Talaka, sauveera, Trikatu, Karanja dwayam, Devadaru, Daru haridra, maricha, spatika, swetha kamala, shankha, Tamra bhasma, Naga bhasma, Abraka bhasma, Kantha loha bhasma, Raktha manahshila, pippali, lavana, samudra phena, Gyrika and shoulded be grinded with vata, shunthi, bringaraj rasa to prepare vati for anjana with Honey or ghee in Timira and Netra srava.

**14) Nayanaamrutam :-** Tuttha, saindhava lavan, Ksheera tuttha, samudra phena, Rasanjan, Tankan, maricha, should be grinded with lemon juice in a copper vessel for 3 days to prepare anjana in Arma and Timira.

**16) Karparyadyanjan :-** Kaphari, Tuttha, Rasanjan, Samudra phena, shankha manahshila, punarnava, Triphala, and should be grinded with lemon juice to prepare vati for anjan with water in Timira Arma.

**17) Tila Pushpanjan :-** Maricha 2 parts, Kaphari 4 parts, Tila pashpa 8 parts, and shoulded be grinded with lemonjuice to prepare vati for anjan in Timira Arma.

**18) Marichanjan :-** Maricha 1 part, Amalaki 2 parts, Karanja beeja 3 parts, should be grinded with Bringaraj swarasa and vati prepared for anjan in Timira etc.

**19) Netra Prabhanjan :-**Samudra phena, Loha bhasma, Kataka, skull of human, Kukkutanda twak, manahshila and should be grinded with jeerakaKashaya for vati anjan in Timira

**20) Chandro daya Varthi :-** Haridra, Nimba pallava, pippali, maricha, vibheetaki, Karanja beeja, shankha, vatsanabhi, manahshilla, should be grinded with Aja, pureesha for vati anjana with water in Arma and Timira.

**21) Darvyadyanjan :-** Application of Rasanjan in Arjuna, Arma, and Timira

**22) Girikarnikanjan :-** Swetha Girikarni root, seeds and flowers, shankha, Haridra, Hareetaki, shunthi, should be grinded with girikarni moola rasa and applied as varthianjan.

**23) Kumarika vari :-**80 tila pushpa, maricha 16, Jathi pushpa 50, pippali 60 used as Vati anjan.

**24) Shiladyanjan :-** Manahshila, pippali, Karpoora, Tinthinee phala, Karanja beeja, should be grinded with water for Varthi anjan in Timira.

**25) Narikelanjan :-**
Triphala, Daruharidra, Yastimadu each 1 phala, (Triphala 3 phala); add Narikela jala and the decoction is prepared then Karpoora, saindhava lavana and madhu added for anjana. in Timira Arma.

## 26) Maha Narikelanjan :-

Yastimadu, Triphala, Darauharidra each 1 phala ; 1 prasta narikela jala, added 1/8 Residual decoction; prepared and Tuttha, karpoora, samudra phena, Gyrika, saindhava lavan, Rasanjan, Maricha, and madhu added for Anjana.

## 21) Shankhadi Vatika anjana :-

Shankha 4 parts, manahshila 2 parts, maricha 1 part saindhava lavan 5 parts, should be grinded with Aja ksheera and used as Anjana in Timira Naktandya.

## 28) Pushpanjan :-

Manijista, Yastimadu, uthphala, Dadhi, pippali twak, chavya, Gorochan, jatamamsi. chandana, shankha, kangiri, Tuttha, pushpanjan, is used in Netra srava Abhishyanda shukra and Netra shoola.

## 29) Godanthadyanjan :-

Go dantha, Kukkutanda twak, makara dantha, shankha choorna, varata churna, samudra phena, Tamra churna, Tuttha, Karpoor, Rasna, chandra kanth Ratna, Madhucchista - all should be grinded and heated, then anjan is used with lemon juice in Timira Arma, Arjuna etc.

## 30) Dhatranjan :-

Triphala should be grinded with lemon juice and is used as Anjan in Netra srava and Timira .

## 31) Uthphaladyanjan :-

Uthphala, saindhavalavan, chandan, Triphala, should be grinded with Lemon juice and is used as anjan in Timira Naktandya.

## 32) Artha Chandrodaya Anjan :-

Karpoora, spatika, shankha, chandana, Yastimadu, Madhuka, sariba, Manjista, Haridra, Daruharidra, Kataka beeja, Gyrika, in equal quantity and add equally purfied Tuttha and grinded with lemon juice and is used for anjana in Timira, Naktandya, Varthma roga.

# ANJANA YOGAS FROM NETRA DARPAN

**1) Laakshaanjan :-**

Laksha, Daruharidra, Rakta manashila, vidanga, and gyrika, should be grinded with stanya in Abhishyanda - netra srava .

**2) Akshanjan :-**

Tuttha, Yastimadu, Amalaki, vidbheetaki and maricha grinded with water for anjana in Timira.

**3) Sudarshananjan :-**

Chandana, manahshila, saindhava lavan, Haritala, shankha, Yastimadu, maricha and spatica, grinded with water for anjanan in Timira and shukra .

**4) Shastra Vallabhaanjan :-**

Shankha, Shigrubeeja, Saindhava lavan, Kukkutanda twak, samudraphena, grinded with water for Anjana with shigru pushpa rasa. in Timira shukra.

**5) Aamalakaanjan :-**

Aamalaki, maricha, karanja beeja, grinded with Bringaraj swarasa for anjana in Timira, kamala etc.

**6) Shankhanjan :-**

Saindhava lavana 1 part, maricha 2 parts, manashila 4 parts shankha 8 parts should be grinded with aja ksheera, for anjana in Timira Arma etc.

**7) Shashi Prabhaanjan :-**

80 Tila pushpa, 50 Jathi pushpa, 16 maricha and 6 pippali - anjana is given in Timira.

**8) Spatikaanjan :-**

Spatika, Lodra, Trikatu, Rasanjan, Ksheera tutta, Saindhava lavan, Tuttha, Yastimadu, vidanga, Karanja beeja, Hareetaki, Vanga bhasma, Naga bhasma, grinded with Lemon Juice or Bringaraj swarasa for anjana in Timira Arma.

**9) Amrutaanjan :-**

Karpoora, samudraphena, vatsanabhi, Tuttha, Yastimadu, Katuki, chandan, Daruharidra, Trikatu, Kaphardik bhasma, Neelanjan, Garudanjan, grinded with madiphala ras for vati anjana with Honey or Ghee.

**10) Bhujangaanjan :-**
Naga bhasma, Manahshila 1 part; Tuttha 2 parts.
Slightly Karpoora - grinded with Dronipashpa swarasa for anjana.

**Tutthaanjan :-**
Tuttha, vata, Yastimadu, shankha, Daruharidra, Trikatu, Karanja beeja, Gandak ,Talaka, parada, Vidanga, Ksheera tuttha, Kataka, Amalaki, Tamra and Loha bhasma - grinded with madiphala rasa for vati anjan.

**Nishaanjan :-**
Vacha, maricha, Daruharidra, Pippali, Saindhava lavana, grinded with Bringaraj swarasa, for anjana

**Laghu marichaanjan :-**
Maricha grinded with Bile of black goat and used for vati anjan.

**Tamraanjan -**
Tamra bhasma, Hareetaki masi, bhallatak beeja masi, grinded with Navaeetha in a copper vessel and used as anjan .

**Rajathanjan :-**
Rajatha bhasma, Varaha shrunga, Gaja nakha, Kukkata Gala asti, grinded with Honey for anjan

**Trikatukaanjan :-**
Trikatu, Triphala, grinded with Aja pureesha for anjana.

## ANJANA YOGA FROM BHAISHAJYA RATNAVALI

**1) Nishadi Netra bindu :-**
Haridra, musta, Hareetaki, vibheetaki, Amalaki, Daru haridra, sharkara, yastimadu, Draksha - Devadaru, (equally), 64 times water is added and arka extracted for Aashchyotan in Abhishyanda - netra shoola, daha etc.

**2) Chandra prabha Varthi :-**
Swetha maricha, Krishnanjan, Pippali, Yastimadu, shankhanabhi, manahshila, Hareetaki, grinded with Aja ksheera for varthi anjan. in Timira, Arma, Nakthandya etc.

**3) Haridra varthi :-**
Haridra, Nimba pallava, maricha, shunthi, methi, vidanga, grinded with Gomutra for varthi anjana in timira Nakthandya etc.

**4) Vyoshadi Varthi :-**

Trikatu, Kamala, Hareetaki, Kusta, Daru haridra used as varthi anjan in Timira arma etc.

**5) Pippalyadi varthi :-**

Pippali, Tagara, Kamala patra, Yastimadu, Haridra used as varthi anjan in Abhishyanda .

**6) Pancha Shataka Varthi :-**

1) Neela Kamal patra 100 parts 2) Mudga 100 parts 3) Nistusha Yava 100 parts 4) malathi pushapa 100 parts 5) Pippali 100 parts - varthi anjan should be given with ghritha in Timira Ashruasrava etc diseases.

**7) Drustiprada varthi :-**

Triphala, Kukkudanda twak, Kaseesa, Loha bhasma, Neela Kamal, vidanga samudra phena, grinded with Aja Ksheera in a copper vessel for 7 days and used as varthi anjan in Blindness.

**8) Kokila Varthi :-**

Trikatu, Loha churna, saindhava Lavana, Triphala, anjana, used as varthi anjan in Timira.

**9) Bruhath Chandrodaya varthi :-**

Rasnajan, sukshma ela, Kumkuma, manahsila, Shankhanabhi, shigru beeja, sharkara used as varthi anjan, in Timira.

## ANJANA YOGA FROM SARANGDHAR SAMHITHA

**1) Karanja Varthi :-**

Karanja beeja + phalasha pashpa swarasa used as varthi anjan.

**2) Samudra phenadi Varthi :-**

Samudra phena, saindhava lavan, shankha, Kukkatanda twak, Shigru beeja, used as varthi anjan in shukra vyadhi.

**3) Dantha Varthi :-**

Animals teeth, shankha, muktha, Samudra phena, used as varthi anjan in Shukra vyadhi.

**4) Atinidranashini Varthi :-**

Neelothphala, shigrubeeja, Nagakesar, used as varthi anjan in Atinidra

## 5) Pushpa Varthi :-

Tila pushpa 80, pippali beeja 60, jathi pushpa 50, maricha 16 - grinded with water varthi prepared and used for anjana in Timira shukra etc.

## 6) Naktandyanashini Varthi :-

Rasanjan, Haridra, Daruharidra, Jathi pushpa, Nimba patra, - grinded with Gomaya ras Varthi is prepared and used for anjana in Naktandya.

## 7) NetraSravahara Varthi :-

Triphala majja + Water used as varthi anjan in Netra Srava

## 8) Tutthadi rasa Kriya :-

Tuttha, swarna makshika, saindhava lavana, shankha, manahsila, sugar, Gyrica samudra phena, maricha. The fine powder + madhu - given as anjan in Timira shukra etc .

## 9) Karpooranjan (Pushpahara Rasakriya )

Karpoora choorna + Vata Ksheera used as anjan in Shukra.

## 10) Atinidraaghna Anjan :-

Maricha got bhavana in Ashwa lala srava + madhu - powdered and anjana given to control sleep.

## 11) Tandraghna anjan :-

Jathipushpa, pravala, maricha kataka, vacha, saindhava lavan, - grinded with Aja mutra and anjana given to control yawnings.

## 12) Daarvyadi Rasanjan :-

Daruharidra, patola, Yastimadu, Nimba, padmakaasta, Neelothphala, prapoundareeka, rasa Kriya prepared and used for anjana in Daha raga paka srava Raktaadikya and shoola of eye.

## 13) Rasanjanadi Rasa kriya :-

Rasanjan, Sarja ras, Jathi pushpa, Manahshila, Samudra phena, saindhava lavan, Gyrica, maricha. grinded with Honey and used as anjana in praklinna varthm .

## 14) Guduchi rasakriya :-

Guduchi Swarasa 12 grams, madhu 1 gram, saindhava lavan 1 gram - Rasa kriya anjan is used  in Timira shukra etc.

15) Punar nava rasakrianjan

| Punarnava | + | milk | in | Netra kanda |
|---|---|---|---|---|
| " | + | madhu | in | Netra srava |
| " | + | Ghritha | in | Shukra |
| " | + | Taila | in | Timira |
| " | + | Kanji | in | Naktandya |

16)  Babboola patra Rasa Kiryanjan with madu in Netra srava.

17)  Ghritha + Madhu as anjan - in sirothpatha .

18)  Krishna Sarpa vasa, shankha, Kathaka, and Rasanjan, the prepared rasa Kri yanjan is used in Blindness.

19)  Saindhava lavana, maricha, each 1/2 part; pippali - samudra phena, sauveeranjan, each 1 part ; choorna anjana is given in Kandu, Kacha.

20)  Sauveera Choornanjan (Bhavana in Triphala Kashaya ) is used in most of the eye diseases.

21)  The pippali of yakruth pippali yoga (Pakwa) + madhu as anjan in Nakthandya .

22)  Kukkutanda twak, manahshila, kacha, shankha, chandan, saindhava lavana,  grinded in water for anjan in Arma disease.

23)  Nayanamrutanjan :-
Melted Naga + Parada + Krishnanjan (equalaly) + 1/10 Karpoora - well grinded and used for anjana in most of the eye diseases.

24)  Sarpa Visha hara anjan :-
Jayapal beeja majja - grinded (Bhavan) in Lemon juice for 21 times and varthi is prepared and used as anjan with saliva of human, it is useful  in snake bites.

26)  Kataka phala - grinded in water and Honey, Karpoora is added, pefectly mixed and used as anjan for netra Prasadan.

# EXAMINATION OF EYE BALL

Eye ball is an important sensory organ for visual perception, a simple mistake may cause blindness so  only while handling diagnosis and treatment of ophthalmic case definite principles should be followed.

The examination of eye ball chiefly contain 3 headings.

**1) History taking** :- the detailed, present, past history and family history, some times give a clue for the diagnosis.

## 2) Objective examination :-
a) Examination of the appendages and anterior segment of the eye ball (eyelids, lacrimal gland, Lacrimal apparatus, conjunctiva, cornea, sclera, Anterior chamber, Iris, pupil and Lens)

b) Examination of posterior segment of eye ball with ophthalmo scope ex :- vitreous, retina, choroid, optic, disc etc.

c) Examination of eye ball with special optical instruments like corneal micro scope, slit lamp, gonioscope, Transilluminator etc.

## 3) FUNCTIONAL EXAMINATION OF EYE BALL

Recording or estimating of function of eyes separately.

**a) Acuity of vision :-**
Both the distant and near vision are tested, Distant vision is recorded with snellen's chart and Near vision is recorded with jaeger's test types etc.

**b) Colour vision test :-**
Test of colour vision is essential for certain occupations such as sailors, Railway engine driver etc. This can be tested by various methods but the most common method is by means of Isihara chart.

**c) Field of Vision :-**
The Examination of Central field and peripheral field of vision is essential. Central field is estimated by Bjerrum's screen and peripheral field of vision is estimated by perimeter.

## A) HISTORY TAKING :-

History taking is extremely important, the patient should be encouraged to narrate his complaints, enquiry should be made about certain complaints and definite questions are put as indicated below .

1) Age sex occupation and address should be asked, it is help ful for the diagnosis.

**Ex :-** a) After 40 yrs of age some diseases comes like senile cataract, presbyopia and also retinopathies.
b) Styes & meibomian cyst are common in the young
c) Styes & allegic blepharitis common in the female (Allergy due to Anjana )
d) Visual problems, corneal opacties etc are common in welders and in the labour working in chemical factories.
e) Xerosis and vitamin deficiences are common in the poor.

2) cheif complaints, aasociated complaints, previous illness, Family history, personal history etc should be asked indetail to assess the disease and to put furthur relavent questions.

## 3) Questions in relation to vision :-
a) Mode of onset of the disease whether gradual or sudden.
b) Duration of the disease whether fresh or chronic
c) Whether it is primary or secondary.
d) Before the visual problems if any head injury happened or not.
e) Whether it is uniocular or Binocular.
f) Whether visual problem is constantly present or getting occasionally.
g) Dim vision whether in day time ( Hemeralopia) or at nights (Nyctalopia)
h) Any glasses (Spectacles ) used before.
i) Any double vision (Diplopia), or multi vision (Polyopia)
j) Any haloes around the light ( Commonly seen in Acute or sub accute conjunctivitis, closed angle glaucoma and in Lenticular opacities)
k) Any spots or floating objects seen infront of eye ( in Aqueous precipitations, Keratic precipitates and in Vitreous haemorrhages)
l) Any distortion of objects ( known as Metamorphopsia, seen in choroiditis and retiinitis)

m) Whether objects appearing smaller than the normal ( known as micropsia, seen in choroiditis and retinitis)

n) Whether objects appearing bigger than the normal (Known as macropsia, seen in Choroiditis and Retinitis)

o) Any subjective flashes of light are seen (Known as photopsia, seen in choroiditis due to retinal irritation)

p) Whether defective vision present in central field or in peripheral field or for colour things.

q) If colour blindness present that is uniocular or Binocular . Whether total or partial If only one colour factor seen among the 3 colours (Red green blue) in known as **monochromics** if two colour factors are seen among the three it is known as **dichromics** (**Protanopes** - red blind, **deuteranopes** - green blind, **Tritanopes**- Blue blind)

r) Whether difficulty in vision for distant objects (myopia), or near objects (Hyper metropia)

s) Whether having the habbit of Tobacco, alcohol and any other toxic things (Produce amblyopia)

t) Any eye strain, head ache, red eyes while reading sewing etc.

4) Questions with regard pain in the eye ball.
      a) Mode of onset b) Duration
      c) Mild moderate or severe
      d) Time of the day when worse
      e) Relation to close work
      f) Any associated nausea vomiting giddiness and fall of vision.

5) Head ache :-
      a)     Location b) whether the site of pain is fixed or altering
      c)     Time of the day when worse d) Mild or moderate or severe
      e)     Whether constant, interupted or intermittent
      f)     Frequency of the pain.
      g)     Relation to close work.
      h)     Any associated nausea vomiting giddiness or fall of vision.

## 6) Watering of the eyes :-
a) Duration
b) Constant or intermittent
c) Relation to close work, travelling on /in fast vehicles, after cinema show, after reading or sewing, after seeing bright things etc.
d) Any associated redness
e) Time of the day when worse
f) Any lesion in lacrimal apparatus (catarrhal dacrocystitis)
g) Stenosis or Obstruction in puncta (epiphora)
h) excessive stimulation of Lacrimal gland (Lacrimation) .

## 7) Discharge of the eyes :-
a)Nature of the discharge whether mucoid, muco purulent or purulent.
b) Onset.
c) duration.
d) Any stickiness of lids or margins in the mornings on waking (in conjunctival lesions and lesions of Lacrimal apparatus this condition is seen.).

## 8) With regard to glasses (Spectacles)
a) Has the patient worn the glasses, is so for what pupose and the glasses relieved the symptoms or not.

## 9) Photophobia ( dislike for light ) present or not .

## 10) History of injury :-
a) Direct or indirect (penetrating types of foreign bodies ) b) Whether dimvision started after the injury c) whether the dim vision agravated after the injury

## 11) Past history :-
a) Past history of the diseases, Hypertension, diabetes, Tuberculosis syphilis, leprosy, thyroid dysfunction, general debility etc.

b) Past medical and sugical history should also enquired for the proper diagnosis.

## 12) While the answering of the patient, the Doctor should observe for the ptosis, proptosis, screwing up of the eye ball, axis of the eye ball, watering, palpebral fissure, head posture etc.

# OBJECTIVE EXAMINATION

B) Examination of the head, for its.
a) Configuration b) its position. ie. head tilt or head turn.

C) Examination of the face,
a) Any asymetry b) Signs of paralysis c) skin changes

D) Examination of eye brows, for
a) Loss of hair b) Depigmentation
c) Any elevation from hyperaction of frontalis muscle.

E) Examination of palpebral fissure
(The wide gap between upper and lower lid margins when the eyes are opened.)
a) Normal    b) Wide    c) Narrow    d) Absent.

F) Examination of orbit for
a) Deformity b) Fullness in any part etc.

G) Examination for the position of eye ball in the orbit for the following
a) Smaller eye ball (microphthalmos)
b) Bigger eye ball (Buphthalmos)
c) shrinken eye ball (Phthisis bulbi)
d) Sunken eye ball (Enophthalmos)
f) Protruded eye ball (Exophthalmos)
g) Deviated axis of eye (Squint or strabismus)
h) Oscillating or pulsating eye ball (nystagmus)
i) Congestion or discolouration should also be noted.
k)

## EXAMINATION OF EYE LASHES (PAKSHMA)

In general the colour of the eye lashes cannot become grey or white (Depigmentation of eye lashes). Normal eye lashes are fresh regular soft blackish and arranged in 2 or 3 rows, the upper eye lashes project forward and upward, lower eye lashes project forward and slight down wards. These prevent the entry of foreign bodies into the eye.

Eye lashes should be examined for the following :-
1) Absence of eye lashes is known as madarosis (pakshma shatha)
a) Partial or total absence, b) Congenital or acquired should be noted.

2) Irregular hard and misdirected eye lashes, is known as trichiasis (pakshma kopa)

3) Irregular misdirected eye lashes if congenitally present is known as distichiasis.

4) Depigmentation ( grey or white) of hair is known as vitiligo (very rare)

5) eye lashes should be examined for nits parasites at its root.

6) Any matting of eye lashes with conjunctival sticky discharge should be noted.

7) Any cracking of the lashes should be noted.

# EXAMINATION OF EYE LID MARGIN
## (PAKSHMA VARTHMA SANDHI)

The lid margins should be normal in thickness, colour and in position (without in-rolling or outrolling.)

1) Inflammation of eye lid margin is known as Blepharitis (Krimi grandhi) " The lid margin appears with ulcers, crusts, scales etc. "

2) Thickening of eye lid margin is known as Tylosis .

3) Hyperaemia of eye lid margin is known as milphosis.

4) Inversion ( in rolling) of lid margin or is known as entropion ( it causes scratches or ulcers on cornea due to constant pricking of eye lashes).

5) Eversion (out rolling) of eye lid margin is known as Ectropion (Due to evertion of lid margin, eye lids cannot closed perfectly, so cause exposure keratitis etc).

6) Small cystic swellings develops at the root of the eye lashes ( on the lid margin ) due to the obstruction in the channels of zeis gland, it is known as zeis cyst or stye or External hordeolum.

7) Puncta should be examination whether it is stenosed, obstructed closed or everted ( puncta is a hole present on the eye lid margin at the inner canthas, through which lacrimal fluid enters into lacrimal apparatus and inferior meatus of nose  1) if puncta is closed causes epiphora ( watering of eyes) 2) and in dacryocystitis, by pressing over the sac area pus regurgitates out through the puncta)

8) Posterior sharp edge of lid margin should be examined for the series of white dots, they are the normal openings of meibomian glands.

# EXAMINATION OF EYE LID PROPER

Eye lid is formed of the following layers. from out to inwards.

1) Skin 2) Loose aeriolar tissue ( no fat) 3) Muscle layer 4) Tarsal plate
5) Palpebral Conjunctiva.

**Note :-** The Lesions of the skin and palpebral conjunctiva can be examined directly where as the other parts lesions are estimated functionally.

1) Examination of the skin of the eye lid.
    a) It is very thin, loose without subcutaneous fat so having more scope for oedema of eye lid due to trauma.
    b) Ulcers, scars, depigmented lesions, burns etc are examined.
    c) Trauma to eye lid may cause swelling and ecchymosis or Black eye lid
    d) Vertical wounds of eye lid may produce a notch on lid margin (Trau matic coloboma)

2) Applied Examination of muscles of eye lid.
    a) Facial nerve palsy causes Lagophthalmos (improper closure of eye lid) due to failure of the function of orbicularis oculi muscle.
    b) Oculomotor nerve Palsy causes ptosis ( improper opening of eye lid or Droopping of eye lid) due to failure of the function of Levator palpebrae superioris muscle ( a) and b) can be corelated to vata hatha varthma).
    c) Over action of muller's muscle (Supplied by cervical sympathetic nerves) causes vigorous blinking of eye lids. (Nimesha)

## 3) Examination of the glands of eye lid.

    a) Zeis gland inflammatory condition is seen due to obstruction in its duct, by which a small cystic swelling is seen in the lid margin, is known as zeis cyst or External hordeolum or stye ( Anjana namika - Kumbheeka ) These commonly resolute naturally if not by pulling the affected eye lash or by giving a tiny Horizontal incision pus should be drained.

### b) Meibomian glands

These present in the tarsal plate of eye lid, a cyst may form due to obstruction in the gland or its duct, is known as meibomian cyst or Tarsal cyst or chalazian (utsangini or lagana or Bahala varthma) . A cyst develops above the lid margin merely in the centre of the eye lid, swelling can be felt through the skin but its pus point, red ness and suppuration seen through the palpebral conjunctiva and for treatment Incission drainage is done by giving a small vertical incission on palpebral conjunctiva. ( small cysts resolute naturally, suppurated cysts are treated by I/D, and hard cyst are treated by Excision. )

# EXAMINATION OF CONJUNCTIVA

Conjunctiva is a thin smooth transparant serous layer that cover under surface ( internal surface) of eye lids and Anterior part of (bulbar) conjunctiva. Different names are given to it according to it's site, they are as follows

**1) Palpebral conjunctiva.**

    **a)** Marginal - The conjunctiva which is at the eye lid margin. **b)** Tarsal conjunctiva - the conjunctiva which covers Tarsal plate of eye lid.**c)** Orbital part - rest of the palpebral conjunctiva beyond the lid posteriorly .

**2) Fornix :-** It is the fold of conjunctiva formed by the reflexion of conjunctiva from eye lid to the eye ball.

**3) Bulbar conjunctiva -** the conjunctiva that covers the anterior part of sclera upto Limbus.

**4) Limbal conjunctiva-**it covers around the limbus (Sclero corneal junction).

**5) Plica semilunaris-** it is the crescentic fold of conjunctiva at the inner canthus which forms boundary for Lacrimal Lake to preserve the tears.

**Note :-** Marginal - Tarsal and Limbal conjunctiva firmly attached to the subjacent tissues but conjunctiva of fornix, orbital conjunctiva and Bulbar conjunctiva are lossely attached to the subjacent tissues.

    1) Bulbar conjunctiva, Limbal conjunctiva, plica semi lunaris can be easily inspected because they present in palpebral fissure, and in the Horizontal meridian.

    2) Lower palpebral conjunctiva and formix should be examined by pressing down the eye lid against the orbital bone.

    3) Upper palpebral conjunctiva and fornix should be examined by everting the eye lid  it is slight difficult than the others.

    4) In general the following lesions should be detected in the conjunctiva.

**a) Examination of the Fornix and palpebral conjunctival lesions:-**

**1)** Hyperaemia (Red ness - due to increased vascularity followed by some lesion inflammatory or traumatic), **2)** Anaemia (loss of blood - pale conjunctiva) **3)** Follicles (Sand particles like eruptions, localised aggregation of lymphocytes in the sub epithelial adenoid layer of the conjunctiva), **4)** Papillae (Hyper trophic Folded epithelium with core of blood vessels by which conjunctiva appears velvety), **5)** True membrane formation as in diphtheria (un separatable layer  if tried to separate causes bleeding), **6)**  False membrane formation (Which can be easily separated from its base without bleeding), **7)** Foreign bodies, **8)** Cicatrical changes (contraction of the tissue due to scar tissue formation  **9)** sub conjunctival haemorrages. **10)** Haemorrhagic lesions.**11)**  Congestion **12)** Discharge (Watery mucoid, mucopurulent, purulent etc).**13)** Adhesions. **14)**  Inflammatory changes (Conjunctivitis) **15)** Congenital lesions etc should be examined.

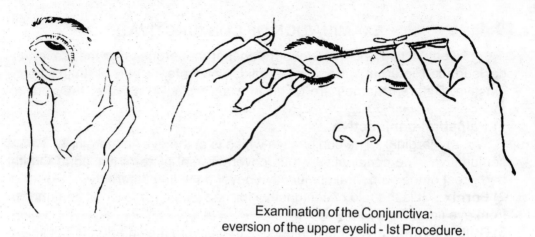

Examination of the Conjunctiva:
eversion of the upper eyelid - Ist Procedure.

Examination of the conjunctiva:
eversion of the lower eyelid

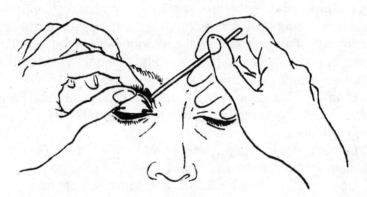

Examination of the Conjunctiva:
eversion of the upper eyelid - Second Procedure

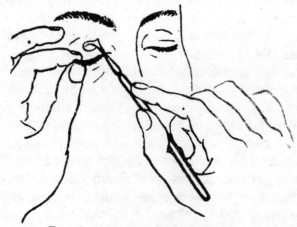

Examination of the Conjunctiva:
eversion of the eyelid for examination of super palpebral fold.

362

**Note:-** a1) Follicles, papillae, cicatrical changes, pannus are the common signs of **Trachoma** (Pothaki)

a2) True membrane formation, congestion, hyperaemia, foreign body sensation, are the common signs of true mebranous conjunctivitis due to diphtherial infection.

a3) Follicles formation,Foreign body sensation, congestion,hyperaemia of conjunctiva are the common signs of follicular conjunctivitis .

a4) Frank pus discharge with inflammatory signs of conjunctiva are seen in purulent conjunctivitis commonly due to Gonococcal infection

a5) The common signs & symptoms of conjunctivitis (Abhishyanda). are conjunctival discharge, hyperaemia (Red ness), chemosis, Foreign body sensation and other constitutional symptoms.

## b) Examination of  Bulbar Conjunctival lesions :-

The following lesions to be noted.

1) Hyperaemia, 2) chemosis; 3) Anaemia, 4) Foreign bodies 5) sub conjunctival haemorrhage (Arjuna) 6) congestion 7) discharge (Watery, mucoid, mucopurulent and purulent ) 8) Follicles, 9) papillae, 10) Truemembrane or False membrane formation, 11) phlycten formation at near limbus due to tubercular infection(phlyctenular conjunctivitis -parvani) 12) Triangular sub-conjunctival layer formation towards cornea do to diegenerative changes is known as pterigium (Arma), 13) A small raised yellowish white nodule occuring in bulbar conjunctiva in Horizontal meridian a little distance away from Limbus occurs due to Allergy and degenerative changes  is known as pinguecula (Pistaka, Balasa graditha),

( A phlycten may ulcerate but pinguecula cannot , Dry lustreless conjunctiva with bitods spots arises a little distance to limbus in horizontal meridian is known as Xerosis or xerophthalmia due to vitamin A deficiency, Adhesion between palpebral and bulbar conjunctiva either due to congenital or acquired causes is known as symblepharon, and any other allergic inflammatory traumatic or degenerative lesion of bulbar conjunctiva should be noted.

## c) EXAMINATION OF LIMBAL CONJUNCTIVA

Ciliary or circumcorneal congestion, (sirajala) and presence of any nodules should be examined.

**(Summary -** conjunctiva should be examined for.

1) Hyperaemia 2) Anaemia 3) Pigmentory changes 4) chemosis 5) collections of foreign bodies 6) Haemorrhagic lesions. 7) sub conjunctival haemorrhages 8) xerotic changes 9) Extra growths (layers, nodules cysts tumours etc) 10) Follicles, papillae 11) discharge 12) Cicatrical changes 13) Congestion 14) Adhesions 15) Inflammatory traumatic degenerative and allergic signs should be noted.)

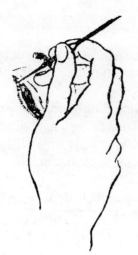

Probing of the lacrimal passages:
Insertion or probe into the lacrimal punctum.

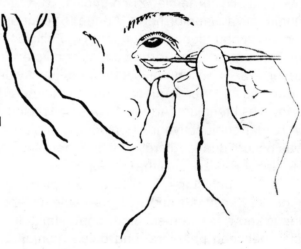

Probing of the lacrimal passages:
Insertion of probe into the lacrimal
canaliculus

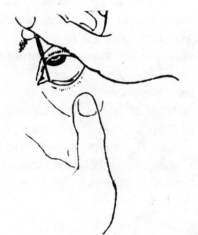

Probing of the lacrimal Passages:
Insertion of probe into the lacrimal sac.

## Examination of Lacrimal apparatus :-

1) Lacrimal sac area (just below the inner canthus) should be examined for any swelling or fistula that may be due to dacryocystitis (inflammation of Lacrimal Sac).

2) By Pressing over the sac area if pus regurgitates through punctum it is of Dacryocystitis.

3) In acute dacryocystitis some times Lacrimal fistula also seen at the same site.

4) Watering of eyes if occurs due to obstruction in lacrimal apparatus is known as epiphora (Netra srava).

## EXAMINATION OF EXTRA OCULAR MUSCLES

The six extra ocular muscles are responsible for the movement of eye ball. So the movement of eye ball should be examinaed in all the directions to check the function of the muscles. (The deviation of the visual axis is knownas squint, the oscillatory movement of eye ball is known as Nystagmus).

## EXAMINATION OF CORNEA

Cornea is the Anterior 1/6th Part of Fibrous coat which is colourless transparent and the first part of the refractiva media, it appears black due to the iris which is placed exactly at behind. it is Avascular but highly sensiitive due to rich nerve supply. The regular arrangement of corneal components keep it's transparency.

### 1) Size of the Cornea :-

Normal :- Approximately 10.5 to 11 mm in diameter, the horizontal diameter is slight more than vertical diameter.

If the size of cornea is smaller. Known as **micro cornea** , If the size of cornea is bigger known as **megalo cornea** or **macro cornea**

### 2) Shape of the Cornea :-

It is sperical anteriorly and circular posteriorly, the anterior surface is smooth regular and with uniform thickness for the refractive purpose, due to congenital abnormalities cornea may present in oval shape, conical shape and in irregular shape.

### 3) Position of Cornea :-

It occupies central position in the eye ball and well fitted in the anterior scleral aperture like the watch glass. its position is well maintained by extra ocular muscles if not cause squint.

## 4) Surface of Cornea :-

The anterior surface of cornea is smooth and uniform for optical purpose, if not leads to visual problems (Astigmatism develops due to uneven surface of cornea) .

## 5) Colour of the Cornea :-

In normal, it is colourless but appears Black due to Iris behind. But in some abnormal conditions it may become red brown white or in multi colours.

## 6) Thicknes of Cornea :-

Normal central corneal thickness is 0.5 mm, normal peripheral corneal thickness is 0.8. mm, The central zone is more thinner for optical purpose. If the thickness varies due to traumatic or inflammatory causes, that should be noted.

## 7) Position of cornea :-

whether Normal in the position or with Anterior synechia Should be noted (Adheson of Iris with cornea is known as anterior synechia.

8) Cornea should be examined whether it is Normal in the position or with Anterior staphyloma (Protrusion of Iris through sclera or cornea .

9) Whether cornea is intact or with Iris prolapse, should be noted (Ajakajatha)

10) Examination of minute corneal ulcers, scratches, Foreign bodies etc. should be examined in bright room with magnifying corneal loupe If they are not visualised by corneal loupe, by the following methods those should be detected.

a) 2% fluorescein drops should put in the eye, normal corneal epithelium cannot respond to the above medicine but the injured epithelium (2nd layer exposure happens) responds and be come green colour, like this the smallest scratches, ulcers, penetrating type of Foreign bodies are detected.

b) An Instrument known as placidos disc is used to detect the scratches or smallest, invisible injuries of cornea those derange the surface of cornea.

Placidos disc contain a round plate with central perforation, one surface is painted with concentrical lines equidistantly around the perforation and painted alternatively (one area with black next area white (no colour) this round plate is given support with a handle.

The patient is asked to sit in front of the doctor with light source at the head level of the patient and to words the left side. The doctor should handle the placidos disc in his hand Facing the painted surface to wards the patient and has to see through the central perforation. The painted surface is illuminated with light source and the corneal surface should be examined through the central perforation of placidos disc.

1) If cornea is as smooth as mirror the placido's image is seen as it is in the mirror

2) If any where corneal tissue is injured in that area the concentrical lines of disc shows some irregularity, so image of placidos disc is seen irregular on the affected site of the cornea.

By above two methods, the smallest scratches, injuries, penetrating type of Foreign bodies etc can be detected to assess whether cornea is transparent or affected.

11) If any corneal ulcer (ulcerative keratitis) or opacity (non ulcerative keratitis) or pentetrating type of foreign bodies presnet, the following details should be collected for the perfect diagnosis .

1) Size of the lesion (smaller or wide) 2) Shape of the lesion. 3) Position of the lesion (Whether central or peripheral) (central corneal opacity obstruct the vision ) 4) Number of lesions 5) progressive or stationary 6) Drylesion or with discharge 7) depth of the lesion 8) Margins of the lesion to know whether healing type or progressive type 9) Alone or with any adhesions or protrusions or prolapse 10) Colour of the lesion.

**Note :-** Smaller single, marginal is stationary, dry, superficial, hyperaemic margins without adhesion protrusion prolapse is non complicative.

**Examination of corneal Vascularisation.:-**
Normally cornea is avascular, except it s 1-2 mm peripheral area. But in some conditions, as a complication cornea may become vascularised or opaque, that should be noted.

Ex:- In trachoma 3rd stage the upper part of cornea is vascularised in triangular shape, is known as pannus formation.

2) In anterior synechia, Anterior staphyloma , Iris prolaps etc diseases due to contact of iris with cornea,  there are chances for Vascularisation. of cornea.

13) The colour and depth of corneal opacity should be estimated.

a) Slight discolouration with involvement of superficial epithelium of cornea is known as Nebula.

b) Brown discolouration with moderate thickness of the corneal opacity is known as macula.

c) White conreal opacity with maximum thickness is known as Leucoma.

**14) Examination of Corneal sensitivity** :- Cornea is having rich nerve supply to have perfect sensitivity to realise the smallest dust particles which collects on cornea, if not the foreign bodies may damage the cornea. But in some Nerve lesions of cornea some part of corneal tissue become insensitive, that affected area should be diagnosed to prevent furthur corneal damge.

## CAUSES FOR LOSS OF CONREAL SENSATION

1) Herpes infection 2) Acute congestive glaucoma 3) Absolute glaucoma 4) Leucoma 5) Leprosy 6) Following alcohol injection in the gasserian ganglian 7) Tumour pressing on 5th Nerve etc.

**Estimation of corneal sensitivity :-**
It is elicited by touching the cornea with a wisp of cotton wool, if the patient do blepharospasm that indicate the cornea is sensitive and if the patient doses not do blepharospasm that indicate some area of cornea is insensitive.

15) Cornea should be examined for any superficial inflammatory changes (superficial keratitis) or deep inflammatory changes (deep keratitis), oedema vesicles or bullae on the epithelium,

16) Corneal endothelium should be examined for any inflammatory deposits known as keratic precipitates.

# EXAMINATION OF SCLERA AND EPISCLERA

Sclera is the white opaque, the 5/6th part of outer fibrous coat , it is responsible to maintain the shape of the eye ball. It is covered by episclera and bulbar conjunctiva anteriorly and episclera and Tenons capsule posteriorly (conjunctival covering present only in anterior part of eye ball, that is replaced by Tenons capsule posteriorly).

The lesions of Sclera and  Episclera are not common.(very rare)
1) Inflammation of sclera is known as scleritis.
2) Inflammation of episclera is known as episcleritis.
3) Thinning of sclera at limbal area may cause scleral staphyloma through which Iris protrudes out.
4) Thinning of sclera at posterior pole of eye ball ( posterior scleral staphyloma) is the commonest cause for axial myopia .
5) Sclera should be checked for foreign bodies. congestion oedema and pigmentory changes.

# EXAMINATION OF LIMBUS

Limbus is a small transitional zone present between cornea and sclera (sclero corneal junction). It contain circular canal of schlemm, having importance in aqueous circulation.

a) LImbus should be examined for any traumatic or surgical scars.
b) Congestion of vessels ( ciliary congestion seen radially)
c) Pterigium, pinguecula, phlycten, Bitods spots, Xerotic changes, Vascularisation.  Staphyloma etc should be examined which are commonly observed at limbus.

**Examination of Anterior Chamber :-**
It is a small chamber (2.5 mm depth centrally) present in between cornea and Anterior uvea (Iris, ciliary body), it contain aqueous humour, through this chamber the aqueous circulate in to schlemm's canal of Limbus, by this normal intra ocular pressure is maintained. Aqueous chamber should be examined (Trans illumination) for the following points.

1) Depth  of the Anterior chamber whether.
a) Normal b) Shallow ( may cause glaucoma due to obstruction in aqueous circulation). c) deep (Commonly in Aphakia)

2) Aqueous fluid should be checked for the inflammatory precipitates.

a) Collection of pus in Aqueous chamber is known as Hypopyon .

b) Collection of blood in Aqueous chamber is known as Hyphaema .

c) Collection of Keratic precipitates on endothelium of cornea.

All these commonly seen in uveitis etc inflammatory lesions.

d) Examination of Angle of anterior chamber is important for the con firmation of glaucoma, it is possible with the instrument known as gonioscope.

## EXAMINATION OF IRIS

Iris is a coloured circular diaphragm present in between cornea and lens. on either sides it continues with ciliary body and chorroid. It contains a central perforation known as pupil, the constriction and dilatation of pupil is regulated by the sphinctre pupillae and dilator pupillae muscles of iris. The anterior surface of Iris is uneven and shows many crypts and fissures. The cornea appears black or brown due to iris which is exactly behind . The following points should be examined.

1) Whether Iris present or absent (congenitally Absence of Iris is known as Aniridia.

2) Iris is a pigmented diaphragm, if the pigment reduces causes photo phobia, blurring of vision and nystagmus, that is known as Albinism .

3) The colours of both Irides or All the sectors of Iris should be in uniform colour,if not called Heterochromia of Iris.

4) Size shape of the iris should be noted .

5) Position of the iris should be noted whether it is central or displaced

a) Adhesion of Iris with cornea is known as anterior synechia .

b) Adhesion of Iris with lens is known as posterior synechia .

c) Bulging of Iris anteriorlly in secclusio pupillae due to the pressure of aqueous humour on iris, is known as Iris bombi

6) Iris vessels are not visible in general but in Rubeosis iridis disease, new vessels are formed and seen.

7) Surface of Iris, should be examined to see the colour crysts and fissure etc, in Iritis the surface appears in uniform mud colour, (no crypts and fissures.)

8) Iris should be examined for its unifolm colour but the lesions of atrophic patches (depigmented) are seen some times, those should be noted.

9) Gapping of Iris (Coloboma) seen in congenital lesions, after iridectomy and by penetrating injuries.

10) The tremulousness ( Shaking or moving Iris) of Iris if elicited by the movment of eye ball, it is known as Iriododonesis. it is observed in the aphakia and in Subluxation of lens etc.

11) Tearing of Iris from it's attachment (ciliary body) and giving the pupil D shape, is known as Iridodialysis .

12) Inflammation of Iris is known as        Iritis.
    "        Ciliary body            "        Cyclitis
    '        Choroid                 "        Choroiditis (Posterior uveitis)

    "        Iris and ciliary body   "        Iridocyclitis or Anterior Uveitis

    "        Iris, ciliary body, choroid      Total Uveitis.

    " The infection of one part easily spreads to other and cause compete Uveitis.

13) Iris can be seen and examined directly through cornea but ciliary body and choroid direct examination is not possible, it can be estimated by the following signs and symptoms.

## COMMON CLINICAL FEATURES OF UVEITIS

1) Hypopyon 2) Hyphaema 3) Keratic precipitates 4) Posterior synechia 5) formation of cyclitic membrane behind the lens 6) retinal detachment 7) Pain and redness of eye 8) moving spots beofre the eye 9) Hazy vision 10) Metamorphopsia (distortion of objects) 11) Micropsia (objects appears maller) 12) Macropsia (Objects seen bigger) 13) Photopsia (Flashes of light seen due to retinal irritation) 14) ciliary congestion 15) ciliary tenderness 16) cloudy aqueous 17) deep anterior chamber 18) muddy Iris 19) Irregular pupil with sluggished reaction. 20) Iris bombi 21) secclusio pupillae and occulusio pupillae 22) secondary glaucoma 23) Finally may cause Hypotony or Phthisis bubi.

## EXAMINATION OF PUPIL

It is the central perforation of the Iris meant for regulating the entry of light rays into the retina by the constriction and dilatation. The following points should be noted while the examination of pupil .

1) Size :- Normal  3 to 4 mm (Bigger in the adults and smaller in the old; constrict in bright illumination and dilates in the dim illumination; pupil constric tors are known as miotics and pupil dilators are known as mydriotics. Mydriotics' or used for fundoscopy and to prevent anterior synechia, miotics used to treat glaucoma).

2) Shape :- Normally circular but seen irregular in Uveal tract lesions and synechia .

3) Position of pupil - Normally present in centre but seen eccentric or drawn to front or back or sides in Uveitis and synechia .

4) Pupillary margin - It should be regular but may become irregular in synechia, Uveitis, seclusio pupillae, and occlusio pupillae .

5) Pupillary aperture should be clear without any occlusion, but following abnormalities should be noted.

    a) Inflammatory exudates collects and cause occlusio pupilae, it causes obstruction to vision.

    b) the pupillary margin completely attached to the lens capsule and produce secclusio pupillae, it causes visual obstruction and iris bombi.

**6) Pupillary reaction to light :-**

    a) Driect method - Light should be focussed and removed alternatively and the constriction and dilatation of the pupil should be noted respectively.

    b) Consensual method - light should be focussed in the one eye and pupillary reaction (constriction and dilatation) should observe in the other eye.

    3) Pupil reaction to accommodation or convergence

    Patient is asked to look at a near object and his pupil should be observed for constriction.

## EXAMINATION OF THE CRYSTALLINE LENS

Lens is a traasparent, Bi convex structure present in the eye ball to converge and focuss the light rays on fovea of macula of retina for visual perception. its dioptric power is + 17.5 . on either sides it is supported by suspensary ligaments or zonule and it is situated in between Iris and vitreous humour.

    In transillumination test a) When the lens is transparant nothing can be seen behind the pupil except a black shade .

    b) When lens become opaque, Brown or white colour opacities are seen behind the pupil.

    c) In Senile Lental Sclerosis also lens appears brown or white in transillumination test.

It should be confirmed by ophtholmoscopic examination.

The findings of ophthalmoscopy.

a1) Lental opacities (cataract) appears as black spots in front of red reflex of the retina -.

a2) In normal condition the red reflex of retina, macula, optic disc and vessels are seen perfectly (no black dots seen)

a3) In immature cataract the red reflex and contents of retina are seen partially.

a4) In mature cataract red reflex is absent, media is obstructed and appears black,

B) In senile Lental sclerosis though lens appears in brown externally, media appears clear by opthalmoscopic examinatiion .

"The different types of cataracts can be easily diagnosed by ophthalm oscopy "

The follwing features should be examined by ophthalmoscopy.

1) Colour of the lens, place of the opacity (central - marginal or total) 3) Displacement of lens (sub luxation - partial dis placement of lens, luxation total displacement of lens) should be noted 4) presence or absence of lens (Aphakia ) should be noted.

During the examination of retinal vessels, the narrowing, tortuosity, dilatation, sheathing, venous compression at the arterio venous crossings and light reflex from the vessels should be noted. when retinal pigment is deficient choroidal vessels seen as pinkish flat ribbons which do not show any light reflex.

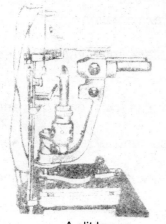

A slit lamp

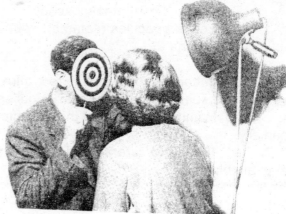

Placido's disc

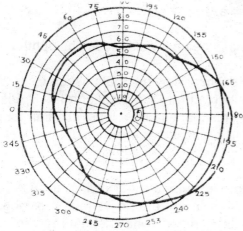

Extent of normal visual field of
the right eye

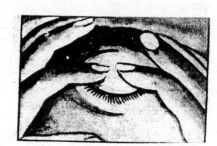

Digital tonometry

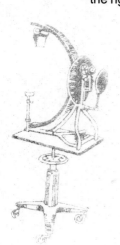

Projection perimeter

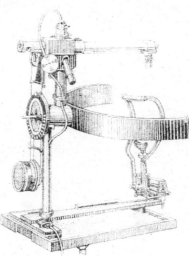

A diagram of gonioscopy

# ESTIMATION OF INTRA OCULAR PRESSURE

## 1) Digital tonometry :-

It is by palpation of the eyes with fingers, patient is asked to look down then the sclera is palpated through the upper lid beyond the tarsal plate. The tension is judged by the amount of fluctuation obtained.

## 2) By Schiotz tonometer :-

The patient is asked to liedown on a table, local anaesthesia is given, the eye lids are separated with fingers or with universal eye speculum. Now the cornea is properly exposed, later the foot plate of tonometer is kept on the cornea then the deflection of the pointer on the scale should be recorded, like the deflextion reading should be recorded for different weight. Later on the deflection should be interpreted in terms of intra ocular tension from the chart accompanying the tonometer. the normal intra ocular pressure is 18 to 25 mm Hg. if it increases causes a dreadful disease known as glaucoma.

## THE FUNCTIONAL EXAMINATION OF EYE BALL

## 1) Visual acuity :-

Central or direct vision

a) Distrant central vision is estimated with snellen's chart.

b) Near central vision is estimated with jaeger's test types, snellen's test types, printer's type of N serives.

## a) Estimationof central distant vision with the help of snellen's chart :-

The snellen's chart is placed 6 meters or 20 feet distance from the patient, the patient is asked to sit on a stool facing the chart from 6 meters distance and asked to read the prints of the chart by closing one eye. The chart contain different sized prints in 7 or 8 Lines, from Bigger size to smaller From Top to down wards.

The each line is marked with some specific number. they are (from top to bottom) 60, 36, 24, 18, 12, 9, 6,5.

If the patient is able to read upto 6 number row, his vision is 6/6 - Normal.

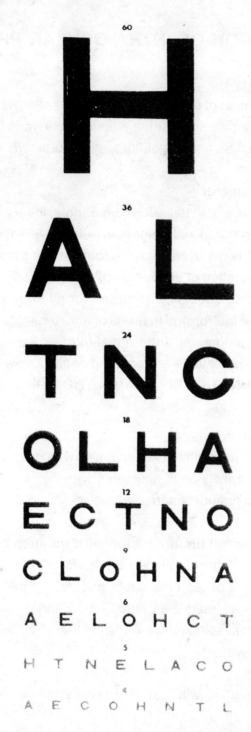

Snellen's Distant Test Types (reduced). The lines, from above downwards, should be read at 60, 26,24,18,12,9,6,5 and 4 m, respectively, i.e., at these distances the letters subtend a visual angle of 5.

| If the patient able to read only 1st line | His vision is | 6/60 |
|---|---|---|
| "    "    2nd line ' | | 6/36 |
| "    "    3rd line " | | 6/24 |
| "    "    4th line " | | 6/18 |
| "    "    5th line " | | 6/12 |
| "    "    6th line " | | 6/9 |
| "    "    7th line " | | 6/6 normal vision |
| "    "    8th  line " | | 6/5 |

**Note :-**
1) 6/6 is normal
2) 6/5 the Best vision.
3) In 6/6 the upper six is the fixed distance between the patient and chart, thelower six is the marking of the 7th line of the Snellen's chart..

**Models of snellens chart prints.**

1) One surace contain English alphabets .

2) 2nd surface contain the letters of different Local language.

3) 3rd surface contain Black dots in squares asked to count the black circles in each square ( for illiterates)

4th surface of the snellen's chast contain E or C shaped pictures, patients are asked to find out the direction of or gap of E or C (This is also for illiterates).

If the patient is not able to recorgnise even the first letter of the chart (vision less than 6/60), than the distance between the chart and patient should be reduced .

| If the patient can see the top letter from 5 meters his vision is | 5/60 |
|---|---|
| "    "    "    4 Meters    " | 4/60 |
| "    "    "    3 meters    " | 3/60 |
| "    "    "    2 meters    " | 2/60 |
| "    "    "    1 meter    " | 1/60 |

If the patient is not able to recognise the top letter of the chart even from 1 meter, he is asked to count the fingers from 3/2/1 feet distance, finally the patient is asked to recognise the projection of light (Directions of light) and perception of light (identificationof Brightness of Light).

Like this the distant central vision can be estimated accurately.

**Note :-** After completion of the examination of one eye, the other eye should be examined.

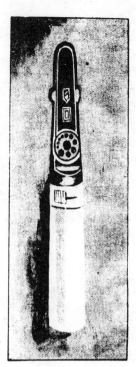

Direct Ophthalmoscope

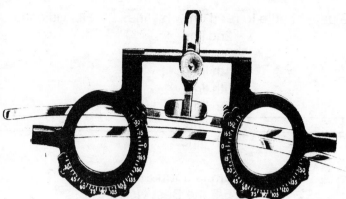

Trial frame (By courtesy of Keeler)

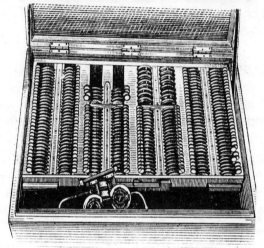

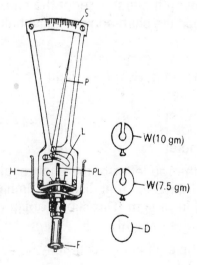

Schiotz Tonometer

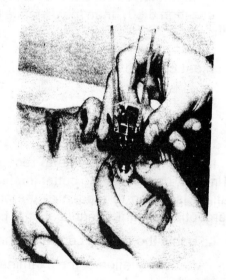

Schiotz tonometer (by courtesy of

# OPHTHALMOSCOPY

Ophthalmoscope is used for the examination of posterior segment of the eye ball, ophthalmoscopy is highly important diagnostic procedure not only in the diseases of eye but also in the many diseases of visceral organs (systemic lesions).

Ophthalmoscope contain a handle and head piece. handle is for handling the instrument to put cells inside, it also contain on - off switch. The head piece contain a central perforation with the arrangement of mini bulb to focuss the light rays into fundus and concave and convex lenes to see the fundus and in addition to above there is arrangement for producing different types of light beams to see the different parts. (Macular beam, fundus beam, Retinal beam, slit beam etc),

Before ophthalmoscopy, pupil dilatation of the patient is neeeded for clear and camplete view of fundus (but pupil dilatation is contra indicated in glaucoma). Right eye of the patient should be examined with the right eye of the examiner by handling the instrument in right hand - and vice versa

**Note :-** 1) In indirect ophthalmoscopy 5 times magnification of the fundus can be seen with inverted image and with Direct ophthalmoscopy 10 times magnification of the fundus can be seen with errect image.
2) Regular practice is needed for conducting ophthalmosopy.

## Direct ophthalmoscopy :-
1) In a dark room patient is asked to sit comfortablly, a red bulb should be arranged above the head level and facing opposite to the patient.

2) While the examination, the doctor should sit infront of the patient and should place the ophthalmoscope close to the patient's eye without hurting him (only one inch gap between 2 faces).

3) The eye is illuminated by the light reflected from the ophthalmoscope.
4) The lenses should adjust to see the media and fundus clearly through the hole of the ophthalmoscope.

5) if both the examiner and the patient are emmetropic a clear view of the fundus can be seen without any adjustment of lens if not by adjusting the lenses ophthalmoscopy should be don.

6) If the refractive media is clear (cornea, aqueous Lens vitreous ) the red reflex of retina is seen brightly at the pupil in ophthalmoscopy.

7) If any opacities are present in the media those appear as black spots (fixed or floating) against the red back ground of fundus of retina.

8) If the media is partially opaque, the red reflex seen partially and if media completely opaque the red reflex cannot be seen.

9) The moving opacities situate in vitreous or aqueous, and the fixed opacities situate in cornea and Lens .

10) When the eye ball is moved if the the opacities move in the same direction those present in the anterior plane, and if move in opposite direction those prasent in the posterior plane.

11) Dots or spots if disappears when closely approached, thay are lental, if persist they are corneal.

12) While the examination of the macula the patient is asked to see straight into the hole of ophthalmoscope.

13) While the examination of optic disc the patient is asked to see towards the opposite shoulder or ear of the examiner to expose the optic disc.

14) If the patient is myopic by adjusting concave lenses, if Hyper metropic by adjusting convex Lenses, fundus should be examined for the following points.
1) Optic disc 2) macula 3) Periphery of retina and 4) Vessels of retina.

**Examination of optic disc :-**
It is a round or oval structure , pale pink in colour, stuated at the poste-. rior part of fundus, medial to macula (Posterior pole) it is also known as optic nerve head. There is excavation at the central part of disc known as the physiological cup, whose dept and extent varies in different subjects. The margins of the disc are normally sharp and distinct so during the examinationof the fundus, the colour shape, margins, physiological cup, presence of abnormal vessels and any other lesions should be noted.

In optic atrophy disc become pale or white with blurred margins, in oedema and raised intra cranial pressure (papilloedema) discbulges and protrudes with blurred margins, in papillitis disc become hyperaemic margin be come blurred and later on disc swells, in chronic glaucoma cupping of the disc seen.

**Examination of macula :-**

It present at the posterior pole cones are tightly packed so only it is responsible for the perception of bright and colour vision, it contain a central depression known as fovea centralis where the light rays are focussed for the visual sensation. During ophthalmoscopic examination fovea appears as a bright reflex, but in degenerative condtitions, burns and in the other lesions the brightness of macula reduces and lead to blindness.

**Examination of Retinal vesels :-**

The arteries and veins radiate from the optic disc and spread all over the fundus. arteries appear in bright red colour and venins in purplish red.

## EXAMINATION OF CENTRAL NEAR VISION

It is carried out with the help of snellen's prints or jaeger's prints or printer's type of N series.

Patient is asked to sit comfortably, the test types should be properly illuminated from behind the head of the patient, each eye is to be tested separately at a distance of about 25 cm or 30 cm . The test types are present from smaller print to Bigger gradually. A person with normal accommodation can read the smallest types also. if he cannot read the smallest types, the types which he can read should be noted,  N/10 , N/12 etc or J/10, J/12 etc.

# EXAMINATION OF COLOUR VISION

The human eye can distinguish seven or eight colour of spectrum (Red - Blue and green are 3 primary colours ). Normal colour perception is essential in some occupations such as the Railway, steamship services, Navy and airforces. There are several methods for tesing colur vsion. Among them the common one is Ishihara ISO chromatic chart.

Ishihara Iso chromatic hart contains bold numerals which are represented in dots of different tints, which are very confusing to the colour blind persons. when he can see all the colours then only he can Identify the numerals of the chart.

**Field of vision :-**

It is a space within an object can be seen when the eye remains fixed on some point. The extent of the field can be roughly estimated by con frontation method, more accurately by the perimeter.

**Confrontation Method :-**

The patient is asked to sit infront of the examiner at a distance of about 2 feet, light is being placed above and behind the head of the patient. To examine the patients Right eye he is asked to close his left eye with his leftpalm and should fix his right eye on the examiner's left eye.

The examiner has to close his right eye and bring his hand with extended fingers in midway between the patient and himselft, from periphery to inward and the patient is asked to indicate when he first see the fingers, the same test is repeated in all the directions. like this the doctor should examine the patients field of vision by comparing to his own vision.

**Perimetry ;-**

Perimeter records the field of vision accurately, this method is known as perimetry. This instrument contain a metallic semi circle which can be rotated in any direction, the arc is marked in degrees "O". at the cnetre and 90 on each end. The patients head should be supported on chin rest of the instrument 33 cm away from the middle of tthe arc one eye should be covered and other fixes on an object placed at the centre of the arc. A test object is a white or coloured disc of varying sizes is carried along the inner surface of arc and the points at which it is first observed in the different meridians should be recorded on a specially designed chart- in routine work the extent of the field should be recorded with two different sized white objects one a 3 mm and other 1 mm, some times coloured test object may also be used.
Extent of normal field of vision for 5 mm test object

The visual field extends $100^0$ on temporal side, $60^0$ on nasal side, 55 to $60^0$ Above and $75^0$ below.

(Within the visual field there may be areas of defect which are known as scotomata ( no perceptive elements )

## Scotometry of Central and paracentral visual field with Bjerrum's screen:-

Bjerrum screen is used to detect central and para central visual field, within a radious of $30^0$. It consist of a black curtain of 2 meters square, which is fixed on a wodden frame work. The patient is seated at a two meters distance. The test object consists of round white disc mounted to a black rod. ( There are various sizes of test objects both white and coloured) with one eye closed, the patient should fix the other eye on white spot which in the centre of the screen. At first blind spot should be mapped out on the screen using a 10 mm white test object, then the extent of the visual field is determined with one or two mm white test objects and finally working systematically over the field the presence of any scotoma should be detected. while recording the extent of a scotoma it is advisable to move the test object from the blind to the seeing area. when the scotoma is relative it may not be detected until a coloured test object is used.

All these findings are marked out by inserting black headed pins on the screen . The result is then transferred on a printed chart for record.

# OPHTHALMIC INSTRUMENTS

Plate No. I

**1) a) Universal eye speculum:-**. It can be used for either eye, it has a spring two limbs to keep the eye lids separate. As there is no guard more space is obtained during the operation (The eye lashes protrude in the field of operation due the absence of guard).

**I) b) Guarded eye speculum :-** There are two instruments one for right eye and another for left eye. it has a spring and two limbs. the upper limb has a guard to keep the eye lashes away from the field of operation.

**2) Fixation Forceps :-** It has 2 to 5 teeth and used to fix the eye ball through the conjunctiva and episcleral tissue during the operation.

**3) Von graefe's Cataract Knife :-**
It has a long narrow thin straight blade with a sharp point and sharp cutting edge, used for making section for cataract operation, iridectomy and for paracentesis .

**4) Elschnigs intra capsular Forceps:-**
Each limb of the forceps has a double curve and blunt point without teeth, it is used to hold the anterior Lens capsule at 6 0 clock position in intra capsular Lens extraction.

**5) Capsulotome or Cystitome :-**
It has a tiny sharp and bent point at the end of a straight narrow limb, it is used to tear the capsule of lens in Extra capsular Lens extraction.

**8) Capsule forceps:-** used to hold the capsule of lens during lens extraction.

**7) Mc namara Spoon :-**
it has two tiny spoons at the ends of a metal handle, used to apply counter presssure beyond the limbus, during extraction of lens and to re-move dislocated lens.

**8) Lens expressor :-**
It has a flat corrugaged metal handle with a curved knob pointed limb it is used to apply pressure with Knob point of the curved limb on the Limbus, druing the extraction of Lens.

**Pate II**

**9) Iris forceps** - The shape of the forceps are of various types (Straight angular curved ) It is used for holding the iris for iridectomy.

**10) Iris scissors :-** The blades vary in shape and used for Iridectomy.

**11) Iris repositor :-** It is used to reposit the iris by clearing it from the wound after iridectomy .

**12) Anterior chamber washing canula :-**
It is used to clean the anterior chamber from various precipitants.

**13) Bowmans discission needle:-** It is straight sharp triangular needle with gaurd, used for discission of congenital or traumatic cataract and for needling of an after catract.

**14) Ordinary discission needle :-**
Same as above but the needle dosen't contain gaurd.

**15) Keratome :-**
It has a triangular bloade with a sharp cutting edges, used for Limbus incision and for paracentesis.

**16) Zeigler's Knife :-**
It has a tiny curved blade with a sharp point at the end of a narrow limb, attached to a handle. it is used for incising the after cataract in the pupillary area.

**17) Vectis :-**
It is a loope of Wire at the end of a narrow Limb attached to a handle, it is used to remove the subluxation of lens

Plate III

**18) Tooke's Knife :-**
It has a short elongated blade attached to a handle with a semi circular cutting edge, bevelled on both surfaces.It is used for splitting the cornea during elliotis sclero corneal trephening operation.

**19) Elliot's sclero corneal trephine handle with blade :-**
It is used for punching a hole in the wall of the eye ball at Limbus in $12^0$ Clock position during Trephine operation.

**20) Disc holding Foceps :-**
It is used for catching the disc of sclero corneal tissue made by the trephine blade.

**21) Broad needle or Paracentesis needle.:-** It is used for paracentesis to drain the aqueous, to reduce the intra ocular prssure.

## 22) Thermo Cautery :-

The cautery is heated in the flame of a spirit lamp and then applied, used for cauterizing tiny iris prolapse, progressive margin of corneal ulcer, and bleeding points.

## 23) Epilation forceps :-

It is used for epilation of eye lashes in trichiasis.

## 24) Des marrie's upper lid retracter :-

It is used for examination of eye in a child and in blepharospasm

## 25) Enucleation scissors :-

It is used to cut optic nerve etc, during enucleation operation.

## 26) Eviscleration scoop of mule :-

It is used for scooping out the contents of eye ball during eviscleration operation.

## 27) Sac knife :-

It is used for incising of skin subcutaneous tissue and for removal of lacrimal sac or for dacryocystorhinostomy operation .

## 28) Muller's Retractor :-

It is used to retract the skin edges during dacryo cystectomy or dacryo-cystorhinostomy operation.

## 29) Rougine :-

It is used for separating the lacrimal sac from lacrimal fossa during dacryo cystectomy operation.

## 30) Lang's dissector with scoop :-

It is used for following the removal of the sac, the scoope is used to scrape off the epithelium from the upper end of the naso lacrimal duct for drainage purpose.

Plate IV

## 31) Nettleship's puctum dilator :-

It is used for dilatation of puncta in case of stenosis of punctum .

**32) Lacrimal canula :-** It is used to test the pateny of the lacrimal sac.

**33) Chalazion forceps :-** It is used for the fixation of chalazian cyst during the operation

## 34) Beer's Knife :-

It is used for incising a chalazian (Vertical incision)

## 34) Chalazian Scoope :-

It is used for scooping out the granulation tissue of the chalazian after incision with Beer's Knife.

## 36) Strabismus hook or Squint hook :-

It is used for catching the extra ocular muscles during squint operation, enucleation operation or operation for detachment of retina.

## 37) Strabismus Scissors ;-

It is used to cut the extra ocular muscles during the operation.

## 38) Foreign body spud and Needle :-

It is used to remove the corneal foreign bodies.

## 39) Sinclair's Cyclodialysis spatula :-

It is used to separate the ciliary body from its attachment to the scleral spur during cyclodialysis operation for aphakic glaucoma.

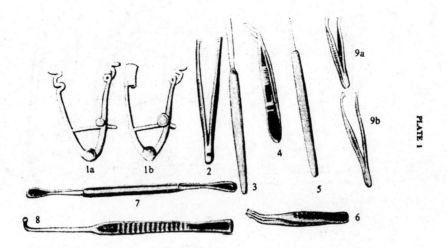

PLATE I

(1a) Universal Eye Speculum (1b) Guarded Eye Speculum (2) Fixation Forceps. (3) Von Graefe's Cataract Knife. (4) Elschnig's Intra-Capsular Forceps. (5) Capsulotome or Cystitome (6) Capsule Forceps. (7) MacNamara Spoon. (8) Lens Expressor (9a) Iris Forceps-Angular. (9b) Iris Forceps-Curved.

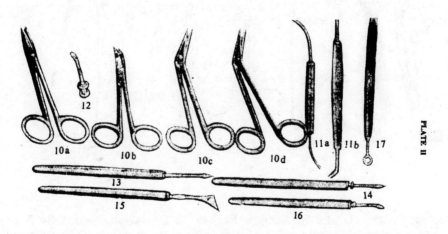

PLATE II

(10a) Iris Scissors-Straight and Sharp-pointed. (10b) Iris Scissors-Curved on flat and sharp-pointed. (10c) Iris Scissors-Angular and sharp-pointed. (10d) Iris Scissors-Angular and Knob-pointed, (11a) Iris Repositor-'S' shaped. (11b) Iris Repositor-Angular. (12) Anterior Chamber Washing canula. (13) Bowman's Discission Needle. (14) Ordinary Discission Needle. (15) Keratome (16) Zeigler's Knife. (17) Vectis

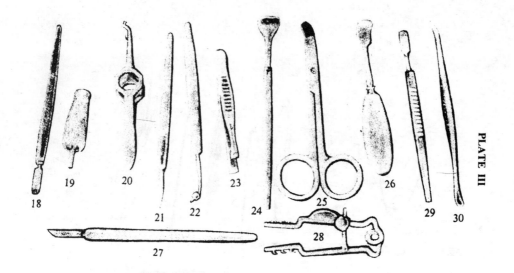

PLATE III

18. Tooke's Knife. 19. Elliot's Sclero-Corneal Trephine Handle with Blade.
20. Disc-Holding Forecepts. 21. Broad Needle or Paracentesis Needle.
22. Thermo-cautery 23.Epilation Forceps. 24. Desmarre's Upper Lid Retractor. 25.
Enucleation Scissors. 26. Evisceration Scoop of Mule. 27 Sac Knife.
28. Muller's Retractor. 29. Rougine 30. Lang's

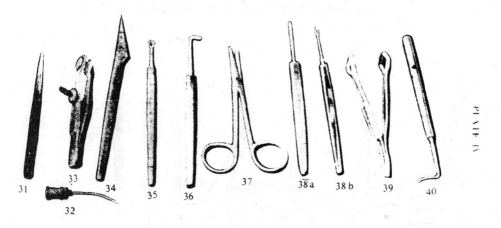

PLATE IV

Nettleships Punctum Dilator. 32. Lacrimal Canula, 33. Chalazion Forceps. 34. Beer's
Knife. 35. Chalazion Scoop. 36. Strabismus Hook or Squint Hook. 37. Strabismus
Scissors. 38a. Foreign Body Spud. 38b. Foreign Body Needle. 39. Knapp's Roller
Forceps. 40. Sinclair's Cyclodialysis Spatula.

# C.S.S.

# N.K.J. AYURVEDIC MEDICAL COLLEGE HOSPITAL - BIDAR.

**AFFLIATED TO RAJIVGANDHI HEALTH UNIVERSITY - KARNATAKA**
**SHALAKYA I CASE SHEET**
**DEPARTMENT OF SHALYA SHALAKYA**

1

1) Name of the Patient      2) Age     3) Sex

4) Caste                  5) Occupation

6) Address            7) Registration No.

                               O.P.D. No.

                               I.P.D. No.

                               Bed No.

8) Date                  9) Provisional diagnosis

---

ii)     1) Patient's chief Complaints, duration.


      2) Associated complaints, duration :


      3) History of Present illness :


      4) History of Previous illness :


      5) Personal history :


      6) Family history :

## III) Asta sthana pareeksha :-

1) Nadi                     2) Mutra

3) Malam                4) Jihwa

5) Shabda               6) Sparsha

7) Druk                    8) Akruthi

## IV) Dasha - vidha pareeksha :-

1) prakruthi            2) Vikruthi

3) Sara                   4) Samhanana

5) Pramana           6) Satmya

7) Satwa                8) Ahara Shakthi

9) Vyayama Shakthi     10) Vayas

## V) Anga pratyanga Pareeksha :-

1) Heart                 3) Liver

2) Lungs                4) Spleen

Other ;-

## VI) Samsthanika - pareeksha : - (Systemic Examination)

## VII. General Examination of FACE -ORBIT and EYE BALL

1. Face whether bilateral symmetrical (     ) or not. (     )
2. Protrusion of eye ball (Exophthalmos)                (     )
3. Sunken eye ball (Anophthalmos)                       (     )
4. Shrinken eye ball (Phthisis bulbi )                  (     )
5. Smaller eye ball (microphthalmos )                   (     )
6. Bigger eye ball (Buphthalmos)                        (     )
7. Deviated axis of eye ball (Squint or strabismus)     (     )
8. Oscillatory eye ball (Nystagmus)                     (     )
9. Congenital abnormalities if any:-                    (     )

## VIII), Examination of appendages of eye ball (lacrimal apparatus etc

## IX) Examination of PAKSHMA MANDALA (Eye Lashes)

1. Normal eye lashes (Fresh, regular, soft, normal
   in colour, position and number.)                     (     )

2. ABNORMAL :-
a) Absence of eye lashes (Pakshma, Shaatha - madarosis   (     )
b) irregular hard eye lashes (Pakshma kopa, Trichiasis)  (     )
c) Depigmented eye lashes (Greyish - whitish)            (     )
d) Eye lashes with parasites (     ) e) Matting of eye lashes (     )
f)
g) Description :-

## x). Examination of PAKSHMA VARTHMA SANDHI (Eye lid margins)

1) NORMAL :-
Normal in colour size, thickness, position and function, without any abnormalities .

2) ABNORMAL :-
a) Inflammation of eye lid margin (krimigrandhi - Blepharitis)   (     )
b) Hyperaemia of eye lid margin (Ragatwam-Milphosis)            (     )
c) Thickening of eye lid margin (Sthulatwam-Tylosis)           (     )
d) Cystic swelling at the root of cilia (Anjana namika
kumbhipitika- zeiscyst or stye)
e) Inversion of eye lid margin (entropion)                     (     )
f) Eversion of eye lid margin (ectropion)                      (     )
g) Adhesions of lid margins, if any.                           (     )
h)
j) Description :

## XI Examination of Varthma Mandala (Eye lids)

1.size :    (a) Normal    b) Abnormal    (   )
2.Shape :    (a) Normal    b) Abnormal    (   )
3.Colour:    (a) Normal    b) Abnormal    (   )
4.Skin surface : a) Normal b) Scars c) Burns d) Injuries    (   )
5.Oedema ;   a) Partial    b) Total    (   )
6.Cyst (Grandhi ) : Chalazian (Utsangini)    (   )
7.Polyps (Arsha) ( ) 8. Abscess (Vidradi ) ( ) 9. Tumour (Arbuda)(   )

10). Varthmakriya (function of eye lids)
    a) Normal    b) Abnormal
A) Lagophthalmos (improper closure of eye lids ) ⎤(Vatahatvarthma) (   )
B) Ptosis (improper opening of eye lids)    ⎦
C) Increased blinking of eye lids (Nimesha)

11.    Varthantah sleshma Kala (Palpebral conjunctiva)
    A) NORMAL :-
    Conjunctiva is bright transparent without any inflammatory,
    degenerative and traumatic lesions.    (   )
B)    ABNORMAL :-
    a) Hyperaemia b) Anaemia c) Follicles d) Papillae
    e) True membrane f) Falsemembrane g Foreign bodies
    h) Cicatrical changes j) Haemorrhagic lesions j) ...............
    k) congestion I) Discharge, m) Adhesions n) .....................
12)    Description :-

## XII)    Examination of Varthma Shukla Sandhi (Fornix)
    1) NORMAL :-

    2) ABNORMAL :-
    a) Hyperaemia b) Anaemia c) Foillicles d) Papillae
    e) True membrane f) False membrane g) Foreign bodies
    h) Cicatrical changes i) Haemorrhagic lesions j) inflammatory lesions
    k) Congestion I) Discharge m) Adesions n) ...................
    Description :-

## XIII) Examination of Shukla Mandala (Sclera - bulbar conjunctiva).
    A ) NORMAL    (   )
    B) ABNORMAL :
    a) Hyperaemia b Anaemia c) Papillae d) Follicles e) True membrane f)
False membrane g) Phlycten h) Pterigium i) Pinguecula j) Haemorrhagic lesions. k) Congestion I) Discharge..................................m) Allergic changes.
n) Inflammatory changes p) Degenerative changes p) Episcleritis. q) Sclertis.
C) Description.

**XIV.)** **Examination of KRISHNA MANDALA (Cornea - Iris)**

A) Examination of cornea :

1) Size :
NORMAL approximately II mm in diameter      (    )
ABNORMAL : a) Micro cornea b) Megalo cornea etc.   (    )

2) Shape
Normal :-Sperical, Horizontal diameter is slight     (    )
More than Vertical diameter
Abnormal :- a) Oval b) Conical c) irreular d)...........   (    )

3) Surface
Normal :- Smooth uniform , Convex anteriorly
Abnormal a) Rough b) irregular c) Flat d)...............   (    )

4) Colour
Normal : Colour less. bright : transparent
Abnormal : a) Brown b) White cO Red d)................   (    )

5) Thickness
Normal : Central thin zone, peripheral thicker zone   (    )
Abnormal :..........................................................   (    )

6) Transparent                       (    )

7) Opaque
a) Corneal opacities b) Uicers c) Scratches d) Foreignbodies   (    )
Central /marginal; Superficial /Deep;     single/ Multiple;
                               Smaller /Wider

8) Vascularisation
9) Sensitivity a) normal b) Partial loss c) Total loss   (    )
10) Congenital abnormalities if any...........................
11)
12) Description :

**B) Examination of Iris :-**
1) size : a) Normal b) Abnormal ( ) 2) Shape : a) Normal b) Abnormal( )    2 )
Surface : a) Normal b) Abnormal (Adhesions, inflammatory lesions.
Injuries etc )                               (    )—
3) Colour :a) Normal  b) Abnormal ( ) 4) Thickness a) Normal b) Abnormal (    )
5) Position :  Normal b) Abnormal (Synechia)         (    )
6) Gaping : a) congenltal (Coloboma) b) Acquired (Iridectomy)  (    )
7) a) Iridencleosis b) Iridodialysis c) Presence of vessels     (    )
8) Description ;-

**C)     Examination of Anterior Chamber and Aqueous humour**
1) Depth of Anterior chamber a) Normal b) Deep c) Shallow          (          )
2) Angle of Anterior chmaber a) Open b) Closed          (          )
3) Aqueous humour
    a) Transparent          c) Hyphaema (with blood)
    b) Hypopyon (with pus)    d) Other precipitants          (          )

4) Intra ocular pressure :
5) Description :-

XV) Examination of Krishna Drusti Sandhi (Limbus)

XVI.) Examination of Drusti  Sandhi
A). Examination of Pupil
      1. size a) Normal (3 to 4 mm dia meter) b) Abnormal          (          )
      2. Shape :- a) Normal (circular) b) Abnormal          (          )
      3. Position ; a) Normal b) Deviated <u>Anterior synechia</u>          (          )
                               posterior synechia
      4. Margin a) Normal b) Abnormal          (          )
      5. Aperture : a) Normal b) Occluded          (          )
      6. Reaction : a) Reactive b) Sluggished c) Absent          (          )
      7. Description :-

B. Lens :-
1.      a) Transparent b) Opaque
2.      Opacity :- a) Capsular b) Cortical c) nuclear          (          )
3.      a) Partial /Total b) Dotlike/Diffused c) Congenital/Acquired          (          )
4.      a) Immature b) Mature c) Hypermature          (          )
5.      Description :-

C). Retina :-
      1. Optic disc
      2. Macula
      3. Fundus
      4. Examination of Refractive media
      5.
      6. Description .

D). Vision Examination          R.EYE          L. EYE
      1. Distant. Vision.
      2) Near Vision.
      3) Colour Vision.
      4) Field of vision.

E) Instrumental Examination

F) Description

**XVII Differential Diagnosis :**

**VIII)    Final diagnosis**

**XIX)    Pancha Lakshana Nidanam**

1. Nidana :

2. Poorva rupa

3. Rupa

4. Upashaya :

5. Samprapthi

6. Dosha Vikruthi

7. Dushya Vikruthi

8. Sroto vikruthi

9. Rogi balam.

10. Roga balam

11. Sadhyaa Sadhyatha

**XX) A.  Chikitsa Sutra**

B.  Pathya :

C. Apathya :

**D. Aushada chikitsa :**

    1. Sthanika chikitsa

    II. Saarva dehika chikitsa

**E.  Shastra Chikitsa ;**

    I.  Poorva Karma

    II.  Pradhana Karma

    III.  Paschaat Karma

**XXI)**  Result

**XXII)**  Advises

Signature of the
Student

signature of the
lecturer

# BIBLIOGRAPHY

1.   Bruhattraya

2.   Laghutraya

3.   Basavarajeeya

4.   Chakradattha

5.   Hareetha Samhitha

6.   Vangasena

7.   Sachitra Shalakya by Dr. Ravindra Chandra Chaudari

8.   Shalakya tantra by Dr. Ramnath Dwivedi

9.   Shalakya tantra by Dr. Vishwanath Dwivedi

10.  Shalakya Tantra by Dr. K.V. Prabhakaram (Telugu)

11.  Parson's ophthalmology

12.  May & worth Ophthalmology

13.  A Short book on Ophthalmology by B. M. Chattergee

14.  A Guide to Ophthalmology by Dhanraj Singh

15.  Notes on Ophthalmology by Experienced teachers.

# Contents

बाल आंजनेय स्वामि (शेषु) प्रसन्न
गणेश स्तुति
शुक्लाम्बरधरं विष्णुं शशिवर्णम चतुर्बुजम्
प्रसन वदनम ध्ययेतसर्व विघ्नोपशांतये


**धन्वंतरि प्रार्थन**
नमामि धन्वंतरि मादिदेवम
सुरा सुरैर्वन्दित पाद पद्मम
लोके जारा रुग्भय मृत्युनाशम
दातार मीशं विविधौशधीनाम


रागादि रोगा: सहजा: समूला
येनाशु सर्वे जगातोप्यपास्त:
तमेक वैद्यं शिरसा नमामि
वैद्याग मझांशचा पितामहादीन

# SHIRO ROGA
# DISEASES OF HEAD

# शिरोरोग

प्राणाः प्राणभृतां यत्र श्रिताः सर्वेन्द्रियाणि च।
यदुत्तमाङ्गमङ्गानां शिरस्तदभिधीयते॥

(च. सू. अ. 17)

शिरो रुजति मर्त्यानां वातापित्तकफैस्त्रिभिः॥

(सु. उ. अ. 25)

हृदये मूर्ध्नि वस्तौ च नृणां प्राणाः प्रतिष्ठिताः।
तस्मात्तेषां सदा यत्नं कुर्वीत परिपालने॥
आवाधवर्जनं नित्यं स्वस्थवृत्तानुवर्त्तनम्।
उत्पन्नार्त्तिविघातश्च मर्मणां परिपालनम्॥

(च. सि. अ.9)

## सुश्रुत के मत से शिरोरोग

शिरो रुजति मर्त्यानां वातापित्तकफै स्त्रिभिः
सन्निपातेन रक्तेन क्षयेन क्रिमिभिस्तथा॥
सूर्यावर्त्तानन्तवाताार्धावभेदकशङ्कुकैः।
एकादशप्रकारस्य लक्षणं सम्प्रवक्ष्यते॥

## शिरोरोग के कारण

धूमातपतुषाराम्बुक्रीडातिस्वप्नजागरैः।
उत्स्वेदाधिपुरोवातवाष्पनिग्रहरोदनैः॥
अत्यम्बुमद्यपानेन क्रिमिभिर्वेगधारणैः।
उपधानमृजाभ्यङ्गद्वेषाधःप्रततेक्षणैः॥
असात्म्यगन्धदुष्टामभाष्याद्यैश्च शिरोगताः।
जनयन्त्यामयान् दोषाः

(अ. ह. उ. अ. 23)

## 1. वातिक शिरोरोग लक्षण

यस्यानिमित्तं शिरसो रुजश्च भवन्ति तीव्रा निशि चातिमात्रम्।
वन्धोपतापैश्च भवेद्विशेषः शिरसोभितापः स समीरणेन॥

(सु. उ. अ. 25/5)

3

तत्रमारुतकोपतः ॥

निस्तुद्येते भृशं शंखौ घाटा सम्भिद्यते तथा ।
भ्रुवोर्मध्यं ललाटं च पततीवातिवेदनम् ॥

वाध्येते स्वनतः श्रोत्रे निष्कृष्येते इवाक्षिणी ।
घूर्णतीव शिरः सर्व सन्निधभ्य इव मुच्यते ॥

स्फुरत्यति सिराजालं कन्धराहनुसांग्रहः ।
प्रकाशासहता घ्राणस्रावोकस्माद् व्याथाशमौ ॥

मार्दवं मर्दनस्नेहस्वेदबन्धैश्च जायते ।
शिरस्तापोयम्

(अ. हृ. उ. अ. २३)

## 2. पैत्तिक शिरोरोग

यस्योष्णमङ्गारचितं यथैव दह्येत धूप्येत शिरोक्षिनासम् ।
शीतेन रात्रौ च भवैद् विशेषः शिरोभिताप: सतु पित्तकोपात् ॥

(सु. उ. अ. 25/6)

शिरोभितापे पितोत्थे शिरोधूमायनं ज्वरः ।
स्वेदोदिहनं मूर्च्छा निशि शीतैश्च मार्दवम् ॥

(अ. हृ. उ. अ. २३)

## 3. कफज शिरोरोग

शिरोगलं यस्य कफोपदिग्धं गुरुप्रतिष्टब्धमथो हिमं च ।
शूनाक्षिकूटं वदनं च यस्य शिरोभिताप: स कफप्रकोपात् ॥

(सु. उ. अ. 25/7)

## 4. रक्तज शिरोरोग

रक्तात्मकः पित्तसमानलिङ्गः स्पर्शासहत्वं शिरसो भवेच्च ॥

(सु. उ. अ. 25/8)

## 5. त्रिदोषज शिरोरोग

शिरोभितापे त्रितयप्रवृत्ते सर्वाणि लिङ्गानि समुद्भवन्ति ॥

(सु. उ. अ. 25/8)

## 6. क्षयज शिरोरोग

बसाबलासक्षतसम्भवानां शिरोगतानामिह संक्षयेण।
क्षयप्रवृत्त: शिरसोभिताप: कष्टो भवेदुग्ररुजोतिमात्रम्॥
संस्वेदनच्छर्दनधूमनस्येरसृग्विमोक्षैश्च विवृद्धिमेति।

(सु. उ. अ. 25/9)

## 7. कृमिज शिरोरोग

निस्तुद्यते यस्य शिरोतिमात्रं संभक्ष्यमाणं स्फुदतीव चान्त:।
घ्राणाच्च गच्छेत् सलिलं सरक्तं शिरोभिताप: कृमिभि: स घोर:
संकीर्णैभोजनैमूर्ध्नि क्लेदिते रुधिरामिषे।
कोपिते सन्निपाते च जयन्ते मूर्ध्नि जन्तव:॥
शिरसस्ते पिबन्तोस्रं घोरा: कुर्वन्ति वेदना:
चित्तविभ्रंशजननीर्ज्वर: कासो बलक्षय:॥
रौक्ष्यशोफव्यधच्छेददाहस्फुरणपूतिता:।
कपाते तालुशिरसो: कण्डू: शोफ: प्रमीलक:॥
ताम्राच्छसिङ्घाणकता कर्णनादश्च जन्तुजे।

(अ. ह. उ. अ. २३)

## 8. सूर्यावर्त्त

सूर्योदयं या प्रतिमन्दमन्दमाक्षभुवं रुक् समुपैति गाढम्॥
विवर्धते चांशुमता सहैव सूर्यापवृत्तो विनिवर्त्तते च।
शीतेन शान्तिं लभते कदाचिदुष्णेन जन्तु: सुखमाप्नुयाच्च॥
तं भास्करावर्त्तमुदाहरन्ति सर्वात्मकं कष्टतमं विकारम्।

## चरक का मत से सूर्यावर्त्त-निदान और समप्राप्ति

सन्धारणादजीर्णाद्यैर्मस्तिष्कं रक्तमारुतौ।
दुष्टौ दूषयतस्तच्च दुष्टं ताभ्यां विमूर्च्छितमू
सूर्योदयेशुंमंतापाद्रवम विष्यन्दते शनै:।
ततो दिने शिर:शूलं दिनवृद्ध्या विवर्धते॥
दिनक्षय तत: स्याने मस्तिष्के संप्रशाम्यति।
सूर्यावर्त: स तत्र स्यात्

(च. सि. अ.९)

## विदेहमत में सूर्यावर्त्त-विपर्यय

तत्र वातानुगं पित्तं चिते शिरसि तिष्ठति ।

मध्याह्ने तेजसार्कस्य तद् विवृद्धं शिरोरुजम् ॥

करोति पैत्तिकीं घोरां सम्प्रशाम्यति दिनक्षये ।

अस्तं गते प्रभाहीने सूर्ये वायुर्विवर्धते ॥

पित्तं शान्तिमवाप्नोति तत: शाम्यति वेदना ।

एष पित्तानिलकृत: सूर्यावर्त्त-विपर्यय: ॥

## वाग्भट के मत से सूर्यावर्त्ता

पित्तानुबद्ध: शंखास्थिभ्रूललाटेषु मारुत: ।

रुजं सस्पन्दनां कुर्यादनुसूर्योदयोदयाम् ॥

आमध्याह्नं विवार्धिष्णु: क्षुद्धत: सा विशेषत: ।

अव्यवस्थितशीतोष्णसुखा शाम्यत्यत: परम् ॥

सुर्यावर्त्त: स इत्युक्का दश रोगा शिरोगता: ।

(अ. ह. उ. अ. २३)

## 9. अनन्तवात

दोषास्तु दुष्टास्त्रय एव मन्यां संपीड्य घाटासु रुजां सुतीव्राम् ॥

कुर्वन्ति साक्षिभ्रुवि शंखदेशे स्थितिं करोत्याशु विशेषतस्तु ।

गण्डस्य पार्श्वे तु करोति कम्पं हनुग्रहं लोचनाजांश्च रोगान् ॥

अनन्तवातं तमुदाहरन्ति दोषत्रयोत्थं शिरसो विकारम्

(सु. उ. अ. 25/13,14)

(उपवासातिशोकातिरूक्षशीताल्पभोजनै:)

दुष्टा दोषास्त्रयोमन्यापश्चाद्घाटासु वेदनाम् ॥

तीव्रां कुर्वन्ति सा चाक्षिभ्रूशंखेष्ववतिष्ठते ।

स्पन्दनं गण्डपार्श्वस्य नेत्ररोगं हनुग्रहम् ॥

सोनन्तवातस्तं हन्यात्

(च. सि. अ.९)

## 10. अर्धावभेदक या अर्धभेद

यस्योत्तमाङ्गार्धमतीव जन्तो: संभेदतोद्भ्रमशूलजुष्टम्॥

पक्षाद्शाहादथवाप्यकस्मात्तस्यार्धभेदं त्रितयाद् व्यवस्थेत्।

(सु. उ. अ. 25/15)

पक्षात् कुप्यति मासाद् वा स्वयमेव च शाम्यति।

अतिवृद्धस्तु नयनं श्रवणं वा विनाशयेत्॥

(अ. हृ. उ. अ. 23)

## 11. शङ्खकरोग

शंखाश्रितो वायुरुदीर्णवेग: कृतानुचात्र: कफपित्तरकै:॥

रुज: सुतीव्रा: प्रतनोति मूर्ध्नि विशेषतश्चापि हि शंखयोस्तु।

सुकष्टमेनं खलु शंखकाख्यं महर्षयो बेदविद: पुराणा:॥

व्याधिं वदन्त्युद्गतमृत्युकल्पं भिषक्सहस्रैरपि दुर्निवारम्।

(सु. उ. अ. 25/16,17)

## चरक:

रक्तपित्तानिला दुष्टा: शंखदेशे विमूर्छिता:।

तीव्ररुग्दाहरागं हि शोफं कुर्वन्ति दारुणम्॥

स शिरो विषवद्वेगी निरूध्याशु गलं तथा।

त्रिरात्राज्जीवितं हन्ति शंखको नाम नामत: ॥

परं त्र्यहाजीवति चेत् प्रत्याख्यायाचरेत् क्रियाम्।

(च. सि. अ.९)

7

# DISEASES OF HEAD
## (SHIRO ROGAS.)

**Synonyms of Shiras :-** Mastaka 2) Urdwa Kaya 3) Urdwanga 4) utthamanga 5) Munda 6) Sheersha 7) urdwa Hrudaya 9) Urdwa Kaphaashaya 9) Urdwajathru 10) Deva kosha 11) Manomaya kosha 12) Shiro hrudaya.

**Importance of Shiras :-**
Shiras (head) is known as utthamanga for Existing vital organs like prana, Indria, Prana vaha srotas, sadyo pranahara marma, pranavata, sadaka pitta, Aalochaka pitta, Tarpaka sleshma and it is the seat for all gyanavah (sensory) Chestavah (motor) prayatna etc,

## REFERENCES EXPLAINING THE IMPORTANCE OF SHIRAS :-

1)  It is the seat of prana and all indrias (prana = Agni + soma + Vayu + Satwaguna + Rajoguna + Tamoguna + Indrias + Pancha maha bhootha)
                                            (Charak Sutra Sthana.)
2)  Description of purusha sooktha starts with shiras.
3)  In "Atharvana veda" shiras is explained as " Devakosha".
4)  In "Thiitthareya upanishad" shiras is explained as " Manomaya Kosha".
5)  "Shakthyopanishad" explained the importance of the Bhru of Shiras.
6)  In yoga shastra, shiras is explained as the seat of " Sahasrara Chakra"
7)  In "Amarkosha"for shiras synonyms like " Utthamanga, Sheersha, shira" are given.
8)  According the Bhela samhitha shiras is named as " Shiro Hrudaya".
9)  Shiras is the seat for pranavata, sadaka pitta, Alochaka pitta and Tarpaka Sleshma.
10) Shiras is the controlling Centre for

    Prana ,
    3 Shareera dosha,    -    3 Mano dosha
    Ekadasha Indria,     -    Pancha maha bhuta

11) While explaining the importance of Shiras, Vagbhata described the body as Urdwa moola (Shiras), Adah shaaka (Limbs Trunk), If root is destructed plant also destructed like wise. If head is injured the Death proceeds. So only it is advised to protect the head from diseases and injuries.

12) In general while praying the God, Respecting the Teachers eldere etc.the head is bended sincerely to thank them, even for extream punishments Shiromundana was implemented (Removing the hair from the head) and when defeated used to present their shiro vestana, These incidents also prooves the utmost importance of Shiras.

**Defination of Shiro Roga:-**
" Shiro roga shabdena shirogath shoola rupa ruja abhideeyatha"

The diseases in which head ache (shirah shoola) is the prime symptom Those are named as shiro roga. The name is given not according to the site of the disease, like other, so only sushrutha not mentioned 9 Kapala rogas in Shiro Roga for not existingShirah shoola But Vagbhata explained these 9 diseases in shiro roga as Kapala roga.

**Classification of Shiro Roga :-**
1) According to Sushrutha, 11 diseases, they are

| | | | |
|---|---|---|---|
| 1) | Vataja Shiro Roga | 2) | Pittaja Shiro Roga |
| 3) | Kaphaja    " | 4) | Raktaja" |
| 5) | Sannipataja   " | 6) | Krimija " |
| 7) | Kshayaja    " | 8) | Suryaavartha" |
| 9) | Anantha Vata  " | 10) | Arthavabhedak. |
| 11) | Shankhaka | | |

2) According to Vagbhat 19 diseases, 10 Shiro roga + 9 Kaphala roga.

**a) 10 Shiro Rogas :-** among 11 diseases of sushrutha. Vagbhata not explained the Kshayaja Shira shoola and Anantha Vata (so 11-2=9 ) And added Shiro Kampa as 10th disease.

**b) 9 Kapala rogas :-**These are not explained by Sushrutha in Shiro roga they are

| | | |
|---|---|---|
| 1) | Upa Sheershak | 2) Aroomshika |
| 3) | Darunaka | 4) Indraluptha |
| 5) | Khalithya | 6) Phalitha |
| 7) | Shiro grandhi | 8) Shiro Arbuda |
| 9) | Shiro vidradi | |

**3) According to Charak**, 5 diseases, they are :

| | | |
|---|---|---|
| 1) | Vataja Shira shoola | 2) Pittaja Shira shoola |
| 3) | Kaphaja Shira shoola | 4) Tridoshaja Shira shoola |
| 5) | Krimija Shira shoola. | |

**Note:** Charaka explained suryavartha, Anantha Vata, Arthaava bhedak, shankhark etc., diseases in charak siddhistana.

4) According to some other authors shiro Rogas are 10 only
From sushrutha's classification they have omitted "Ananthavata" for having similarity with Anyatho vata of sarvagath netra roga.

# NIDANA - SAMPRAPTHI OF SHIRO ROGAS.

| Sl. No. | Lakshanas | Description | Vitiation |
|---|---|---|---|
| 1) | Dhooma paana | smoking or exposure to smoke | Pitta Raktha and allergic disorders |
| 2) | Rajo sevan | Exposing to dust | -do- |
| 3) | Aatapa Sevan | Exposing to sun light | -do- |
| 4) | Atisweda | Excessive sudation | -do- |
| 5) | Jala Kreeda | Swimming or diving or staying in water for long time | Kapha vitiation head injury. |
| 6) | Tushaara Sevan | Exposing to snow Or Moisture | -do- |
| 7) | Diwa Swapna | Sleeping in day time | -do- |
| 8) | Poorva Vata Sevan | Exposure to Air coming from east | -do- |
| 9) | Nishi Jaagara | night arousal | Vata Vitiation. |
| 10) | Bhashpa Nigrah | Suppression of tears | |
| 11) | Ati rodan | Excessive weeping | -do- |
| 12) | Vegadharan | Supression of natural urges | -do- |
| 13) | Pralapa | prolonged irrelavant talking | -do- |
| 14) | Ucchiir bhashana | Loud talking | -do- |
| 15) | Urdwa-Adah Pratatekshaniihi | Looking Upwards Or down wards for a long time. | -do- |
| 16) | Ati Vyayama | Excessive exercise | -do- |
| 17) | Ati Vyavaya (Miithuna) | Indulging more sex | Shukra, Ojo Kshaya Tridosha vitiation. |
| 18) | Abhighata | Head injury | Vata vitiation, death |
| 19) | Atyambu paana | ExcessiveFluids in take | Malnutrition |
| 20) | Atimadya paana | Excessive intake of alcoholic drinks | Dhathu, Ojo kshaya |
| 21) | Aama | Indigested infected food | Obstruction of tissue channels. |
| 22) | Krimi | Worm infestation | Infection. |

| 23. | Asatmya gandha sevan | Inhaling bad or unsuitable smell | Nasal allergy |
| 24. | Abhyanga dwesha | Rajecting head massage | Neuralgias |
| 25. | Dusta pratishyaya | nasal paranasal Chronic infections. | a) Meningeal |
| 26. | Atiyoga Or Ayoga of Nasya | Excess Or Inada quate Nasya | b) Non Meningeal |
| 27. | Karna Vikar | Middle, and internal ear complication. | c) Neurological<br>d) Vascular. |
| 28. | Vatanadi Vikar | Cranial neuralgias | Complications arises |
| 29. | Raktha Vikar | Vascular problems. | |
| 30. | Not wearing shirastrana | Not wearing cap to the head. | Head injury |
| 31. | By not conducting Shirah shodhan | Rejecting shodhan karma | Tridosha vitiation. |
| 32 | Mano Klesha | mental worries | Vitiation of mano dosha |
| 33. | Bhaya, Krodha | Fear and anger | Stress strain aggravates pitta. |
| 34. | Other diseases | Eye problems, Crainal, Nasal etc., Disorders. | Tridosha vitiation |

Due to above causes vatadi doshas vitiate, reaches the shiras and produces different types of diseases in the Shiras.

# SHIRO ROGA SAMANYA CHIKITSA

## Common treatment Principles of Shiro Rogas:-

1) Nidana Parivarjan (Avoiding the causative factors)
   Exposure to dust smoke moisture causes allergic disorders - so care should be taken to prevent the diseases.

2) Wearing of Shiro strana (helmet Or Cap) is needed to protect the head from injuries especially in open air, cool places. early mornings and while travelling etc.

3) Regular practice of Shiro Abhyanga (head massage with Oils) can prevent the diseases of head, Eye, Nose, hair etc.,

4) Care should be taken about Nasal paranasal infections, allergic conditions, stress strain, ophthalmic problems etc those cause shiro rogas.

5) To prevent the seasonal doshic variations, shira shodhan (Nasya) should practice, regularly.

6) Nasya karma is having utmost importance in the preservation of health Or treating the Shiro rogas why because Nose is the only gate way to elimi nate the doshas outside form the shiras.

7) Nose is the major source for the infection to enter in to the Shiras, so care should be taken against dust cold smoke etc., allergic factors.

8) Vitiated Dosha should be identified for giving treatment primarily.
Ex. Vataja Kaphaj disorders get relief by hot therapy and pittaja Rakthaja disorders get relief by cool therapy.

9) Treatment principle.

Sneha (bahya, Abhyantar) sweda, Lepa, nasya, dhooma pana, vaman, Virechan, Vasti, gandoosha, Kavalagrah and Rakthamokshan.

## 10) Some common external Applications (Lepa)

a) Gunjadi lepam:- Gunja,Karanja, Brungaraj Maricha + Water, should be grinded and applid to the shiras. b) Marichadi Lepam -Krishna Maricha, rakta Maricha + Snuhiksheera - Should be grinded and applied to the shiras. c) Muchakunda pushpa should grind with water and applied to the shiras. d) Pathaadi Lepam :- Patha, Patola Patra, shunti, Erenda moola, Shigrubeeja, Chakramarda beeja, and Kusta.e) Agaru, neelotphala, swetha chandan, Kusta + Ghritha.f) Prapoundareeka, suradaaru, Kusta, Yastimadu Ela. Rakta Kamala, Neelakamala + ghritha. g) Navasagar + Water.

## II) Some important common Nasya Yoga.

Fine powders of a) 250 mg. Yastimadu+ 250 mg Vatasanaabhi, should be used for pradaman nasya. b) Navasagar + sudha Churna + water-should inhale. c) Nasya with Karanja, shigrubeeja, Patri, Twak, and swetha sarshapa. d) Guda, ardraka, pippali, saindhava lavan + water, for nasya.e) Kumkuma fry in ghritha, add sugar and used for nasya. f) Guda + Shunthi, for nasya. g) The medicated oil prepared with Neela uthphala, pippali, Yastimadu,chandana, pundareeka, Amalaki,tila taila - is used. for nasya. h) Karpasabeeja, Dalchini, Musta, Jathi patra and pushpa Avapeedan Nasya. i) Aparajitha moola, phala swa rasa nasya. j) Shunti 3 Grams, Milk 192 grams - Bhavana and then Nasya. k) Artha naareeshwara rasa disolved in water and used for Nasya. l) Spatica churna + Karpoora as Nasya.

## Ghrita and Taila.:-

1) Shat bindu taila for nasya 2) Doshamoola taila (Tila taila Ajaksheera each 1kgs, Brungaraj swaras 4 kg, kalka drugs total 250 gram, ( Erenda mola, tagara, shata pushpi, Jeevanthi, Rasna, Lavana, dalchini, vidanga - Yastimadu shunthi) for abhyanga and Nasya- (Sarshapa taila 2 kg , Dashamoola quatha 8 kg cow milk 8 kg, dashamoola Kalka 1/2 kg - oil should prepare according to taila paka vidhi) **3) Dathura taila** for abhyanga ( Sarshapa taila 2kg , Dathura quath 8 kg, dathura Kalka 1/2 Kg and oil should prepare according to Taila paka vidhi) **4) Gunja taila** for a bhyanga and Nasya ( Tila taila, Kanji, Brungaaraj swarasa each 375 grams, gunja kalka 95 grams - oil should prepare according to Taila paka vidhi) **5) Himamshu taila 6) Kumari taila 7) Kanak Taila 8) Rudra taila 9) Brungaraj taila 10) Mayuradya ghrita 11) Maha Mayaradya ghrita** etc. are used for abhyanga and Nasya

## 12) Kwatha.

## Pathya Shadanga Kwata.

Haretaki, Vibheetaki, Amalaki, Kiratatikta, Nimba, Amruta - 8 times water added and is boiled and reduced to half, Then it is used for oral administration.

## 13) Rasa Aushada - Vati - Capsules and churna :-

1) Shira shooladri vajra ras 2) Maha Lakshmi Vilas ras 3) Lagu suthasekara ras, 4) Swarna sutha sekara ras , 5) Chandra Kantha ras, 6) Chandanadi vati, 7) Siddhamruta ras, 8) Suryavarthi ras, 9) Triphala guggulu, 10) Kanchanara guggulu

## Churnas :-

| | |
|---|---|
| 1. Ashwagandhadi churna | 7. Triphala Churna |
| 2. Shatavaryadi Churnam | 8. Trikatu Churna |
| 3. Talisadi Churnam | 9. Shunti Churna |
| 4. Sitophaladi churna | 10. Haridra Khanda |
| 5. Chopachenyadi Churna | 11. Nimbadi Churna |
| 6. Yastimadhu Churna | 12. Vyshwanar churna etc. |

**Pathya :-** Shiro abhyanga, shiro vestana, sheetajala shira snana, sweda, nasya , Dhoomapana, Virechan, Lepa, Seka, Upavasa, Shiro Vasti, Raktamokshan, Agnikarma, Upanaha, puranaghritha, shalidhaanya, Shastika dhaanya, Yusha, Ksheera, Jangala Mamsa, patola, Shigru, Drakasha, Vastuka, Kaaravellak, Godanthi, Amra phala, Amalaki, Trikatu, Dadima Phala , Mathulunga, Haridra, Yastimadu, Tulasi, Vasa, Dathura, Taila, Takra, Kaanji, Narikela, hareetaki, Kusta, Brungaraj, Dashamoola., Kumari, Musta, usheera, Chandana, Karpoora, Chandrakiran, Hingu, Navasagar etc.,

**Apathya :-** Abhyanga-dwesha, shiro abhighata, Shiro abhitapa Vegavarodha (Supressing natural urges), Viruddha bhojana (eating the uncompatible food), Jala Kreeda (Swimming Or Exposure to water), Diwa Swapna (Daytime sleeping), Nishi jagara (Night arousal), Ajeerna (Indigestion), Exposure to dust, smoke etc., neglecting the Nasal, ear, teeth and eye diseases etc.,

# 1) VATAJ SHIRA SHOOLA (NEURALGIC HEAD ACHE)

## Aetiology By Charak:-

Supressing the natural urges, talking Loudly, Night arousal, indulging moresex, exposure to cold. alcoholism, head injury, fasting, weeping, wait lifting, fear, anxiety, Atigoya of shodhan Karma etc., Causes the vitiation of Vata dosha, that propogates towards the head and causes vataj shiro Roga.

## Description :-

The Vitiated vata dosha causes head ache without obvious cause, the pain becomes more at nights and reduces by Oleation (Sneha Karma), sudation (Sweda Karma), mardana (Gentle compression), Abhyanga (Oil massage), Bandana (tieing the cloth Or rope around the head), Hot therapy (ushnopachar) and with other Vata hara treatment principles.

## Vagbhata:-

In addition to above description, he explained the affecting site and nature of the head ache in detail as follows.

Severe pricking pain, is experienced at temporal region, back of the neck, Frontal region and at the root of the nose, Associated symptoms are otaligia (Karna shoola), Tinnitus (karna Nada), Pain in the eye ball, vertigo, pulsation of the vessels, neck rigidity, Lock jaw, Photophobia, dislocation of joints, Rhinorrhoea and discomfort in the body.

## Treatment of Vataj Shira shoola.

1) Shiro abhyanga (Head massage) 2) Sneha pana (Oral intake of Oleous substances). 3) Upanaha sweda (hot applications to head) 4) Seka (pouring the medicine on the head) 5) Lepa (medicated applications to head) 6) Shiro Vasti (keeping of Sneha drugs on the head by special procedure) 7) Vasti (Anuvasan Vasti) 8) Snehika Dhooma pana 9) Snehika Nasya 10) Vata hara Aahara and Vihara.

1. Charak suggested sneha - Sweda and nasya.
2. Sushrutha and Vagbhata suggested - Vata Vyadhi chikitsa and Snehan Nasya.
3. Chakradatta suggested - Shiro vasti.

**1) Abhyanga -** (Massage)

With Narayan tail, mashadi taila, prasarini taila, Trivruth taila, Bala taila etc.,

**2) Sneha paana** (Oral administration of Sneha dravyas). Chathur sneha (sarpi, Taila, vasa and Majja), Varunadi ghrita Or taila, Kakolyadi ghrita Or taila, Mayuradya ghrita, Maha Mayuradya ghrita, Bala taila, Trivruth taila, cow milk and ghee should be given at nights.

**3) Upanaha sweda** (Application of Medicated paste in hot condition)

1) Agaru, should be fried in Oil and applied. 2) Application of Jeevak, Rushabhak, Meda, Maha Meda, Kakoli, Ksheera Kakoli, mashaparni, mudga parni, Jeevanthi, Yastimadu etc. 3) Fried flesh of fish (Matsya mamsa) 4) Payasa Krushara and saindhava lavana 5) Other vata hara dravya.

**4) Lepa (External applications)**

1) **Kustadi lepam** (Kusta, erenda moola grinded with Kanji Or takra). 2) **Muchakunda pushpa kalka** (Paste) 3) Kusta, erenda moola shunthi + takra. 4) **Devadarvyadi Lepa** (Devadaru, Tagara, Kusta, jatamamsi, Shunthi + Kanji Or Ghee). 5) **Chandanadi Lepa** (Chandan, Kamala, Kusta, Pippali + water) 6) Erenda beeja, Chakra marda beeja + Kanji.

**5) Nasya Yogas.**

1) Snehan Or Brumhana nasya. 2) Anu taila, 3) Shatbindu taila, 4) Swaskutar rasa + water. 5) Rasnadi Taila. 6) Mayur- Maha Mayura Ghrita 7) Bruhat pancha moola Ksheera 8) Varunadi Ksheera sarpi 9) Karpasabeeja, lavanga, Musta, Jathipatra + Hot water 10) The medicated oil prepared with yastimadu madhuksar, vidari, chandana Neelothphala, jeevak, rushabhak, Draksha, Ksheera, Mamsa, Sharkara, Taila.

**6) Dhooma Pana -** Snehika dhooma pana.

**7) Shiro Vasti** and **anuvasan vasti** with vata hara taila Or ghritha.

**8) Seka** : - With Bhadradharvyadi Ksheera

**9) Oral remedies** Like Rasnadiguggulu Triphala guggulu vata vidwamsini , Neurotics like bala, Ashwagandha, shatavari, Erenda, Nigundi, Rasna, Devadaru shigru, Yastimadu, Dashamoola, Masha, Rasona, Sariba, Tila Brahmi etc., are benificial

**10) Vata hara Aahara And Vihara should be given**

## 2) PITTAJA SHIRAH SHOOLA.

A person who takes katu Amla kshara food excessively, and have the anger and fear, exposure to over heat etc. causes the pitta dosha vitiation and manifest severe burning pain in the head eyes nose and throat " Dhoomayan Agnidagdha Vath Peeda". The patient feels comfort by cool therapy (Sheetopachar) and at nights.

**Additional points of Vabhata**-Burning pain, Fever, Virtigo, Sweating and Finally causes unconsciousness.

**Treatment : -**

**Note:-** Pittaja and Raktaja shirah shoola contain similar treatment principles.
1) Rakta and pltta dosha hara Chikitsa .
2) Panchakarma except Vamana.
3) **Seka:-** with ghee Or Milk Or sugar cane juice Or Honey Or sugarwater Or Kanji Or decoctions of Sheetha Veerya Aushada Like uthpaladi, Kakolyadi drugs.

4) **Lepa :-** (External application of the medicine)

a) Amalakyadi Lepa. b) With the paste of Nala, Vetas, Uthphala, musta Swetha chandan, Padmaka, Vamshi, Doorva, Yastimadu, Kamala + Water + Ghee. c) With the paste of Chandana Yastimadu, Bala, VYaghranakhee, usheera, Kamala + Water + Milk. d) With the paste of Shatavari, Kusta, Krishna tila, yastimadu, Kamala, punarnava + Milk. e) With the paste of Lamajjak, usheera, Chandana, Anjan, muktha, gyrica + Water. f) with the paste of Kusta, Tagara, uthphala, chandana, + Ghritha.
5) Aastapana Vasti Or Niruha Vasti, with the Milk prepared with uthphaladi drugs.
6) Anuvasan Vasti Or sneha Vasti. a) with Ksheera sarpi b) Kakolyadi Ghritha

**7) Mrudu Virchan : -**
By the oral administration of Ghee prepared with Draksha, Triphala, Ikshurasa and Milk.
**8) Shiro Abhyanga.** With Himamshu taila, Himasagar taila and Shatadhoutha Ghritha.
**9) Shiro Vasti:-** With Ghee Or milk. (Plain or medicated)

**10) Panaka ( Drinks)**

a) Kesara, Mishree, Ghee and Milk. b) Parpataka 6 grams, dhaniya 6 grams. draksha 6 grams, mishree 48 grams, water 120 grams. and 12 grams Gulab arka. c) Shadanga Paneeya + Sugar. d) Sheeta Kashaya of Draksha Or Kharjura and Sugar.

**11) Nasya Yogas.**

1) Ksheeri Sarpi. 2) Kakolyadi Ghritha Or taila. 3) Uthphaladi ghritha Or taila. 4) medicated ghee prepared with Vasa of Jangala Animals. 5) Yastimadu Chandan Sariba ksheera Ghritha. 6) Yastimadu Ksheera sarpi., 7) Yastimadu, Draksha, Mishree and Ghee. 8) Shaman Nasya with Brumhana, Sheeta Veerya drugs.

## 12) Oral Remedies.

1) Swarna Malini Vasant ras. 2) Chandra Kala ras. 3) muktabhasma. 4) Shunthi bhasma. 6) Makshika bhasma 7) Varata bhasma, 8) The medicated ghee prepared with Sharkara, Kumkum, ghrita etc. 9). Sheetha kashaya prepared with Chandana Or useera Or Draksha etc. 10). Triphala Guggulu 11) Amrutadi Guggulu. 12) Nimbadi guggulu. 13) Lagusuthasekararas. 14) Chandanadi Vati. 15) Yastimadu churna, Aamalaki churna, Triphala Churna, Pancha Valkala Churna, Truna Panchamoola, Vasa, Nimba, Usheera, musta, amrutha, Chandan, Nagakshara Draksha Parpataka, Padmak, uthphala etc. drugs can be used according to the necessity.

## 3) KAPHAJ SHIRAH SHOOLA.
(Headache due to Cold and Sinusitis.)

Excessive sleeping, sitting, intake of heavy bulk oily food etc. causes the Kapha dosha vitiation. The Vitiated Kapha dosha causes headache, heavyness, rigidity, coldness of hands and body, Oedema of Face and eye ball. The head and throat appears as lined with thick sputum.

The disease (headache) is severe at nights and minimum at day time . it is controlled by Hot therapy (ushnopachar) and by kapha hara treatment principles.

**Charak added** - Tandra - Alasya and Aruchi

**Vagbhat added** - Mandaruja, karnaKandooyan and Vaman.

## Treatment Principles :-

1) Ghrita pana 2) Upavasa, 3) Ruksha Ushna Sweda, 4) Vaman with Katu Dravya. 5) Pradaman nasya 6) Teekshna Gandoosha 7) Teekshna dhooma pana. 8) Anjan, 9) Lepa, 10) Rakthamokshan 11) Daha Karma, 12) Kapha hara Aahara Vihar (Trikatu, Yava, Yavakshara, Patola, yoosha, Kulutta, Mudga, Purana Ghritha, honey, intake of light non-oleus and hot food, intake of katu Tikta Kashayarasa, doing exercise, avoiding of diva swapna, IceCreams, fridge items, sweets and curd etc. 13) Teekshna Vasti.

## I) External applications (Lepa)

1) Saraladi Lepam (sarala Kusta, Devadaru, lata karanja, rohisha truna, Apamarga, Lavan should be grinded with water). 2) Pathyadi, Lepam (Hareetaki shunthi, musta, yastimadu, shatapushpi, neelkamal + water). 3) Devadarvyadi lepam (Devadaru, Tagara, Kusta, jatamamsi, shunthi + Taila Or Kanji). 4) Shunthyadi Lepam (Shunthi, Kusta, Devadaru, Chakramarada beeja + mahisha Mootra). 5) Krushnadi Lepam (Pippali, Shunthi, musta, Yastimadu shatapushpa, Neelkamal , Kusta + Water). 6) Harenu, Tagara, shilajith, Musta, Agaru, Ela, Devadaru, jatamamsi, Rasna, Erenda Moola.

17

**II) Nasya Yoga :-** Or pradaman Nasya (Teekshna Rechan Nasya) with madhuk sar, churna 2), Ingudi Twacha churna 3) Katphala churna, 4) Mesha Srungi Churna, 5) Arkadi Churna, 6) Trikatu Churna, 7) Vidanga Churna.

**III) Dhooma Pana:-**

with the varthi prepared from 1) Ingudee 2) Meshashrungi 3) Erenda moola Agaru, guggulu, chandan, Jatamamsi and kshouma Vastra.

**IV) Gandoosha :-** with teekshna ushna kaphahara decoctions like Trikatu Kashaya.

**V) Daha Karma:-** In vataj and Kaphaj disorders daha Karma is suggested at Bhru Shankha and Lalata.

**IV) Anjan:-**

Teekshna Anjan Or Lekhana anjan Like Chandrodaya varthi is used.

**In Brief :-**

1) Purana ghritha pana, 2) Ruksha Sweda, 3) Vamana, 4) Teekshna nasya, 5) Teekshna vasti , 6) Teekshna Gandoosha, 7) Dhooma pana 8) Anjan, 9) Daha karma 10) Local applications.

**Common Remedies :-**

1) Kanchanara guggulu 2) Nimbadi guggulu 3) Triphala guugulu 4) vidangadi guggulu 5) Khadhiradi Vati, 6) Trijathakadi Vati, 7) Eladivati, 8) Ekangaveer Ras , 9) Maha lakshmi vilas ras 10) Sutasekar ras, 11) Godanthi Bhasma + Spatica bhasma. 12) Talisadi Churna 13) Shrungyadi Bhasma 14) Tankan bhasma 15) Arka Lavan, 16) Seetamshu ras, 17) Anand bhiiravi ras , 18) Mruthyumjaya ras, 19) Tribhuvan Keerti ras, 20) Kaphahara Kshara- Lavana - Bhasma etc.,

## 4) RAKTAJ SHIRAH SHOOLA
(Headache due to acute alcoholism and Hypertension.)

The Vitiated raktha dosha causes the terrific head ache. The signs symptoms and treatment is similar to pittaja shirah shoola. The seveority of the symptoms is more than pittaja shirah shoola (Severe burning pain in the head eyes nose and throat) the additional symptom is tenderness of the head (Sparshasahishnutha) and occassionally epistaxis also occurs. The patient feels comfort by cool therapy and at nights.

**Treatment :-**

**A) External applications :-**1) Like Pittaja shirah shoola. 2) Ksheeri sarpi. 3) Shigru patra swarasa + Maricha Churna, 4) Pippali, Shunthi, Yastimadu, Shatavari, Musta, Uthphala, Kuruveru + water. 5) Kantakari Phala swarasa 6) Amalaki, Dhava, Khaskhas, Sariba, Kamala, Draksha + Gulabjal.

**B) Nasya ;-** 1) Pippali saindhavalavan + Ghee. 2) Ksheeri sarpi 3) Yastyadi Ghrita Or taila 4) Shatbindu taila 5) Yastimadu, Aamalaki swarasa + Honey 6) Shunthi + Milk 7) Dadima Pushpa Swarasa + Doorva Swarasa 8) Karpoora - milk and Honey 9) Uthphaladi ghritha. 10) Vidarigandhadi Ghritha. 11) Doorvadi ghritha.

## C) Oral remedies :-

1) Udumbara Phala ghritha + Ela + Pippali + Maricha + Sita, 2) nimbadi guggulu 3) Amrutadi gugulu 4) Triphala guggulu 5) uthphaladi ghritha 6) Vidari gandhadi ghritha. 7) Dooravadi ghriitha. 8) Vasadi ghritha. 9) Patoladya ghritha. 10) Triphala ghritha 11) Purana ghritha 12) ksheeri Sarpi 13) Lagusutha sekara ras. 14) Chandanadi Vati 15) Chandanasav 16) usheerasav 17) Muktha, Pravala, shankha, Kaphardak, makshika, Vykranth. bhasma and pisti. 18) Tandulodak + Mishri 19) Draksha, chandan, usheera, yastimadu, kamala, Uthphala pundareeka, Vasa, parpataka, dhanyaka, ghritha, mishri etc., 20) Sheeta veerya, Brumhana, Raktha stambana and shaman drugs should be give.

## 5) SANNIPATHAJ SHIRAH SHOOLA.

All the mixed signs and symptoms of Tridosha present.

**Chikitsa :-**
**1)** Tridosha hara Chikitsa **2)** Oral intake of purana ghritha Or Triphala Ghritha.

## 3) Nasya yoga.

1) Hot milk + Shunthi 2) Jeevakadi - Shatahvadi Taila 3) Madan Phala, shigru beeja, Kusta, Tila, jatamamsi, Tutta etc., drugs 4) Karanja, Shunthi, Shigrubeeja, vacha, milk and sugar.

**4) Lepa** (Luke warm applications) with,
1) Swetha chandana, karpoora, sariba, priyang, haridra, shunthi and Old rice.2) Priyang, Ananthmool, Nishotha, Shunthi, Chandan. 3) Kusta, shunthi, Yastimadu, Shatapushpi, kamal, Pippali.

## 6) KSHAYAJA SHIRO ROGA (SHIRAH SHOOLA )

The Kapha dosha, Raktha dosha and Vasa get reduced (kshayam),head is injured and produces a terrific complicated headache known as Kshayaja shirah shoola.

The disease aggravates by sweda (Sudation), Vaman ( Emesis), Nasya, Rakthamokshan (Blood letting process) and Dhoompana (medicated smoking) why because all these are shodhan karma cause depletion of dosha and dhathu, allready there is dhathu kshaya in this disease, so only all the above pancha karma therapies are contra indicated.

**According to Charak :-**

Vata pitta kapha doshas are depleted and cause derangement of the normal functions of Shiras, so only produces terrific headache.

The common symptoms are, headache, bodypains, vertigo, lightness in the head and body, general debility and unconsciousness.

**Treatment :-**

1) Brumhana Chikitsa. 2) Oral intake of ghee and milk. 3) Oral administration of Ashwagandadi ghritha,vasaghritha, Pancha tikta Ghritha, Brahmi ghritha, Ghee + Guda or sharkara.

4) Brumhana or shamana Nasya with Ksheeri Sarpi, Vidarigandhadi, uthphaladi, Kakolyadi ghritha.

5) Kshayaja Kasa - kshaya (raja yakshma) treatment should be give.

**6) Oral remedies :  -**

Muktha bhasma, pravala bhasma, Vajra bhasma, Vykranth bhasma, Makshika bhasma, Godanthi bhasma, Abraka bhasma, Vasanth Malathi ras, Vasantha Kusumakar ras, Ekangaveeras, Swarna and maha Lakshmi Vilas ras, shilajith, Arogyavardiniras and other Rasayan yogas should be give.

**Churna -Ghritha - Avalehya Aasava Arista etc  : -**

Ashwagandha Churna, shatavari Churna, Vidarikand Churna, Chopacheenyadi Churna, Amrutha Satwa, Kapikacchu Churna, Yastimadu Churna Triphala Churna etc. Neurotic drugs; Vasavalehya Ashagandhava lehya, Herakaprash, chyavanaprash Avalehya; Draksha Khajura etc., mantha; Vasa Patola Ashwagandhadi etc ghritas; usheera Chandana Dhanyaka etc. Sheeta kashaya; Ashwagandharista, Balarista, Rasnadi guath etc. will correct the debilitative factors and promote immunity to the body.

### 7) KRIMIJA SHIRO ROGA

A person who is habitated to take the food which is  uncompatible, indigested undigested, excessive, un hygienic, sweety, sticky, like Tila Guda dadhi Oleus substances etc, causes tridosha vitiation. The vitiated Tridosha produce Krimi in the shiras and causes terrific headache by eroding the soft tissue flesh and blood of shiras.

**Sushrutha ;-**  A person experiences pricking and cutting type of pain in the head and also experiences that Krimi is eroding or eating the brain tissue. The associated symptoms are nasal blood stained discharge and discomfort.

**Vagbhata :-** Tridosha vitiate and produces the krimi in the shiras that destructs the flesh, soft tissue and blood and causes terrific pain in the head. The associated symptoms are Manovibrama (confusion state) Fever, cough, general debility, Oedema, roughness of body, cutting pricking throbbing burning type of pain, itching sensation at head palate and the scalp, Tinnitus, Foul smel and blood stained nasal discharge etc.

**Treatment :-**

1) Krimi hara chikitsa 2) Nasya with blood, the Krimi get unconscious and come out through nose, by special techniques Krimi should be removed. 3) Rechan Nasya with a) Vidangadi Taila (Vidanga, Sarjaras, Danthi, Hing, gomutra and tila Taila). b) with vidanga, maricha, shigru beeja, Apamarga beeja + Go mutra. c) with Trikatu, shigru, Tulsi + Go mutra Or Aja Mutra. d) Nasyam with Vidanga + Aja Ksheera 4) Dhoopan with Krimighna drugs, dried Fish etc., 5) Raktha Mokshana is contra indicated.

## 8) SURYAAVARTHA OR BHAASKARAAVARTHA (FRONTAL SINUSITIS - MIGRAINE)

It is a special type of headache (Shirah shoola) that changes according to the intensity of the sun rays, The headache is directly proportionate to the intensity of the sun rays so only named as Suryaavartha. The headache starts in the morning, gradually increases upto noon (miximum at noon or mid day) then gradually decreases upto night (minimum at night). The pain is experienced more at Eye, root of the nose (bhru), Temporal (Shankha) and frontal region (Lalata).

1) Sushrutha explained it as Tridoshaja disease.
2) Vagbhata and madhava charya explained it as pitta predominent, Vata Associated, Tridoshaja diseases (it subsides naturally).
3) Charaka explained it as due to the suppression of natural urges, indigestion etc., causes Vata and Raktha doshas vitiate, affects the Mastulunga and causes the disease.
4) Videha explained **"Suryaavartha Viparyaya"** in which symptoms are same as suryavartha but it is Vata predominent, pitta associated sannipataj disease.
5) The Author of Gadanigrah explained the "**Dwandaja suryavartha**" in which the symptoms are opposite to suryaavartha (Pain maxi mum at night and minimum at day time)

**Description :-**
1. The seviority of the disease reduces some times with hot therapy and some times with cool therapy, this indicates the vata and pitta predominence in tridoshas.

2. The seviority of the disease should be judged according to the pitta dosha, at night due to pitta shaman pain is reducing and at day time due to pitta prakopa pain is aggravating.

**Note :-** Avapeedan Nasya with Shireesha moola, pippali moola, vacha etc., drugs reducing the disease though the medicines are pitta kara why because the drugs are effective not according to dosha karma But according to prabhava (Vyadhi Prathyaaneeka. ).

3) At night pain is reducing why because the aggravated Kapha not accumulating due to widely opened srotas but at day time due to narrow - Closed srotas Kapha is accumlating and obstructing the channels, so only pain is aggravating (**Contraversial description**).

**4). According to Charak.**

The pain is aggravating in day time due to the vitiation of Rakta, Vata and liquification of Mastulunga and the pain is reducing at night due to solidification of mastulunga.

5)     Explaination of the Aetio pathology of the disease according to dosha is very difficult.

**A) Treatment Principles :-**
1. Tridosha hara chikitsa (especially pitta - vata hara chikitsa) 2) Oral intake of Ghee + Guda. 3) Oral administration of Ghritha after meals. 4) Meals with milk or milk products. 5) Meals with the Jangala Mamsa rasa. 6) Shiro Vasti with chathur Snehas sarpi (ghee), Taila (Oil). Vasa (Fat,) Majja (bone marrow). 7) Lepa (Local applications). 8) Seka with ghee or milk. 9) Kavalagrah (medicated gargles) 10) Virechan (Purgation therapy) 11). Vasti. (medicated enema) 12) Shiro Virechan. (nasya) 13) Upanaha sweda with jangala Mamsa. (Hot applications) 14) Raktha Mokshan, (Blood letting process)

**B) Nasya yogas for Suryaavartha**
1) Ksheeri sarpi (Ghee prepared from milk) 2). Brungaraj swarsa + goat's milk. 3) apamarga swarasa 4) Shireesha moola, pippalimoola, vacha, Avapeadan Nasya 5) Jeevaneeya Ghritha Nasya. 6) Katphala churna pradamanNasya. 7) Vacha + Pippali 8) Yastimadu + Honey. 9) Manahshila +Water. 10) Chandan + Honey. 11) Shireesha beeja + Moolak beeja + water . 12) Vamshi beeja + Moolak beeja + Karpoora.13) Inhalation of gas releasing from Navasagar + Sudha churna. 14) Masha Moola, swetha aparajitha moola, Gunja moola, Shireesha beeja and moola, Rasona Swarasa, Chakramarda beeja, Tulasi beeja Trikatu - Separately Or mixed can be used as nasya 15) Dashamoola kashaya + Saindhava Lavana. + ghee
16) Sita (sharkara) + madhanphala churna + cow milk. etc. are used as Nasya in suryaavartha.

**C) Lepas (External applications)**
1) Suryamukhee beeja + Suryamukhee Swarasa. 2) sarivadi Lepa (Sariva,) uthphala, Kusta, Yastimadhu, Should be grinded with Kanji and applied to the shiras. 3) Tila + milk.

**D) Rasaushadhies (oral remedies)**
1) Suryavarthiras 2) Danthi bhasma 1 gram. + Praval bhasma 125 mg with ghee. 3) Shira shooladri Vajra ras tablets. 4) Guggulu Preparations. 5) Chandanadi Vati 6) Godanthi Bhasma+ spatica bhasma, equally.

7) Vata roga hara yogas like Vata Vidwamsini etc., 8) Strength, promoting medicines like Ashwagandha, Shatavari, Vidarikand, Bala , Yastimadu, draksha, mukta, Pravala, Guduchi etc.

**Note :-** It is not possible for the exact modern co-relation of Suryaavartha to the present existing science.

## 9) ANANTHA VATA
### (Trigeminal neuralgia - sinusitis - Referred headache etc.)

It is a disease in which tridoshas vitiate the manya or Greeva parshwa (The two nadies on either sides of neck) (due to excessive weeping, anger - Rough and cool items eating, fasting or taking less food etc., Causes) and produces severe untolerable pain at the back of the neck, in the eyeball, in the frontal region (Lalata), root of the nose (Bhru) and in temporal region (shankha). It also causes lockjaw (hanugraha), Eye diseases and shivering of Jaws (Ganda Paarshwa Kampa).

**Note : -** Some authors not mentioned this disease in shiro rogas for having similarity with anyathovata of sarvagatha netra disease. But by the following explanation it is clear that they are different not one.

| Anantha Vata | Anyathovata |
|---|---|
| 1. Shiro Roga | 1. Netra roga |
| 2. Headache is the main symptom | 2. Eye problem is the main symptom. |
| 3. Tridoshaj disease | 3. Vataj disease. |
| 4. Common symptoms are vitiation of manya and pain radiating to temporal & Orbital region. | 4. Common symptoms are vitiation of manya and pain rediating to Temporal and orbital region. |
| 5. Additional Lesions are Lockjaw, Shivering of jaws. | 5. These symptoms are absent |
| 6. Tridosha hara, Suryavartha Treatment should be given. | 6. Vata hara, Netra Brumhana Treatment should be given. |

**Treatment Principles:-**

1) Like Suryaavartha, 2) Tridosha hara Chikitsa, especially Vata and Pitta dosha chikitsa. 3) Meals with milk, Ghee and its products. 4) Oral administration of Ghee after meals. 5) Upanaha Sweda (Hot applications) 6) Snehika dhooma pana (medicated smoking) 7) Mrudu Virechana (Light Purgation) 8) Sneha Vasti (Anuvasan Vasti). 9) Shiro Vasti (Keeping of Oleus substances on head by special procedure). 10) Raktha mokshan (Blood letting process). 11) Lepa (External Applications). 12) Periseka- (Pouring medicated Warm liquids). 13) Gandoosha (Gargling with medicated liquids). 14) Snehan Nasya. (Nasal drops) 15) Anjan (application of collirium) 16) Daha Karma. (Cauterisation) 17) Oral intake of sweets, Oleus substances and nutritive food .

**A)      Nasya Yogas for Anantha Vata :-**
         1) Snehan Nasya 2) Ksheeri Sarpi (Ghee prepared from milk) 3) Dhanwantari tail 4) Ksheera bala taila 5) Shatbindu tail 6) Anutaila 7) Nasya with Jeevaneeya ghritha 8) Shunti + Aja Ksheera

**B)      Anjana yogas :-**
1) Chandrodaya Varthi 2) Nagarjuna Varthi
**C) Lepa yogas** (External Applications)
1) Paste of Suryamukhee beeja + Suryamukhee Swarasa. 2) Sarivadi Lepam 3) haridradi Lepam

**D)      Oral Remedies. :-**
1) Shira Shoooladri Vajra ras. 2) Ekaanga veer ras 3) Sudhanidhi ras, 4) Godanthi Bhasma + Spatica bhasma (equally) 5) Guggulu preparations 6) Sapthamruta loha. 7) Vata Vidwamsini Ras etc., Vatahar Aushadas 8) mayura ghritha 9) Triphala ghritha 10) Patoladya ghritha 11) Pathyadi quath 12) Maha Rasnadi quath 13) Neurotic drugs like Ashwagandha shatavari Yastimadu Bala Rasna Kapikacchu Vidarikand Devadaru Nirgundi etc., drug preparations can be given.
**Note :-** It can be corlated to Trigeminal neuralgia, referred head ache upto some extent.

# 10)   Arthaavabhedak (Migraine)
         It is termed as Half head ache by the common public, it is a severe inter-rupted head ache, teases once in 3-5- 10-15 or 30 days.
1) According to charak and Madhavacharya, it is Vataj or Vata Kaphaj disease.
2) According to sushrutha It is Tridoshaj disease.
3) According ot vagbhata- It is vataj disease (in Vataj shira shoola head ache is wide spread in the head but in Arthavabhedak it is only in the half part of the head)

**Aetiological factors and Symptoms-According to Charak.**
         Suppression of Natural Urges, indulging more exercise and sex, exces-sive in take of dry rough food. fasting, exposure to fog or cold, talking loudly - irrelavantly. Due to all these causes Vata or Vata Kapha doshas vitiate, affects the shiras and produces head ache in posterio lateral aspect of head (Manya), Tem-poral region (Shankha), frontal region (Lalata), root of the Nose (Bhru), ear, eye-ball, and finally causes blindness and deafness as a complication.

**According to Sushrutha :-**
         Tridoshas vitiate, affects the half part of the head and causes different types of pain (head ache ) (pricking, cutting, stabbing, tearing, burning type) for a short duration and reccur in 3-5-10-15 -30 days (inturrupted pain), It associates with vertigo.

**Vagbhata :-**

He said it is a part of Vataja shira shoola.

**Treatment Principles :-**

1) Like suryavartha. 2) Shiro abhyanga 3) Sneha pana - Oral intake of Chatur sneha or 10 years Old ghee. 4) Upanaha Sweda Or Nadi Sweda. 5) Shiro Vasti 6) Virechan, 7) Nasya 8) Vasti . 9) Dhooma Pana 10) Oral intake of Milk and Ghee after meals. 11) Oral intake of Milk and Ghee products. 12) Food with Jangala Mamsa rasa. 13). Pratishyaya, chikitsa 14) Shavaasan daily 15 to 30 minutes. 15) Regular practice of Pranayaama 16) Lepa. 17) Seka 18) Raktha Mokshan 19) Agni Karma at Bhru Lalata and Shankha in Vataj and Kaphaj disorders. 20) Physical and mental rest 21) Vata - Kapha hara Chikitsa.

**A)      Nasya Yogas :-**

## AVAPEEDAN NASYA WITH

1) Shireesha Moola Or Phala. 2) Vamshi moola, Karpoora + Water, 3) Vacha Pippali + water. 4) Yastimadhu + Honey, 5) Vidanga Krishnatila + Aja Ksheera. 6) Milk + Sugar. 7) Chandana, manashila + Honey. 8) Katphala churna. 9) Arka patraswarasa. 10) Yastimadu, Yava, Vacha, Pippali + Water + Honey . 11) Shireesha beeja, Apamarga moola, Bidalavan 12) girikarnee phala Or moola + Water. 13) Madhura Brumhana Ghritha. 14) Tuvareedala + Doorva Swaras. 15) Gandhaathee + Jatamamsi + Ghritha (Pakwa.) 16) Kumkum + Ghee. After shodhan nasya - Shaman nasya should be given with.

1) Kakolyadi Ghritha 2) Moorvadi Ghritha 3) Ksheera bala taila 4) Dhanvantari taila 5) Anu taila 6) Shatbindu taila etc.,

**B)      Lepa yogas - (External Applications):-**

1) Sarivadi Lepam (Sariva, Neelkamal, Kusta, Yastimadu Vacha, Pippali, Kanji, Taila and ghee.) 2) Vidanga, Krishna tila + Aja Ksheera. 3) Tiladi Lepam (Tila, Jatamamsi, Saindhava Lavan, Shrunga bhasma + Honey.4) Application of Haridra Or Sariva. 5) maricha + Brungaraja Swarasa. 6) Shunti + Water.

# II) SHANKHAKA
## ( Lateral Sinus thrombosis, Mastoid abscess, Encephalitis)

**1) Charak :-** Raktha, pitta and Vata doshas Vitiate and produces a painful red swelling at temporal region with severe burning sensation, it spreads very quickly like the poison, obstruct the chanels of head throat and kills the person within 3 days.

**2) Sushrutha** : - Vata predominent Tridoshas and Raktha vitiate and produces unbearable pain in the head, especially at temporal region, it is incurable and kills the person within 3 days.

26

**3) Vagbhata :-** Pitta Predominent tridoshas and Raktha vitiate and produces a Terrific Painful swelling at temporal region, associated with burning sensation fever thirst vertigo yellowish face, bitter taste of mouth, with irrelavant talking and kills the person within 3 days.

**4) Madhava Kara : -** It is due to the vitiation of Raktha, pitta and Vata. doshas.

1.  Charak :-  Raktha predominent, pitta and Vata associated.

2.  Sushrutha :-  Vata predominent, pitta Kapha and Raktha associated.

3.  Vagbhata :-  Pitta predominent ; Vata kapha and Rakta associated.

4.  Madhava Kara :- Raktha predominent, pitta and Vata associated.

All the people accepted it as a terrific disease that kills the person within 3 days.

**Treatment Principle :-**
It is incurable but can try like suryavartha. 2) Oral intake of Ghee and milk products. 3) Oral intake of ghee and milk after meals. 4) Food with Jangala mamsa rasa 5) Ushna Sweda is not advisable. 6) Sira Vyadana at (Shankha) temporal region. 7) Local applications as follows.

a) Shatavari, Tila, Yastimadu, Neelothphala, Doorva, punarnava with Kanji Or milk. b) Vidarigandhadi Or Kakolyadi Or uthphaladi Lepa Or seka. C) Daru haridra, Manjista, Nimba Twak, Ushera, Padmaka. d) Sariba, Nishotha, Priyang, Sarpagandha, with Kanji, e) Bala Moola, Neela Kamal, Dhoorva, Krishna tila, Punarnava with Water. f) Ksheeri Vruksha Lepam.

**8) Nasya ;-**  1)  Avapeedan Nasya those explained in Suryaavartha.
        2)  Girikarna Moola or phala Swarasa nasya.

## SHIRO KAMPAM

It is explained by vagbhata in shiro roga. Vata Predominent. Tridoshas vitiate and produces (Kampam) shivering in the shiras, is known as shiro Kampa.

**Treatment :-** Like Vataj Shiro Roga.

## ADDITIONAL 9 DISEASES OF VAGBHATA (KAPAALA ROGA).

### 1) Upasheershak.

During the pregnancy a painless, same coloured Oedema Or cyst develops on the head of the foetus by the vitiation of Vata dosha, it is known as upasheershaka, (Vata vitiates due to Midyaahaara vihara of the pregnant mother).

It can be co-related to 1) Cephal **haematoma** (effusion of the blood between the skull and pericranium in the vertex presentation, during delivary, gives rise to soft fluctuant tumour on the parietal bone or occiput) 2) **Caput succedenum** (Oedema due to compression of superficial vessls during delivary) 3) **Hydro cephaly** (increased intra cranial pressure gives abnormal big head.)

Among these 3 diseases No. 1-2 doesn't need any treatment they resolute naturally inshort time but No. 3 want specific treatment.

**Treatment :-**

1)      In Non suppurative stage (apakwa grandhi).
        Treatment should be given like Vata Vyadhi.
a)      Abhyanga- Gentle massage with medicated Oils etc.
b)      Upanaha Sweda- application of the warm paste of the medicines for light Fomentation effect.
        **Ex:-** 1. Warm paste of Yava-Gudhuma-Mudga+Ghee.
               2. Warm paste of Panchavalkala should be applied to the lesion.

**2) a) Pariseka :-**
        Luke warm Dasha moola quath + Ghee should be poured on the affected area from 2 to 4 inches height.

**3) Bandana:-**
        Tight compression bandage.
4)      Symptomatic treatment like analgesics, anit inflammatory and Antibiotic drugs.
5)      If cyst is infected due to contageous infections, the cyst may suppurate (Pakwa grandhi) with pus collection. Bhedhana puyanirharan and Vrana chikitsa should be done (incision Drainage and wound healing therapy).
But         suppuration of this cyst is uncommon.

### 2) Shiro Grandhi Or Pitica (Cyst)

It is of 5 tyes 1) Vataj 2) Pittaj 3) Kaphaj 4) Siraja 5) Medoja Grandhi.

### 3) Shiro Vidradi (Abscess)

It is of 6 types 1) Vataj 2) Pittaj 3) Kaphaj 4) Tridoshaj 5) Kshataja 6) Raktaj Vidradi.

### 4) Shiro Arbuda (Tumours)

It is of 6 types 1) Vataj 2) Pittaj 3) Kaphaj 4) Raktaj 5) Mamsaja 6) Medoja Arbuda.

**Note :-** The aetiology - Pathology - Clinical features and Treatment of Shiro grandhi, Shiro Vidradi and Shiro arbuda is like Shareeraja grandhi arbuda and Vidradi.

## 5) AROOMSHIKA

Multiple exudative small cysts arise on the scalp by the vitiation of pitta, Kapha, Raktha dosha and Krimi, it is an irritative disease, discharges yellowish foul sticky secretion, produces inflammatory skin lessions and hair loss.

**Treatment Principles :-**

1) Jalaukaavacharan to remove impure blood. 2) Cleaning the scalp with the decoction of Nimba etc. drugs. 3) Application of Lavan + Ashwa Pureesha. 4) Application of the paste of Patola patra, Nimba patra and Haridra. 5) Application of Paste prepared with Gomutra, Pinyaka and Kukkuta puressha. 6) Application of the Fried powder of Kusta + Taila. 7) Application of the paste of Khadhira nimba and Jambu. 8) Application of Jathyadi Tailam. 9) Application of the paste of Neelothphala Kesar, Aamalaki + Yastimadu.10) Application of Triphaladi Taila (Triphala, Yastimadu Brungaraj, uthphala,, sariba, saindhavalavana, Taila).11) Shareer shodhan with vaman virechan etc., 12) Shiro shodhan with Nasya.

## 6) DARUNAKA

The Vitiated vata and Kapha doshas deranges the skin of the scalp and changes it into dry rough with severe itching sensation and pain . The dried skin of the scalp fall in small pieces, causes loss of sensitivity and hair loss.

**Treatment Principles :-**

Prakshalana - Seka-Lepa-Abhyanga-Shirovasti Nasya and Rakthamokshana.
1) Cleaning the head with warm water and allow it to dry properly. 2) Raktha mokshan at frontal region. 3) Shiro abhyanga-Oil application to head to bring the Oleusness in the scalp. 4) Shiro Vasti with Vata Kapha hara sneha 5) Local application of the Paste of Priyala beeja, Yastimadu, Kusta, Masha Sarshapa and Honey. 6) Seka Or pariseka (pouring of Medicine) with the solution of the Kshara Prepared with Kodrava and Truna. 7) Application of the paste of Taila, Khas Khas Beeja + Milk, to the scalp. 8) Application of the paste of Kantakari phala ras Or japa Pushpa rasa + Taila to the scalp. 9) Application of the medicated oil prepared with Brungaraj swarara + Loha Kitta + Triphala + Sariba + Taila, to the scalp. 10) Nasya Karma with Brungaraj taila etc.

## 7) INDRALUPTHA

1) **Madhavakara** explained the Indraluptha, Khalithya,and Ruhya as synonyms. 2) According to **Kartheeka,** if hair of scalp fall down  known as Khalithya, hair of the body fall down known as ruhya and hair of mushtaches fall down known as Indraluptha. 3) But **vagbhata** explained that sudden fall of hair is Known as Indralupta and gradual fall of hair is Known as khalithya. 4) vagbhata said that Indraluptha is also called as chacha. 5) **Madhava Kara** said that Khalithya Or Indralupta doesn't occur in ladies because the the vitiation of the blood is corrected by menstruation in every month. So only If hair fall down that grows without any obstructing lesions.

## INDRALUPTHA :-

The Vitiated Vata and Pitta affects the hair roots and causes loss of hair, then the vitiated Kapha and Raktha obstructs the hair roots, so there is no chance for the regrowth of hair (if hair roots are partially closed, by the proper treatment there is scope for regrowth of hair).

**Treatment Principles : -**

1) Sira vyadan at the nearer site and application of the paste of Kaseesa Manashila Tutta and maricha Or pippali to the head.
2) Application of Brungaraja taila.
3) Application of the paste of Bruhatiphala + Gunja moola.
4) "              "        Black cow urine + Japa pushpa,
5) "              "        Brungaraj swarasa + Taila (Pakwa)
6)                         root and fruit of Gunja.
7) "              "        Langali root + Milk.
8) "              "        Karaveera Patra Swarasa.
9) "              "        Kantakari Swarasa + Honey.
10) "              "        Dathura Patra Swrasa with Honey Or Ghee.
11) "              "        Bhallatak ras with Honey Or Ghee.
12) "              "        Tila pushpa, gokshura with Honey Or Ghee.
13) "              "        Hastidantha Masi + Taila (Tila Taila)
14) Upto the completion of the treatment bathing is not advised (Water contact aggravates the vitiation).

## 8) KHALITHYA OR KHALATHI

Aetiology and pathology of khalithya is like Indraluptha. i.e. Vata and pitta causes hairfall, kapha and Raktha obstructs the hair roots so No chances of regrowth of Hair But in Khalithya hairfall is gradual Or Slow, Not sudden as in Indraluptha.

1) If Vata dosha vitiation is predominent , the Skin of the scalp becomes thicker like the scar of burns. (Dagha charma).

2) If pitta dosha vitiation is predominent, in the the Skin of the scalp is with venous congestion and sweating.

3) If Kapha dosha vitiation is predominent the Skin of the scalp be comes more thicker.

4). If Tridoshas vitiates all the symptoms appears (If the scalp Skin is like the nail, burnt scar and with tridosha vitiation it is said as asadya.).

**Treatment :-**

Positive result Or improvement is not adequate but can try with the following principles.

1) Mukha and shiro Abhyanga. 2) Shodhan therapy - Vaman Virechan and Nasya etc., 3) Oral intake of milk daily. 4) Avoiding of Sex (Brahmacharya) 5) Local application of the paste of Jatamamsi, Kusta Tila Krishna Sariva, Neelothphala + Cow Milk + Honey. 6) Nasya Karma with nimba taila for a month. 7) Nasya with Bruhatyadigana taila Or jeevaneeyagana taila for a month. 8) Laghu panchamoladi taila nasya for a month.

**Note :-** Falling of the hair, occur due to so many aetiological factors but exact cause is obscure.

1) Genetic factors 2) emotional factors. 3) Mental Worries.4) Chronic head ache. 5) Refusing regular head massage with nutrient oils 6) Repeated head bath. 7) Changes in the sebasious secretions of scalp. 8) Skin lesions of scalp (connective tissue disorders). 9) Unhygienic conditions of scalp. 10) Irritative inflammatory lesions of scalp. 11) Fungus infective lesions of scalp. 12) Ulcerative lesions of scalp by alcolies, acids, injuries, contagious infections, burns, drug toxicity, allergic disorders and chronic diseases etc., causes the hair loss.

## 9) PHALITHA OR PHALITHYA

Depigmentation of the hair occuring due to physical strain, mental strain, exessive anger, weeping etc., the over heat is produced in the body that propogates towards the head along with vitiated pitta dosha, affects the hair roots and causes the disease, known as phalitha, 1) In Vata predominence hair becomes rough dry brittle and brownish, 2) In pitta predominence hair becomes Yellowish with burning sensation, 3) In Kapha predominence hair becomes whitish Oily thicker and Lengthy, 4) In Tridoshaja vitiation all the above symptoms togetherly present and it is said as Asadya.

**Note :-** 1) Phalitha - If occurs due to headache contain tendernes of the scalp,
2) Phalitha if occurs due to Old age, is Yapya and need Rasayana Therapy.
3) Tridoshaja Phalitha is said as Asadya.

**Phalitha Chikitsa :-**

1) sannipathaj Phalitha is Asadya. 2) Phalitha of Old age is Yapya. 3) Shiro Abhyanaga (Oil applications) 4) Shiro lepa (Medicine application) 5) Shodhan Karma (Vaman Virechan-Nasya). 6) Oral intake of Cow Milk, 7) Avoiding of Sex (Brahmacharya) etc are benificial.

**A)	Nasya Togas : -**

1) Bruhatyadi Jeevaneeya taila nasya. 2) Nimba taila nasya for a month. 3) Prapoundareekadi taila nasya. (Medicated oil prepared with Amalaki, Tila taila, prapoundareeka, Yastimadu pippali, chandana, Neelothphala, Taila, has to prepare according to taila paka vidhi) 4) Shatavaryadi taila Nasya. (medicated oil prepared from Shatavari, Jeevanthi decoctions, cow milk, yamaka sneha, Jeevaneeya Kalka - taila). 5) Neelinyadi taila nasya.

6) Ksheeradi taila Nasya. (medicated oil prepared from cow milk, sahachara, Brungaraja, Tulasi swarasa, tila taila and Yastimadu taila,) 7) Mundee taila for oral and for nasya. 8) Mayuradi ghritha nasya. 9) Shatbindu ghritha nasya. (medicated ghritha prepared from yastimadhu, Vidanga, shunti, bringaraj, madhuka and ghritha.)

**B)      External applications (Lepa).**
1) Haridra, daruharidra + Navaneetha. 2) Neelothphala, Tila, Yastimadu , sarshapa, nagakesar, and Aamalaki. 3) Aja Shrunga masi + Tila taila. 4) Karpasa beeja majja + Arka ksheera. 5) Dugdika, Karaveera + Cow Milk, 6) Priyaladi Lepam. (Priyala, Yastimadu, Jeevaneeya dravya, tila taila and Cow milk) 7) Tila, Amalaki, Padmakinjalka, Yastimadu + Honey. 8) Jatamamsadi Lepam. (Jatamamsi, Kusta, Krishna Tila, Krishna sariba, Neelothphala + Cow Milk + Honey.) 9) Aayushchurnadi lepam (loha Churna, Brungaraja, Triphala, Krishna Mruttika, ikshurasa - should kept for a month and applied.) 10) Mashadi Lepam, (Masha, Kodrava, Kanji, Kept for 3 days then Lohachurna added and applied) 11) Kantakari phala rasa + taila. 12) Application of the swarasa of Japapushpa .

**C)      Ghritha yogas :-**
Mayuradya ghritha, maha mayuradya ghritha etc., can be used for oral administration, massage, vasti and Nasya.

# HEAD ACHE

Head ache is a term commonly used for "Pain felt anywhere in the head". It is observed as a symptom in most of the diseases. The signs, symptoms, nature, seviority, duration and prognosis of the diseases etc., depends upon the aetiological factors and affected part. Some of the factors responsible for producing headache are hereunder.
1) Referred pain 2) Extra cranial Lesions.  3) Cranial neuralgias 4) Meningeal irritation. 5) Vascular changes 6) Traction and distortion, of the intra Cranial structures. 7) Psychogenic 8) Headache in association with other, systemic diseases.

**I) Reffered Head Ache :-**
Pain in the head experienced because of the lesions of peripheral structures like ear, nose, paranasal sinuses, teeth, tonsils etc.,

### a) Head Ache in Frontal Area Of the Head :-
Frontal head ache Occurs in glaucoma, iritis, frontal and maxillary sinusitis (behind the eyes in ethmoidal sinusitis) Chronic Rhinitis, ice cream head ache due to Cold stimulus to palate, in Temparo mandibular joint lesion (Facial neuraliga) and in the the involvement of ophthalmic branch of Trigeminal nerve in Trigeminal neuralgia.

## B) HEADACHE IN OCCIPITAL AREA OF THE HEAD

In cervical spondylosis, sphenoidal sinusitis (to the vertex also pain radiates), in refractive errors with high lesions, Meningitis, encephalitis and in sub arachnoid haemorrhages.

## C) HEAD ACHE IN TEMPORAL AREA OF THE HEAD.

In cranial, vascular, dental and Aural lesions.

## D) IN QUINSY (PERITONSILAR ABSCESS )

Hemicranial headache occurs.

### 2) Head Ache Due to extra Cranial Lesions. :-

Spastic contractions of neck and scalp muscles.

### 3) Head Ache Due to Cranial Lessions.

(Cranial Neuralgia)

Extordinary stimulus Or pressure exertion, Or due to un Known causes, severe head ache occurs due to the affection of 5-7-9-10 cranial nerves and cervical 1-2-3 nerves.

a)     **Trigeminal neuralgia -** Paraxysmal and sharp pain confined to the distribution of 5th Cranial nerve.

b)     **Glosso pharyngeal neuralgia -**
Stabbing pain in pharynx and deep into the ear that aggravates by eating and swallowing.

c)     **Facial Neuralgia :-**
Pain radiates to the Frontal and Temporal region by the involvement of facial nerve at temporo mandibular joint.

### 4) Head Ache due to Meningeal Irritation :-

Encephalitis meningitis and sub -arachnoid haemorrhage causes occipital head ache with photo phobia, drowsiness, pyrexia and neck stiffness.

### 5) Vascular Changes

Throbing type of head ache at temporal area due to the dilatation of intra cranial and extra cranial vessels.

**Ex:-**  In migraine, unilateral periodic cluster head ache occurs.

### 6) Traction on the intra cranial structures. :-

Cerebral tumours, sub dural haematoma causes increased intra cranial pressure, lumbar puncture causes decreased intra cranial pressure - these two produces severe head ache.The condition aggravates by strain, coughing and Bending.

**7)	Psychogenic Head ache :-**

In schizophrenia like disorders head ache is assoicated with anxiety and depression etc.

**8)	Head Ache In Systemic Diseases :-**

1) Chronic nephritis. 2) Uraemia. 3) Hypertension. 4) Hypotension. (low B.P.) 5) Polycythemia 6) Anaemia. 7) Acidosis. 8) Alcolosis. 9) Alcoholism 10) Congestive heart failure. 11) Hyperacidity. 12) Lead Poisoning. 13) Liver disorders. 14) Sun Stroke. 15) Syphilis. 16) Disorders of uterus. 17) Disorders of Testicles. 18) Vataj and Kshayajja Kasa (Dry cough with debilitative diseases.) 19) Vata balasak jwara, 20) Vishama Jwara. 21) Antrika Jwara. 22) Masurika Jwara. 23) Peetha Jwara. 24) Constipation. 25) Apasmara. 26) Vata Raktha. 27) Madhu meha. 28) Raktha pitta poorva rupa. 29) Vata roga. etc. 30) Dusta Pratishyaya etc.

# TRIGEMINAL NEURALGIA

It is commonly observed in middle age group, the exact aetiology is obscure but it may be due to Neurological vascular muscular problems, commonly follows after chronic contageous infections, pyogenic infections, Cold wind attacks, genetic and debilitated conditions.

The pain is paroxysmal, sharp and confined to the distribution of 5th nerve. The nerve get stimulated by talking - coldwind- washing and chewing etc., First maxillary and mandibular branches affects then ophthalmic branch. Each paroxysm lasts for only few seconds, with shooting cutting burning and stabbing type of pain. The stab of the pain may be followed by a dull aching. The Pain is precipitated by touching localised trigger zones on the affected side of the face. Paroxysms continue for days or weeks. remission become shorter and less frequent as the disease progresses. On examination of 5th nerve no functional abnormality is observed.

**Treatment :-**

1) Carbamazepine 200mg tabs tid. 2) Phenytoin 100 mg. tid. 3) Clonazepam 1-2mg tid. 4) Alcohol injection into the branch of the nerve Or into Gasserian ganglian.

# MIGRAINE

Migraine is characterised by periodic headache which is typically unilateral and offen associate with visual disturbance and vomiting. The attacks occur at intervals which vary from a few days to several months.

34

It is believed to be due to disturbance in the carotid Or vertebro basilar vascular tree by the sudden contraction and dilatation of the vessels. First Vaso constriction causes ischaemic symptoms and followed vaso dilatation, exerts pressure on the nerve endings of vessels of intra Or extra cranial arteries, causes throbing pain in the head. Pain may be prolonged by Secondary muscular contractions.

Most of the cases of migraine are observed with the Family history (genetic) it is stimulated Or aggravated during menstruation, exposure to flash lights, stress strain, anxiety, eating of Chacolate cheese and usage of medicines like reserpine, tyramine etc.,

The common symptoms are paraesthesiae Or weekness of One half of the body, severe throbing pain in the half part of the head (The affected side is not constant with each attach) With Vomiting, Photophobia, pallor, sweating and prostration which may necessitate the patient taking to bed in a dark room. The attack may last from few hours to several days and leaves the patient weak and exhausted, In rare cases hemiplegic migraine occurs.

**Treatment :-**
1) Anti anxiety drugs. 2) Sleep inducing drugs. 3) pain killers. 4) Brain tonics.

## EXAMINATION OF HEAD (SHIRAS)
Sushrutha explained 11 shiro rogas those contain shirashoola (Headache) as the Prime symptom. but vagbhata explained 19 diseases including the scalp and hair lesions. The lesions of scalp and hair can be easily diagnosed. but diagnosis of Head ache is not so easy for containing so many aetiological factors like the following.

1) Disorders of scalp and Hair 2) Brain and Meninges 3) Cranial nerves 4) Intra and Extra cranial blood vessels. 5) Muscles of neck face and scalp 6) Diseases of Eye ear nose sinuses teeth and throat 7) Psycological factors. etc. So, for the proper diagnosis of head ache detailed histry of the case and complete investigations are needed

While taking histry the following points are helpful for the diagnosis.

**1)    Size and Shape of Head :-**
a)    Normal - Abnormal b) Bilateral Symmetrical or not
c)    Normal Or bigger Or smaller.

**Note :-** In congenital abnormalities, Hormonal disorders, the lesions in the size and shape of the head can be noted.

**2)     Examination of the scalp.**

Whether normal Or abnormal, if abnormal for the following lesions of scalp should be checked.

a) Wounds, b) Scars c) Dandruff d) Inflammatory lesions e) Allergic lesions f) Cysts g) Tumours h) Abscess i) Pigmentory changes of Skin of the Scalp etc.

**3)     Examination of the Hair.**

a) Whether lengthy, thicker Or with loss of hair (Partial or Total)

b) Normal Pigmentation Or depigmentation.

**4)     Head Ache (Shira Shoola)**

(A) Collection of the associated symptoms of headache

a) Burning sensation b) Itching sensation. c) Heavyness of head d) Nausea - Vomitings. e) Drowsiness f) Photophobia g) Neck pain h) Body pains i) Otalgia j) Eye strain K) Tinnitus l) Hypertension m) Hypotension n) Rhinitis o) Sinusitis p) Carious teeth q) Neck stiffness r) Giddiness s) Indigestion t) Constipation u) Hyer acidity v) Dysphagia w) Gas abdomen x) Nasal Obstruction. y) Palpitation. z) Oedema of face limbs etc.,

**Ex :-** 1) In cranial lesions associated symptoms are Drowsiness, photophobia and Neck stiffness.

2) In Refractive errors - Eye strain. is associated.

3) In Nasal lesions - Nasal Obstruction - rhinitis. etc associated.

4) In Hyper tension - Burning sensation, giddiness, pulsation of Vessels. etc associated.

5) In ear disorders - Otalgia, Tinnitus. etc. assoicated.

6) In G.I.T. lesions - Gas abdomen, constipation, Hyperacidity- indigestion etc., associated.

7) Cold allergy - Heavyness of head, itching sensation etc. are associated.

**B)     Differentiation of Head Ache for Proper Diagnosis :-**

The following data give idea for the diagnosis.

1) Head ache partial Or Localised Or Total

2) Fixed Or spreading.

3) Continuous Or interrupted.

4) Regular Or Irregular.

5) Site of the Pain :- Whether at Frontal region, temporal. parietal, occipital vertex, retrobulbar area of eye. etc.,

**6)     Seveority of head ache :-**

a) Whether Mild - Moderate or severe b) In the morning - Noon or night
c) In summer - Winter or Rainy season. d) Irrelavant or irregular.

**7)     Nature of Pain :-**

Pricking pain-cutting pain-tearing pain, stabbling pain or churning pain etc.,

**8) Duration of Pain :-**

For - seconds, minutes, hours, days weeks or months etc.,
Duration of recurrence for 3 days -5-10-15-30 days. Duration of remission of pain
short, moderate or Long.

**9) Aggravating Factors :-**
By Stress and strain, coughing, sitting, sleeping, Reading, bending, Talking, Night arousal, Hot therapy, Hot exposure, Cold therapy, Cold wind exposure,
dust exposure smoke exposure, swallowing, at mornings, Noon or at Nights. Psychological etc.,

**10) Relieving factors :-**
Naturally - seasonally - by rest, Cold therapy - Hot therapy, Oleation, sudation - Pancha Karma therapy- Drugs etc.,

**11) Investigations :-**

a)     Urine In general

b)     Blood for Hb%, CBP, ESR and seriological examination.

c)     Stools for Ova and Microbs.

d)     X ray - for Nasal sinus - Brain and ear.

e)     CT scan of Brain & E.E.G.

f)     E.C.G. and Echo.

g)     Vision tests - Ophthalmo scopic examinations.

h)     Audio metry

i)     Rhinoscopy

j)     Pharynogo scopy- Laryngo scopy.

k)     Systemic examinations etc.

# KARNA ROGA
# DISEASES OF THE EAR

## कर्णरोगों की सम्प्राप्ति और निदान

अवश्यायजलक्रीड़ाकर्णकण्डूयनैर्मरुत्

मिथ्यायोगेन शस्त्रस्य कुपितोन्यैश्च कोपनैः ॥

प्राप्य श्रोत्रशिराः कुर्याच्छूलं स्रोतसि वेगावान् ।

ते वै कर्णगता रोगा अष्टाविंशतिरीरिताः ॥

(यो॰ : कर्ण)

## कर्णरोगों के भेद

कर्णशूलं प्रणादश्च वाधिर्यं क्ष्वेड एव च ॥

कर्णस्रावः कर्णकण्डुः कर्णवर्चस्तथैव च ॥

कृमिकर्णप्रतिनाहौ विद्रधिर्द्विविधस्तथा ॥

कर्णपाकः पूतिकर्णस्तथैवार्शश्चतुर्विधम् ।

काण्णार्बुदं सप्तविधं शोफश्चापि चतुर्विधः ।

एते कर्णगता रोगा अष्टाविंशतिरीरिताः ॥

(सु. उ. 20/3,4,5)

## 1. कर्णशूल

समीरणः श्रोत्रगतोन्यथा चरः समन्ततः शूलमतीव कर्णयोः ।

करोति दोषैश्च यथास्वभावृतः स कर्णशूलः कथितो दुराचरः ॥

(सु. उ. 20/6)

## वातिक कर्णशूल

प्रतिश्यायजलक्रीड़ाकर्णकण्डूयनैर्मरुत् ।

मिथ्यायोगेन शब्दस्य कुपितोन्यैश्च कोपनैः ॥

प्राप्य श्रोत्रसिराः कुर्याच्छूलं स्रोतसि वेगवत् ।

अर्धावभेदकं स्तम्भं शिशिरानभिनन्दनम् ॥

चिराच्च पाकं पक्वं तु लसीकामल्पशः स्रवेत् ।

श्रोत्रं शून्यमकस्माच्च स्यात् संचारविचारवत् ॥

(अ॰ हृ॰ उ॰ अ॰ १७)

## पित्तज कर्णशूल

शूलं पित्तात् सदाहोषाशीतेच्छाश्वयथुज्व रम् ।
आशुपाकं प्रपक्वं च सपीतलसिकास्त्रुति: ॥
सा लसीका स्पृशेद् यद्वत् तत्तत्पाकमुपेति च ।

(अ॰ हृ॰ उ॰ अ॰ १७)

## कफज कर्णशूल

कफाच्छिरोहनुग्रीवागौरवमन्दतारुज: ।
कण्डूश्वयथुष्णेच्छा पाकाच्छ्वेतघनस्त्रुति: ।

(अ॰ हृ॰ उ॰ अ॰ १७)

## रक्तज कर्णशूल

करोति श्रवणे शूलमभिघातादिदूषितम् ॥
रक्तं पित्तसमानार्ति किंचिद् व्याधिकलक्षणम् ।

(अ॰ हृ॰ उ॰ अ॰ १७)

## सन्निपातज कर्णशूल

शूलं समुदितैर्दोषै: सशोफज्वरतीव्ररुक् ॥
पर्यायादुष्णशीतेच्छं जायते श्रुतिजाड्यवत्
पक्वं सितासितरक्तघ्रनपूयप्रवाहि च ॥

(अ॰ हृ॰ उ॰ अ॰ १७)

## 2. बाधिर्य

स एव शब्दानुवहा यदा सिरा: कफानुयातो व्यनुसृत्य तिष्ठति ।
तदा नरस्याप्रतिकारसेविनो भवेतु वाधिर्यमसंशयं खलु ॥

(सु॰ उ॰ अ॰ 20/8)

श्लेष्मणानुगतो वायुर्नादो वा समुपेक्षित: ।
उच्चै: कृच्छ्राच्छ्रुतिं कुर्याद् वधिरत्वं क्रमेण च ॥

(अ॰ हृ॰ उ॰ अ॰ १७)

## 3. कर्णनाद

यदातु नाडीषु विमार्गमागत: स एव शब्दाभिवहासु तिष्ठति ।
श्रृणोति शब्दान् विविधांस्तदा नर: प्रणादमेनं कथ्यन्ति चामयम् ॥

(सु॰ उ॰ अ॰ 20)

शब्दवाहिसिरासंस्थे शृणोति पवने मुहुः।
नादानकस्माद् विविधान् कर्णनादं वदन्ति॥

(अ॰ हृ॰ उ॰ अ॰ १७)

## 4. कर्णक्ष्वेड

श्रमात् क्षयाद्रूक्षकषायभोजनात्
समीरणः शब्दपथे प्रतिष्ठितः॥
विरिक्तशीर्षस्थं च शीतसेविनः
करोति हि क्ष्वेडमतीव कर्णयो:

(सु॰ उ॰ अ॰ 20)

## 5. कर्णस्राव या कर्णसंस्राव

शिरोभिघातादथवा निमज्जतो
जले प्रपाकादथवापि विद्रधेः॥
स्रवेतु पूयं श्रवणोनिलावृतः
स कर्णसंस्राव इति प्रकीर्तितः॥

(सु॰ उ॰ अ॰ 20)

## 6. कर्णकण्डू

कफेन कण्डूः प्रचितेन कर्णयो:
भृशं भवत् स्रोतसि कर्णसंज्ञिते॥

(सु॰ उ॰ अ॰ 20)

## 7. कर्णगूथक

विशोषिते श्लेष्मणि पित्ततेजसा नृणां भवेत् स्रोतसि कर्णगूथकः॥

(सु॰ उ॰ अ॰ 20)

## 8. कर्ण-प्रतिनाह

सकर्णविट्को द्रवतां यदा गतो
विलायितो घ्राणमुखं प्रपद्यते।
तदा स कर्णप्रतिनाहसंज्ञितो
भवेद् विकारः शिरसोभितापनः॥

(सु॰ उ॰ अ॰ 20/12)

वातेन शोषित: श्लेष्मा स्रोतो लिम्पेत्ततो भवेत्।

रुग्गौरवं पिधानं च स प्रितिनाहसंज्ञित: ॥

(अ॰ हृ॰ उ॰ अ॰ १७)

## 9. कृमिकर्ण

यदातु मूर्च्छन्त्यथवापिजन्तव:

सृजन्त्यपत्यान्यथवापि मक्षिका:

तदंजनत्वाच्छ्रवणो निरुच्यते

भिषग्भिराद्यै: कृमिकर्णको गद: ॥

(सु॰ उ॰ अ॰ 20/13)

वातादिदूषितं श्रोत्रं मांसासृक्क्लेदजारुजम्॥

खादन्तो जन्तव: कुर्युस्तीव्रां सकृमिकर्णक:

(अ॰ हृ॰ उ॰ अ॰ १७)

## 10,11) कर्णविद्रधि

क्षताभिघातप्रभवस्तु विद्रधिर्भवेत्तथा दोषकृतोपर: पुन:।

सरक्त पीतारुणमस्त्रमास्त्रवेत् प्रतोदधूमायनदाहचोषवान् ॥

(सु॰ उ॰ अ॰ 20/14)

श्रोत्रकण्डूयनाज्जाते क्षते स्यात् पूर्वलक्षण: ॥

विद्रधि: पूर्ववच्चान्य:

(अ॰ हृ॰ उ॰ अ॰ १७)

## 12. कर्णपाक

भवेत् प्रपाक: खलु पित्तकोपतो

विकोथविक्लेदकरश्च कर्णयो: ॥

(सु॰ उ॰ अ॰ 20)

## 13. पूतिकर्ण

स्थिते कफे स्रोतसि पित्ततेजसां विलाय्यमाने भृशसंप्रतापवान्।

अवेदनो वाप्यथवा सवेदनो घनं स्रवेत् पूति च पूतिकर्णक:

(सु॰ उ॰ अ॰ 20)

कफो विदग्धः पित्तेन सरुजं नीरुजं त्वपि ॥
घनपूतिबहुक्लेदं कुरुते पूतिकर्णम्

(अ॰ हृ॰ उ॰ अ॰ १७)

# 14 से 17) चत्वारि अर्शा
# 18 से 21) चत्वारि शोफा
# 22 से 28) सप्तार्बुदानिच

(सु॰ उ॰ अ॰ 20)

## 1. कुचिकर्णक और     2. कर्णपिप्पली
गर्भेनिलात् संकुचिता शष्कुली कुचिकर्णकः ।
एकोनीरुगनेको वा गर्भे मांसाङ्कुरः स्थिरः ॥
पिप्पली पिप्पलीमानः

(अ॰ हृ॰ उ॰ १७)

## 3. विदारिका
सवर्णः सरुजः स्तब्धः श्वथुः, स उपेक्षितः ॥
कटुतैलनिभं पक्वः स्रवेत् कृच्छ्रेण रोहति ।
संकोचयति रूढा च सा ध्रुवं कर्णशष्कुलीम् ॥

(अ॰ हृ॰ उ॰ अ॰ १७)

## 4. पालीशोष
सिरास्थः कुरुते वायुः पालीशोषं तदाह्वयम् ।

(अ॰ हृ॰ उ॰ अ॰ १७)

## 5. तन्त्रिका
कृशा दृढ़ा च तन्त्रीवत् पाली वातेन तन्त्रिका ॥

(अ॰ हृ॰ उ॰ अ॰ १७)

## 6. परिपोट
सुकुमारे चिरोत्सर्गात् सहसैव प्रवर्धिते ।
कर्णशोफः सरुक्पाल्यामरुणः परिपोटवान् ॥
परिपोटः स पवनात्

(अ॰ हृ॰ उ॰ अ॰ १७)

## 7. उत्पात

गुर्वाभरणभाराद्यै श्यावोरुग्दाहपाकवान् ।
श्वयथुः स्फोटपिटिकारागोषाक्लेदसंयुतः ॥

(अ॰ हृ॰ उ॰ अ॰ 27)

## 8. उन्मन्थ

पाल्या शोफोनिलकफात्सर्वतो निर्व्यथः स्थिरः ।
स्तब्धः सकर्णः कण्डुमान् उन्मन्थो गल्लिरश्च सः ।

(अ॰ हृ॰ उ॰ अ॰ 27)

## 9. दुःख वर्द्धन

दुर्विद्धे वर्धिते कर्णे सकण्डुदाहपाकरुक् ।
श्वयथुः सन्निपातोत्थः स नाम्ना दुःखवर्धन ।

(अ॰ हृ॰ उ॰ अ॰ 27)

## 10. लेह पिटिका

कफासृक्कृमिजाः सूक्ष्माः सकण्डूक्लेदवेदनाः ।
लेह्याख्याः पिटिकास्ता हि लिह्युः पालीमुपेक्षिताः ।

# EAR DISEASES

**KARNA SHAREERA.**
(Anatomy of ear According to Ayurveda)

In Ayurvedic samhitas detailed Anatomical description of ear is not available, some description is here under.

| | | | | |
|---|---|---|---|---|
| 1) | Shrotram | = | Indrium -1 (Invisible) |
| 2) | Karnam | = | Indria Adhistaanam |
| | | | (Visible 2 ears) |
| 3) | Aakasham | = | Indria dravyam. |
| 4) | Shabdam (sound) | = | Indriaartham |
| 5) | Shroto buddhi | = | Indria buddhi.(Auditory centre) |
| 6) | Dikh | = | Indria Devata. |
| 7) | 2 ear are grouped under " Nava Dwara" |
| 8) | Shravanendrium is one among " Panchendrias " |

**9. Karna Pali (Karna Lathika)**
It is lobule of external ear, karna vyadana is done (in the diiva krutha Chidra of pali) to it.

**10) Karna Peetham** (Putrikopari Pradesham).
It is the seat of auricle.

**11) Karna Putrika** (Bahya Karnaavyava)
It is the auricle or pinna

**12) Karna Shaskuli** (karna Gatha Aavarthaka)
It is the external auditory meatus.

**13) Karna patah** (Tympanic Membrane)

14.   The distance between karna and apanga is 5 angula.

15.   It is supplied by 2 damani and 10 sira.

16.   
| | | |
|---|---|---|
| Bahya Karna | = | External ear. |
| Madyama Karna | = | Middle ear |
| Antah Karna | = | Internal ear. |
| Shabdanadi | = | Auditory Nerve |

# ANATOMY OF EAR

Ear is the organ of hearing and equilibrium. Anatomically it can be divided into 3 parts. 1) External ear 2) Middle ear 3) Internal ear.

## 1)     External Ear :-
It consists of a) Pinna (Auricle ) and
b) External auditory canal.

## a)     Pinna (Auricle)
The pinna is composed of a skin covered yellow elastic cartilage. The posterior surface is convex, smooth and with loose skin, the anterior surface is concave with folds and hollows (Scaphoid fossa superiorly and concha medially at the centre) here the skin is directly adherent to the perichondrium .

The anterior external margin of pinna is known as helix, the parallel ridge which is infront is known as anti helix, the protruding cartilage over the external auditory meatus is named as tragus, the parallel protruding cartilage at the lower end of antihelix is known as Anti tragus, at the bottom of pinna there is lobule which is devoid of cartilage and there is another part which is devoid of cartilage is at the junction of root of helix and tragus known as Incisura terminalis (formed by fibrous tissue ) it is utilised for Endaural incision for mastoid surgery .

### Blood Supply ;-
1) Anterior surface of pinna is supplied by the branches of the superficial temporal artery. 2) Posterior surface is supplied by posterior auricular artery, a branch of external carotid.

### Nerve Supply ;-
1) Upper 2/3 of Anterior surface of Pinna is supplied by auriculotemporal nerve.
2) Lower 1/3 of Anterior surface of Pinna is supplied by Greater auricular nerve.
3) Lower 2/3 of posterior surface of Pinna is supplied by Greater auricular nerve.
4) Upper 1/3 of posterior surface of Pinna is supplied by lesser occipital nerve.

## b) External auditory Canal:-
It is a tortuous canal, extending from bottom of concha to lateral surface of tympanic membrane (ear drum), approximately 2.4cm. (24mm) in length. The outer 1/3 (8mm area) is cartilagenous portion and inner 2/3 (16mm area) is bony portion. The direction of cartilagenous meatus is inwards upwards and backwards while the bony meatus is inwards downwards and forwards, in total S shape is produced in the meatus. So while examining the ear meatus the pinna must be pulled backwards and upwards in adults and downwards and outwards in children to straighten the canal to visualise the canal and tympanic membrane properly. The walls of the meatus are lined with skin, The skin of the cartilaginous part has hair follicles, sebaceous and ceruminous glands which secrete the ear wax or cerumin, for the protection of ear drum.

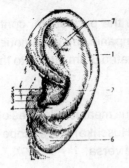

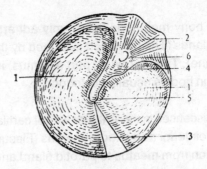

**Auricle:**
*1*—helix, *2*—anthelix, *3*—tragus, *4*—antitragus, *5*—concha, *6*—lobule, *7*—crus of the anthelix, *8*—acoustic meatus

**Tympanic membrane:**
*1*—pars tensa, *2*—pars flaccida, *3*—cone of light, *4*—manubrium of the malleus, *5*—umbo, *6*—mallear prominence

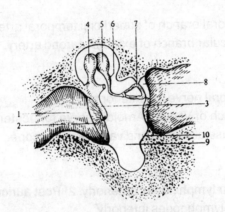

**Tympanic cavity:**
*1*—acoustic meatus, *2*—tympanic membrane, *3*—manubrium of the malleus, *4*—head of the malleus, *5*—anvil (incus), *6*—long process of the anvil, *7*—stapes, *8*—oval (vestibular) window, *9*—tympanic cavity, *10*—round window

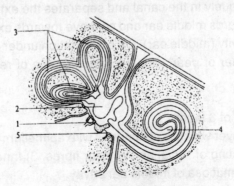

**Internal ear:**
*1*—oval window, *2*—vestibule, *3*—semicircular canals, *4*—cochlea, *5*—round window

The skin of bony meatus is thin, firmly adherent to the periostium, contain no hair follicles or glands (The bony part is formed by the tympanic and squamous portions of temporal bone). The narrowest part (isthmus) is situated 5mm lateral to the ear drum where foreign bodies usually get lodged.

Dehiscences in the Anterior wall of cartilaginous meatus (Fissures of Santorini), and at Anteroinferior part of bony meatus (Fissure of Huschke) gives scope for spreading of infection from meatus to parotid gland and vice versa.

Anteriorly meatus is related to temparomandibular joint hence infection of external auditory canal may cause Trismus (Painful Opening of mouth.)

**Blood Supply : -**
1) Auriculo temporal branch of superficial temporal artery.
2) Posterior auricular branch of external carotid artery.

**Nerve Supply :-**
1) Auriculo temporal nerve for anterior half.
2) Auricular branch of Vagus - Arnold's nerve for posterior half stimulation this nerve may cause coughing and vasovagal syncope.

**Lymphatic Drainage :**
1) Pre auricular lymph nodes anteriorly. 2) Post auricular lymphnodes posteriorly . 3) Infra auricular lymphnodes inferiorly

**Tympanic membrane (Ear Drum)**
Tympanic membrane is a thin freely mobile, translucent elliptical, greyish white membrane, set obliquely in the canal and separates the external ear from the middle ear. It is convex towards middle ear and concave towards external ear. It is the lateral wall of tympanic cavity (middle ear). On examination under illumination it appears as pearly grey or mother of pearl with a triangular cone of reflected light in its antero inferior quadrant.

**Layers :-** It consist of 3 layers.
1) Outer epithelial layer which is continuous with epithelium of external ear. 2) Middle fibrous layer, consisting of radial and circular fibres. 3) Inner mucous layer which is continuous with the mucosa of middle ear cavity.

**Note : -** The upper smallest zone of tympanic membrane (Pars flaccida) contain only 2 layers (devoid of middle fibrous layer).

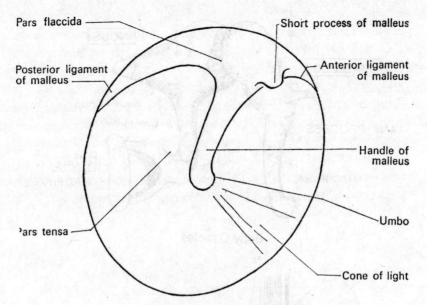

Normal Tympanic membrane.

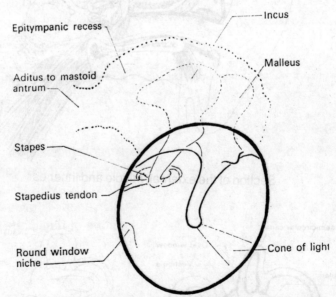

Diagram of Rt. Tympanic membrane showing the relationship
of the auditory ossicles.

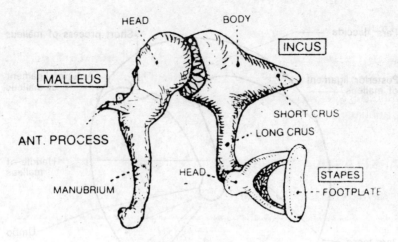

Bony Ossicles

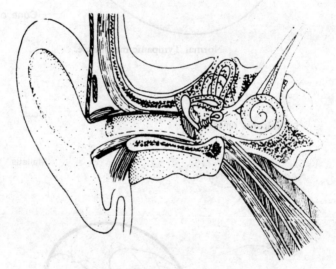

Section of the external, middle and inner ear

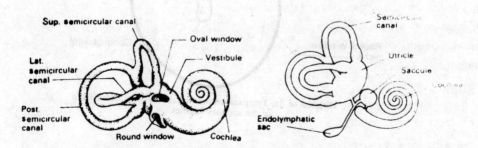

Bony labyrinth

Membranous labyrinth

**Parts of Ear Drum :-** 2 parts

### 1) Pars Tensa :-

It is the largest tense part of tympanic membrane, thickened peripherally into fibro cartilaginous annulus which fits into the bony ring or tympanic sulcus. The sulcus is grooved to receive the annulus.

### 2) PARS FLACCIDA OR SHRAPNELL'S MEMBRANE OR ATTIC PART

It is is devoid of fibrous layer and annulus, it fits into the notch of Rivinus. It is lax or flaccid part.

### Size :-

Approximately 10mm in vertical diameter and 8mm in horizontal diameter.

### Shape :-

It is oval or elliptical in shape.

### Position :-

The drum is placed obliquely at an angle of $55^0$ with the floor

**Surfaces:-**
1) Lateral surface is free and concave.
2) Medial surface is convex.

### Features : -

On examination ear drum appears pearlygrey translucent and concave, pars tensa shows vertical handle of malleus attached to the tympanic membrane at medial surface which passes downwards and backwards from the short or lateral process of malleus to the umbo at thecentre of the drum, the conical light reflex extend from Umbo to the antero inferior quadrant of ear drum, the long process of incus may be visible through the ear drum behind and parallel to handle of malleus. The anterior and posterior. Malleolar folds run forwards and backwards from short process of Malleus by which it is divided into two, smaller above part pars flaccida and larger below part is pars tensa. The pars tensa is divisible into four quadrants by drawing the imaginary lines from Umbo vertically and horizontally, they are 1) antero superior quadrant 2) antero inferior quadrant 3) Postero superior quadrant 4) postero inferior quadrant This description is beneficial for discription of tympanic lesions.

### Blood Suply ;-

1) External surface is supplied by auricular branch of maxillary artery. 2) Inner surface is supplied by

a) Anterior tympanic branch of maxillary artery b) Posterior tympanic branch of stylomastoid branch of posterior auricular artery. c) Inferior tympanic artery a branch of ascending pharyngeal artery. d) Arteria nutricia incudo mallei a twig of middle meningeal artery.

## Nerve supply :-

Outer suface as like external auditory meatus, inner surface is supplied by tympanic plexus.

## Middle Ear Anatomy ;-
(Tympanum)

The entire middle ear cavity is lined with respiratory mucous membrane which is an extension of mucosa of Nasopharynx. It is extending from medial suface of tympanic membrane to cochlear promontory of internal ear. (It lies in between external ear and inner ear) it is shaped like a biconcave disc. The vertical and antero posterior diameters are 15mm and transverse diameter is 6mm at upper part, 2 mm at the centre and 4 mm at the lower.

## Tympanic Cavity :-
1)       **6 walls**
        1) Roof 2) Floor 3) Anterior Wall 4) Posterior wall 5) Medial wall 6) Lateral wall.
2)       **4 Chambers :-**
        1) Meso tympanum 2) Epitympanum 3) Hypo tympanum 4) Posterior tympanum.
3)       **Contents :-**
        Typanum contaiins 1) Air 2) Ossicles 3) Tympanic plexus 4) Intra tympanic muscles (tenden of Tensor tympani and stapedious muscles) 5) Chorda tympani nerve 6) Ligaments 7) Arteries and veins.
**4) Communication :-**
        1) Anteriorly to naso pharynx through Eustachian tube 2) Posteriorly to mastoid antrum through the aditus.

1) Walls of the tympanum - 6 They are
**1) Roof or tegmental Wall :-**
        Roof separates the tympanum from the middle cranial fossa by a thin bony plate known as Tegmen tympani chronic inflammatory conditions of middle ear may spread through the tegmen to the meninges of brain.

**2) Floor :-**
        The middle ear cavity is separated from the jugular bulb by a thin bony plate (it is known as jugular wall ) chronic inflammatory conditions of middle ear may spread to jugular vein and may cause thrombosis.

**3) Lateral Wall :-**
It is formed by the tympanic membrane and partly by bone above behind and below.

**4) Anterior Wall or Carotid Wall :-**

From above down wards the following openings are present on the anterior wall.
1) Cannal for chorda tympani nerve (canal of Huguier) 2) Canal for tensor tympani muscle.
3) Eustachian tube opening. 4) Giaserian fissure transmit the tympanic artery and the anterior ligament of the malleus. 5) A thin bony plate known as carotid canal wall separates the middle ear cavity from internal carotid artery.

## 5) Posterior wall or Mastoid Wall :-

1) Aditus antrum connects the epitympanum with the mastoid antrum. 2) Below to aditus a bony projection known as pyramid present through the tip of it stapedius tendon passes and inserts into the neck of stapes. 3) lateral to the pyramid is the opening for the chorda tympani nerve of facial nerve.

## 6) Medial Wall or Labyrinthine Wall :-
It separtes middle ear cavity from internal ear.

1) Most obvious feature is promontory of cochlea formed by the turn of cochlea. 2) Above and behind the promontory there is fenestra ovalis (Oval window) that is closed by foot plate of stapes and annular ligament. It lies between middle ear and scala vestibuli of the cochlea. 3) Below and behind the promontory Round window present that is closed by Secondary tympanic membrane which separates middle ear from scala tympani of the cochlea (Sinus tympani a depression between the two openings Oval and round ) 4) Above and posterior to promontory Fallopian canal with facial Nerve present. 5) Lateral Semi circular canal Prominence present just above the facial Nerve.

## TYMPANIC CAVITY :-
Middle ear cavity can be divided in to 4, they are

1) **Meso tympanum :-** It is the middle ear proper and the biggest of the 4 , it corre sponds with the pars tensa of tympanic membrane.
2) **Epitympanum :-** It is also known as epitympanic recess or Attic, the area above to meso tympanum (the upper part of tympanum)
3) **Hypo tympanum :-** The lower part lying below the tympanic membrane (Or below the meso tympanum).
4) **Posterior Tympanum :-** The posterior part lying behind the level of tympanum.

## COMMUNICATIONS OF MIDDLE EAR CAVITY
(Anteriorly it is having communication with Eustachian tube.)

### Eustachian Tube :-
It is about 3.5cm in length connects the middle ear with Naso pharynx. The outer third of this is bony, that adjoins with middle ear, The inner 2/3 is cartilagenous and leads in to Nasopharynx. The naso pharyngeal opening lies behind and on a level with the posterior end of inferior turbinate, at rest it remains closed and during Yawning or swallowing opens. In adults the tube is Obliquely placed where as in infants it is short, wide and horizontally placed so Naso pharyngeal infections easily spread to middle ear in infants.

## 2) Mastoid :-

Posteriorly middle ear cavity communicates with mastoid antrum through aditus.

a) Aditus ad antrum - a short canal connecting epitympanum with mastoid antrum.

b) Mastoid antrum :- It is the largest air cell in mastoid bone.

**Anteriorly :-** It recieves the aditus medialy related to horizontal semicircularcanal

**Laterally :-** formed by the cortex of mastoid bone.

**Roof :-** Is formed by tegmen plate, postero inferiorly antrum communicates with numerous mastoid air cells.

**c)      Mastoid Air Cells :-**

Variable in number, size and distribution, these communicate with the matoid antrum, 3 types of mastoid processes are

1) Cellular 2) Diploctic 3) Sclerotic.

**Contents of middle Ear :-**

3 Ossicles (3 tiny bones ) they are

1) Malleus (Hammer) 2) Incus (Anvil ) 3) Stapes (Stirrup)

**1)      Malleus (Hammer)**

Largest and most lateral ossicle, measuring 8mm in length It has a head, neck, handle, anterior and lateral processes Handle is firmly attached to the pars tensa of ear drum, head is situated in the epitympanum and articulate with body of incus.

**2)      Incus (Anvil)**

It has a body, a short process and long process. Body articulates with head of malleus, short process projects backwards in the attic, long process projects down wards behind the handle of malleus and articulates with the head of stapes.

**3)      Stapes (Stirrup)**

Smallest Ossicle measuring about 3.5 mm and consists of a head neck, foot plate and also anterior and posterior crura. Head articulates with long process of in cus and Foot plate of stapes is held to the Oval window by the annular ligament.

**Muscles :-**

1)      Tensor tympani is inserted into neck of malleus

2)      The stapedius is inserted into neck of stapes.

These muscles decrease the movements of Ossicles.

**Relations of the Middle Ear Cavity :-**

Laterally External ear and medially inner ear.

1) Tegmen plate (Roof) separate the tympanum from Temporal Lobe of brain and meninges. 3) Cere bellum is postero medial to mastoid air cells. 3) Horizontal semi Circular canal lies postero superior to facial Nerve. 4) 5-6-th cranial nerves lie close to the Apex of petrouse pyramid. 5) Horizontal part of facial Nerve present back of medial wall. 6) Lateral Sinus is posterior to mastoid cell. 7) Jugular bulb close with Floor of tympanum. 8) Internal carotid artery is anterior to tympanum.

So middle ear chronic inflammatory lesions easily spread to above parts and cause severe complications.

**Blood supply :-**1) Middle meningeal artery 2) Maxillary artery 3) Ascending pharyngeal artery 4) Stylo mastoid branch of posterior auricular artery.

**Nerve Supply :-**
**Sensory :-** Tympanic branch of Glosso pharyngeal nerve.
**Motor :-** Tensor tympani by mandibular Nerve, stapedius by facial nerve.
**Lymphatic Drainage :-**1) Pre auricular lymph nodes. 2) Retro pharyngeal lymph nodes.

**Inner Ear (Labyrinth)**
Inner ear is a structure of winding passage, it is also named as labyrinth situated in the temporal bone, consists of 2 parts. 1) Bony Labyrinth 2) Membranous labyrinth (Mambranous labyrinth is covered by bony Labyrinth) Membranous Labyrinth contains endolymph and perilymph is present in between bony and membranous labyrinth.

**Bony Labyrinth :-**
It has 3 parts.
1) Vestibule 2) Cochlea 3) Semicirular canals.

**1) Vestibule :-**
It lies in the centre of bony Labyrinth on its lateral wall is the opening of Oval window which is closed by foot plate of stapes. Postero medially there is an opening for the aqueduct of the vestibule.

**2) Bony Cochlea :-**
It lies infront of the vestibule and is like a snail shell. It has 2 3/4 turn around a central pillar known as modiolus, an ossco membranous lamina divides the tube lumen into two, the upper one scala vestibuli which communicates with vestibule, the lower one is scala tympani which communicates with tympanic cavity through round window these two cavties are filled with perilymph and are communicated at the apex through a small opening known as Helicotrema.

**3) Bony Semicircular Canals:-**
These are 3in number 1) Horizontal 2) Superior and 3) Posterior semicircular canals are set at right angles to each other. The 3 canals open by five openings into the vestibule posteriorly.

**Membranous Labyrinth :-**
Membranous labyrinth present in the bony Labyrinth, filled with endolymph and comprises the following .
1) Saccule and utricle present in bony vestibule 2) Membranous semicircular ducts present within the corresponding bony canals. 3) Ductus cochlearis present in the bony cochlea.

**1) Saccule and Utricle :-**
Utricle lies in the upper part of vestibule and is connected with 3 semicircular ducts by five openings while the saccule lies below and infront of utricle and communicate with duct of cochlea. These two join to form endo lymphatic duct which ocupies the bony aqueduct of vestibule. There is specialised neuro epithelium known as Macula which is end organ for gravitational pull and Linear accele ration.

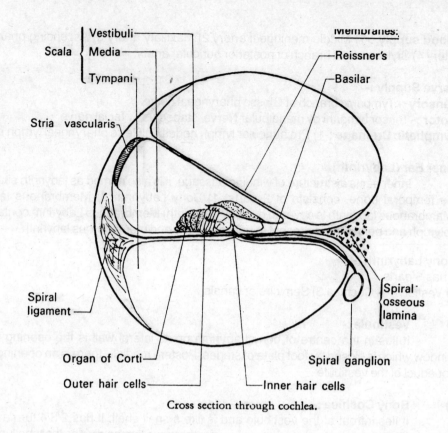

Cross section through cochlea.

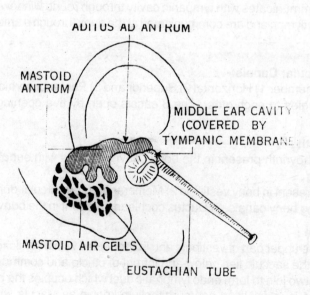

ADITUS AD ANTRUM

MASTOID
ANTRUM

MIDDLE EAR CAVITY
(COVERED BY
TYMPANIC MEMBRANE)

MASTOID AIR CELLS

EUSTACHIAN TUBE

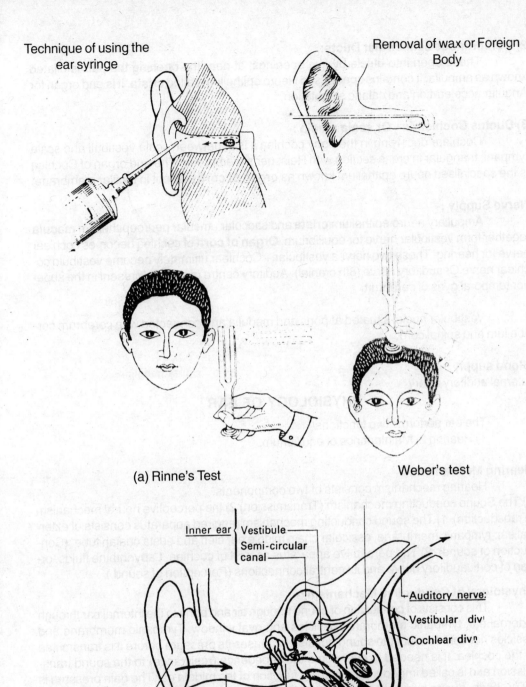

Technique of using the
ear syringe

Removal of wax or Foreign
Body

(a) Rinne's Test

Weber's test

Inner ear {
Vestibule
Semi-circular
canal

Auditory nerve:
Vestibular div[n]
Cochlear div[n]

Auricle

Middle ear

Scala tympani

Scala vestibuli

External auditory canal

Conduction of sound through the ear.

57

## 2) Membranous semicirular Ducts:

These open into utricle by five openings, at near the opening the part is dilated known as ampulla, it contains specialised Neuro epithelium called **crista**, it is end organ for Angular acceleration and calaric stimulation.

## 3) Ductus Cochlearis - Or scala media :-

Cochlear duct lying in the bony cochlea it is in between scala vestibuli and scala tympani, triangular in cross section with Reissner's membrane. The end organ of Cochlea is the specialised neuro epithelium known as **organ of corti** present in basilar membrane.

## Nerve Supply :-

Ampullary neuro epithelium **crista** and saccular utricular neuroepithelium **macula** together form vestibular nerve for equilibrium. **Organ of corti** of cochlea becomes cochlear nerve for hearing. These two nerves vestibular + Cochlear ultimately become vestibulo cochlear nerve Or auditory nerve (8th cranial). Auditory centre of hearing present in the superior temporal gyris of cerebrum.

Vestibular nuclei situated at pons and medulla and connected with cerebrum cerebellum and spinal cord.

## Blood supply :-
Internal auditory artery

# PHYSIOLOGY OF EAR

The ear performs two functions
1) Hearing 2) Maintenance of equilibrium.

## Hearing Mechanism:-

Hearing mechanism consists of two components.
1) The Sound conducting mechanism (Transmission) 2) the perceptive neural mechanism (Transduction) 1) The sound conducting mechanism required apparatus consists of external ear, tympanic membrane, ossicular chain middle ear cleft and eusta chaian tube. (Conduction of sound). 2) The perceptive apparatus consist of cochlea, Labyrinthine fluids, organ of corti, auditory nerve and its central connections (Perception of sound.)

## Physiology of Conductive Mechanism :-

This consists of conduction of sound through air and bone to the internal ear through external ear, tympanic membrane, ossicles and oval window. Tympanic membrane and ossicles not only conduct the sound but also increases its pressure before it is transmitted to the cochlea. It is needed to over come the impedence (resistance) to the sound transmission and is called impedence matching function of the middle ear. The gain pressure is 22 or 28 db, due to hydraulic effects of middle ear and lever effect of ossicles. Hydraulic effect is due to difference in the vibrating surface area of the drum (55 Sq.m.m. ) and foot plate of stapes (3.5 sq. m.m ) which is approximately 17. Lever effect of Ossicles is due to relative difference 1:1.3. Total gain sound pressure transformer ratio is 17 x 1.3 = 22.

This is how the middle ear functions as the sound pressure transformation mechanism helps in impedence matching of sound.

## IMPORTANCE OF ROUND WINDOW :-

The soundwaves which are transmitted through tympanic membrane ossicular chain reaches the Oval window and vibrate the perilymph of cochlea for the stimulation of organ of corti and gives protection to round window (when tympanic membrane is intact) from the direct impact of sound waves thus allow it to function as a release point necessary for fluid displacement of the inner ear (to give phase difference between oval and round window).

## Importance of Tympanic Muscles :-

The muscles restrict the ossicular movement to save the delicate inner ear from loud sounds.

## Functions of Eustachian Tube :-

1) It is useful for the aeration of middle ear cleft for the proper function. 2) For providing hypo tympanic air bubble for the movement of the membrane of round window. 3) To equalise the air pressure on either sides of tympanic membrane.

**Ex :-** When atmospheric pressure is reduced as during ascent in an aeroplane the air in the middle ear cavity gets absorbed and a negative pressure develops in side the middle ear cavity that can be equalised by frequent swallowing movements by which eustachian tubes open. Failure to open the tubes causes tympanic rupture and serous otitis media.

## Function of Mastoid Aircells :-

It is not clear but may serve the following functions.
1) Air reservoir for middle ear cavity. 2) Protect the Labyrinth from temperature variations. 3) provide resonance to sound.

## Bone conduction of sounds :-

Besides air conduction the sound is also transmitted by bone conduction by the vibration of skull bones. Perceptive neural mechanism and apparatus. the sound waves normally enters the cochlea through the Oval windows (through round window and also by skull bones).

Propogation of sound within the cochlea is controversial But it is clear that the foot plate of stapes causes movement of cochlear fluids, an energy displaces the basilar membrane, the organ of corti gets stimulated which results in generation of cochlear microphonics and the nerve impulses are carried to the central connection.

## 1)      Hydrodynamics. :-

Sound vibration through stapes movemet will produce a flow of perilymph from scala vestibuli - Helicotrema -scala tympani and vice versa. Accoustic energy displaces the basilar membrane to and fro between the two scaleae.

## 2)      Mechanical Excitation of The Hair Cells :-

Vibration of basilar membrane results in a sliding or shearing movement between the tectorial membrane and haircells. This results in the development of cochlear microphonic due to electrical potential difference in endolymph. perilymph and organ of corti which help accoustic impulse to be transmitted as neural impulse.

**Theories of Hearing :-**
1) Resonance theory or place theory of Helmholtz:- The perception of pitch of sound depends upon the selective vibratory action of the basilar membrane.
2) Rutherford's telphone theroy or Telephone diaphragm theory:-.
Whole basilar membrane vibrates with each sound and perception of pitch is related to the rate of firing of individual nerve fibres.
3) Volley theory Or Waver's Theroy.

Combined theory of above both.
a) higher frequencies are perceived by place theory.
b) Lower frequencies are perceived by telephonic theory.
c) Intermediate frequencies are perceived by both theories.

4) Travelling wave theory or Bekesy's theory. Sound waves travel from basilar membrane to the apex of cochlea, The point of maximum amplitude on the basilar membrane depends upon the frequency of sound, and the final perception of sound occurs in the cerebrum.

**Physiology of Equilibrium :-**
Vestibule is very important end organ of the proprioceptive mechanism. Other proprioceptors of the body are in muscles tendons, joints, skin and eyes These end organs are connected to cerebellum and cerebrum where the final perception of the sense of equilibrium occurs.

**The Vestibular Apparatus :-**
It supplies information to the brain about the position and movement of head as a basis for postural adjustments.

**1) Utricle and Saccule :-**
The macule of utricle and saccule get stimulated due to linear acceleration or gravitational pull and in static posture (Rest.

**2) SEMI CIRCULAR CANALS:-** The crista of ampulla of semicircular canals gets stimulated by angular acceleration (Kinetic posture produced during movements.)
The three canals on each side of body are arranged at right angles to each other and thus stimulated by movements.

**HISTORY TAKING AND SYMPTOMATOLOGY.-**
Before otoscopy and and functional examination of ear, knowing the History of the patient with common symptomatology is very important and gives scope for correct diagnosis.
1) Age of the patient (for senile degenerative lesion)
2) Placeof living (At dusty crowdy areas allergic disorders are common).
3) Occupation (Labours working in noisy surroundings are commonly prone to deafness etc., disorders).
4) Personal history - (Smoking, tobacco chewing, swimming and diving, eating of cold items, fridged items, scratching the ear canal with match sticks, Lower socio economic and un hygienic living habits etc.,).

5)       Past history of diseases like diabetes, hypertension, syphilis, Tuberculosis, habit of Ototoxic drugs. injuries, operations etc.,

6)       Family histroy of deafness otosclerosis etc.,

7)       History of drug intake like salicylates, aminoglycosides, quinine and cytotoxic drugs.

8)       History about the present condition or Chief complaint & associated complaints.

Origin, duration, severity, progress, nature of the disease, aggravating factors, focal lesions of referred lesions, continuous problem or intermittent, sudden onset or gradual, fixed lesion or spreading type, unilateral or bilateral, congenital or hereditory or developmental Or degenerative, or traumatic or inflammatory or Neoplastic or metabolic or Aliergic or idiopathic - in all these angles case study should be carried that gives perfect scope for diagnosis.

**The common symptoms of ear diseases are :-**
1) Earache 2) Itching sensation in the ear canal
3) Deafness , 4) Otorrhoea. 5) Tinnitus 6) Vertigo

**General Symptoms :-**
1) Head ache. 2) Body pains. 3) Fever 4) Nausea. 5) Vomitting. 6) Common Cold and cough. 7) Upper respiratory symptoms. 8) CNS (Central nervous system). 9) Allergic symptoms etc.,

**Note :** - Enquiry about each symptom indetail is explained in their concerned topics.

**Physical Examination of Ear.**
**Auricle or Pinna :-**

1)       a) Appearance - Congenital deformities, inflammatory changes, ulcers, swellings, scars are observed.

2)       Mastoid region should be examined for abscess swelling and fistula (Mastoiditis).

3)       Position of Pinna - It is pushed outwards forwards and downwards by a mastiod abscess.

4)       Tenderness - in Acute otitis externa the movements of pinna and tragus are extremely tender.

5)       Post auricular groove gets obliterated and auricle stands out prominently in furunculosis.

**Otoscopy :-**
Examination of external auditory canal and tympanic membrane with the help of an ear speculum or electric otoscope is known as otoscopy.

1)       Electric Otoscope is self illuminated with ear speculum easy for handling and examination but difficult for manipulations with instruments etc.,

2)       Ear speculum needs the support of bright illumination (Bull's eye condensor ) and forehead mirror to focuss the light rays into the ear canal.

3)       Forehead mirror with light also available for Otoscopy.

**Procedure of Otoscopy :-**

1) Doctor should sit slightly lower than the patient.
2) Patient should sit in a chiair facing the doctor.
3) Bull's eye condensor (illuminator) should be placed close to the left side of the patient on a level with patient's head.
4) The Doctor should adjust the head mirror and through the central aperture of mirror only he should visualise the ear canal with his right eye.
5) Children should be properly examined with the aid of an assistant.
6) According to the size and diameter of ear canal only proper sized speculum should be selected, the dilated part of speculum is held between thumb and forefinger, it is then carefully introduced into the meatus up to 8mm depth without touching the bony part (causes pain and irritability).
7) At the same time of insertion of speculum the pinna is pulled upwards and back wards in adults and downwards and backwards in infants to straighten the canal to visualise the contents and tympanic mambrane properly,.
8) In the ear canal there may be wax, fungus, foreign bodies, furuncles, polyps, swellings ,cysts, inflammatory changes and ear discharge etc., The nature of the contents should be observed and for deeper examination (tympanic membrane ) wax and discharge etc., should be cleaned with wax removing probe and cotton tippped applicator.

9) **Tympanic membrane**
   **Norma Findings :-**
   Greyish white transluscent Obliquely set membrane through which handle of malleus short process of mallus, Anterior and posterior malleolar folds, short and long process of incus, umbo and cone of light are seen.

**Abnormal Findings :-**
A) **Integrity of Membrane Should be Examined.**
a) Whether it is intact or perforated.
b) **If perforated :-** Site (Central or safe, mariginal or unsafe, attic or complicative with cholesteatoma,), Shape (Round or oval or irregular), Size (Small or big,) Number (Single or multiple,) with discharge or without discharge and whether middle ear contents are visible or not (the visible contents are ossicles, or polyps or cholesteatoma or granulations etc.,).

**B) Colour of tympanic membrane :-**
Normally greyish white, pale, lustreless in secretory otitis media, congested in Acute otitis media, Bluish in haemotympanum etc.,

**C) Position of tympanic membrane :-**
Bulged in effusions of middle ear.
Retracted in Eustachian block, serous otitis media and Adhesive otitis media with reduced mobility.

## D) Mobility of tympanic Mebrane :-

Restricted in Adhesive otitis media or effusions of middle ear, Hyper mobile in scarring etc., (The mobility of tympanic membrance is examined with siegle's neumatic speculum. It contains a ear speculum attached with rubber bulb and tube ear speculum is inserted into the ear canal and rubber bulb is pressed for air pressure to cause mobility of ear drum that should be visualised with ear speculum in bright illumination)

E)    Eardrum should be examined for fluid Levels like in serous otitis media.
A test for examine the patency of eustachian tube -

a)    Ear drops if reaches the throat is the significance of tympanic performation with patent eustachian tube.

b)    Air bubblles in ear discharge suggests the perforated ear drum and patent eusta chian tube.

c)    While closing the mouth and nose if patient is asked to blow out and if the patient hears the air rushing into the middle ear with mobility of ear drum suggestsa patent eustachian tube.

d)    **Politzerisation :-** The nozzle of the politzer bag is inseted into one nostril and the both nostril should be closed by the patient and asked to make a swallowing movement and the bag is pressed simultaneously if the patient feels air rushing into his ears it is significant of patent eustachian tube (By swallowing movement Estachian tubes open so the released air from politzer's bag enters into middle ear through the patent eustachian tube).

**e) Eustachian Catheterisation :-** Eustachian catheter is attached to rubber bulb, the tip of catheter is inserted at the opening of eustachian tube through Nasopharynx and the bulb is pressed, if the Eustachian tube is patent air rushes into middle ear and causes movement of eardrum.

## 11) Radigoraphy Confirms the diagnosis.

# FUNCTIONAL EXAMINATION OF EAR :-

The hearing may be tested in number of ways.
1) Voice test.
    a) Conversational voice
    b) Whispered Voice.
2) Watch test.
3) Tuning fork test
4) Audiometry.

## 1) Voice Test :-

a) Conversational Voice test (C.V)
b) Whispered Voice (W.V.) each ear is tested separetely while the other ear should be masked. These tests are performed in a sound proof quiet room.
a) Normal Conversational Voice can be heard upto a distance of 20 to 40 feet or 12 meters.
b) Normal whispered Voice can be heard upto a distance of 12 feet or 4 meters.

### 2) Watch Test :-
This test is carried out with the help of watches, a normal person hears the ticking sound of watch.

Above 2 types of methods are not for an accurate assessment of hearing.

### 3) Tuning fork Test :-
These test are carried out by the vibration of tuning forks of Varying frequencies 256, 512, 1024 etc.,

The most useful fork is the 512 CPS (cycles per second)

### 1) Air conduction (A/C)
The vibrating tuning fork is placed opposite to the ear canal (Sound conduction through air and tympano ossicular chain)

### 2) Bone Conduction (BC)
The vibrating tuning fork is placed on the mastoid bone or forehead (Sound conduction through skull, cochlea, auditory nerve and central connections).

**Note :-** For vibrating the tuning fork, handle the stem of the fork and strick slightly against knee or Elbow or on soft surfaces like rubber pad or on hypo thenar eminence of palm etc.,

### (A) Rinne's Test :-
The comparative assessment of Air conduction with Bone conduction.

Strike the tuning fork and place before the external auditory meatus to hear the vibration of sound through air, ask the patient to raise the finger when he can no longer hear the vibrations, after the signal place the base of the of the fork on mastoid process and ask him if he again hears the vibrations Rinne's test is Negative, if he cannot hear the vibrations at mastoid Rinne's postive.

### Interpretation :-
1) In Normal hearing Air conduction is longer than Bone conduction, this is called Rinne positive.

Normal hearing            = A.C. More than B.C.
Rinne positive

2) when Bone conduction is longer than Air conduction it is called Rinne negative - Suggests conductive deafness.

Rinne negative
Conductive deafness       = B.C. More than A.C.

3) Air conduction is more than Bone conduction but low volume and shorter duration is called as low positive Rinne, suggests sensori neural deafness.

Low Rinne positive.
Sensori neural deafness       A.C. more than B.C.

4) Rinne equivocal - Air conduction and Bone conduction are equall suggests Low or mild conductive deafness.            A.C. = BC

5) False Rinne negative - Suggests unilateral sensori neural deafness. AC and BC are markedly reduced on the diseased side. But B.C appears normal though reduced because the Bone conduction is heard normally by spreading to the normal opposite side, soonly explained as false Rinne negative (to avoid this masking of the ear is needed)

a)    A.C. > B.C. -    Normal
b)    A.C. > B.C.      But both reduced, mild perceptive deafness.
c)    B.C. > A.C.      Conductive deafness.
d)    AC = BC          Mild conductive deafness.
e)    Only AC,         No, B.C. - Severe perceptive deafness
f)    Only BC,         No. A.C. - Severe conductive deafness.

**(B) Weber's Test :-**
1)      It is useful for testing the unilateral deafness or when there is marked difference between the two ear.
2)      Bone conduction of two ear are compared.
3)      Air conduction is not examined.

**Procedure :-**
This test is performed by placing the base of vibrating tuning fork at the centre of fore head or vertex or on the upper incissor, the patient is asked in which ear the sound is best heard a) Better hearing on one side b) Equal on both sides c) Not hearing at all, this may be expressed as the Lateralisation of Sound (lateralisation occur when there is difference of bone conduction by more than 5 db.)

**Interpretation :-**
1) Normal Person hears equally on both sides.
2) Conductive deafness.
a) Bilaterally equal conductive deafness centralisation of sound.
b) Bilaterally unequal conductive deafness, sound lateralisation towards more deaf side.
c) In unilateral conductive deafness, sound Lateralisation occur towards affected side.
3) Sensori neural deafness.
a) In bilaterally equal nerve deafness Centralisation of sound.
b) In bilaterally unequal nerve deafness, Lateralisation of sound towards better ear.
c) In unilateral nerve deafness sound lateralisation towards normal ear.

**c) Absolute Bone Conduction Test (A.B.C.) :-**
The bone conduction of the patient is campared with that of the examiner, assuming that the examiner has a normal hearing.
For testing A.B.C. the ear canal is blocked by a finger, the vibrating tunic fork is placed on the mastoid process of the patient, As soon as he stops hearing it is transferred to themastoid of the examiner. The process may be tried again in a reverse manner.
1) In Normal and Conductive deafness A B C of patient is equal to ABC of examiner.
2) In Sensori nerve deafness ABC of patient is reduced.

**D) Schwabach Test :-** This is as like A.B.C. but the test is performed without occluding the meatus, it is less reliable than A.B.C.

# TUNIING FORK TEST ANALYSIS

|  | Rinne | Weber | A.B.C. |
|---|---|---|---|
| A) Normal hearing. | Rinne postive | Central heard equally on both sides. | Normal |
| B) Conductive deafness. | | | |
| a) Right side | RT ear negative LT ear positive | Lateralised to right | Normal |
| b) Left side | RT ear positive LT ear Negative | lateralised to left. | Normal |
| c) Bilateral | Both ears Negative | Lateralised to deafer side or central if equal on either sides. | |
| C.) Sensori Neural deafness | | | |
| a) Right ear | Right ear Positive (Low ) Left ear Positive | lateralisation to left ear | RT ear reduced. |
| b) Left ear | Left ear positive (low) Right ear positive | Lateralisation to right ear. | Left ear reduced. |
| c) Bilateral | Both ear Positive (Low) | lateralisation to better side or central if equally deaf. | both ear. reduced |

## 4) Audiometry.

Audiometer is an electronic instrument providing uniform standard graphical measurement of hearing qualitatively and quantitatively. It is capable of producing pure tone sounds of different frequencies at variable intensities, pure tones are delivered to the ears by a head phone for A.C. and by a vibrator for B.C.

The frequency ranges from 125 C.P.S. to 8000 C.P.S. (Mainly 500 to 2000). The intensity is measured in decible (dB), ranging from O.dB to 110 dB,

The intensity of sound is increased or decreased for each frequency in A.C. and B.C. is plotted on a graph called audiogram.

66

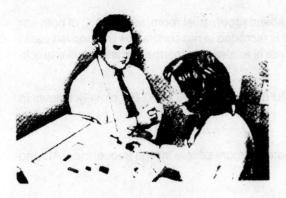

Taking an audiogram

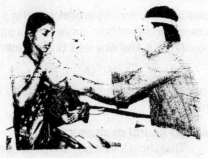

Technique of holding the child for E.N.T. examination

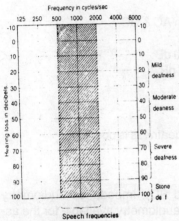

fig. 4-5   Audiogram chart.

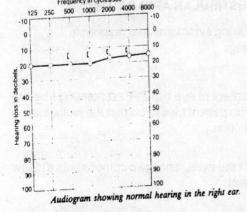

Audiogram showing normal hearing in the right ear.

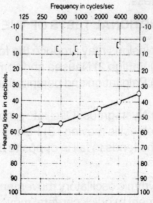

z. 4-7:   Audiogram showing sensorineural deafness in the right ear

Audiogram showing conductive deafness in the right ear.

**Procedure :-** Audimetry is performed in a sound proof, quiet room, initially A.C of both ear is recorded, the threshold curve of right ear is recorded in red continuous line and left ear in blue continuous line whereas B.C. of both ear is recorded in interrupted lines or like brackets.

**1) Normal -** A threshold between O to 20 dB is normal, AC and BC closely follows in normal limits.

**2) Sensori neural deafness :-**
Threshold levels beyond 20bB, deafness more severe in high frequencies. AC and BC are reduced.

**3) Conductive deafness :**
Threshold levels - AC is beyond 20dB, but BC is within normal limits. Loss of hearing by AC is more in lower frequencies - wide gap between AC and BC.

**4) Mixed Deafness :-**
AC reduced, BC partially reduced with some gap between AC & BC.
5)      Mild deafness. hearing loss between 20 to 30 dB.
6)      Moderate deafness hearing loss between 30 to 60 dB.
7)      Severe deafness, hearing loss between 60 to 110 dB.

# Use :-
1)      Permanent record is obtained
2)      Diagnosis of qualitative and quantitative deafness is possible,
3)      For fitting aproper type of hearing aid.
4)      For special test of recruitment.

**Note :-** Other types like speech Audiometry (SRT and SD), Impedance audiometry (Tympanometry), Bekesy Audiometry, Evoked response audiometry available for the assessment of deafness.

## FUNCTIONAL TESTS OF THE VESTIBULAR APPARATUS.

Vestibular lesions may produce the following symptoms and response.
A. Symptoms -  1) Vertigo 2) Nausea and vomiting,
                3) Palpitation and perspiration.

**B. Response :-** 1) Nystagmus (Oscillatoy movement of eye ball 2) Fast pointing (the patient feels that the object is moving ) 3) Falling (The patient tries to correct the hallucination of movement and he tends to fall in opposite direction.),

**Nystagmus :-**
It is the rhythmic oscillatory movement of the eyes, it has two components a) Slow labyrinthine movement b) quick cerebral movement.

**It is of 3 types.**
1)      Central        -       associated with intra cranial lesions.
2)      Ocular         -       associated with eye lesions.
3)      Vestibular     -       due to vestibular lesions.

**Vestibular nystagmus is of 2 types.**:- 1) Spontaneous   2) Induced

1) Spontaneous
 a)Ist degree-nystagmus produced when a patient looks in the direction of quick component
b) 2nd degree Nystagmus produced on looking straight.
c) 3rd degree - Nystagmus produced on looking in the direction of slow component.

2)        Induced - Due to stimulant  like in caloric test, rotation test, etc.,

**1) Caloric Test** (Hallpike Test)
        Caloric test is a test of the vestibular function based on the principle of stimulating Labyrinth by temperature differences. Patient is placed in supine position with the head raised $30^0$ from horizontal level to bring the horizontal semi circular canal into vertical position. Nearly 200 to300 CC water with $30^0$ C and $44^0$ C(Separately) is flushed into external ear upto 40 seconds with enema can - Nystagmus and vertigo develops, the duration of Nystagmus in measured. it is approximately 1 minute and 20 seconds to 2 minutes in normal labyrinth.

In every ear two readings should be measured one with Cold water ($30 C^0$) and another with hot water ($44 C^0$), cold water causes Nystagmus to opposite side where as hot water causes Nystagmus to the same side. The 4 Values commonly equal.

        In canal paresis the duration of induced Nystagmus is reduced this  is observed in menieres disease, post aural vertigo and vestibular neuronitis. Unilateral hypo activity of a Labyrinth with perceptive deafness is highly suggestive of acoustic neuroma. Sometimes calaric responses are enhanced in one particular direction that is known as Directional preponderance of Nystagmus.

**2) Cold Caloric Test (Kobrak's Test )**
        About 5CC of Ice cold water is injected into external auditory meatus, Labyrinth is stimulated and nystagmus occurs with 2 minutes duration. (Rough method for testing).

**3) Cold Air Caloric Test.**
        In perforated ear drum of the patients, Cold water instillation causes complications so in such cases only cold air is supplied by Dundas Grant apparatus.

**4) Fistula Test :-**
        It is used to detect a fistula in the bony wall of the Labyrinth, on increasing the air pressure in external auditory meatus and middle ear with Siegle pneumatic speculum that is transmitted into Labyrinth through the fistula and causes vertigo and Nystsgmus it suggests fistula test positivie.

**5) Rotation test :-**
        Patient is placed on a revolving baranys chair which is roated at the rate of 10 revolutions per second (10 rps) the chair is then stopped and patient is observed for post rotational nystagmus.

**6) Romberg's Test :-**
        Patient is asked to stand with his feet together and arms at his side. He is asked to close the eyes- The patient falls on the side of the lesion in vestibular paresis.

**7) Opkokinetic Test :-**
        A white rotating drum with black vertical lines is rotated horizontally and stopped normal person get Nystagmus of both side. but unilateral Nystagmus suggests central vestibular Lesion.

# SAMANYA NIDANA OF KARNA ROGA
## (Common aetiological factors of ear diseases)

**1) Avashyaya - Exposure to snow Or Cold Items:-** Exposure to Cold items gives scope for infection, fungus development, common Cold, pressure differences on either sides of tympanic membrane, and so many cold wind allergic manifestations of External and middle ear.

**2) Jalakreeda -** Diving or swmming Or exposure to polluted water.

Water enters into external ear and causes infection, fungus collections and trauma to tympanic membrane.

**3) Karna Kandooyaya :-** Picking Or Probing the external auditory canal.

It is common habit to get relief from itching sensation. But it causes scratches, ulcers and inflammation in the external auditory canal, which leads to many complications.

**4) Mithya yogena Shastrasya ;-** Improper instrumentation during the examination and treatment.

Improper use of ear wax removing probes, Foreign body removing hooks, syringes Or forceps by untrained persons. It causes severe complications. like tympanic perforation, otitis externa etc.,

**5) Sound Pollution ;-** Hearing (high frequency) loud sounds, this causes problems like tympanic rupture (conductive deafness) etc.,

**6) Abhighata :-** Injury to head especially to the temporal bone may cause severe complications of ear and even death.

**7) Regular Head Bath (Shira snana)**

The water if entered in to the ears, easily cannot come out side because of curved external auditory canal, some water by retaining in side causes fungus infection etc., complications.

8) All the aetiological factors explained for Nasal diseases also applicable to ear diseases.

9) Peripheral or adjacent lesions like scalp infection, pharyngeal lesions and lesions of face may cause ear problems.

10) Chronic systemic infections like Tuberculosis, Leprosy, syphilis etc may cause ear problems.

11) Congential (Atresia of external auditory canal), Hereditory, Psychological, Professional (Labour working in mills with sound and dust pollution), Vascular, Neurolgical, Drug induced (Streptomycaetin induced deafness), degenerative by age (senile deafness), Allergic and Idiopathic causes can produce ear diseases.

# SAMANYA SAMPRAPTHI OF EAR DISEASES

**Samprapthi :-** 1) Doshaj 2) Aaganthuja.

1) By above causes vatadi doshas vitiate the Shabda vaha srotas and cause ear diseases like Karna shoola, Karnanada, Badirya etc.,

2) Due to traumatic causes also in short time ear diseases like deafnees (Badirya), Tinnitus (Karna Pranada), karna Pratinaha (Tympanic perforation) may be produced.

## CLASSIFICATION OF EAR DISEASES

I)    According to Sushrutha and Yogaratnakar ear diseases are = 28
II)   According to vagbhata = 25 ear diseases
III)  According to Charaka = 4 Diseases.

## I) Sushrutha's classification of ear diseases = 28, they are,

1) Karna shoola         (Otalgia - Pain in the ear)

2) Karna pranaada       (Noises in the ear - Tinnitus)

3) Karna Kshweda        ( -do-                  )

4) Badirya              ( Deafness              )

5) Karna Srava          ( Otorrhoea             )

6) Karna Kandu          (Itching Sensation in the ear canal )

7) Karna gootha Or Varcha ( wax in the external auditory canal)

8) Karna Pratinaha      (Tympanic perforations)

9) Krimi Karna          (Maggots in the ear)

10) Karna Paka          ( Furunculosis)

11) Poothi Karna        ( Suppurative otitis media)

12) and 13). 2 types of Vidradi (Abscess)

(14 to 17 ) . 4 types of Arsha (Polyps of ear)

(18 To 21) . 4 types of shopha (Oedema Or Swellings)

(22 To 28 ) 7 Types of Arbuda (Tumours)

## II Vagbhata's classification of ear diseases = 25

15 diseases of ear canal (Karna sroto rogas)
10 external ear diseases (Bahya Karna rogas)

The 15 Dieseases of Karna srotas are,
1 to 5, 5 Types of Karna shoola (Otalgia)

| | |
|---|---|
| 6) Karna Nada | (Tinnitus) |
| 7) Badirya | (Deafness) |
| 8) Karna pratinaha | (Tympanic perforations) |
| 9) Karna Kandu | (Itching sensation in the ear canal) |
| 10) Poothi Karna | (Suppurative Otitis media) |
| 11) Krimi Karna | (Maggots of ear) |
| 12) Karna shopha | (Oedema Or swelling of ear) |
| 13) Karna arsha | (Polyps of the ear) |
| 14) Karna vidradi | (Ear abscess) |
| 15) Karna arbuda | (Tumours of ear) |

**Bahya Karna Rogas** = 10, They are,
1) Kuchi Karnika
2) Karna Pippali
3) Vidarika
4) Pali sosha
5) Tantrika
6) Paripotha
7) Uthpatha
8) Unmatta Or Gallire
9) Dukha Vardana
10) Lehyaa.

**Asadya Karna rogas According to Vagbhata are 4 in number, they are.**
1) Karna Pippali
2) Sannipataj Karna shoola
3) Vidari
4) Kuchi Karnika.

## III) Charaka's Classification of ear diseases 4 in number they are.
1) Vataj Karna roga
2) Pittaja Karna roga
3) Kaphaj Karna roga
4) Sannipataj Karna roga.

# Description of Ear Diseases According to Charaka - 4, they are

## 1) Vataja Karna Roga.

The patient complains of different types of sounds in the ear, pain, deafness, dried wax and with scanty thin blackish ear discharge.

## 2) Pittaja Karna Roga.

The patient complains of red coloured oedema, crustformation, burning sensation and with yellowish foul ear discharge.

## 3) Kaphaja Karna Roga :-

The patient complains of deafness, deformity of ear, itching sensation in the ear canal, light pain, immobile swellings and with whitish sticky ear discharge.

## 4) Sannipathaja Karna Roga :-

All the above (mixed type) symptoms are present

# 1) KARNA SHOOLA
## (Otalgia Or Earache)

1)      Sushrutha explained it without any sub divisions.
2)      Charaka explained 4 sub divisions they are.

     1) Vataja Karna shoola      2) Pittaja karna shoola
     3) Kaphaja Karna shoola      4) Sannipataj Karna Shoola.

3) Vagbhata explained 5 sub divisions.

     1) Vataj Karna shoola 2) Pittaj Karna Shoola 3) Kaphaja Karna shoola
     4) Raktaja Karna Shoola 5) Sannipataj Karna Shoola.

## a) Karna Shoola according to sushruta.

In the ear canal the vitiated Vata dosha is encircled (Aavarana) by pitta Kapha Rakta and other types of Vata, and causes improper circulation of vata (Vata viloma gathi) and produces untolerable pain in the ear, is known as Karna shoola which is explained as difficult to treatment (Kasta sadya).

## 1a) Vataja Karna shoola according to Charak :-

Vitiated Vata causes Noises in ear, pain, dried scanty thin ear discharge and deafness.

## I.b) Vataj Karna Shoola According to vagbhata :-

Pratishyaya (Rhinitis), jala kreeda (Swimming or diving ), Karna Kandooyan (Scratching of ear canal with sticks etc), hearing loud sounds, rest lessness and dieting etc, causes vata vitiation in the auditory canal (shabda vaha srotas)., and causes severe pain in ear. The associated symptoms are Ardhaava bhedak (Migraine), Hanustamba (Lock jaw), loss of appetite, disinterest in cool things, ulceration of ear with watery discharge and intermittent deafness etc.

It can be co-related to Acute otitis externa, Acute serous otitis media etc diseases.

## 2 a) Pittaja Karna Shoola By Charak :-

Vitiated pitta causes reddish oedema, cutting and burning type of pain and yellowish foul discharge from the ear.

## 2. b) Pittaja karna Shoola By Vagbhata :-

Vitiated pitta dosha causes pain,fever, burning sensation, quickly suppurative oedema with yellowish watery discharge and shows interest in cool things. (By sticking of the discharge to the other normal site causes progression of the disease).

It can be co-related to Acute otitis externa (Furunclosis) Acute serous otitis media etc diseases.

## 3 a) Kaphaj Karna Shoola by Charak :-
The vitiated Kapha dosha causes deformity, deafness, itching sensation, light pain and bigger oedema with whitish sticky discharge from the ear.

## 3. b) Kaphaj Karna Shoola by Vagbhata :-
The vitiated Kapha dosha causes light pain in the ear, Heavyness in the head, jaws and neck, itching sensation, sticky white discharge from ear and the patient desires hot things

It can be co-related to chronic otitis externa and chronic otitis media.

## 4) Sannipaaja Karna Shoola By Charak and Vagbhata :-
The tridoshas vitiate and produces terrific pain, swelling and multi coloured pus discharge from ear with fever. Symptoms are fluctuating according to dosha predominence. It can be co-related to Acute/chronic otitis media.

## 5) Rakthaja Karna Shoola By Vagbhata, it is not Explaind By Charak.
Raktha dosha vitiates due to injuries (Trauma to ear or head) and produces bleeding ulcer in the ear canal or blood stained ear discharge and signs and symptoms of pittaja karna shoola (signs and symptoms are more severe than pitta Karna shoola).

It can be co-related to traumatic acute otiitis.

## Complications of Karna Shoola :-
If Karna shoola associates with following complications it becomes incurable (Asadya).

1) Moorcha, 2) Burning sensation, 3) Jwara, 4) Kasa, 5) Klama, 6) Vamana.

# OTALGIA (Pain in ear)

The pain in ear occurs due to lesions of ear and also due to referred causes in the lesions of the organs which have the same nerve supply.

**A)    Local Causes of otalgia**
**a) External ear Lesions which cause Otalgia :-**
1) Furunculosis, 2) Impacted wax in the external ear canal. 3) Foreign bodies, especially Animate Foreign bodies, 4) Perichondritis, 5) Acute otitis externa, 6) Otomycosis, 7) Myringitis, 8) Trauma, 9) Tumours, 10) Ramsay - Hunt's Syndrome.

**b) Middle ear Lesions which cause Otalgia :-**
1) Eustachian catarrh, 2) Acute otitis media, 3) Acute mastoiditis, 4) Complications of otitis media, 5) Trauma, 6) Barotrauma, 7) Tumours.

**B) Referred Otalgia :-**
Referred otalgia occurs in the lesions of the organs having following nerves supply
**1)** 5th (Trigeminal), **2)** 7th (Facial ), **3)** 9th (Glossopharyngeal), **4)** 10th (Vagus ), **5)** Cervical 2nd, **6)** Cervical 3rd,

**1) Via Trigeminal Nerve :-**
The auriculotemporal nerve (the branch of mandibular of Trigeminal nerve) supplies to external ear and also to the oral cavity, teeth, nasopharynx, nose, para nasal sinuses and tempero mandibular joint, so in the lesions of these parts, pain referred to ear throgh auriculotemporal nerve.

**Ex :-** in caries teeth, alvoeolar abscess, impacted wisdom tooth, traumatic and inflammatory lesions of mouth, tongue and salivary glands, tempero mandibular joint arthritis, deviated nasal septum, sinustitis and malignancy.

**2)     Via Facial Nerve :-**
This nerve supplies face and some sensory fibres to the ear, so in herpes zoster like lesions pain radiates to the ear through facial nerve fibres.

**3)     Via Glossopharyngeal Nerve : -**
Tympanic branch of glossopharyngeal nerve supplies to the middle ear and also to oropharynx, tonsils etc., so in

a) Acute ulcerative tonsilitis b) Peri tonsilar abscess
c) Retropharyngeal abscess d) Para pharyngeal abscess
e) Neuralgia etc, lesions pain refers to ear.

## 4) Via Vags Nerve :-

Auricular branch of Vagus supplies to the external auditory canal, eardrum pharynx, Larynx, crico pharynx etc, in these lesions pain radiates to ear.

## 5) Via Cervical 2-3 Nerves :-

Lesser occipital and great auricular nerve supply to the external ear and also to the cervical region, so in cervical lesions like a) Spondylosis b) Fibrositis c) Myositis d) Herpes - Pain refers to the ear.

## 6) Neuralgia also cause pain In the ear.

Treatment :-

A) For Local otalgia

1) Avoid the causative factor.
2) Cleaning of wax from external audiotroy canal.
3) Removing of Foreign bodies if any.
4) Broad spectrum antibiotics Or fungicides, Local and systemic.
5) Oral Anti inflammatory drugs and analgesics.
6) Anti histamine drugs (Systemic)

B) For referred Otalgia -

The causative disease should be treated.

## 2) KARNA NADA OR KARNA PRANAADA.

(Tinnitus Aurium)

Vitiated Vata dosha either entering into other channels (Vimaarga gaman) or encircled by Kaphadi doshas in shabda vaha srotas (auditory canal) produces defferent types of sounds in the ear like Bheri, mrudanga, shankha etc, is known as karnanada or Karna Pranaada.

## 3) KARNA KSHWEDA

Tinnitus Aurium

The vata etc doshas are vitiated due to Dhaathu Kashaya , taking of cold water after excessive Nasya karma etc, causes the vitiation in the auditory canal (shabda vaha srotas) and produces noises like Flute, in the ear, is known as karna kshweda

(It is not explained by vagbhata)

# DIFFERENTIAL DIAGNOSIS OF KARNA NADA AND KARNA KSHWEDA.

| Sl. No. | Karna Nada | Karna Kshweda. |
|---|---|---|
| 1. | Vata dosha only vitiates | 1) Vata and other doshas vitiate (Vata pitta Kapha and Raktha). |
| 2. | Different types of sounds are heard. | 2) Only flute noise is heard. |
| 3. | It arises due to obstructive lesions of shabda vaha srotas ( external and middle ear) | 3) It arises due to degenerative lesions (Dhathu Kshaya etc) of shabda vaha srotas ( internal ear). |
| 4. | Treating the Vata dosha cures the disease. | 4) Vata etc doshas should be treated for improvement. |

## TINNITUS

Tinnitus is defined as an auditory sensation or adventitious sound heard in one or both ears in the absence of any relevant external stimulus to cause it. The sounds are of different types like whistling, hissing, buzzing, steaming ringing, roaring, clicking etc.

**Types** A)  1) Unilateral   2) bilateral
B)  1) Central       2) Peripheral (Functional types.)
C)  1) Subjective tinnitus (Sounds heard only by patient)
2) Objective tinnitus (sounds heard by patient and examiner or Doctor
D)  1) Intermittent - Tinnitus with gaping
2) Continuous - without gaping
3) Fluctuant - Not uniform with the changes in intensity.
4) Changes in the pitch of tinnitus.

### Causes of Tinnitus :-
**A)     Subjective Tinnitus.**
I) Tinnitus with deafness.
All the causative factors responsible for the deafess also produce tinnitus.
Ex :- 1) Impacted wax Or Foreign bodies in ear
2) Secretory otitis media 3) Aero otitis media. 4) Oto Sclerosis 5) Acoustic trauma.

**II)     Tinnitus without Deafness ;-**
Ex :- 1) Anaemia 2) Hypertension 3) Hypotension 4) Caries teeth Or impacted wisdom teeth.

### III) Functional Tinnitus :-
Due to emotional factors.
### IV)    Idiopathic causes

## B) Objective Tinnitus causes.
1) Clicking tempero madibular joint,2) Clonic contractions of palatal and tympanic muscles, 3) Patulous eustachian tube, 4) Live insects in the ear canal, 5) Vascular pathology Ex:-Arterio venous shunt, Glomus jugulare tumour, Aneurism of occipital, superficial temporal vessels and arch of Aorta (Around the ear).
6) Intra cranial vascular tumours.

### Investigations :-
Otological, neurological, cardio vascular, audiological, vestibular and Radiological examination are needed for the diagnosis

### Treatment ;-
1) Cause should be treated 2) Mild sedatives, anxiolytics, vasodilators, Carbamazepine, vitamins are useful. 3) Reassurance to the patient explaining that it is not dangerous. 4) Masking of  the sounds with alarm clock Or radio etc. 5) Surgical treatment -sectioning of cochlear nerve, but is not so beneficial

## 4) KARNA BADIRYA.
### (Deafness )
The vitiated vata dosha or vata kapha doshas by deranging or obstructing the shabda vaha srotas (Auditory canal ) or shabda Vaha sira (Vessels) and nerves of the ear or neglecting Karna nada etc. diseases causes difficulty in hearing or in capability of hearing is known as Badirya.
1)      Kaphaj Badirya can be co-related to conductive deafness
2)      Vataj Badirya can be co-related to perceptive deafness
3)      Vata kaphaj Badirya can be corelated to mixed deafness.

### Deafness ;-
The deafness means impairment of hearing. It can occur at any age, congenital or acquired, and it varies in degree "mild to servere". (Congenital deafness is commonly associate with dumbness).
**Types :-** 1) Conductive deafness 2) Perceptive deafness 3) Mixed deafness.

### I) Conductive Deafness :-
It is due to defect in the conducting mechanism of the ear (External and middle ears) from external auditory canal to the oval window.
### Causative Factors of Conductive Deafness :-
### a) Causes of External Ear :-
1) Congenital causes (Atresia or Microtia),
2) Acquired causes like Wax or cerumin, impacted foreign bodies, otomycosis, Otitis externa, Polyps, tumours, myringitis or Tympanic perforations.

## b) Causes of Middle Ear :-

1. Congenital defects of ear drum and ossicles, ossicular discontinuity, Haemotympanum,
2. Traumatic lesions like fracture of Base of skull and Barotrauma
3. Inflammatory lesions like acute otitis media, chronic otitis media, serous otitis media, adhesive otitis media, secretory otitis media, barotraumatic otitis media, tympano sclerosis, specific otitis media.
4. Neoplasms
5. Miscellaneous like otosclerosis.

## c) Causes of eustachian tube and nasopharynx :-

Eustachian catarrh or obstruction, Eustachian tube dysfunction, Barotrauma, enlarged, adenoids and growths in nasopharynx.

## II) Sensory neural deafness or Perceptive deafness.

The deafness is due to the lesions of Labyrinth (internal ear) , 8th cranial nerve (auditory nerve) and central connections. (It includes psychogenic deafness).

## The Causative factors of sensory neural deafness :-

## 1) Congenital causes :-

Hereditary developmental defects, consanguineous marriages, Rh incompatability, diseases affecting the pregnant mother (like german measles, diabetes, syphilis, hypertension, pre eclampsia), intake of ototoxic drugs by pregnant women (like thalidomide quinine, streptomycin, kanamycin or gentamycin etc.,) Major surgery under general anaesthesia during pregnancy, prolonged and difficult labour, forceps delivery with head injury, premature delivery, post natal kernicterus, encephalitis, meningitis, ototoxic drugs, viral infections, head injury etc.,

## 2) Acquired Local Causes :-

a) Trauma :- Head injury, surgical injury to Labyrinth, loud sounds producing concussion, contusion or laceration of the labyrinth.

b) Infection ;- Like mumps, syphilis Tuberculosis, measles, chicken pox, influenza, meningitis, enteric fever, labyrinthitis, herpes etc.,

c) Ototoxic Drugs :- Streptomycin, Gentamycin, quinine, salicylates, frusemide etc.,

d) Tumours - Acoustic neuroma

e) Meniere's Disease :- Ramsay Hunt syndrome etc.,

f) Degenerative :- Senile deafness or presbyacusis.

## 3) Acquired General Causes :-

Athero sclerosis, Hypertension, Vasospasm of C.N.S., Labyrinthine artery disseminated sclerosis, cerebro vascular insufficiency due to thrombosis, embolism and haemorrhages, cerebello potine angle tumour.

Diabetes, Hypothyroidism, Avitaminosis, Smoking, Alcoholism, Psychological etc.,

**III) Mixed Deafnes :-** If both conductive and perceptive deafness are present that is known as mixed deafness.

**Causes :-** Blast injuries, Acoustic trauma, Head injuries, Chronic suppurative otitis media with Labyrinthitis, senility (Presbyacusis) and otosclerosis.

**IV) Psychogenic Deafness :-** There is no organic cause for this deafness.

**1) Hysterical :-** The deafness is outside conscious control. The patient ceases to listen and so fails to hear. Patients are usually female (Functional or emotional).

**2) Malingering :-** Patient is conscious of deception. He or she listens intently but endeavours not to respond. (Pretends to be deaf for personal gains).

**Causes of sudden Sensory Neural Deafness :-**
      **1) Vascular : -** Spasm, thrombosis, embolism, haemorrhage,
      **2) Trauma :-** Head injury, acoustic trauma, rupture of round window membrane.
      **3) Infection :-** Viral Labyrinthitis, mumps.
      **4)** Meniere's disease. **5)** Ototoxicity **6)** Central nervous system :- meningitis encephalitis.vascular lesions, trauma. **7)** Functional.

## DIFFERENTIAL DIAGNOSIS OF CONDUCTIVE AND PERCEPTIVE DEAFNESS.

|  | Conductive deafness | Perceptive deafness. |
|---|---|---|
| 1. Congenital | Less Common mainly progressive | More common Sudden as well as progressive |
| 2. History of Viral fevers, exanthematous fevers, prolonged medication, sound trauma. | Nil | More Common. |
| 4. History of head injury, vertigo | Less Common | More Common |
| 5. History of Otorrhoea | Often | Nil |
| 6. Voice | Speaks in Low Voice | Speaks Loudly |
| 7. Noise intolerance | No | Yes |
| 8. Speach discrimination | Good | Poor |
| 9, Recruitment | Absent | present in Cochlear lesion |
| 10. Site of Lesion | External and Middle ears. | Inner ear, 8th nerve with central connections |
| 11. Rinne test | Rinne(-), BC> AC | Rinne positive AC>BC But reduced. |
| 12. Weber test | Lateralised to the worse ear | Lateralised to better ear |
| 13. Pure tone Audiometry | BC threshold normal AC " increased, good AC, BC gap. | AC, BC thresholds both increased. |
| 14. Hearing loss | Not more than 60 dB. | May be more than 60 dB. |

### Degres of Deafness :-
1) Mild deafness 20 to 30 dB.
2) Moderate deafness 30 to 60. dB.
3) Severe deafness :- Above 60. dB.

### Investigations.
1) Hearing tests. 2) Audiometry. 3) Caloric tests. 4) V.D.R.L., Blood sugar, serum cholesterol. 5) Radiography. 6) Blood pressure. 7) Neurological examination etc.

### Treatment ;-
A) Conductive deafness ;-
1) Treating the causative factor
2) Hearing aids.

### B) Sensory Neural Deafness :-
1)     Treating the specific causative disease if any like syphilis, Diabetes etc.
2)     Vaso dilators for menier's disease like disorders. .
3)     Vitamines - B1, B6, B12, A,C,E,
4)     Steroid therapy in sudden perceptive deafness.
5)     Tranquilizers, Antidepressants for Tinnitus with deafness.
6)     Hearing aids.
7)     Conversation should be slow, clear and not loud wih the patient.
8)     Auditory training and Lip reading.

# Presbyacusis :- Senile deafness.
It is a type of sansorineural deafness due to old age, speech discrimination is poor
and don't tolerate loud sounds,

# Meniere's Disease
This disease is characterised by a triad of symptoms consisting of 1) Vertigo 2)
Deafness 3) Tinnitus, which occur at irregular and unpredictable intervals. This occurs due
to failure of the mechanism regulating the production and absorption of endo lymph.

### Aetiology ;-
1) Exact cause is unknown  2) Vaso spasm (Reduced circulation to Labyrinth)
3) Endo lymphatic hydrops (Increased tension in the endo-lymph of Labyrinth).
4) Emotional factors.5) Sympathetic system over activity causes vasospasm.
6) Hormonal disturbances may cause water and electrolyte imbalance in the endo lymph.
7) B. Complex deficiency. 8) Allergy and septic focus.

### Pathology ;-
Increased tension of endo lymph causes distention of membranous labyrinth with
degeneration of Labyrinth leads to rupture of mebranous labyrinth, mixing of perymph and
endolymph and damage to organ of corti and vestibular neuro epithelium.

## Clinical Features :-

1) Rotatory type of giddiness of varying intensity duration and intervals. 2) Fluctuating type of sensori neural deafness, and intolerance to loud sounds. 3) Continuous or interrupted Tinnitus.4) Nausea and Vomitting present if giddiness is more.. 5) Perspiration, Gastric upset and diarrhoea due to vagal stimulation. 6) Fullness in the affected ear. 7) Head ache 8) Nystagmus. 9) Anxiety 10) First unilateral then becomes Bilateral,

## Diagnostic Criteria ;-

1) Sensori neural deafness.2) At first deafness present in lower frequencies, latter on at higher frequency. 3) Recruitment present . 4) Speech discrimination reduces. 5) Conal paresis present. 6) Spantaneous nystagmus 7) Directional preponderance present.

## Treatment ;-

1) Reassurance regarding the nature of the disease, 2) Labyrinthine sedatives like prochlorperazine or Dimenhydrinate. 3) Vaso dilators. 4) Vitamines. 5) Diuretics and Low salt diet,. 6) Tranquillizers and antidepressants. 7) Avoiding smoking, alcohol, septic focus.

## Surgery :-

1) Decompression or shunt operation of the endo lymphatic sac. 2) Partial destruction of Vestibule 3) Vestibular nerve section. 4) Labyrinthectomy.

**(Lermoyez Syndrome ;- Similar to meniere's syndrome but deafness dominates thevertigo).**

# OTO SCLEROSIS

Fixation of the stapes to the oval window due to development of new bone in the annular ligament of stapes. This gives rise to conductive deafness, aetiology is not clear.

**Symptoms ;-** 1) Deafness 2) Tinnitus 3) Giddiness
**Signs :-**

Flamingo tint - a pink patch may be present on the promontory and may be visible through the drum.

**Investigations -** Tuning fork test, Gelle test, Audiometry, impedance audiogram confirm the diagnosis

**Treatment :-** Stapedectomy operation.

# VERTIGO :

Vertigo or Giddiness is a disturbance of the sense equilibrium and movements. It is a sense of turning one's body (Subjective vertigo) or the environment (Objective vertigo). Severe vertigo may be accompanied by nausea, vomiting, nystagmus, perspiration, gastric upset and diarrhoea due to vagal stimulation.

The maintenance of equilibrium depends upon the co-ordination of informations from various parts of the vestibular apparatus, muscles, joints, tendons, cutaneous touch receptors and visual source. If there is interference with co-ordination of information in the brain stem and cerebellum, then vertigo is experienced.

## Causes ;-
### A) Lesions of Ear :-
Wax ,furuncle in the external ear due to vagus stimulation ,Eustachian catarrh due to transmission of negative pressure to inner ear, Labyrinthitis due to A.S.O.M. or, C.S.O.M. head injury with fracture of Temporal bone and Labyrinth, surgical trauma to vestibule, acoustic trauma, perilymph fistula due to rupture or viral infections, Vascular changes due to thrombosis or embolism disease, motion sickness and ototoxic drugs.

### b) Causes other than Ear :-
1) hypertension, hypotension, atherosclerosis, aortic stenosis ,mitral regurgitation, etc., cardiovascular lesions diminish blood supply to Labyrinth ,cerebellum and cerebrum and cause vertigo.

2) Neurological lesions like vertebro basilar artery syndrome, disseminated sclerosis, tumour or abscess of cerebellum and brain stem, epilepsy, increased intra -cranial tension, and head injuries causes vertigo.

3) Metabolic disorders like 8th nerve neuritis due to diabetes, Hypoglycemia etc reduces glucose supply to the vital parts leads to vertigo.

4) Anaemia - Reduced Oxygen supply to Labyrinth and brain stem causes vertigo.

5) Opthalmic lesions like diplopia refractive errors and glaucoma cause vertigo.

6) Cervical spondylosis causes vertigo.

### c) Non Patholgical vertigo
1)      Height- Due to unusual visual stimulation from heights causes vertigo.
2)      Spinning movements cause vertigo due to stimulation of semicircular canals.
3)      Sudden changes of Floor texture.

### d) Functional vertigo - The causes are still unknown
### E) Other causes :
| | | |
|---|---|---|
| V | = | Vascular causes |
| E | = | Epilepsy - Hypoglycemia and diabetes (endocrine lesion) |
| R | = | Remedies (Ototoxic drugs) |
| T | = | Trauma, Tumours, Hypothyroidism |
| I | = | Infection to Labyrinth |
| G | = | Glial disease (Multiple sclerosis) |
| O | = | Ocular diseases, other like menier's diseases. |

### Investigations ;-
1) History about above lesions. 2) Otoscopy and functional examination of ear. 3) Vascular Examination 4) Radiological Examination. 5) E.C.G. 6) C.T. Scan 7) Pathological investigations.

### Treatment ;-
1) Cause should be treated
2) Similar toTinnitus and meniere's syndrome.

# OTOTOXICITY

Ototoxicity is the damage caused by the toxic effects of certain drugs to the inner ear.

## Ototoxic Drugs :-
1) Aminoglycoside antibiotics
a) Cochleo toxic - Neomycin, Kanamycin, Framycetin tobramycin
b) Vestibulo toxic - Streptomycin, gentamycin.
2) Diuretics - Frusemide, elthacrymic acid
3) Salicylates
4) Cytotoxic agents - Nitrogen mustard cisplatinum.
5) Antiprotozoal - Quinine
6) Anti epileptic drugs - Phenytoin sodium
7) Anti heparinzing agents.
8) Beta blockers - Propranolol.

## Clinical Features :-
Tinnitus, deafness and vertigo.

**Treatment ;-** Withdrawl of the medicines.

# POSITIONAL VERTIGO

It is the momentary Vertigo which occurs only in certain positions of the head while changing the position.

Aetiology - Head injury, Labyrinthitis and idiopathic causes.

Pathology - there may be changes in maculae of the utricle or sacule on one side, the otolyth membrane may be damaged. or due to certain brain stem lesions like demyelination or malignant metastasis.

## Clinical Features :-
1) Momentary or positional giddiness .
2) No - nausea, Vomiting, deafness and tinnitus.

**Treatment -** Similar to meniere's disease.

## Vestibular neuronitis.

It is the acute inflammatory condition of the vestibular nerve due to viral infection.

**Clinical features :-** 1) Giddiness, nausea, vomiting present 2) No deafness, tinnitus and recurrence of the disease.

**Treatment :-** Similar to meniere's disease.

## Acoustic Neuroma.

It is the neurofibroma arising from the neurilemma sheath of the 8th cranial nerve in or near the internal auditory meatus.

## Clinical Features :-
1) Unilateral sensori neural deafness and tinnitus 2) Chronic unsteadiness. 3) Trigeminal symptoms 4) Facial paralysis 5) Late Symptoms like intra cranial tumour and headache. 6) Nausea and vomiting absent

# LABYRINTHITIS

Inflammation of inner ear is known as Labyrinthitis, the infection may affect the Labyrinth in 3 stages.

1) Circumscribed Labyrinthitis or fistula formation or perilabyrinthine inflammatory process, the infection doesnot reach upto membranous labyrinth.
2) Diffuse serous labyrinthitis with reversible clinical features. (Mild inflammatory change in perilymphatic space)
3) Diffuse purulent labyrinthitis. Massive purulent infection of perilymph and endo lymphatic space with permanent deafness and loss of vestibular function.
4) Dead Labyrinth

**Clinical Features :-**
1) Vertigo. 2) Deafness. 3) Nystagmus. 4) Nausea Vomitings. 5) Fistula test positive. 6) Tinnitus.

**Treatment :-** Labyrinthotomy for the drainage of pus from the labyrinth.

**Infective Labyrinthitis :-**
Infection spread from meningeal route Or haematogenous route.

**Viral Labyrinthitis**
Certain viral infections such as measles, mumps, influenza etc may cause destruction of organ of corti and vestibule.

**Tox ic Labyrinthitis.**
Layrinthitis occurs by intake of ototoxic drugs like streptomycetin, quinine, diuretics, Tobacco, alchohol etc.,

**Traumatic Labyrinthitis.**
Labyrinthitis due to fracture of skull or temporal bone or due to surgical trauma follows stapedectomy.

**Ottic Labyrinthitis**
Labyrinthitis due to middle ear infections.

# COMMON TREATMENT PRINCIPLES OF EAR DISEASES
# (KARNA ROGA)

1) Oral intake of cow ghee with luke warm milk, especially at night.
2) Regular usage of Rasayan Yogas like Chyavan prash, Triphala churna with Tila taila, ghritha Or madhu etc.,
3) Taking rest Or avoiding excessive exertion or strain (Avyaayama ).
4) Avoiding head bath
5) Brahmacharya
6) Avoiding loud or prolonged or irrelavant talking (Pralapa causes vata vitiation so only mita bhaashan is suggested)
7) Avoiding the aetiological factors of pratishyaya.
8) All the treatment principles of pratishyaya.
9) Vrana hara (ulcer healing therapy) treatment is suggested.
10) Advised to take mamsa rasa in the meals.

11) Advised to take Vata hara, kapha hara ghrithas at nights.

12) Vegetables like Varthaka, patola, shighru, Karavellaka and food grains like Goduma, shali, Yava, mugda etc are advised to use.

13) Systemic treatment principles (Deha shodhan), Abhyanga, sneha pana, shirovasti, Swedan(nadi Sweda and pinda Sweda), Vaman, virechan, Nasya, vasti, Dhooma and Raktamokshan. etc.

14) Karna shodhan (local treatment principles):- karna mala nirharana (Removing wax), Karna prakshalana (Ear wash), Karna dhoopana (Fumi gation), Avadhoolana (Dusting the medicated powders), Karna poorana (instillation of ear drops) and karna pramarjana (Dry mopping method).

15 Apathya (contra indications)
a) Head bath b) Excessive Exercise c) Loud and irrelevant talking (pralapa)
d) Swimming Or diving ) Scratching the skin of external auditory canal (karna Kandooyana). f) Oral intake of heavy bulk food items. g) usage of sticks for brushing the teeth h) Foods or habits which cause pratishyaya. i) Vata, Kapha dosha vitiating foods or habits. j) Head injury. k) improper instrumental manupulations. l) Rejecting the head masage. m) Drinking cold water or cool drinks. h) Hearing loud sounds.

1) **Karna shoola**
2) **Karna nada**
3) **Badirya**      These 4 diseases contain similar treatment principles.
4) **Karna Kshweda.**

## A) The Treatment Principles of Vataj Karna Shoola :-

1) Vata hara sneha (Oleus) drugs, for oral administration and for the external applications (Abhyanga- Shiro vasti etc.)

2) Nadi sweda Or pinda Sweda with Vata hara drugs.

3) Snehika Nasya, virechan, Vasti, Dhoomapana and Karna pooran.

4) According to necessity Dosha elimination process (shodhan karma) like Vaman Virechan Nasya Vasti and Rakta mokshan - has to be selected for the therapy.

5) According to necessity Local therapies like a) Karna pooran (Filling or dropping the medicine into external ear canal ). b) Karna dhoopan (fumi gation of external ear canal with medicated smoke).
c) karna prakshalan (Ear wash.) d) karna mala nirharan (removing wax etc waste material from the ear canal) e) karna pramarjan (Dry mopping with cotton tipped sticks or probes), etc has to select for the therapy.

6) Common treatment principles which are explained are also beneficial,

7) The following Oleus preparations are advised for oral administration .
a) cow ghee with Luke warm Milk, especially at night b) Shata Paka Bala taila c) Vata hara snehas like Rasnadighritha, Dashamool taila etc.,

8) Bala taila is advised for external applications, Oral administration, Nasya Shiro Vasti and for Karna pooran

**9) Nasya Yogas :-** Bala taila, Anu taila, Ksheera bala taila, Narayan taila etc.,
10) The common drugs used for NADI SWEDA are
Bilwa, Erenda, Arka, Punarnava, Kapittha, Dathura, Shighru, Agnimantha, Ashwagandha, Tarkeri, Vamshaankur, etc., should grind with Amla Varga drugs like Kaanji, decoction is prepared and is used for Nadi Sweda in Vataj and Kaphaj Karna shoola.

11) Pinda sweda is done with the hot bolus of Flesh, packed in cloth pieces (fish hen, Lavak etc., or with hot solid milk products,)

12) Karna dhoopan with the Kshauma Vastra, guggulu, Agaru and ghritha etc., drugs, The smoke is exposed to the affected site with Dhooma Yantra to dry the infection like fungus.

**13) Karna mala nirharan :-**
Wax, Fungus (Karna gootha), Disintegrated foreign bodies (krimi ) etc., should be cleaned with cotton tipped shalaka, ear probe, foreign body remover etc., instruments.

**14) Karna Prakshalan (ear wash):-**
To remove deeply seated foreign bodies, Or to flush out dried ear debris, ear syringing is done with Lukewarm water Or medicated decoctions like Triphala Kashaya etc., drugs.

**15) Karna Pramarjan (Dry mopping).**
The Oozing ear secretion or Wet ear canal is cleaned Or dried with cotton tipped stick or probe.

**16) Karna pooran Yogas :-**
a)The extracts of following wet medicines (Swarasa) should put in the ear,

Lashuna, Aardraka, Shigrubeeja, Moolaka, Kadaliphala, Kapittha, Mathulunga, Arkapatra, Suryamukhee, Tila parnee, shyonaka etc., drugs individually or in combination.

b) Puta paka Swarasa of
Ashwatha, Bilwa, Arka, Erenda, Moolaka, shyonaka etc., the drugs are used individually. by the application of lavan and taila the leaves are heated and the juice is extracted by special process and is used for karna pooran

c)    Oil prepared with above 2 groups of drugs, is used (either individually or in combination) for Karna pooran.

d)    The following Oil preparation are used for karna pooran.

Nirgundee taila, Kshara taila, Bilwa taila, Ksheera bala taila, Hingwadi taila, Apamarga Kshar taila, Katu taila, Kakajangha taila, Nagaradi taila, Dashamoola taila, Lashunadya taila, Tila taila, ghritha, Ashwatta patra Khalla taila, Karnabindu taila etc.,

e)    Milk or stanya (Breast Milk) or Kaanji are used for karna pooran

f)    Karna pooran with Lukewaram urine of the 8 types of Animals like 1) cow 2) Sheep 3) Goat 4) Buffallo 5) camel 6) Elephant 7) Horse 8) Donkey etc. (individually)

g)    Karna pooran with the oil prepared with Hingu. tumburu, shunthi and Sarshapa taila etc drugs.

h)    Karna pooran with the Oil prepared with Devadaru, shunthi, Vacha, shatahwa, Kusta, saindhava Lavan, sarshap, Aja mutra, taila etc drugs.

i)    Karna pooran with Oil prepared with Varata bhasma. agaru (scented items) Rasanjan, Shunthi, Tila taila etc drugs.

j)    Karna pooran with the Oil prepared with decoction of vatahara drugs, 8 types of animals urine, amala varga drugs, and chathur Sneha (Sarpi - Taila - Vasa- Majja).

k)    Karna pooran with the Oil prepared with Hingu, Shunthi, Saindhava Lavan, Sarshapa taila etc drugs.

l)    Karna pooran with the Oil prepared with Samudraphena, Vacha, Shunthi Saindhava lavan, Aardraka Swarasa and Tila taila .

m)    Karna pooran with the Ghee prepared with goat's urine, vamsha twak and cow's ghee.

n)    Karna pooran with goat's milk and saindhava Lavan (in Luke warm State).

o)    Karna pooran with the compound formed by Kantakari moola 1 phala, Goat's milk 8 phala, Kukkuta Vasa and heated again this can be used for Karna pooran.

g)    Karna pooran with Deepika taila.

Bruhat pancha moola or Devadaru or Kusta Or sarala etc, drugs 18" Length root is taken and covered with Kshauma Vastra (Malmal Cloth ) is dipped in medicated Oil and the Lower end of the root is burnt and the drops which are dribling from the flame should be collected for karna pooran.

17)    Vataja pratishyaya Chikitsa - should be given.
18)    Vata Vyadhi Chikitsa should be given.
19)    Nidana parivarjana (Avoiding the causative factors or predisposing factor).

20)     Giving, shoola hara shotha hara yogas like Triphala guggulu Kanchanara guggulu, Ekangaveer ras, saribadi vati, Induvati, Lakshmivilas ras, Lagusutha sekara ras, Khadhiradi Vati, etc drugs are beneficial

## B) Treatment principles of Pittaja Karna Shoola.

1)     Most of the drugs of Vataja karna shoola are effective for this disease also in addition to these the following principles are also helpful.
2)     Pittaja pratishyaya Chikitsa,
3)     Vata Vyadhi chikitsa,
4)     Abhyanga Nasya and shiro Vasti are advised with sheeta Veerya snehas.
5)     Sneha virechana, Or mrudu Virechana, shaman Nasya, Virechanika dhooma, shaman gandoosha etc., are useful.
6)     The Oil prepared with the decoction of Yastimadu and Milk (1and 2 prasta), Tila Taila 1 Kudava, and semi solid paste (kalka) of Yastimadu, Guduchi, chandana, usheera, kakoli, Lodra, jeevak, Manjista, Sariva, kamal nala etc., This Oil is beneficial for abhyanga, Nasya and Karna pooran.
7)     Lepa or external application of the paste of above drugs with ghee is ef fective.

**8) Nasya Yogas :**
a) Vidari gandhadi ghritha. b) Kakolyadi ghritha. c)  Panchavalkala ghritha (leaves of ficus group), d) Chandanadi ghritha. e) Yastimadu ghritha, f) Ksheera Bala taila, g) Shata paka Bala taila, h) Anu taila, i) Ksheeri sarpi.

**9) Karna Pooran Yogas :-**
Karna pooran is done with any of these
          a) Stanya (Breast milk) b) Ghritha (Old ghee) c) Ksheeri sarpi.d) Ashwatha patra Khallasta tail Or ghritha. e) Kanji. f)  Deepika taila. g) Ghee prepared with Yastimadu chandan Trivruth Sugar and Chatur snehas. h) Yastika ghritha i) Chandanadi ghrita,  j) Maha Tiktha ghritha. k) Ksheeri Vruksha pallava ghritha l) Kakolyadi Ksheera (According to ksheera Paka) m) Kakolyadi ghritha. n) Vidarigandhadi ghritha. o) the decoction of Draksha Yastimadu and stanya p) Asta mutra with saindhava lavan or samudra Phena churna. q) Aja ksheera + Saindhava Lavan or samudra phena churna. r) with leaves extract (Swarasa) like Arka, Tulasi, Vasa, Lashuna, Aardraka.

## C) Treatment Principles of Kaphaja Karna Shoola.

          Most of the above yogas are useful, in addition the following principles are also helpful.
1) Abhyanga with ushna veerya sneha like pippalyadi ghritha. 2) Rooksha sweda. 3) Vaman. 4) virechana 5) Rechan Nasya. 6) Teekshna dhooma pana & Gandoosha. 7) Kaphahara lepa, Shiro Vasti and Karna pooran.

## 8) Karna Pooran Yogas :-

a) Ingudi and sarshapa taila,

b) Lukewarm sarshapa taila. c) Surasadi taila. d) Bruhath panchamoola taila.
e) The extracts (Swarasa) of Aardraka, Kapitha, matulunga, shyonaka, Tulasi moolaka, Kadali kanda, shirgru, (either individually Or in combination. f) Oil prepared with above drugs.g) Arka patra puta paka swarasa h) Kanji and samudra phena or saindhava lavan. i) Sarshapadi Taila - prepared with vamsha twak, Aja or avi mootra (Goat or sheep Urine), Tila taila, hing, shunthi, Sarshapa taila.

## D) Treatment principle of Raktaja Karna shoola

1) Like pittaj karnashoola 2) in addition sira mokshana is suggested by Vagbhata.

## E) Treatment Principles of sannipataj Karna Shoola

1) Tridosha hara Chikitsa
2) All the above principles are beneficial.

## SPECIAL TREATMENT PRINCIPLES OF KARNA NADA AND KARNA KSHWEDA.

1) Karna shoola treatment, 2) Pratishyaya treatment. 3) If kapha dosha is associated, first Vamana Karma is advised. 4) Vata dosha Chikitsa should be done, 4) karna pooran with a) katu taila or sarshapa taila b) Vachadi taila (the Oil prepared with vacha Hingu jatamamsi Lavanga twak Sarjakshara, Pippali tila taila), c) Karna nada hara taila (prepared with Erenda varuna shigru moolaka etc drugs leaves extracts 4 parts, cow milk 8 parts, tila taila 1 part, other drugs are Yastimadu Kakoli Ksheera kakoli etc. drugs.) d) Shambhooka taila e) Lashunadya taila f) Nagaradi taila, g) Apamarga Kshar taila. h) Bilwa taila etc are useful.
5) Oral administration of drugs like.
a) Sarivadi Vati.b) Rasnadi guggulu. c) kanchanara guggulu. d) Triphala guggulu .e) Ekangaveer ras f) Vatavidwamsini vati h) Induvati with Amalaki Swarara i) Chopacheenyadi Choorna j) Krauncha beeja choorna k) Ashwagandha rista or l) Balarista m) Drakshasav n) maha Rasnadi quath o) Shankha Pushpi syrup p) Saraswatarista q) Brahmi Vati. r) Lakshmivilasras with Gold. s) Susthasekara ras, etc are benificial.

## SPECIAL TREATMENT PRINCIPLES FOR KARNA BADIRYA.

1) Like, Vataj Karna shoola, Vataj pratishyaya and Vata Vyadhi treatment.
2) Vaman etc shodhan Karmas to eliminate Kapha etc doshas, to purify the body.

## 3) Karna Pooran Yogas.:-

a) Lashunadya taila (Lashuna Amalaki Haritala each 25 gram, Tila taila 250grams, Milk 1 litre, 4 times water, Oil should be prepared according to taila paka vidhi)
b) Nagaradi taila :- Should prepare with shunthi saindhavalavan pippali musta Hingu Vacha Lashun each 1 Tola,Arka patra swarasa 1kg, phalasha patra swarasa 1kg, Tila taila 250 grams.

c) Dashamoola taila (oil prepared with Dashamoola - Tila taila )
d) Kakajangha taila (oil prepared with Kakajangha - Tila taila )
e) Apamarga Kshara taila (oil prepared with Aparnarga Kshara Tila taila ).
f) Bilwa taila :- Bilwa majja 250 grams should be grinded in 1kg gomutra, add 1kg cowmilk and 1kg tila tail - Oil should prepare.
g) Shambhooka taila
4) Raktha mokshan is suggested by vagbhata.
5) oral administration of Indu Vati with Amalaki Swaras.
6) Rasayan, Brumhan, Nadibalya Aushadas should be given.
7) Deafness if occurs to children (due to congenital Or hereditory causes) Aged or old or existing since long time is said to be Asadya.

## 5) KARNA SRAVA OR KARNA SAMSRAVA
(Chronic suppurative Otitis media (C.S.O.M.) Otitis externa-Otorrhoea).

Vitiated Vata dosha causes pus discharge from the ear due to head injuries (Shirobhighatha), diving in water (Jala nimajjana), inflammation of aural mucosa (karna Paka), and ear abscesses (karna Vidradi) etc causes, is named as karna srava or Karna Samsrava.

### 1) Head injuries (Shirobhighata)
Traumatic lesion of external ear (otitis externa) and middle ear (Otitis media) causes foul pus discharge from ear due to suppurative inflammatory processes of Aural mucosa.

### 2) Diving in water (jalanimajjana)
It causes forcible entry of polluted water into the ear canal, that may cause tympanic rupture along with Aural inflammation (Otitis externa- otitis media - myringitis and tympanic perforation or rupture).

### 3) ULCERATION OR INFLAMMATION OF AURAL MUCOSA (KARNA PAKA)
It is the main factor for the suppurative inflammation of external or middle ear in which infection spreads to the ear through external auditory canal, eustachian tube, blood stream or due to traumatic lesions.

### 4) Ear Abscesses (karna Vidradi)
Suppuration of abscess of external ear Or middle ear may causes pus discharge from ear.

**Note :-** By above discription it is clear that, Karna srava is one of the clinical features of the suppurative lesions of the external and middle ear like,
Otitis externa (furunculosis - diffuse otitis externa) suppurative otitis media, etc.,

## 6) POOTHI KARNA
### (Supurative Otitis media - Otitis externa Foul Otorrhoea.)

The painful or painless foul discharge from the ear is known as poothi karna.

**According to Sushrutha ;-**

The kapha of Karna Srotas (The mucosal lining of the ear) is melted by pittoshma (Acute inflammatory process)and causes foul sticky ear discharge with or without pain, is known as poothi karna.

The painful condition with profuse sticky foul discharge from the ear is the significance of acute inflammatory process. The painless scanty foul discharge from the ear is due to the chronic inflammatory process of ear, either middle or external ear, So poothi karna is a clinical feature observed in suppurative lesions of middle ear (Suppurative otitis media )and external ear (Otitis externa).

## 7) KRIMI KARNA
### (Maggots in the ear)

It is a curable disease of the ear occurs by the vitiation of Tridoshas in which a single or multiple small insects are Visualised with severe otalgia (ear pain).

(1)The maggots (flies, mosquitoes ants etc., may enter into the ear canal from outside, erode the tissue of the ear canal and so causes severe earache with ulcerative lesions.

(2) Unhygienic conditions, impaction of ear wax, ulcerative lesions suppurative conditions etc., may vitiate vatadi doshas that deranges the Twak, Rakta, Mamsa of the ear canal and small infective organisms are produced from the excreta (dead tissue wax exudations pus etc) these also cause destructive process and associate with severe earache.

(1)Vitiated Kapha causes - Collection of debris or exudates causes itching, foul smell and animate Foreign body sensation.

(2)Vitiated pitta causes tissue degeneration (Dhathu Paka ) Putrifaction and tissue necrosis.

(3) Vitiated Vata Causes severe earache.

## Treatment principles of Karna Srava - Poothi Karna and Krimi Karna.

1)   Karna Srava - Poothi Karna and Krimi Karna are having Similar treatment principles.

2)   Common treatment principles of Karna roga are also applicable here.

(3) The common treatment procedures for these 3 diseases are
- a) Shiro Virechana
- b) Dhooma Pana
- c) Swedana
- d) Gandoosha
- e) Dusta Vrana Chikitsa
- f) Karna prakshalan
- g) Karna Pramarjan
- h) Karna dhoopan
- i) Karna Pooran
- j) Karna Avachoorana

## SPECIAL REMEDIES FOR THE TREATMENT OF KARNA SRAVA OR KARNA SAMSRAVA

(1) The ear discharge (mucoid, mucopurulent, purulent Blood stained discharges ) should be cleaned by ear wash (karna Prakshalana Or Karna dhavan) with the following decoctions.

(a) Triphala Kashaya b) Yastimadu Kashaya c) Shunthi Kashaya,(b) Nimbadi Kashaya (e) Pancha Valkala Kashaya (f) Dashamoola Kashaya (g) Trikatu Kashaya(h) Aaragwadadi Kashaya i) Raja Vrukshadi Kashaya j) Surasadi Kashaya k) Manjista, Khadira Sariva, Patola, Guduchi, Rasna, shigru, etc decoctions.

The decoctions are taken in the ear syringe for ear wash, while syringing the nozzle of the syringe should face the walls of the ear canal and piston should be pressed with gentle pressure.

2) After Karna prakshaalan the ear canal should be cleaned with cotton buds known as karna pramarjana (Dry mopping)

3) The Residual exudations should be dried by inserting medicated smoke or fumes is known as Karna dhoopan, it is done with Vrana dhoopan Yantra. The common remedies which are used for dhoopan are guggulu, Agaru, kshauma Vastra, rasanjan, Hingu, Varthaka Phala, Vidanga etc. drugs.

4) Karna pooran - Putting the ear drops or Dusting the medicated fine powder into the external auditory canal is known as Karna pooran.

### Some Remedies of Karna Pooran :-

a) With Triphala Kashaya or Aaragwadadi Kashaya etc., decoctions which are used for ear wash.b) Tindukadi pancha Kashaya (Tinduka Abhaya Aamalaki Lodhra Manjista).c) Sarja Twak + Vana Karpasa phala swarasa + honey d) Tindukadi Pancha Kashaya + Kapittha Swarasa + Honey. e) Sarja kshara + Lemon Juice. f) Pancha Valkala Kashaya + Kapittha swarasa + Honey. g) Dusting the fine medicated powders into the ear canal (Karna avachoornan with the following medicines.

A) Samudra phena Churna    E) Rasanjan
B) Sphatic bhasma          F) Sarjarasa
C) Tankan bhasma         G) haridra Churna
D) Laksha Choorna

**H) Quatha Churnas** of pancha Kashaya, panchavalkala kasahya,Triphala Kashaya, Nimbadi Kashaya, Aragwadadi Kasaya, Surasadi Kashaya, Raja Vrukshadi Kashaya etc.,

h)       Karna pooran with the Oils prepared with above decoctions.

i)        Karna pooran with the oil prepared from Amrapallava, Kapittha pallava, Madhuka, dhava, shalatwak and taila.)

j)       Karna Pooran with Priyangwadi taila (Priyangu, Yastimadu, Patha, Dhataki, uthphala, Shalaparni, Manjista, Lodra, Laksha, Kapittha and taila.

k)       Karna Pooran with the oil prepared from Doorva, snuhi, Jambu, Amra patra, Karkatak Shrungi, Manduka Parni, Honey and Taila.

l)       Rechana Nasya (Apamarga beeja churna Or Katphala Churna) Dhoomapan, Swedan, Gandoosha etc,has to do according to the condition of the patient.

## SPECIAL REMEDIES FOR TREATMENT OF POOTHI KARNA.

1) The common treatment principles and remedies are merely like Karna srava.

2) The order of treatment procedures are like the following

      a) Karna Prakshalan        -        Ear wash

      b)      " Pramarjan         -        Dry mopping

      c)      " Dhoopan          -        Fumigation

      d)      " Pooran            -        Filling the medicated drops.

3) Some remedies of Karna pooran -

     **a)** Most of the preparations are as like Karna Srava. **b)** Stanya + ghritha + madhu + Rasanjan. **c)** Jambu, Amra, Kapittha, Karpasaphala swarasa + madhu. **d)** Oil prepared with above drugs + Sarshapa, Nimba, Karanja + Taila. **e)** Oil prepared with Amra, Jambu, Yastimadu, Vata patra, Jathi patra + Taila. **f)** Oil prepared with Nirgundi patra, Saindhava Lavan, Gruha dhooma, guda, madhu and Taila. **g)** Kustadi taila prepared with, Tila Taila 1kg, Ajamutra 4 Kg, Kalka dravyas - Kusta, Hingu, Vacha, Devadaru, Shunthi, Saindhava Lavan - Total 250 grams. **h)** Jathi patra Swarasa + Honey. **i)** Gomutra + 125mg. Haritala. **j)** Nishataila - Prepared with 8 phala sarshapa taila, Haridra and Gandhak each 1 phala, Dathura swarasa 10 phala. **k)** Nasya Gandoosha, Dhoomapana, swedan etc., according to the condition.

**Special Remedies For Tretment of Krimi Karna :-**

1) Treatment principles and most of the remedies are as like Karna srava and poothi Karna.
2) Dusta Vrana and Krimi hara treatment should give.
3) The order of treatment procedures is

   1) Karna prakshalan        -      Ear wash
   2)     " Pramarjana       -      Dry mopping
   3)     " Dhoopan        -      Fumigation.
      (with guggulu, Agaru Hingu, Vidanga Rasanjan, Kshauma Vastra, Varthaka phala etc.)
   4) Karna Pooran

4) Additional Karna pooran preparations for the treatment of Krimi Karna are:
a) Sarshapa Taila. b) Gomutra + 125 mg Manahshila. c) Gomutra + Vidanga Churna. d) Oil prepared with Nimba Kashaya 12 grams, haridra Churna 1gram, Sarshapa taila. e) The extracts of Langali moola, Phalasha moola, Trikatu, Suryamukhee, Sindhuvar, etc drugs.

5) The visible alive or dead insects should be removed by special skillfull techniques.

## CONGENITAL ABNORMALITIES OF EAR :-

### A) External Ear Defects :-

1) Pre auricular sinus - it is due to improper fusion of the auricular tubercles during the developmental stage. The exact site of the sinus is near the tragus and root of helix.
2) Small elevations of Skin with cartilage at tragus and helix.(accessary auricles)
3) Anotia :- Absence of Pinna
4) Microtia :- Small deformed Pinna
5) Macrotia :- Abnormally big sized pinna
6) Coll aural fistulae :- A fistula in between external auditory canal and angle of jaw at theanterior border of sterno mastoid.
7) Dermoid Cysts :- Develop on the Pinna.
8) Darwin's tubercle :- A small elevation on the postero superior part of helix.
9) Wilder muth's Ear :- Anti helix is more prominent than helix, lobule may be absent or adherent to the side of the ear.
10) Bat ear :- Abormal outward protrusion of pinna with absence of anti helix.
11) Atresia of external auditory canal.
12) Changes in the curvature of the external auditory canal.
13 Treacher collin's syndrome - hypo plasia of external ear, middle ear, eyes, malar bones, maxillae and mandible.

### Treatment :-

1) Plastic surgery in minor defects.
2) Prosthesis in major deformities.
3) Excision of Sinuses and cysts.

## B) Middle ear defects (Congenital)

1) Ossicular deformities

     a) Fusion of malleus with incus Or malleos adherent to the walls of epitympanum.
b) Fusion of incus with malleus or stapes. c) Fusion of Foot plate of stapes to oval window etc.,

2)     Abnormal coarse of Facial nerve in its bony canal.

3)     Treacher collins syndrome.

### Treatment :-

     Surgical exploration to reconstruct the parts for the maintenance of normal hearing mechanism.

### C) Internal Ear :-

     1) Abnormalities of Bony or membranous Labyrinth.

     2) Deaf mutism.

     3) Sensori neural deafness (cochlear and auditory nerve lesions).

     4) Labyrinthine lesions with the symptoms like vertigo Tinnitus develops.

# DISEASES OF EXTERNAL EAR

## 1) Haematoma of Pinna :-

     Collection of blood on the outer suface of the pinna under the perichondrium

### Treatment :-

1) Aspiration and pressure bandage. 2) Antibiotics. 3) Analgesics and Anti inflammatory drugs.

## 2) PERICHONDRITIS OF AURICLE :-

     Perichondritis is the inflammation of cartilage of Pinna. It may follow haematoma injury to pinna as a complication of furnculosis and mastoid surgery.

     The causative organisms are staphylo cocal aureus, Bacillus pyocyaneus. It is a very painful condition with acute inflammatory features and leads to necrosis and deformity of pinna.

### Treatment :-

     1) Antibiotics. 2) Incision and drainage of pus. 3) Pressure bandage. 4) Plastic surgery for the correction of the deformity.

## 3)     Frost Bite of the Pinna :-

     It is the lesion of pinna for being exposed to temperature variations like cold affect and produces pain, burningsensation, oedema, blebs and necrotic changes.

### Treatment :-

1) Slow thawing.2) Vaso dilator drugs. 3) Treatment like gangrene. 4) Burns of Pinna - should treat by surgical methods.

## 4) Burns of Pinna :- Should be treated as per surgical methods.

5) **Pseudo cysts of Pinna :-**
Should treat by 1) Aspiration 2) Incision and drainage 3) Pressure bandage 4) Wound therapy.

6) **Otitis Externa :-**
It is the inflammation of mocosa of the external ear It may be Acute or chronic, Localised Or diffuse, infective or reactive.

## CLINICAL TYPES OF OTITIS EXTERNA
### A) Due to Infection.
a) Bacteria 1) Localised otitis extena Or furunculosis. 2) Generalised " or Diffuse otitis externa 3) Erysepelas.

b) fungal      1) Otomycosis

c) Viral      1) Herpes Simplex 2) Herpes Zoster
           3) Bullous Myringitis.

B) Reactive       1) Eczematous Otitis externa
                   2) Seborrhoeic Otitis externa
                   3) Myringitis
                   4) Malignant Otitis extena
                   5) Keratosis Obturans etc.

1) **Localised Otitis Externa Or Aural Furunculosis.**
It is a staphylococcal infection of root of hair follicle and sebaceous gland in the cartilagenous portion of external auditory canal.

The infection usually follows
1) Injury to canal while cleaning. 2) Affection of ear discharge coming from middle ear. 3) Diabetes.

**Clinical Features :-**
1) Severe pain in the ear that aggravates by the movement of pinna, chewing, yawning and opening the mouth. 2) Swelling and redness of meatus wall. 3) Otorrhoea - When the furuncle ruptures. Blood stained purulent discharge comes. 4) Deafness due to occlusion of meatus with furuncle. 5) Tinnitus at night. 6) Severe itching sensation. 7) Trismus. 8) On examination meatus appears congested, oedematous, stenosed and with pus collection. 9) Infection by spreading backwards causes cellulitis in the post aural region, by obliterating post aural groove and the auricle stands out forwards and outwards. 10) The infection may cause perichondritis and post aural Lymphadenitis etc. 11) The infection spreads forwards into parotid region through the fissures of santorini and inwards into tympanic cavity through the notch of Rivinus.

**Treatment :-**
1) Packing of the canal with gauze soaked in 10% Ichthyol in glycerine, glycerine reduces oedema and pain where as Ichthyol is an antiseptic. 2) Antibiotic drops. 3) Antibiotic drops with steroids. 4) Ear toilet by cleaning the secretions. 5) Incision and drainage of Furuncle may be performed for prompt relief from pain. 6) Systemic Antibiotics, analgesics and anti inflammatory drugs. 7) Diabetes if present should be treated.

## 2) Generalised Or Diffuse Otitis Externa.

Generalised infection involving the entire skin of external auditory canal including the surface of tympanic membrane.

The predisposing factors are scratching of the ear canal, water entry into ear canal, unskilled instrumentation and affection of the discharges of Acute or chronic suppurative otitis media. The commonest affecting organisoms are staphylococcus aureus PS. pyocyanea, B. Proteus, E.Coli. etc.,

**The Common clinical features are :-**
1) Irritation discomfort and pain in the ear. 2) Inflammatory changes in External auditory canal. 3) Crusting, desquamation and discharge with stenosis of external auditory canal.

**Treatment :-**
1) Avoidance of predisposing factors. 2) cleaning the ear canal by putting Astringent drops, lubricants, Hydrocortisones and with antibiotics etc drug applications. 3) Systemic antibiotics, Analgesics and anti inflammatory drugs.

## 3) Erysepelas.

It is an acute streptococcal Lymphangitis and dermatitis of ear canal, spreads rapidly which often follows a scratch.

**Treatment :-** Systemic antibiotics, Anti inflammatory drugs.
1) 10% Ichthyol in glycerine application. 2) Ultra Voilet light exposure.

## 4) Oto Mycosis.

It is one of the varieties of Otitis externa which is caused by the fungus. It is common in the damp and rainy seasons, it is very painful infection, fungus causing the infection.

**Clinical Features :-**
1) Severe pain with itching 2) Scanty Brownish Or blackish discharge. 3) Deafness Tinnitus and Trismus may also present. 4) On Examination cotton like growth or wet news paper like mass (Brownish Black ) present with inflammatory changes. 5) Other symptom of otitis externa also present.

**Treatment :-**
1) Cleaning the ear frequently. 2) Instillation of drops of Broad spectrum fungicides. (clotrimazole, tolnaftate, Nystatin etc. 3) Symtomatic treatment.

## 5) Herpes Viral Infection :-
1) Vesicles formation in the external auditory canal. 2) It is a neurotrophic virus causes paralysis of facial nerve (Ramsay hunt syndrome - Deafness vertigo and facial nerve palsy).

## 6) Bullous Myringitis :-

Haemorrhagic vesicles on the external surface of the ear drum. There is severe pain conductive deafness and blood stained otorrhoea.

**Treatment :-**
1) Local and systemic antibiotics. 2) Analgesics and anti inflammatory drugs. 3) Aural toilet. 4) Anti histemine drops.

**7) Eczematous Otitis Externa :-**
This is allergic dematitis of the external auditory canal (allergen may be extrinsic or intrinsic)

**Clinical Features :-**
1) Irritation, redness, oedema follwed by vesication, weeping and curst formation. 2) In chronic stage or with secondary infection fissuring and scaling of external ear canal is observed with fibrosis and stenosis.

**Treatment :-**
1) Steroid or Antibiotic Ointment applications. 2) Systemic antibiotics. 3) Anti histamines. 4) plastic surgery for fibrosed or stenosed external auditory canal.

**8) SEBORRHOEIC OTITIS EXTERNA**

It is similar to seborrhoeic dermatitis of scalp. Characterised by a greasy scaly and crusty skin of the external wall with itching sensation.

**Treatment :-** 1) Steroid or Antibiotic Ointment applications.
2) Aural Toilet 3) Shampooing of Scalp every alternate day.
4) Systemic antibiotics and anti inflammatory drugs.
5) Anti histamine drugs etc.,

# 9) Myringitis :-
Inflammation of external surface of ear drum.

**Clinical Features :-**
Severe pain, deafness, tinnitus and discomfort in the ear canal.

**10) Malignant Otitis Externa :-**
It is a progressive necrotising infection of ear canal and involves the tissues of the base of skull and temporal bone along with cranial nerves. The causative organism is pseudomonas and commonly occurs to the chronic diabetic.

**Clinical Features :-**
1) Rapidly spreading granulations in thejunction of Bony and cartilaginous meatus. 2) Infection spreads to parotid, Base of skull and to cranial nerves (7,9,10.12, ).

**Treatment ;-**
1) Diabetes should be controlled. 2) Local and systemic antibiotics. 3) Surgery to drain the abscess or to remove necrotic tissue.

## II) Keratosis Obturans :-

It is due to abnormal desquamation of the epithelium in the deep external auditory canal, forms similar lesion like cholesteatoma and causes bony erosion with destruction of surrounding tissues.

**Treatment :-** Surgery.

## 12) WAX :-

Wax is a mixture of secretions of the ceruminous glands, sebaceous glands, shedded epithelium and dust particles, etc.

If the wax is impacted in the external auditory canal causes pain, discomfort, conductive deafness, tinnitus, vertigo etc.,

**Treatment :-**
1) Wax removal by the instillation of Lubricant drops etc.,

**Note :-** (detailed explanation given at <u>Karna gootha</u> disease description).

## 13) Foreign Bodies of External Ear.

Various types of Foreign bodies are found in the ear.

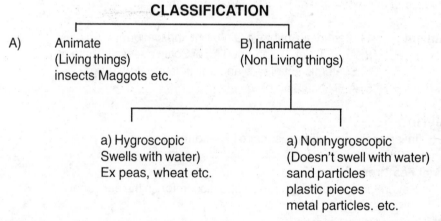

Treatment :-

**1) Animate Foreign bodies :-** Instilling of oil or water into the ear to suffocate the insect then by syringing or Forceps or with foreign body removing hook ,probe etc. Foreign body should be removed.

**2) Hygroscopic Foreign bodies :-**

These swell with water so syrining causes impaction of foreign body by increased size instilling glycerin or alcohol is advisable to shrink and lubricate the foreign body then with the help of Forcep Foreign body should be removed.

**3) Non hygroscopic Foreign bodies** can be removed by ear syrining with water etc.,

**4) In Non co-operative patients** like children general anaesthesia should be given to remove Foreign bodies.

### 14) Tympanic Membrane Rupture or Perforations :-

Rupture follows trauma and the perforation follows pathological lesions

### Aetiology of tympanic rupture :-

1) Picking the ear with matchsticks pencil etc. 2) Improper instrumentation while removing foreign bodies 3) Improper syringing of ear 4) Air compression due to sudden atmospheric changes 5) inflammation of Eustachian tube 6) head injury especially to petrous part of temporal bone.

In traumatic ruture of tympanic membrane the lesion is irregular and not easy for repair.

The tympanic perforation is commonly due to middle ear pathology, these are

1) Central perforation (heals quickly)
2) Marginal perforation (Difficult for healing)
3) Attic perforation (Complicative)

### Clinical Features ;-

Deafness, Tinnitus, earache, vertigo, otorrhoea, inflammatory changes and with tympanic perforation.

### Treatment :-

1) Swimming, head bath, syringing of the ear, mopping of the external auditory canal etc should be avoided.
2) Aural toilet
3) Systemic Broad spectrum antibiotics like pencillin.
4) Treatment for associated symptoms.
5) If treatment doesn't respond.
   Myringo plasty operation is the only alternative.

## DISEASES OF MIDDLE EAR CAVITY ;-

### Otitis media :-

It is an inflammatory condition of mucosa of middle ear cavity

## CLASSIFICATION

1) Suppurative otitis media     a) Acute
   b) Chronic
2) non Suppurative otitis media     a) Acute
   b) Chronic
3) Specific otitis media - Ex. TUberculous, syphilitic.
4) Adhesive otitis media

## 1) ACUTE SUPPURATIVE OTITIS MEDIA
## (A.S.O.M.)

It is an acute inflammatory condition of middle ear mucosa. The common organisms responsible for this disease are streptococus haemolyticus, staphylococcus aureus, pneumococcus, haemophilus influenzae, Bacillus pyocyneus, Bacillus coli, Bacilllus proteus etc.

**Aetiology :-** 1) it is common in children than adults

**Eustachian tube :-** It is shorter wider and horizontally placed in children, So only most of naso pharyngeal infections easily spread into middle ear and cause the disease. (in majority of cases infection spreads through Eustachian tube).

2)      Infection also spreads in to middle ear through the external ear canal by the rupture of tympanic membrane (improper instrumentation while cleaning, imporper ear syringing, scratching of ear with matchsticks, Forcible entry of water while diving into water etc.)

3)      Head injury may affect the middle ear by the fracture of temporal bone

4)      Blood borne infection rarely reaches the middle cear.

5)      Predisposing factors are

     **a)** Reduced vitality (Resistance power) **b)** Atmospheric pressure changes during Flying, diving etc. **c)** Infections like chronic rhinitis chronic sinusitis, tonsilitis, adenoids exanthematous Fevers like measles scarlet fever chronic or reccurent pharyngitis, etc. **d)** nasopharyngeal polyps, tumours, packing etc. **e)** Eustachian tube block.

**Pathology :-**

     The infection passes through 5 stages

1) Catarrhal state or stage of congestion, occlusion of eustachian tube and congestion in the middle ear

**2) Stage of exudation :-** Exudates collects in the middle ear which is serous at first and later becomes purulent.

**3) Stage of Suppuration :-**

     The collected pus in the middle ear stretches the drum and perforates by presure necrosis and the exudates starts escaping into external auditory canal.

**4) Stage of healing ;-** Depending upon the virulence of the organism, resistance power of the patient and drugs administration the infection clears up completely without complications.

**5) stage of complications ;-**

     If resistance power of patient is less, infecting organism is more virulent and proper antibiotics are not given, the infection progresses and cause complication, like mastoiditis

**Clinical Features :-**

**1) Catarrhal stage :-** Heavyness and pain in the ear, deafness, tinnitus, autophony, fever body pains.

Retraction and congestion of ear drum with loss of light reflex is seen on examination.

**2) Exudative stage ;-** Above symptoms aggravate, and bulging of tympanic membrane by the pressure of exudates of tympanum.

**3) Stage of suppuration :-**

a) At this stage drum perforates and pus starts flowing out b) Pain and other constitutional symptoms reduce after escape of ear discharge c) The type of discharge can range from mucoid to frankly pus

**4) Stage of healing ;-** it may begin from any stage depending upon the virulence of organism, resistance power of patient and administration of antibiotics.

**5) Stage of Complicatins:-**
Infection spreads to mastoid and neighbouring structures.

**Treatment :-**
1)      Systemic antibiotics like erythromycin, ampicillin, pencillin, etc. for 7 days.
2)      Systemic and Local (nasal) decongestants to decongest the mastoid tympanum nasal cavity and eustachian tube
3)      Analgesics and anti inflammatory drugs.
4)      Instillation of antibiotic ear drops.
5)      Aural toilet, ear discharge may be mopped with cotton buds.

# 6) Myringotomy :-
Giving incision to drain the pus from middle ear cavity, in exudative stage under general anaesthesia to avoid irregular tympanic rupture and to promote easy healing.

## MYRINGOTOMY

It is a surgical procedure in which ear drum is incised to drain the exudates of middle ear cavity, in the stage of exudation of Acute suppurative otitis media to prevent tympanic rupture and to relieve from severe earache.
1) Atropinisation to prevent vaso vagal attach. 2) General anaesthesia is given. 3) Patient lies in supine position with the head turned to the opposite side of the affected ear. 4) Under good illumination, with operative microscope with aseptic precautions, with myringo tome, a J shaped incision is given in the postero inferior quadrant mid way between umbo and annulus. 5) The fluid in the middle ear escapes out side or should be aspirated. 6) A strip of gauze is inserted in the ear. 7) Local and systemic antibotics should be given. 8) Analgesics and anti inflammatory drugs. should also be given for proper healing.

**Myringo puncture :-**
It is puncturing of the ear drum with a long thick injection needle to aspirate the middle ear exudates.

**Myringo Plasty**
Myringo plasty is the repair of the perforation of tympanic membrane usually done by temporal fascia or vein graft.

**Tympano Plasty :-**
it is a surgical process in which the reconstruction of the ear drum and the ossicular chain is performed.

**Indications :-**
1) Dry tympanic perforation 2) Benign Perforation 3) Eustachian tube should be functioning. 4) Stapes should be mobile. 5) After getting stamina against upper respiratory infections.

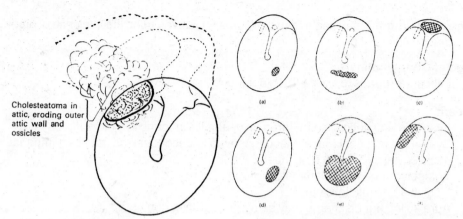

Cholesteatoma in attic, eroding outer attic wall and ossicles

(a)    (b)    (c)

(d)    (e)    (f)

. 16  Small peripheral attic perforation of serious otitis media.

*Different types of perforations of the right tympanic membrane: (a) Acute Otitis media with a small perforation: (b)Traumatic perforation; (c) Attic perforation; (d) and (e) Central perforation; (f) Marginal posterosuperior quadrant perforation.*

ACUTE DISEASES OF THE MIDDLE EAR CLEFT

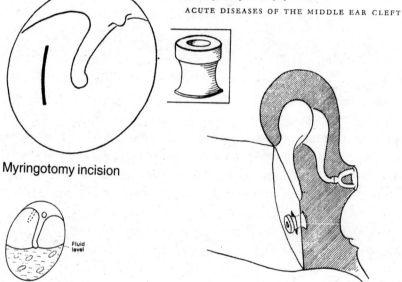

Myringotomy incision

Fluid level

Fluid seen behind the ear drum

Secretory Otitis Media. Grommet inserted in a myringotomy incision. Inset- "Teflon" Grommet.

**Contra Indications :-**

1) Dangerous perforation. 2) Wet perforation with active discharge. 3) with pharyngeal - upper respiratory infections. 4) Eustachian tube dysfunction. 5) Otosclerosis. 6) Bleeding disorders. 7) with diabetes and hyper tension. 8) Sensori neural deafness.

**Method :-**

1) Under general anaesthesia Temporalis facia should be collected in 1.5 c.m. diameter for grafting.

2) Of the three layers of ear drum the outer layer is reflected laterally from the middle fibrous layer along with some portion of the skin of external auditory meatus.

**3) Ossiculoplasty ;-** the ossicular chain is inspected by lifting the layers of ear drum from its attachment at the annulus and corrected by transposition or ossicular grafting.

4) The tympanic perforation is repaired by laying temporalis fascia on the fibrous middle layer of the drum, the ear canal skin and outer layer of the drum are replaced back on the temporalis tascia (onlay technique).

(In inlay technique temporalis fascia is put medial to ear drum by elevating the ear drum from its annulus in the posterior part.)

5) Pressure bandage and plugging of external auditory canal.

6) Administration of proper antibiotics for healing of the lesion.

# CHRONIC SUPPURATIVE OTITIS MEDIA
## (C.S.O.M.)

It is the chronic inflammatory condition of middle ear mucosa, it may remain as benign or may lead to fatal intra cranial complications.

**Types :**

1) Safe or Tubo tympanic type or Benign Type :-
Eustachian tube and tympanum affects central tympanic perforation present with no complications.

2) Unsafe or Dangerous or Attico antral type.
Attic or epitympanic region and antral part is affected, marginal or attic perforation is seen with severe life threatening complications like destructive cholesteatoma and intra cranial complications.

**Aetiology ;-**

1) Failure of the treatment for A.S.O.M. due to recurrent upper respiratory problems and others like Tonsilitis, Adenoids, Rhinitis, sinusitis, pharyngitis, laryngitis, Low resistant power, virulent infection, acute necrotic otitis media with exanthemata, Traumatic rupture, big unhealing perforation of tympanic membrane, Eustachian catarrh and congenital cholesteatoma.

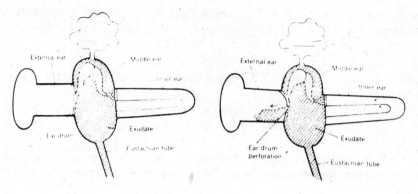

*Acute otitis media, stage of exudation.* ig. 6-2: *Acute otitis media, stage of suppuration.*

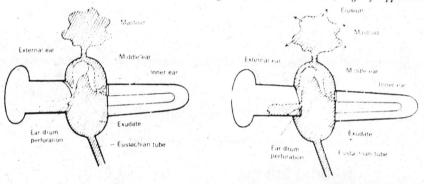

*Acute otitis media with acute mastoiditis.*  *Acute otitis media, stage of complications*

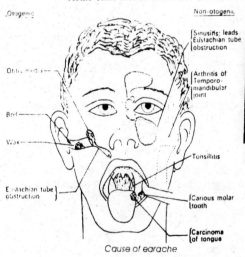

Otogenic

Otitis media

Boil

Wax

Eustachian tube obstruction

Non-otogenic

Sinusitis: leads Eustachian tube obstruction

Arthritis of Temporo-mandibular joint

Tonsillitis

Carious molar tooth

Carcinoma of tongue

*Cause of earache*

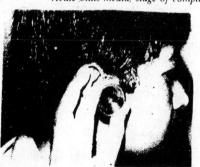

*Examination of the ear with an aural speculum*

## 2) Causative organisms :-

a)      For benign or safe type, are streptococci, staphylococci and pneumococci.

b)      For unsafe or dangerous type, are bacillus pyocyaneus, Bacillus proteus, Bacillus coli and haemolytic streptococci.

## 3) General Factors:-

Unhygienic conditions, recurrent upper respiratory infections, upper respiratory infections, poverty, malnutrition, and Low resistance.

## Pathology :-

1) Tubo tympanic type or Benign type :-

a)      Poor blood supply to tympanic membrane especially at the tip of handle of malleus so more scope for perforation.

b)      Necrosis of ossicular chain (Acute necrotic otitis media)

c)      Persistent mucosal disease.
       Repeated infection of middle ear causes hyper plasia of its mucosa, even leads to polyp formation.

2)      Attico antral type is dangerous by the formation of Cholesterol granuloma (Neither it is a tumour nor contain cholesterol)

Hyper trophy of tympanic mucosa causes obstruction for ventilation from eustachian tube so vaccum is created in the posterior portion of tympanum leads to extravasation of blood into middle ear, this provokes the formation of cholesterol granuloma, Tympanic membrane appears blue in this condition.

Cholesteatoma is a sac lined by Keratinising stratified squamous epithelium in the middle ear cleft and contains desquamated epithelium arranged like onion skin layers. It has the consistency of a tooth paste but it possesses a great bony destroying capacity Hence it is called "Bone destroying disease of ear "

| Symptoms | Benign | Dangerous |
|---|---|---|
| 1) Name of disease | Tubo tympanic | Attico antral |
| 2) Perforation | Central | Attic or marginal |
| 3) Discharge | Intermittent muco purulent or purulent usually without foul smell, white or yellowish Bledding is un common copious | Continuous Always purulent Always foul smelling, yellow or brown or green may be blood stained often scanty. |
| | Increases with upper respiratory tract infections. | Not affected by R.T.I. |

| | | |
|---|---|---|
| 4) Polyp | Occasional | Common |
| 5) Cholesteatoma | Very rare | Common |
| 6) Deafness | Conductive mild to moderate | Conductive or mixed mild to severe |
| 7) Complication | Very rare | Common |
| 8) Radiography of mastoid | Cellular or sclerotic | Sclerotic with erosion |
| 9) Fistula test | Negative | Positive |
| 10) Treatment | Satisfactory | Notsatisfactory. |

## Clinical stages :-
1) Benign perforation 3 stages
   a) Active - discharge actively flowing
   b) Quiescent - ear remains dry for 6 months
   c) Inactive - ear remains dry for more than 6 month.

The perforation may healed completely or may heal with a thin membrane formation. It may associate with tympano sclerosis, ossicular discontinuity due to necrosis or adhesions.

2) Dangerous perforation - Always active stage
investigations - 1) Audiometry 2) Patency of Eustachian tube 3) Radiology of mastoid 4) Otomicroscopy 5) Bacteriological examination of ear discharge.

## Treatment :-
A) Benign perforations:-

## Active stage with otorrhoea.
1) Removal of septic foci 2) Aural toilet to keep the ear canal clean and dry3.) Antibiotic ear drops if there is ear discharge 4) Chemical cautery of perforation with 50% Tri chloracetic acid 5) improvement of nutrition of the patient.

**surgery :-** If conservative treatment fail surgery is advisable
1) Polyps and granulation should be removed 2) Tympano plasty. 3) Myringoplasty

B) Treatment of Attico antral - dangerous perforation.
   1) Same conservative treatment similar to above.
   2) Suction cleaning under the micorscope.
   3) Granulation and polyps should be removed.
   4) Radical mastoidectomy or modified Radical mastoidectomy.
   5) Atticotomy and Attico Antrostomy.
   6) Tympano plasty.

# COMPLICATIONS OF OTITIS MEDIA.

I) Mastoid infection.

A) Mastoiditis.
    1) Acute mastoidits.
    2) Chronic mastoiditis.

B) Matoid abscesses
    1) Sub periosteal abscess
    2) Bezold's abscess.
    3) Zygomatic abscess.
    4) Luc's abscess
    5) Citelli's abscess.

II) Extra cranial complications.
1)     Petrositis
2)     Facial nerve palsy
3)     Labyrinthitis.

III) Intra cranial complications.
    1) Extra dural abscess.
    2) Sub dural abscess.
    3) Meningitis.
    4) Sigmoid sinus thrombo phlebitis.
    5) Brain abscess.
    6) Otitic hydro cephalus
    7) Encephalitis.

**Otorrhoea :-**
    Discharge from the ear is known as otorrhoea. it is due to ear diseases and also due to other external causes.

**A) Causes of Ear**
    1) furunculsis 2) Otitis externa 3) Otomycosis 4) Granulomas 5) myringitis
    6) Tumours 7) A.S.O.M., 8) C.S.O.M. 9) Suppurative Labyrinthitis
    10) Aural abscess

**B) External causes of Otorrhea**
    1) Cerebro spinal fluid otorrhoea
    2) Parotid abscess and Temparo mandibular abscess rupturing into external auditory canal.

**Differential Diagnosis :-**
1) Watery otorrhoea in C.S.F. otorrhoea.
2) Serous otorrhoea in eczematous otitis externa.
3) Mucopurulent otorrhoea, in A.S.O.M. and safe C.S. O.M
4) Purulent otorrhoea in Furuncle, abscess of ear and the parotid abscess and Tempero mandibular joint abscess which open into external ear.
5) Foul otorrhoea in Cholesteatoma
6) Blood stained otorrhoea in aural polyp, granulations, acute otitis media, malignancy.
7) Frank blood otorrhoea in Trauma and glomus tumour.

**Treatment :-**  1) Aural toilet
2) Broad spectrum Local and systemic antibiotics.
3) Symptomatic, according to cause.

# Mastoiditis:-

Inflammation of the mucosa of mastoid antrum and air cells is known as mastoiditis it occurs in two forms.
1) Acute mastoiditis 2) Chronic mastoiditis

**Acute mastoiditis :-** It occurs in cellular type of mastoid bone due to the complication of acute suppurative otitis media.

**Aetiology/pathology :-**
1) Inadequate drainage of exudates and spread of infection to the mastoid.
2) Virulence of the infective organisms.
3) Lowered resistance of the patient.
4) Improper treatment of acute otitis media.
5) Cellular mastoids are more likely to be involved.

**a) Catarrhal mastoiditis :-** Congestion of mastoid mucosa with aggravated symptoms like 1) severe boring type of pain in the ear and at mastoid region 2) creamy yellowish otorrhoea 3) deafness 4) Tenderness on mastoid antrum.

**b) Coalescent mastoiditis :-** Infection proceeds, pus collects in the mastoid antrum, inter cellular septa of mastoid get destructed due to pressure necrosis, the air cells in the mastoid coalesce and mastoid cavity get converted to a bag of pus (empyema). The Clinical features are 1) Severe pain and Fever 2) Otorrhoea may increase or reduce 3) congested ear drum 4) Deafness 5) Tenderness of mastoid antrum 6) Pinna pushed forwards 7) Sagging of postero superior part of external auditory canal 8) Retro auricular oedema or sub periosteal abscess 9) Tachycardia 10) Patient looks ill and anxietic.

**Investigations :-** 1) X-ray of mastoid Air cells are hazy or opaque with coalescence 2) Blood:- polymorpho nuclear lecuco cytosis, increased erythrocytic sedimentation rate.

**Tretament ;-** 1) Surgery is needed, if neglected it causes Trigeminal neuralgia, 6th cranial nerve paralysis and masked mastoiditis etc complications.
2) Cortical mastoidectomy or schwartze operation or simple mastoidectomy is the choice of operation.

**Surgical method (Cortical mastoidectomy ):-** 1) Cortical mastoidectomy is performed to remove the infected air cell of the mastoid process (the middle ear and its contents are not interfered with)

2) General anaesthesia is given.

3) Preparation of the site for giving incision.

4) Postaural incision (wilde's ) is given parallel to the post auricular grooove 1/2 cm behind to it, from the tip of mastoid to the level of upper attachment of the auricle .

5) The incision is deepened up to mastoid bone through skin subcutaneous tissue and periosteum.

6) The soft tissues are elevated from the bone by a periosteum elevator then self retaining mastoid retractor is applied for the exposure of the mastoid and for haemostasis.

7) The supra meatal triangle of Mc Even is identified and in this region the mastoid cortex is removed with a hammer and gouge or with an electric drill until the antrum is reached.

8) The mastoid air cells are removed without injuring the boundaries.

9) Widening of the aditus to antrum to provide drainage of mastoid to the middle ear.

10) Insertion of polyethylene drainage tube at the lower end of the incision and the wound is closed in layers.

11) Drainage tube should be removed after 48 hours and sutures should be removed after 7 days.

12) Suitable antibiotics should be given in adequate dosage for about 7 to 10 days.

## Chronic Mastoiditis

Chronic inflammatory changes of mastoid mucosa is known as chronic mastoiditis.

1) Benign chronic otitis media may produce scanty granulations in the mastoid.

2) Dangerous chronic otitis media with cholesteatoma may erode the mastoid bone gradually.

3) Pus will be scanty and purulent.

4) The patients are usually poor with low standards of hygiene

**Clinical features :-** 1) Otorrhoea - Scanty foul creamy and purulent 2) Deafness 3) Granu-loma formation 4) Other symptoms of Acute mastoiditis.

### Radiological Examination

Sclerotic mastoid with or without erosions

### Treatment :

1) Radical mastoidectomy
2) Modified Radical mastoidectomy.

### Radical mastoidectomy ;-

The mastoid, middle ear and external auditory canal are converted into a single cavity by lowering the wall between the mastoid and tympanum by removal of remnants of ear drum, malleus and incus (Stapes is not removed)

Incision and exposure of mastoid cavity is as like cortical mastoidectomy.

Proper antibiotics are sprinkled in the cavity after operation and the patient is advised for review and for cleaning of the wax debris frequently.

**Complications :-**
1) Facial palsy 2) labyrinthitis 3) conductive deafness 4) Unhealed cavity.

## Modified Radical Mastoidectomy :-

Similar to radical mastoidectony but meso tympanum and hypo tympanum is preserved (only epitympanum is removed along with mastoid air cells).

## Mastoid abscesses
These occur due to acute /Chronic mastoiditis.

### 1) Sub periosteal abscess -
It is the commonest type of abscess due to mastoid infection.
Pain and swelling over the mastoid antrum with all common features of mastoiditis

**2) Zygomatic abscess :-** Pain and swelling infront of and above the external auditory canal

**3) Luc's abscess -** Pus from zygomatic region may track outwards under the periosteum of the roof of the bony canal and reach infra temporal region.

**4) Bezolds abscess -** Perforation of the inner surface of the tip of mastoid, may give rise to an abscess deep to sterno mastoid muscle, it is also known as sinking abscess of neck.

**5) Citelli's abscess -** Extension of abscess to digastric triangle from tip cells.

**6) Apisitis or petrositis :-** extension of the infection to the body and apex of petrous bone.
**Treatment :-** Surgery like mastoiditis.

## Aural Polyp :-
It is a peduculated mass lying in the external auditory canal but can arise from external ear or middle ear.

**Aetiology :-** External ear -
1) Granuoma develops due to constant irritation due to un healed furuncle, traumatic ulcer, wax otitis externa.
2) Tumours
**Middle ear :-**
1) A polyp may arise from the middle ear as a prolapsed mucous membrane or a pedunculated granuloma
2) Tumours.

**Clinical features :-**
Otorrhoea, Bleeding, deafness, pain, itching and presence of pedunculated mass.

**Treatment :-**
1)      Antibiotics
2)      Polypectomy.
3)      Treating the causative factor.

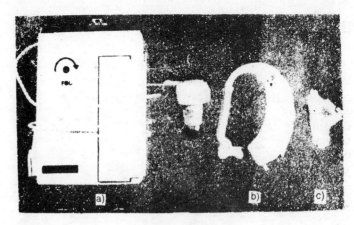

Hearing Aids

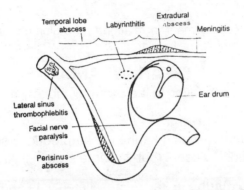

*Diagram showing the possible complications of otitis media*

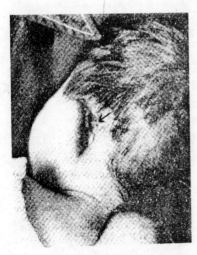

Postaural fistula

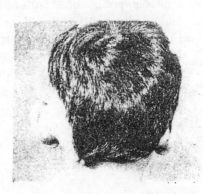

Acute subperiosteal mastoid abscess

## TUMOURS OF EAR :

**External ear :-**
Ceruminoma is a rare benign tumour which may present as a polyp and no malignant lesions are seen .

**Middle ear :-**
1) Benign - Not common
2) Malignant
a) Squamous cell carcinoma (common)
b) Adeno carcinoma
c) Sarcoma      rare
d) Glomus jugulare

**a) Squamous cell carcinoma :** - Common, Blood stained discharge, facial palsy, deafness, pain and bleeds on touch, diagnosis is confirmed by biopsy
**Treatment :-** Excision and radio therapy

**d) Glomus jugulare :-**
It is a rare vascular tumour in relation to the glomus tumour in relation to the glomas bodies. on the dome of the jugularbulb.

# 8) KARNA KANDU
(Itching sensation in the external auditory meatus)

**According to sushrutha :-**
The accumulated, vitiated kapha dosha produces severe itching sensation in the external auditory canal,(bahya karna srotas) is known as karna kandu

**According to madhava kar :-** The vitiated vata and kapha produces severe itching sensation in the external auditory canal is known as karna kandu.

**The common aetiological factors are :-**
1) Collection of polluted water in the external auditory canal due to swimming, head bath etc causes.
2) Fungus infection in the external auditory canal (Otomycosis)
3) Dust, smoke etc exposures may cause allergic reactions that produce itching sensation in the external ear canal.
4) Wax impaction in external auditory canal.
5) Collection of suppurative infective exudates of otitis media and otitis externa.
6) Improper cleaning of ear
7) Putting of impure oils etc in the ear .

**Treatment :-**
1) Nadi sweda
2) Vamana
3) Virechanika dhooma
4) nasya
5) Kapha hara chikitsa
6) Nidana Parivarjan.

114

7) **Karna prakshalan** (ear wash) with Aragwadadi Kashaya, etc decoctions to clean the exudation. 8) **Karna pramarjana** - (dry mopping) the exudates should be cleaned to keep the external auditory canal dry with the cotton buds. 9) **Karna dhoopan** - with guggulu agaru Hingu, Rasanjan etc to dry or burn the vitiated Kapha dosha.10) **Karna Pooran** with sarshapa tail etc oils. 11) Removing of thick sticky collections with shalaka yantra (ear probe or Foreign body remover etc.)12) **Oral remedies** like Lagusuthasekara ras, Khadhiradivati, Trijathakdi vati, Nimbadi guggulu, kanchanara guggulu, Triphala gugulu, Haridra Khandha, chopa cheenyadi churna, yastimadu churna, sitophaladi churna, Talisadi churna, Trikatu churna,

# 9) KARNA GOOTHA OR KARNA VARCHA
### (cerumen or wax in the external auditory canal)

The vitiated or accumulated Kapha dosha get burnt by pittoshma and causes the collection of semi solid or solid material in the external auditory canal, is known as Karna gootha or Karna varcha or Karna vit.

## CERUMEN OR WAX - IN
## EXTERNAL AUDITORY CANAL

The sebaceous glands and ceruminous glands of external auditory canal secrets oily sticky secretion, this secretion and hair protects the external ear from the entry of Foreign bodies.

Sebaceous secretion + Ceruminous secretion + Dust particles + Necrotic tissue and shedded epithelium forms sticky blackish brown wax which is physiological when present in less quantity without producing the symptoms and signs.

This wax collection when packed in the external auditory canal (Without removing in regular intervals) causes deafness, tinnitus, itching sensation, vertigo, pain and inflammation of external ear. (in fungus infection (otomycosis ) wet paper like exudations collected with severe itching sensation)

**Treatment :**
**If the wax is hard :**
1)      Softening of wax by putting oleus ear drops (Karna Pooran
        ( Ex : Nirgundi taila, Kshara taila )

2) Removing the wax with wax probe (karna gootha nirharana shalaka)
3) Swedana to liquify the wax and to reduce pain.
4) Karna pramarjan with cotton buds.
5) karna dhoopan with Guggulu Rasanjan etc drugs.
6) According to modern to soften the wax dewax ear drops -waxsolve eardrops etc are used, then the liquified wax is removed with probe or by ear wash (syringing).
7) Symptomatic treatment to reduce pain and inflammation.

## 10) KARNA PAKA OR KARNA PRAPAKA.
### (Otitis externa (furunculosis or diffused otitis externa )

Vitiated pitta dosha produces ulcerative lesions, tissue necrosis and discharge from the external auditory canal, is known as karna Paka.

The associated symptoms are pain, tenderness, burning sensation and fever, On examination the external auditory meatus appears inflammed with narrow canal and discharge.

**Treatment :-**
1) Pitta hara or pitta visarpa hara treatment should be given. 2) Cool applications and eardrops (shata dhoutha ghritha). 3) Krimi hara chikitsa. 4) Karna Pramarjan and dhoopan to clean and dry the canal. 5) Shoola hara, shotha hara, Krimighna, Vrana ropana, ear drops and oral medicines should be given, 6) Vaman, virechan, nasya, dhooma pana, gandoosha and sweda has to do according to the condition. 7) Amrutadi guggulu, Nimbadi guugulu, chandanadi vati, Lakshudi guggulu, Triphala guugulu, Kancha nara guggulu, Rasnadi guggulu, Lagusuthasekara ras, saribadi vati, Khadhiradi vati, Lakshmi vilas ras etc are beneficial.

## NON SUPPURATIVE OTITIS MEDIA

The disease is characterised by accumulation of non purulent effusion in the middle ear cleft resulting in conductive deafness.

**1) Secretory otitis media :-**

**Synomyms :-** Serous otitis media, catarrhal otitis media, secretory otitis media, glue ear etc.

**Aetiology :-** Not exactly known but following several factors may be concerned.
1) Obstructive cause :- Septal deviation, polyps in nose, enlarged adenoids, tubal occlusion, Nasopharyngial tumours, Adhesions following adenoidectomy etc.

**2) Barotrauma :-**

Collection of serous effusion in the middle ear cleft following atmospheric pressure changes.

**3) Viral infective causes:-** It may produce effusion in middle ear cleft

**4) Allergic changes :-** Allergic disorders of Nose, paranasal sinuses, Nasopharynx may also cause Allergic changes in the middle ear mucosa (Because of anatomical continuity) and produce oedema and effusion.

**5) Un resolved acute Otitis media ;-**

A.S.O.M. Infection is inactivated by the medication but resolution is not complete, sterile effusion present as residue.

6)      Cleft palate or palatal Paralysis.

7)      Disturbances in muco ciliary transport system and secretomotor mechanisms.

**8) Vaccum Theory**

Eustachian tube blockage produces negative pressure in tympanum leads to re-traction of ear drum and extravasation of fluids into middle ear cavity from the vesseles

**9) Hypo gammaglobulinaemia.**

**10) Radiotherapy of head and neck region.**

It is a low grade inflammatory condition of middle ear. Though exact cause is not known it is understood that above factors play an important role in the production of non purulent effusion in the middle ear.

**Clinical Features :-**

Deafness, earache, feeling of fluid in the ear, tinnitus, retracted dull lustreless pinkish ear drum with congested vessels and fluid levels (hair line)

**Diagnosis By :-**1)Clinical features 2) Tuning fork test BC>AC denotes conductive deafness. 3) Pure tone audiometry.4) Tympanometry. 5) Radiotherapy.

**Treatment :-** 1) Medical treatment by decongestant nasal drops, and oral medicine, Anti histamines, steroids, mucolytic agents etc. 2) inflation of eustachian tube by valsalva's manoeurve politzerisation or Eustachian catheterisation may prove helpful.

**3) Surgical Treatment :-**

Myringotomy and suction of glue with the insertion of grommet (plastic tube ) for the aeration of the tympanum.

Surgery for underlying predisposing factor like antral lavage, polypectomy, sub mucous resection of septum, adeno tonsilectomy etc.

## 2) ATELECTASIS OF THE TYMPANUM -
## AND ADHESIVE OTITIS MEDIA :-

Collapse and medial retraction of tympanic membrane following long standing non suppurative otitis media, should pass through various stages like the following.

**1)** Effusion or evidence of fluid in the tympanum **2)** Medial retraction of postero superior Quadrant of ear drum **3)** Atelectatic ear drum :- the entire posterior half of ear drum collapses and drags the ossicles towards medial wall of middle ear **4)** Adhesive otitis media - The entire tympanic membrane (fibrous layer) undergo degeneration and becomes. thinner, Adhesions are formed between eardrum, ossicles and middle ear.

### Treatment :-
1)    Unhealed tympanic perforation is corrected by myringoplasty.
2)    Atelectic ear can be corrected by myringotomy and grommet insertion.
3)    In adhesive changes, Tympanoplasty, ossiculoplasty etc can be tried but results are not encouraging.

### 3) Tympano Sclerosis :-
It is the lesion of the middle ear cleft where there is chalky calcrious deposits on the ear drum and middle ear mucosa with fixation of ossicular chain.

Hyaline degeneration of the fibrous layer of the middle ear mucosa which under goes calcification and appears like snow flakes, symptom is the conductive deafness.

### Treatment :-
1) Tympanoplasty including ossiculoplasty. 2) Stapedectomy 3) Hearing aids.

# 11) KARNA PRATINAHA

According to sushrutha it can be co-related to Tympanic perforation with meningeal Non meningeal complications following Chronic suppurative otitis media.
2) According to vagbhata can be co-related to Eustachian catarrh)

### According to Sushrutha :-
The liquified ear wax or other exudate reaches the mouth and nose, producing severe headache and other complications, is known as karna pratinaha

Unless the tympanic membrane gets ruptured the exudates or wax of external auditory canal can not reach the oropharynx or nasopharynx, so the disease can be corelated to tympanic perforations. It may occur due to traumatic causes or due to otitis media. Sushrutha also explained the severe headache and other complications, these may be the meningeal and Non meningeal complications of chronic suppurative otitis media.

### According to vagbhata :-
The vitiated Kapha dosha is dried by the vitiated vata and sticks to the Karna srotas, produces earache, heavyness and deafness, is known as karna pratinaha, It can be corelated to eustachian catarrh.

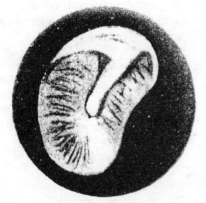

Normal tympanic membrane

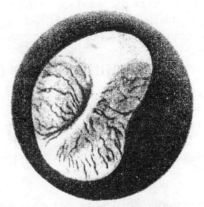

Acute otitis media

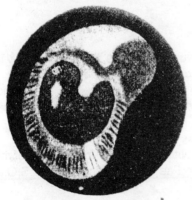

Kldney shaped perforation

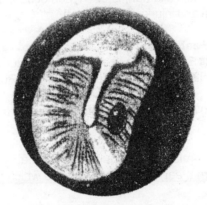

Small central perforation

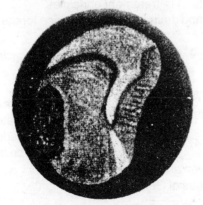

Posterior marginal perforation
(with granulations)

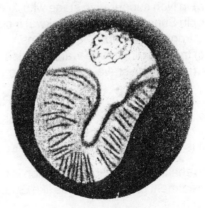

Attic perforation
(with cholesteatoma)

**Tretment :-**

1) Oleation (sneha Karma ), sudation (Sweda karma) and shiro virechana. 2) Karna gootha Nirharan (cleaning of ear wax). 3) Karna pramarjan (drymopping with cotton buds).4) Pratishyaya Chikitsa 5) Dusta Vrana Chikitsa (for healing of tympanic perforation.)6) Karna srava and poothi Karna Chikitsa.7) Teekshna Gandoosha and dhooma pana.

## 12 -13) KARNA VIDRADI (ABSCESS IN THE EAR)

It is of two types

| | |
|---|---|
| 1) Doshaja vidradhi | 2) Aaganthuja vidradhi |
| (1) Vataja, (2) Pittaja, (3) Kaphaja, | 1) Kshataja    2) Abhighataja |
| (4) Sanni pathaja | |

1) Doshaja vidradhi is of 4 types, occurs by the vitiation of vata pitta Kapha and tridoshas. 2) Aaganthuja Vidradhi is of 2 types occurs due to scratching of external auditory canal (kshataja) and injuries (Abhighataj)

**Clinical Features :-**

      1) Either due to doshic vitiation or due to traumatic lesions, the ear canal is vitiated and exhibits different coloured exudations (Reddish ,Yellowish etc ) through the ear.

      2) Associated symptoms are severe and different types of pain, burning sensation, itching sensation , headache. etc.

It can be corelated to suppurative otitis media and otitis externa, (Vrana shopha of middle and external ear) mastoid abscesses which formed as the complication of A.S.O.M. or C.S.O.M.

**Treatment :-**

1) Vidradhi treatment should be given
      a) In Non suppurative stage with Alepa etc "11 " treatment principles.
      b) In Suppurative stage (Pakwa) incision and drainage should be done for the irrigation of impure exudations.
      c) In Exudating stage vrana chikitsa should be done.
      (Like Karna srava and poothi Karna).

## 14-17) KARNA ARSHA
### (Polyps of ear )

It is of 4 types 1)Vataj 2) Pittaj 3) Kaphaj 4) Raktaj.

In shalakya tantra the discription is not given and explained that the aetio- pathology and treatment principles are as like Guda arshas of General medicine.

Polyps in the external and middle ear occur due to stenosed chambers with improper ventillation, constant irritation and chronic collection of exudates. The mucosa is stimulated and gives an elongated mass like structure known as arshas or polyp.

It causes earache, otorrhoea, discomfort and deafness

1) Vataj Arsha - Blackish red, dried rough polyp with pain.
2) Pittaj Arsha - Yellowish red polyp with pain and burning.
3) Kaphaj Arsha - Whitish or pale polyp sticky with severe itching.
4) Raktaj Arsha - Dark red coloured polyp with pain, burning sensation and bleeds on touch.

**Treatment :-**
1) Medical 2) Surgical 3) Kshara karma
(Chemical cauterisation ) 4) Agni karma
(Electric cauterisation)
5) Treatment like Nasa arsha.

## 18 21) KARNA SHOPHA (AURAL OEDEMA)

It is 4 types 1) Vataj 2) Pittaj 3) Kaphaj 4) Sannipathaj (General discription as like in Kaya chikitsa).
It causes pain, discomfort, otorrhoea, and deafness.

**Treatment :-** 1) Like aural polyp or Nasal polyp. 2) Pratishyaya, Karna srava, Poothi Karna and Vrana chikitsa should be done.

## 22-28 ) KARNA ARBUDA
### (Tumours of ear)

Vitiated vatadi doshas by deranging twak, raktha, mamsa etc dhatus produce 7 types of arbudas, they are,
1) Vataj 2) Pittaja 3) Kaphaj 4) Raktaj 5) Medaja 6) Mamsaja 7) Siraja.
" Description is as like in Kaya Chikitsa ."

**Clinical features :-** earache, discomfort, otorrhoea, deafness, vertigo and meningeal, non-meningeal complications.
" Arbudas are commonly non suppurative in nature ( Apakwa) due to the predominence of Kapha and medo dhathu

**Treatment :-**
1) In Non Suppurative stage should treat like shopha.
2) If suppurates should treat by incision and drainage.
3) Vrana chikitsa.
4) Hard non suppurative complicative tumour should be excised.
**Note :-** These can be corelated to benign and malignant tumours of middle ear.

### BAHYA KARNA ROGAS
#### (Diseases of Auricle) by Vagbhata

Additionally vagbhata explained 10 diseases of exteral ear.
1) Diseases of karna Shaskuli are     3
2) Diseases of Karna Pali are     7
    **Total**     =     10

## 1) Kuchi Karnika :-

It is an uncurable, congenital abnormality of the auricle (Karna shaskuli), affects during the pregnancy by the vitiation of vata dosha in which the auricle becomes smaller or contracted, is known as Kuchi Karnika.

**Treatment :-** It is Asadya vyadhi (Uncurable).

## 2) Karna Pippali :-

It is also an uncurable, congenital disease of the ear, affects during the pregnancy by the vitiation of vata dosha, in which a painless immobile growth resembling the pippali develops on auricle (Karna Shaskuli) , is known as Karna Pippali.

**Treatment :-** It is also Asadya vyadhi (uncurable)

## 3) Karna Vidarika :-

It is also an uncurable congenital aswell as acquired disease of the aucricle (karna shaskuli), affects by the vitiation of tridoshas, in which a painfull same coloured suppurative oedema develops with itching sensation, if not treated in time dicharges foul exudate resembling sarshapa taila and causes structural deformity after healing.
**Treatment :-** Asadya vyadhi (uncurable) But can try like Karna vidradi

## 4) Pali sosha :-

The vitiated vata dosha causes atrophy of the Karna Pali (ear lobule).

**Treatment : -** 1) Like the treatment of Vataj Karna shoola.
2) udvarthana (rubbing at the lesion) with the powders of Tila, priyala beeja, yastimadu, Ashwagandha, yava etc.

3) Abhyanga with Brumhana snehas (Oil prepared with shatavari ashwagandha, jeevanthi, Jeevaka, erenda, cow milk and Tila taila) 4) Sweda 5) Lepas 6) nasya 7) Surgery :- The fresh part of the lobule should adjoin to the atrophic part.

## 5) Tankrika :-

The vitiated Vata dosha changes the Karna Pali into a thin hard wire (Tantri) So named as Tantrika.

**Treatment :-** 1) It is Yapya vyadhi 2) Abhyanga and mardana with Vatahara Brumhana snehas to nourish the lobule (karna pali)

## 6) Pari Pota :-

Conducting Karna vyadana to the aged instead of children causes inflammation of the lobule (cracking redness oedema and pain) due to the vitiation of Vata dosha, is known as paripota.

**Treatment :-** 1) Vatahara Chikitsa. 2) Abhyanga and mardana with Brumhana snehas. 3) Shothahara, shoolahara chikitsa.

## 7) Uthpaata :-

It is an inflammatory condition of the lobule (pitta and raktha vitiates) occurs by putting heavy ornaments to the ear lobule. The clinical features are pain, burning sensation. blister formation, blackish discolouration and suppurative oedema with discharge.

**Treatment :-**
1) Jalauka mokshana to remove impure blood from the lesion.
2) Cool applications to the site.
3) Application of medicated pastes, oils, ghee etc which reduce the Raktha and pitta vitiation.
4) Abhyanga with Jambwaditail (the oil is prepared with jambu, amra pallava, Kanji and Tila taila.)
5) Anti inflammatory and wound healing therapy should give.

## 8) Unmantha Or Gallira :-

Vitiated Kapha and Vata produces a painless, immobile, same coloured oedema on Karna pali with itching sensation is Known as unmantha.

**Treatment :-** 1) Abhyanga with the snehas which reduce the vitiation of Kapha and vata (Godhaa Karka Vasadi taila).
2) Nasya with Katphaladi Choorna Or with the oil prepared with Tulasi, Langali, Taila.

## 9) Dukkha vardana :-

Tridoshas vitiate due to improper Karna Vyadana and improper widening of the hole of the lobule causes pain, oedema, burning sensation, itching sensation and discharge.

**Treatment :-** 1) Laksha Vidangadi taila abhyanga.
2) Vrana Chikitsa (Wound healing therapy)

## 10) Lehya or Parilehika :-

Vitiated Kapha Raktha doshas and krimi causes inflammation of the lobule (Pustules pain, itching and exudation) if it is not treated in time causes destruction of the lobule.

**Treatment :-**
1) Vidangadi Lepa with Avi mutra. 2) Application of the paste of kutaja, ingudee, karanja Arogwada valkala + Avi mootra (sheep's urine) 3) Application of the Oil prepared with above drugs + Nimba Patra, maricha, madan phala and sarshapa taila. 4) Sudation (Swedan) with cow's faecal material. 5) Krimighna treatment therapy.

## TREATMENT OF INJURED AND BLEEDING LOBULE :-

1)      Setting of the lobule without irregularities.
2)      Application of Honey and ghee to the lesion .
3)      Dusting the powders of gyrika and Yastimadu.
4)      Bandage (yaugika bandana) upto 7 days.
5)      After healing, Lengthening of the lobule should be done by the application of Karna vardana taila

### 6) Karna Vardana sneha :-

The medicated ghee is prepareed with, jala shooka (algae), swayam guptha, Haridra dwayam, Bruhati dwaya, Ashwagandha, Bala, Gaja pippali, Swetha sarshapa, karaveer, Arka, Saptha parni, the mud house of chuchundari and madhukaree, Laksha, Jalauka, Rasona, Hasti and Ashwa Mootra, Tila taila and Mahisha gritha.

### Karna Vyadana Vidhi ;-

It is done not only for wearing ornaments but also for prevention of the diseases.

It is done in the children at 6th or 7th month of age. in a good day dhatri should hold the child and the doctor while pulling the ear with his left hand has to do karna vyadana with his right hand at Diiva krutha chidra.

(Karna vyadana should do first to the right ear in male child and to the left ear in female child).

In samyak (proper) Karna vyadan pain and bleeding is minimum.

If  Karna vyadana is improperly done it causes 1) Kalika sira viddha (jwara, daha shoola shotha) 2) Marmarika sira viddha (jawara shool and vrana) 3) Lohithik sira viddha (manya stamba, apatanak, shirograh and karna shoola) etc complication.

### Karna Bandhan :-

While wearing the heavy ornaments to the ear or  widening the ear lobule or by the punishments of kings to the victims there were ear abnormalities, for correcting those problems 15 types of Karna bandhanas were explained by sushrutha. They are.

**1) Nemi sandhanak :-** The ear lobule is equally cut but becomes lengthy and thick.

**2) Uthphala bhedak :-** The ear lobule is equally cut but becomes round and thick.

**3) Vallurak :-** The ear lobule get atrophied, but both the halves are equal in size.

**4) Asangima :-** Among the 2 halves of cut lobule only inner lengthy part is existing (outer half gets atrophied).

**5) Ganda Karna :-** Among the 2 halves of cut lobule only outer lenghty part is existing (inner half gets atrophied).

**6) Aaharya :-** Both halves of cut lobule mostly destructed.

**7) Nirvedak :-** Complete lobule get atrophied so karna vyadhan should be done to karna putrika, then karna vardana has to do.

**8) Vyayojima :-** Among the 2 halves of cut lobule one is normal and the other is smaller and irregular.

**9) Kapat Sandhik :-** Among the 2 halves of lobule inner half is lengthy and outer half is smaller.

**10) Artha Kapat Sandhik :-** Among the 2 halves of cut lobule, the outer half is lengthy and inner half is smaller.

**11) Samkshiptha :** Among the 2 halves of cut lobule, outer half is atrophied and inner half becomes smaller.

**12) Heena karna :-** Complete atrophy of lobule with the base.

**13) Valle Karna :-** Very small thin and irregular loubule.

**14) Yasti Karna :-** Hard vascularised very small lobule.

**15) Kakaustak :-** Emaciated constricted small lobule like the beak of crow.

**Treatment for above (15 types of abnormalities).**

## SANDHANA KARMA

A) Ist, 2nd, 3rd types - Both the halves of lobule are in same size so proper setting and bandhana should be done.

B) a) 4th (Asamgima) The inner lenghty half should be cut and joined to the outer half.
b) 5th (Ganda Karna) The outer lengthy half should be cut and joined to the inner half

C) 6th (Aaharya) - Lobule mostly destruicted so the tissue is collected from the cheeks and grafted to the lobule.

D) 7th (Nirvedak) complete lobule gets atrophied so Karna vyadan should do to the karna patrika then Karna Vardana should do.

E) 8th, 9th, 10th, -- In these 3 types one half is lengthy than other- so the lengthy part should adjoin with shorter.

F) 11 to 15 Asadya.
After proper adjoining therapy the irregularities are corrected by
1) Utsadan Karma 2) Avasadan karma 3) Mrudu Karma 4) Daruna Karma 5) Krishna karma
6) Pandu Karma 7) Roma Sanjanan Karma 8) Romapaharan karma etc.,

# NASA ROGA
# DISEASES OF THE NOSE

# नासारोग

## कारण

संधारणाजीर्णरजोतिभाष्यक्रोधर्तुवैषम्यशिरोभितापै: ।
प्रजागरातिस्वपनाम्बुशीतैरवश्यायमैथुनवाष्पधूमै ॥

संस्त्यानदोषे शिरसि प्रवृद्धो वायु: प्रतिश्यायमुदीरयेतु ।

(च॰ चि॰ २६)

नारीप्रसङ्ग:शिरसोभितापो धूमोरज: शीतमतिप्रताप:

संधारणं मूत्रपुरीषयोश्च सद्य: प्रतिश्यायनिदानमुक्तम्

(सु.उ.अ.२४)

अवश्यायानिलरजोभाष्यातिस्वप्नजागरै: ।
नीचात्युच्चोपधानेन पीतेनान्येन वारिणा ॥

अत्युम्बुपानरमणच्छर्दिबाष्पग्रहादिभि: ।
क्रुद्धा वातोल्वणा दोषा नासायां स्त्यानतांगता: ॥

जनयन्ति प्रतिश्यायं वर्धमानं क्षयप्रदम् ॥

(अ.ह.उ.अ.१९)

## नासा रोग संख्या

अपीनस: पूतिनस्यं नासापाकस्तथैव च ।
तथा शोणितपित्तंच पूयशोणितमेव च ॥
क्षवथुभ्रंशथुर्दीप्तो नासानाह: परिस्त्रव: ।
नासाशोषेण सहिता दशैकाश्चेरिता गदा: ॥
चत्वार्यर्शांसि चत्वार: शोफा: सप्तार्बुदानि च ।
प्रतिश्यायाश्च ये पंच वक्ष्यन्ते सचिकित्सिता: ।
एकत्रिंशन्मितास्ते तु नासारोगा: प्रकीर्त्तिता: ॥

(सु.उ.अ.22/3,4,5)

## प्रतिश्याय सम्प्राप्ति

चयं गता मूर्धनि मारुतादय: पृथक् समस्ताश्च तथैव शोणितम् ।
प्रकोप्यमाणा विविधै: प्रकोपणै नृणां प्रतिश्यायकरा भवन्ति ॥

(सु.उ.अ.२४/4)

# प्रतिश्याय का पूर्वरूप

शिरोगुरुत्वं क्षवथो: प्रवर्त्तनं तथाङ्गमर्द: परिहृष्टरोमता।

उपद्रवाश्चाप्यपरे पृथग्विधा नृणां प्रतिश्यायपुर:सरा: स्मृता: ॥

(सु.उ.अ.२४/5)

## 1. वातिकप्रतिश्याय लक्षण

आनद्धा पिहिता नासा तनुस्नावप्रवर्त्तिनी।

गलतात्लवोष्ठशोषश्च निस्तेद: शङ्ख्योस्तथा ॥

स्वरोपघातश्च भवेत् प्रतिश्यायेनिलात्मके।

(सु.उ.अ.२४/6)

तत्र वातात् प्रतिश्याये मुखशोषो भृशं क्षव: ॥

घ्राणोपरोधनिस्तोददन्तशङ्खशिरोव्यथा: ।

कोटिका इव सर्पन्तीर्मन्यते परितो भ्रुवौ ॥

स्वरसादश्चिरात् पाक: शिशिराच्चकफस्रुति:

(अ॰ हृ॰ उ॰ अ॰ १९)

## 2. पैत्तिक प्रतिश्याय

उष्ण: सपीतक: स्नावो घ्राणात् स्नवति पैत्तिके ॥

कृशोतिपाण्डु: सन्तप्तो भवेत्तृष्णानिपीडित: ।

सधूमं सहसा वह्निं वमतीव च मानव: ॥

(सु.उ.अ.२४/7,8)

पित्तात्तृष्णाज्वरघ्राणपिटिकासम्भवभ्रमा: ॥

नासाग्रपाको रुक्षोष्णताम्रपीतकफस्रुति:

अ. हृ. उ. अ. 19

## 3. कफज प्रतिश्याय

कफ: कफकृते घ्राणाच्छुक्ल: शीत: स्रवेन्मुहु: ।

शुक्लावभास: शूनाक्षो भवेद् गुरूशिरोमुख: ॥

शिरोगलौष्ठतालूनां कण्डूयनमतीव च।

(सु.उ.अ.24/9)

कफात् कासोरुचि: श्वासो वमथुर्गात्रकगौरवम् ॥

माधुर्य वदने कण्डु: स्निग्धशुक्लकफस्तुति: ।

(अ॰ हृ॰ उ॰ अ॰ 19)

## 4. त्रिदोषज प्रतिश्याय

भूत्वा भूत्वा प्रतिश्यायो योकस्माद् विनिवर्त्तते ॥

संपक्वो वापक्वो वा स सर्वप्रभव: स्मृत: ।

लिङ्गानि चैव सर्वेषां पीनसानां च सर्वजे ॥

(सु.उ.अ.24/10,11)

सर्वजो लक्षणै: सर्वैरकस्माद् वृद्धिशान्तिमान् ॥

(अ॰ हृ॰ अ॰ 19)

## 5. रक्तजप्रतिश्याय

रक्तजे तु प्रतिश्याये रक्तास्त्राव: प्रवर्त्तते ।

ताम्राक्षश्च भवेज्जन्तुरुरोघातप्रपीडित: ॥

दुर्गन्धोच्छ्वासवदनस्तथा गन्धान् वेत्ति च ।

मूर्च्छन्ति चात्र कृमय: श्वेता: स्निग्धास्तथाणव: ॥

कृमिमूर्ध्विकारेण समानं चास्य लक्षणम् ।

(सु.उ.अ.२४/12,13)

दुष्टं नासासिरा: प्राप्य प्रतिश्यायं करोत्यसृक् ।

उरस: सुप्तता ताम्रनेत्रत्वं श्वासपूतिता ॥

कण्डु: श्रोत्राक्षिनासासु पित्तोक्तं चात्रलक्षणम् ।

(अ॰ हृ॰ उ॰ अ॰ १९)

## दुष्टप्रतिश्याय

प्रक्लिद्यति पुनर्नासा पुनश्च परिशुष्यति ॥

मुहुरानह्यते चापि सुहुर्विव्रियते तथा ।

नि:श्वासोच्छ्वासदौर्गन्ध्यं तथागन्धान् वेत्ति च ॥

एवं दुष्टप्रतिश्यायं जानीयात्कृच्छ्रसाधनम् ।

(सु.उ.अ.२४/14,15)

## प्रतिश्याय के उपद्रव

सर्व एव प्रतिश्याया नरस्याप्रतिकारिण: ॥

कालेन रोगजनना जायन्ते दुष्टपीनसा: ।

बाधिर्यमान्ध्यमघ्राणं घोराँश्च नयनामयान् ॥

कासाग्निसादशोफाँश्च वृद्धा: कुर्वन्ति पीनसा: ॥

(सु॰उ॰अ.24/16,17)

## 6. अपीनस या पीनस

आनह्यते यस्य विधूप्यते च प्रक्लिद्यते शुष्यति चापि नासा ।

न वेत्ति यो गन्धरसाँश्च जन्तुर्जुष्टं व्यवस्येत्तमपीनसेन ॥

तं चानिलश्लेष्मभवं विकारं ब्रूयात् प्रतिश्यायसमानलिङ्गम् ।

(सु॰उ॰अ.२२/6)

कफ: प्रवृद्धो नासायां रुद्ध्वा स्रोताँस्यपीनसम् ।

कुर्यात् सघुर्घुरश्वासं पीनसाधिकवेदनम् ॥

अवेरिव स्रवत्यस्य प्रक्लिन्ना तेन नासिका ।

अजस्रं पिच्छिलं पीतं पक्वं सिङ्घाणकं घनम् ॥

(अ॰ हृ॰ उ॰ प्र॰ १९)

## आम वा अपक्वपीनस

अरुचिर्बिरसं वक्त्रं नासास्रावो रुजारति: ।

शिरोगुरुत्वं क्षवथुर्ज्वरश्रामस्य लक्षणम् ॥

## पक्व पीनस

तनुत्वमामलिङ्गानां शिरोनासास्यलाघवम् ।

घनपीतकफत्वं च पक्वपीनसलक्षणम् ॥

## 7. पूतिनास या पूतिनस्य

दोषैर्विदग्धैर्गलतालुमूले संवासितो यस्य समीरणस्तु ॥

निरेति पूतिमुखनासिकाभ्यां तं पूतिनासं प्रवदन्ति रोगम् ॥

(सु॰ उ॰ अ॰ २२/7)

तालुमूले मलैर्दुष्टैर्मारुतो मुखनासिकात्।
श्लेष्मा च पूतिर्निर्गच्छेत् पूतिनासं वदन्ति तम्॥

(अ॰ हृ॰ उ॰ अ॰ १९/23)

## 8. नासापाक वा नासिकापाक

घ्राणाश्रितं पित्तमरूंषि कुर्याद् यस्मिन् विकारे बलवांश्च पाक:॥
तं नासिकापाकमिति व्यवस्येद् विक्लेदकोथावापि यत्र दृष्टौ॥

(सु॰ उ॰ अ॰ २२/8)

पचेन्नासापुटे पित्तं त्वङ्मांसं दाहशूलवत्॥

(अ॰ हृ॰ उ॰ अ॰ १९)

## 9.नासागत रक्तपित्त

चतुर्विधं द्विप्रभवं द्विमार्गं वक्ष्यामि भूय: खलु रक्तपित्तम्

(सु॰ उ॰)

## 10. पूयरक्त

दोषैर्विदग्धैरथवापि जन्तोर्ललाटदेशेभिहतस्य तैस्तु।
नासा स्रवेत् पूयमसृग्विमिश्रं तं पूयरक्तं प्रवदन्ति रोगम्॥


निचयादभिघाताद्वा पूयासृङ् नासिका स्रवेत्।
तत् पूयरक्त माख्यातं शिरोदाहरुजाकरम्॥

(अ॰ हृ॰ उ॰ अ॰ १९)

## 11. क्षवथु
## दोषज क्षवथु

घ्राणाश्रिते मर्मणि संप्रदुष्टे यस्यानिलो नासिकया निरेति॥
कफानुयातो बहुश: सशब्दस्तं रोगमाहु: क्षवथुं विधिज्ञा:॥

(सु॰ उ॰ २२/अ॰)

## आगन्तुक्षवथु

तीक्ष्णोपयोगादतिजिघ्रतो वा भावान् कटूनर्कनिरीक्षणाद्वा॥
सूत्रादिभिर्वा तरूणास्थिमर्मण्युद्घाटितेन्य: क्षवथु निरेति॥

(सु॰ उ॰ अ॰ 22)

भृषक्षव

तीक्ष्णाग्रणोपयोगार्करशिमसुत्रतृणादिभि: ।
वात्तकोपिभिलरन्यैर्वा नासिकातरूणास्थनि ॥
विघट्टितेनिल: क्रुद्धो रुद्ध: शृङ्गाटकं व्रजेत् ।
निवृत्त: कुस्तेत्यर्थ ज्ञवथुं स भृशज्ञव: ॥

(अ॰ हृ॰ उ॰ १९ अ॰)

## 12. भ्रंशथु

भ्रश्यते नासिकयैव यश्च सान्द्रो विदग्धो लवण: कफस्तु ॥
प्राक्संचितो मूर्धनि पित्ततप्तस्तं भ्रंशथुं व्याधिमुदाहरन्ति ॥

(सु॰ उ॰ अ॰ २२)

## 13. दीप्त

घ्राणे भृशं दाहसमन्विते तु विनि:सरेद् धूम इवेह वायु: ॥
नासा प्रदीप्तेव च यस्य जन्तोव्याधिं तु तं दीप्तमुदाहरन्ति ॥

(सु॰ उ॰ अ॰ २२)

रक्ता नासा दग्धेव बाह्यान्त:स्पर्शनासहा ।
भवेद् धूमोपमोच्छ्वासा सा दीप्तिर्दहतीव च ॥

(अ॰ हृ॰ उ॰ अ॰ १९)

## 14. नासानाह वा नासा प्रतिनाह

कफावृतो वायुरुदानसंज्ञो यदा स्वमार्गे विगुण: स्थित: स्यात् ॥
घ्राणं वृणोतीव तदा स रोगो नासाप्रतीनाह इति प्रदिष्ट ॥

(सु॰ उ॰ अ॰ २२)

नासानाहे तु जायते
नद्धत्वमिव नासाया: श्लेष्मरुद्धेन वायुना ॥
नि:श्वासोच्छ्वाससंरोधात् स्रोतसी संवृते इव ।

(अ॰ हृ॰ उ॰ अ॰ १९)

## 15. नासास्राव

अजस्रमच्छं सलिलप्रकाशं यस्याविवर्ण स्रवतीह नासा ॥
रात्री विशेषेण हि तं विकारं नासापरिस्रावमिति तं व्यवस्येत् ॥

(सु॰ उ॰ अ॰ २२)

स्त्रावस्तु तत्संज्ञः श्लेष्म संभवः
अच्छोजलोपमोजस्त्रं विशेषान्निशि जायते ॥

(अ॰ हृ॰ उ॰ अ॰ १९)

## 16. नासा शोष या नासा परिशोष

घ्राणाश्रिते श्लेष्मणि मारूतेन पित्तेन गाढं परिशोषिते च ॥
समुच्छ्वसित्यूर्ध्वमधश्च कृच्छ्राद्यस्तस्य नासापरिशोष उक्तः ॥

(सु॰ उ॰ २२ अ॰)

शोषयन्नासिकास्त्रोतः कफं च कुरुतेनिलः ।
शूकपूर्णाभनासात्वं कृच्छ्रादुच्छ्वसनं ततः ॥

(अ॰ हृ॰ उ॰ अ॰ १९)

## पुटक रोग

पित्तश्लेष्मावरुद्धोन्तर्नासायां शोषयेन्मरुत् ।
कफं, स शुष्कः पुटतां प्रापनोति पुटकं तु तत् ॥

(अ॰ हृ॰ उ॰ अ॰ १९)

## 17 से 23) अर्बुद

स्त्रोतः पथे यद्विपुलं कोशवच्चाबुंदं भवेत् ॥

(सु॰ उ॰ अ॰ २२)

## 24 से 27) शोफ

शोफास्तु शोफविज्ञाना नासास्त्रोतो व्यवस्थिताः ।
निदानेर्शांसि निर्दिष्टान्येवं तानि विभावयेत् ॥

(सु॰ उ॰ अ॰ २२)

## 28 से 31) अर्श

नामार्शः के लक्षण साधारण अर्शः की तरह हैं। इसके भेद 4

(सु॰ उ॰ अ॰ २२)

# NASA SHAREERA

In Ayurvedic samhitas the detailed description of NASA SHAREERA is not available like in Netra shareera. But the following points are explained in brief.

Ghranendrium is one among pancha Gyanendria. it develops to the foetus in the 3rd month of intra uterine period.

| | |
|---|---|
| Indria | Ghranendria (only one) |
| Indria adhistana | Nasa (2 nostrils) |
| Indrai dravya | Pruthwi Predominent |
| Indriaartha | Gandha |
| Indria buddhi | Ghrana buddhi |

The finalisation of smell sense is by the indria buddhi

1)  Nasa Puta pramanam $1\frac{1}{3}$ or $2\frac{2}{3}$ Angula
2)  It contains Tarunasti (Cartilage) and 3 bones.
3)  It contains 2 Bahya srotas
4)  It contains 2 Peshi (muscles)
5)  It contains 2 phana marma and shrungatak marma
    a) Phana marmas are Sira marma, Vikalya Kara marmas Arthangula pramana,    If damaged causes loss of smell sensation.
    b) shrungatak marma nourishes the nose, if damaged causes immediate death.
6)  It contains 24 Siras  (6 Vata vahini, 6 pitta Vahini 6 Kapha Vahini, and 6 Raktha Vahini.)
    Among 24 Sira 4 are avedhya ,2 are for smell sensation.
7)  It contains 2 Damani for smell sensation.

## SOME WORDS RELATED TO NASA

| | | | |
|---|---|---|---|
| 1) | Nasa, ghrana, nasika are synonyms | | |
| 2) | Nasa nadi,  nasa srotas, ghrana marga, means nasal cavity. | | |
| 3) | Nasa tarunasti | = | Nasal cartilage |
| 4) | Ghrana asti | = | Nasal Bone. |
| 5) | Nasaagra | = | Tip of the nose. |
| 6) | Grana moola | = | Root of the nose. |
| 7) | Nasaasti danda | = | Bridge of the nose. |
| 8) | Ghrana randra | = | Anterior nares |
| 9) | Nasa Pashchaath randra | = | Posterior nares. |
| 10) | Ganda vah damani | = | Olfactory nerves. |
| 11) | Bahya Nasa | = | External nose. |
| 12) | Nasa guha | = | Nasal cavity. |
| 13) | Ganda grahana | = | Olfaction. |

# ANATOMY OF NOSE

**External Nose :-**

The external nose is pyramidal in shape composed of bone ,cartilage, and soft tissue. The base of pyramid is perforated by two orifices, called anteior nares or Nostrils, they are separated by a median partition called columella, The root of the nose is the junction of it with forehead, the tip of the nose is called the apex, the dorsum of the nose is the anterior border joining the root with Apex, the upper bony portion of the dorsum is called the bridge of the nose, the rounded eminences at the lower end of the sides are named ala nasi.

The Bony portion of the Nose is formed by a) Nasal bones, b) Nasal process of maxillae and c) Nasal process of frontal bone. The cartilaginous portion is formed by paired and unpaired cartilages. Paired cartilages are a) upper nasal cartilages b) Lower nasal cartilages or greater alar cartilages c) Lesser alarcartilages or Accessary alar cartilages. d) Vomero nasal cartilages. and un paired cartilage is the septal cartilage.

1) upper nasal cartilages are 2 in number triangular in shape attached above to the Lower borders of the nasal bones and medially to the dorsum of the septal cartilage.

2) Lower Nasal cartilages or greater alar cartilage are bend around to form the contour of the ala and the nasal tip, the medial crus of this cartilage joins with it's opposite to form the columella

3)     smaller alar cartilage situated posterior to the Lateral crus of Lower Nasal cartilage.

4)     Vomero nasal cartilage lie on either side of the postero inferior edge of the septal cartilage and are attached to the vomer bone.

5)     Septal cartilage- septum divides the nasal cavity in to two halves. Anterior Quadrilateral part is septal cartilage and posterior portion is the bony. septum.

Muscles of the external Nose.
1)     Dilators and Compressors of the nostrils
2)     Depressors and elevators of the alaenasi

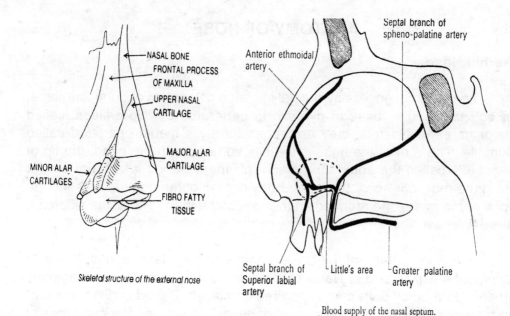

NASAL BONE

FRONTAL PROCESS
OF MAXILLA

UPPER NASAL
CARTILAGE

MINOR ALAR
CARTILAGES

MAJOR ALAR
CARTILAGE

FIBRO FATTY
TISSUE

*Skeletal structure of the external nose*

Anterior ethmoidal
artery

Septal branch of
spheno-palatine artery

Septal branch of
Superior labial
artery

Little's area

Greater palatine
artery

Blood supply of the nasal septum.

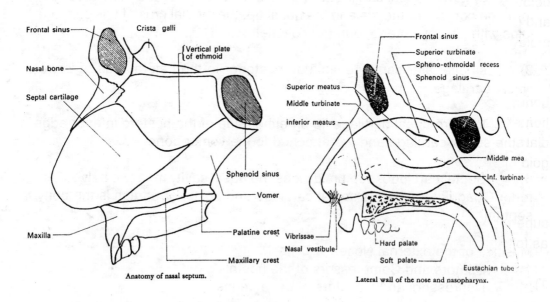

Frontal sinus

Crista galli

Vertical plate
of ethmoid

Nasal bone

Septal cartilage

Sphenoid sinus

Vomer

Maxilla

Palatine crest

Maxillary crest

Anatomy of nasal septum.

Frontal sinus

Superior turbinate

Spheno-ethmoidal recess

Sphenoid sinus

Superior meatus

Middle turbinate

inferior meatus

Middle mea

Inf. turbinat

Vibrissae

Nasal vestibule

Hard palate

Soft palate

Eustachian tube

Lateral wall of the nose and nasopharynx.

136

**Blood Supply of external Nose:-** Facial and Ophthalmic arteries.

**Venous drain :-** In the anterior facial and Ophthalmic veins.

**Lymphatics :-** Drain into sub mandibular and preauricular lymph glands.

## Nasal Cavity :-

It lies below the cranial caivty, above the oral cavity and in between the orbits. Nasal caivty is divided into two halves by Nasal septum. Each Nasal cavity communicates with nasopharynx posteriorly through posterior nares or choana and anteriorly to the atmosphere through anterior nares or choana. it also communicates with paranasal sinuses and nasolacrimal duct.

The Nasal cavity is bounded by 1) Lateral Wall 2) Medial Wall 3) Roof 4) Floor.

### 1) Lateral Wall :-

It is mainly formed by medial wall of maxilla, lateral mass of ethmoid. other smaller parts are formed by Ascending process of maxilla, perpendicular plate of palatine bone and medial pterygoid process of sphenoid bone.

It contains ridges (Turbinates or choncha) and depressions (meatus below to the turbinates.) There are 3 turbinates and 3 meatus superior middle and inferior respectively. Superior and middle turbinates are the part of ethmoid bone while the inferior turbinate is the separate bone.

Anterior part of the lateral wall is formed by the inner aspect of Nasal bones, anterior part of body of maxilla, frontal process of maxilla and a portion of inferior turbinate. Middle part of the lateral wall is formed by the medial surface of ethmoid labyrinth, superior and middle turbinates and the pterygoid plates. In the upper part is the spheno palatine foramin.

Meatus is the depression area below the turbinates, 3 in number - superior middle and inferior meati, various ducts opens in to meati they are as follows.

1)      Naso Lacrimal duct opens into inferior meatus.

## 2) Into Middle Meatus.

a) Frontal sinus, Anterior ethmoidal cells open into anterior part of the meatus.

b) Middle ethmoidal cells open into middle meatus above the haitus semilunaris .

c) Maxillary sinus opens in the posterior part of the haitus semilunaris ( In the middle meatus there is a bulge known as Bulla ethmoidalis and Haitus semilunaris is the semilunar gap below it ).

## 3) In to Superior Meatus :-

Posterior ethmoidal cells open. Above and behind the superior turbinate a small depression known as spheno ethmoidal recess present in which the sphenoid sinus opens.

## II) Medial Wall :-

Nasal septum form the medial wall of the Nasal cavity, it has bony (Posteriorly) and cartilagenous (Anteriorly) parts.

### 1) Bony part of the septum is formed by

a) Postero - inferiorly by the vomer bone.

b) Postero superiorly by perpendicular plate of ethmoid.

c) Nasal spine of frontal bone joins the ethmoid plate.

d) Rostrum of sphenoid between the vomer and ethmoid plate.

e) Nasal crest of two maxillae and palatine bones.

## 2) Cartilaginous part of nasal septum :-

It is quadrilateral cartilage attached postero superiorly to the perpendicular plate of ethmoid bone,posteriorly to the antero- inferior border of vomer, inter nasal crest superiorly and to the nasal crest of the maxilla and anterior nasal spine inferiorly.

## III) Floor :-

The floor of the nasal cavity is formed by palatine process of maxilla and two horizontal plates of palatine bone.

## IV) Roof :-

The roof of the nasal cavity is formed by 2 nasal bones, under surface of nasal spine of frontal bone, cribriform plate of ethmoid bone and under surface of body of sphenoid bone.

**Blood Supply of Septum & Nasal Cavity :-**

(From External and internal carotid artery).

1) Long speno palatine branch of the internal maxillary artery (Main blood supply to septum).

2) Anterior and posterior ethmoidal branches of the ophthalmic artery - supplies to upper part of lateral wall and upper and posterior part of septum.

3) Terminal branches of greater palatine artery supplies to antero inferior part of septum, floor and Lateral Wall.

4) Superior labial artery branch of facial artery supplies to septum and nasal alae .

**Note :-** Most of Blood vessels get anastamosed at anterio inferior part of septum called (keissel- bach's plexus) Little's area. This is the common site of Nasal bleeding.

**Venous drainage :-** Anteriorly into facial vein posteriorly into pharyngeal plexus of veins and middle part into pterygoid plexus. of veins.

**Nerve Supply :-**
**Respiratory Portion :-** Is supplied by
1) Anterior ethmoidal branch of nasociliary nerve 2) Spheno palatione Nerve 3) Greater palatine Nerve 4) Anterior superior dental nerve 5) Sympathetic and parasympathetic nerve fibres.

From the olfactery portion filaments pass through foramina of cribriform plate of ethmoid and end in the olfactery bulb.

**Lymphatic drainage :-**
External and anterior part of Nose into sub mandibular lymph nodes, Rest of the nose into deep cervical lymph nodes.

**Paranasal Sinuses :-**

Paranasal sinuses are the spaces filled up with air in certain skull bones in relation to nose, they are divided into 2 groups as follows

1) **Anterior group :-** a) Maxillary Sinuses (Antrum of high more)
b) Frontal sinuses.
c) Anterior group of ethmoidal sinuses.
these sinuses drains into middle meatus.

2) **Posterior group :-**
a) Posterior group of Ethmoidal sinuses. drains, into superior meatus.
b)Sphenoidal sinuses. drains into spheno ethmoidal recess.

All these sinuses are lined with respiratory epithelium (pseudo strati-fied columnar cilaited epithelium) The movement of the cilia in the para nasal sinuses is directed towards the nasal caivty.

1)    Maxillary sinus (Antrum of Highmore ) This is pyramidal cavity in the maxilla, sinus cavity may be divided into small spaces by bony septa it is the largest of the paranasal sinuses with 15CC capacity, Base lies medially and Apex lies in the zygomatic portion of maxilla. It has 5 walls. 1) Medial wall - Or base of the antrum is the part of lateral wall of Nose. Opening lies beneath the roof of the antrum medially so only un favourably placed for the drainage of cavity  2) Roof of the sinus is formed by the floor of the orbit It is grooved by infraorbital Neve. 3) Floor of the sinus lies about 1cm below the level of nasal cavity and is formed by alveolar process of maxilla - so there is every possibility for spreading of infection from pre molar and molar teeth roots. 4) Anterio lateral wall :- It is formed by anterior part of body of maxilla it contain-ing infra orbital foramin. 5) Posterior wall is formed by posterior surface of maxilla, it separates the sinus from pterigo palitine fossa.

The opening of maxillary sinus is in the posterior part of the haitus semilunaris between bulla ethmoidalis and the uncinate process of ethmoid bone,on the lateral wall of nose.  below. the middle turbinate.
**Blood Supply :-** Infra orbital facial and greater palatine arteries.
**Nerve Supply :-** Infra orbital Nerve and anterior posterior alveolar nerves
**Lymphatic drainage** - sub mandibular and Retro pharngeal Nodes.

## Frontal Sinuses :-
Frontal sinus capacity is Icc, it has 3 walls, the 2 sinuses are unequall is size and are separated by medial wall.

**1)    Anterior wall** Formed by the outer table of frontal bone 2) Posterior wall is thin and seperates the sinus from cranial fossa. 3) Floor is formed by a thin bone separating  the sinus from the orbit.
Frontal sinus is drained by the fronto nasal duct which opens in the anterior part of themiddle meatus.
**Blood Supply :-** Supra orbital artery.
**Nerve Supply :-** Supra orbital nerve.
**Lymphatic drainage :-** Sub mandibular lymph nodes.

## Ethmoidal sinuses :-
There are 3 groups of ethmoidal sinuses having approximately 15 to20 ethmoidal cells on either sides, They occupy the ethmoidal bone. Anterior, middle They occupy the ethmoidal bone. Anterior, middle ethmoidal cells drains in the middle meatus and posterior ethmoidal cells drains into the superior meatus .

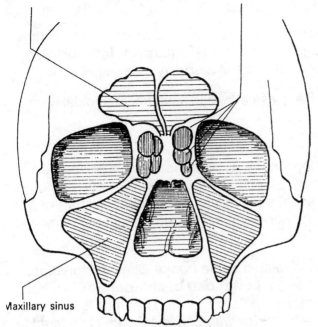

Maxillary sinus

Relationship of nasal sinuses (anterior view)

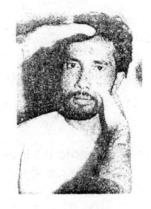

Testing for tenderness of maxillary sinus

Frontal sinus

Ethmoidal sinuses

Sphenoidal sinus

Line of edge of middle turbinate

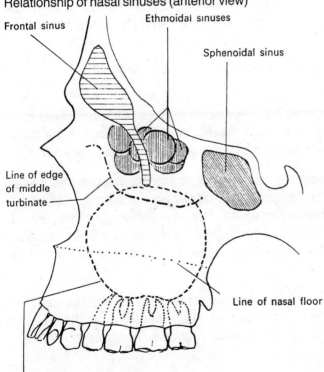

Line of nasal floor

Line of maxillary sinus

Relationship of nasal sinuses. Note relation of tooth roots to maxillary antrum.

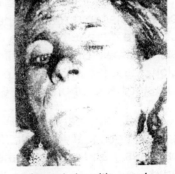

Acute frontal sinusitis causing cellulitis of the eye lids

**Relations :-**
**Superiorly -** Cranial fossa, **laterally** orbit, optic nerve and naso lacrimal duct. **medially** Nasal cavity, superior and middle turbinates. **inferiorly** maxillary sinus, **posteriorly** sphenoidal sinus. **Anteriorly** external nose.

These sinuses are supplied by anterior and posterior ethmoidal Nerves and vessels.

**The Sphenoidal Sinus ;-**
Sphenoid sinuses develops in the body of the spenoid bone, the two sinuses are unequally divided by a septum, the capacity of each sinus is about 1cc. The opening of the sinuses is situated in the upper part of the anterior wall, it drains in the superior meatus through the sphenoethmoidal recess.

**Superiorly :-** The sinus is related to the frontal lobe olfactory tracts, optic chaisma, pitutory body and pons. **Lower part of anterior** wall is related to vessels and nerves from the spheno palatine fossa. **The floor** is related to nasopharynx with **Vidian** nerve. **Posterior wall** or basisphenoid is related to the basilar artery and brain stem. **Lateral wall** is related to the cavernous sinus with intenal carotid artery and optic nerve. **anteriorly** related to Nasal cavity .

## PHYSIOLOGY OF NOSE AND PARANASAL SINUSES

**Functions of the Nose :-**
1) Respiration - inspired air passess upwards in a narrow stream medial to the middle turbinate and then down wards and back wards in the form of an arc,mouth breathing is an acquired lesion due to the nasal obstruction.

2) Olfaction :- The olfactory mucosa is located in roof of the nasal cavity adjacent area to superior turbinate and upper part of septum.Olfactory cells are distributed in the olfactory mucosa. The exact theory of olfaction is still unknown But the odoriferous material reaches the olfactory area by diffusion, the olfactory cells are stimulated and carries the smell sensation to the olfactory bulb of brain.

3) Purification of (Filtration) inspired air carried out by **vibrissae** (Nasal hair ) of nasal vestibule (filter the coarse particles), cilia (remove the smaller particles ) and by lysozyme enzyme of nasal mucosa (Anti bacterial property).

4) Warming and moistening of cold and dry inspired air (Air conditioning occurs) before reaching the lungs by the highly vasculared Nasal mucosa, if not causes damage to the respiratory tract.

5) Resonance is added to the voice by the nasal cavity and paranasal sinuses and there are also responsible for pronouncing the nasal consonants like M. and N.

6) The Nose acts as the out let (Drainage cavity) for paranasal sinuses and lacrimal apparatus.

7) Nose acts as the ventilating shaft for the Eustachian tube for the equalisation of pressure of air between the external atmosphere and the middle ear cavity through the eustachian tube .

8) Reflexes like sneezing have a protective function on exposure to irritaants the respiration may be stopped temporarily to protect the respiratory tract.

## FUNCTIONS OF PARANASAL SINUSES

The exact functions of the paranasal sinuses are uncertain. But perfrom the following functions.

1) Protection to the orbit
2) Reducing the skull weight (lightening)
3) Resonance of Voice.
4) Respiratory and air conditioning function up to some extent.
5) Rapid growth of face due to formation of sinuses.
6) Sinus mucosa acts as donar site for reconstructive procedures.
   Ex. implantation of maxillary sinus mucosa into nasal cavity in atrophic rhinitis
7) Increase surface area for teeth eruption.

# NASA PAREEKSHA

Examination of Nose according to Ayurvedic texts.

According to Ayurveda there is no special description of Nasa pareeksha. But in general the description is available like.

1) Bahir srotopareeksha (Nose and and nasalcanal)

II) Ghrana indria Pareeksha (one among panchendria)

1) Bahir sroto pareeksha includes the common examination of Nose for its size shape position function in this most of points will be covered except.nerve perception.

Ex : -

      1) Nasal secretory lesions (Rhinitis) pratishyaya, peenasa, puthi nasya, Puyaraktha etc.

      2) Obstructive lesions, Nasa pratinaha, Arsha, grandhi, vidradi, arbuda

      3) Inflammatory lessions - (Nasa paka, deepthi)

      4) Atrophic lesions - (Nasa sosha)

      5) Asatmyaja (Allergic) - (kshavathu)

      6) Abhighataja - Traumatic lesions etc.

I) Ghrana indria pareeksha ( test for olfaction)

      a) Normal smell sensation

      b) Reduced smell sensation (Hena yoga) (Hyposmia)

      c) Unpleasant change in smell (Mithyayoga) (Parosmia)

      d) Exaggerated smell sensation (Atiyoga) - (Hyperosmia)

      e) Loss of smell sensation (Ayoga) (Anosmia)

So Indria vikar is explained according to hena midiya Ati and Ayoga but the exact etiological factors and methods of examination are not explained.

## EXAMINATION OF THE NOSE AND PARANASAL SINUSES

An acurate history of the patient is essential for the correct diagnosis , so the origin duration and progress of each of the following nasal symptoms should be enquired and examined to get a fair idea about the disease, among the following symptoms few or total may present according to the condition of the disease they are,

1) Rhinorrhoea (Nasal discharge) 2) Blocking cf Nose.
3)Sneezing 4) Epistaxis 5) Head ache 6) Disorders of olfaction
7) Post nasal drip 8)Speach defects 9) Nasal pain
10)Symptoms due to extention of the disease.

### 1) Rhinorrhoea :-

Discharge from the nose may be unilateral or bilateral, it may be watery, mucoid, muco-purulent, purulent or Blood stained.

a) Watery discharge is usually found in the early stages of common cold, vaso motor rhinitis and C.S.F. Rhinorrhoea.

b) Mucoid discharge is usually a feature of allergic rhinitis.

144

c) Muco purulent discharge is a feature of infective rhinitis and sinusitis.

d) Purulent discharge is a feature of atrophic rhinitis, furunculosis and foreign bodies in the nose.

e) Blood stained nasal discharge usually indicates malignancy, old foreign body, rhinolith, nasal diphtheria, rhinosporidiasis etc.

## AETIOLOGY OF NASAL DISCHARGE

| Unilateral causes | Bilateral causes |
|---|---|
| 1) Old foreign body in the nose in children | 1) Nasal allergy-Vasomotor rhinitis |
| 2) Unilateral sinusitis | 2) Bilateral sinusitis |
| 3) Unilateral choanal atresia | 3) Bilateral choanal atresia |
| 4) Antro choanal Polyp | 4) Ethmoidal polyp |
| 5) Rhinosporidiasis | 5) Atrophic Rhinitis |
| 6) C.S.F. rhinorrhoea | 6) Enlarged adenoids |
| 7) Neoplasms | 7) Diphtheritic rhinitis |
| 8) Rhinolith | 8) Specific Rhinitis |

## 2) BLOCKING OF NOSE

The following points should be enquired and examined.

a) Onset is whether congenital (By birth), or acquired (Polyp - DNS Allergy)

b) If persistent obstruction (Adenoids,D.N.S,polyp) or Temporary obstruction(Allergy)

c) If unilateral or Bilateral

## AETILOGY OF NASAL OBSTRUCTION

| Unilateral obstructive causes | Bilateral obstructive causes |
|---|---|
| 1) Congenital - unilateral choanal atresia, Atresia of Anterior nares. | Congenital - Bilateral choanal atresia. |
| 2) D.N.S. | 2) Ethmoidal polyp |
| 3) Antro choanal polyp | 3) Nasal allergy (vasomotor rhinitis) |
| 4) Foreign body or Rhinolith | 4) Acute rhinitis and sinusitis |
| 5) Unilateral sinusitis | 5) Chronic sinusitis (Bilateral) |
| 6) Synechia | 6) Diphtheritic rhinitis |
| 7) Hypertrophy of inferior turbinate | 7) Atrophic rhinitis |
| 8) Rhinosproridiosis (unilateral) | 8) Enlarged adenoids |
| 9) Neoplasms | 9) NeoPlasms |
| | 10) Rhinosporidiosis (Bilateral) |
| | 11) Antro choanal Polyp (rarely) |
| | 12) Septal abscess |
| | 13) Specific infection. |
| | 14) Rhinitis medicamentosa. |

## 3) Sneezing :-

Sneezing is the normal nasal reflex to clear the secretion from the nose but some times due to constant nasal mucosal irritation with infection, Allergy, exposure to cold, heat, polluted air, noxious gases etc. causes the abnormal sneezing.

**4) Epistaxis :-** Bleeding per Nose occurs due to so many causes, the common causative factors are injury to head or Nose, hypertension Blood dyscrasias ,nasal picking due to nasal irritation, sunstroke etc., The bleeding may be unilateral or Bilateral

(The little's area of nose due to its high vascularity (multi vessels anastamosis) prone to bleeding due to irritative factors)

## 5) Headache :-

Head ache due to nasal and paransal diseases commonly associate with cold, nasal discharge, nasal obstruction etc symptoms

**Ex:-** 1) Vaccum head ache, due to nasal obstruction in which the air is packed in the sinuses and causes pain.

2) In frontal sinusitis in the early morning fore head pain present that reduces after sunrise.

3) Sphenoidal sinusitis causes head ache at occiput

4) maxillary sinusitis and ethmoidal sinusitis causes head ache at their site.

## 6) Disorders of Olfaction :-

a) Hyposmia ;- Diminished smell sensation due to old age, menopause, tobacco habit etc causes.

b) Anosmia ;- Loss of smell snesation due to obstructive lesions of nose, central lesions of brain and Lesions of mucosa, and due to trauma etc.

c) Parosmia - Unpleasant change in smell sensation due to skull fracture, streptomycin therapy etc causes.

d) Hyperosmia - Exaggeration of the olfactory sensitivity due to Epilepsy, pregnancy, hunger, strychnine poisoning etc causes.

e) Cacosmia - perception of foul smell due to the internal causes like maxillary sinusitis, dental sepsis, pus in the middle ear and lung abscess etc. cause.

## 7) Post nasal drip and Hawking -

It is common in adenoids sinusitis (Allergic and infective lesions of Nose and para nasal sinuses ) and produces pharyngeal symptoms.

## 8) Speech defects :-

Disorders of nose and para nasal sinuses may cause loss of resonating function leads to Nasal voice (Nasal intonation or Rhinolalia.)

# AETIOLOGY OF RHINOLALIA

**Rhinolalia clausa**
1) It is due to lesions of Nose,Naso pharynx, & paranasal Sinuses.
2) Nasal obstruction occurs due to
Nasal polyp, Hypertrophied turbinates, DNS, Rhinitis medicamentosa, growths
3) Nasopharyngeal obstruction due to
Adenoids, Nasopharyngeal fibroma, Nasopharyngeal mass.
4) Choanal atresia

**Rhinolalia aperta**
1) It is due to palatal lesions
2) cleft palate
3) Palatal paralysis
4) Sub mucous cleft palate
5) Congenital short palate
6) Some times after adenoidectomy.
7) Palatal Cicatrisation.
8) Palatal perforation

**9)** **Nasal Pain -** due to vestibulitis, trauma furunculosis, cellulitis of Nose, Neuralgia and caries teeth.
**10)** Symptoms due to extension of the disease to the adjacent regions like orbit, cranium, cavernous sinus etc. and produce symptoms of respective parts.

## EXAMINATION OF EXTERNAL NOSE

### Inspection & Palpation :-
Normally Nose appears pyramidal in shape, nasal bridge should be straight, centrally placed on the dorsum of the nose, (bilateral symmetrical) with centrally placed septum, equal size of Anterior nares and nasal cavities
But due to congenital developmental traumatic and inflammatory causes it may become Asymmetrical or deformed, ex:- depressed, bridge, Broadened nose, swellings, polyps, scars and sinus etc.
**Ex :-**
a) Broadened nose - due to congenital developmental Traumatic and due to nasal polyps and malignancy
b) Deformed Nose - Due to congenital, traumatic causes and also due to leprosy
c) Depressed Nasal bridge - due to Congenital traumatic and due to syphilis.
d) Woody feeling of Nose due to Rhinoscleroma
e) Potato nose in Rhinophyma
f) Stenosed anterior nares in Rhino scleroma

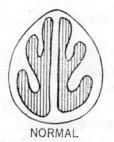
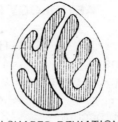

NORMAL          'C' SHAPED DEVIATION

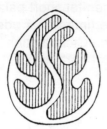
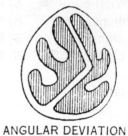

ANGULAR DEVIATION

—Deviation of the Septum.

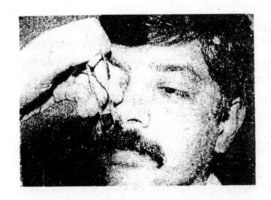

Anterior rhinoscopy with Thudichum nasal speculum

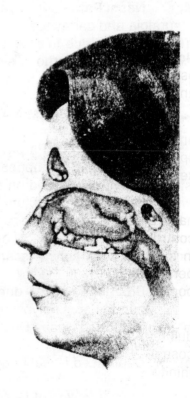

Pus discharge from various paranasal sinuses

g) Scars - Traumatic and surgical
h) A sinus in mid line of Dorsum of Nose is congenital
i) Vestibule should be carefully examined for swellings furuncle ulcer crust etc.
j) Displaced Anterior end of septum may be projecting in to vestibule due to traumatic causes.
k) By Crepitations of Nasal bones fracture can be detected.

## Examination Nasal Cavity

**Anterior Rhinoscopy :-**

Examination of Anterior part of the Nasal vestibule is usually done (without a nasal speculum ) by raising up the tip of the nose for inspection of redness swelling as in furunculosis and dislocated anterior end of the septum projecting into vestibule.

While the examination of Anterior part of Nasal cavity with nasal speculum, the following structures can be seen (by Anterior rhinoscopy)
1) Vestibule of the nose
2) Nasal septum and Little's area
3) Inferior and middle turbinates and meatus (superior turbinate and meatus cannot be seen)
4) Floor of the nasal cavity.

**Note :-** Initial examination of nasal vestibule without nasal speculum is necessary otherwise the blades of speculum may injure the papillomas cysts and bleeding points of the region if any.

The Anterior Rhinoscopy is carried out using a head mirror Light sourse and Thudicum's speculum or st clair Thomsons speculum with a handle. The speculums are in different sizes. the speculum must be held in left hand keeping the right hand free for Manipulations.

The thudicum's speculum is held with the thumb and forefinger of left hand, the middle finger rests on one side and ring finger on the other side to controle the spring of the speculum. The closed speculum should introduced in to nasal canal and the blades of the speculum are gradually opened to permit proper examination of the nose. The floor lateral wall septum and posterior portions of nasal cavity are Veiwed .

The colour of the nasal mucosa should be examined, in normal it is dull red but in inflammatory lesions becomes congested, pale or bluish mucosa in Allergic conditions and dry mucosa with crusting is seen in atrophic rhinitis etc.

Septal deviations or spures and perforations of septum should be examined.

149

Inferior and middle turbinates appear as prominent fleshy, firm and red projections on the lateral wall, these donot move on probing, the turbinates get shrinken or dried in atrophic rhinitis and grossly hypertrophied in chronic rhinitis, vasomotor rhinitis and in allergic rhinitis . The inferior and middle meati should examine for redness, polypi and for discharge, A postural test may be done to note the probable site of origin of discharge (clean the pus from the middle meatus if it reaccumulates quickly it indicates that pus is coming from frontal sinus, if the patients head is turned to the normal side and kept for some time if pus reaccumulates at middle meatus that is coming from maxillary sinus).

The floor of the nasal cavity is seen as a concave tunnel

Nasal cavity is examined whether the space is equall on both sides or obstructed. Assessment of airway is done by Keeping a cold glass slide or metallic tongue deppressor just infront of the nostrils. on expiration the warm air produces an area of condensation on the surface, the difference on the two sides is an indication of nasal obstruction. the air blast can also be compared by watching the degree of movement of wisp of cotton woool held infront of the nostril

**Abnormal findings in Anterior Rhinoscopy :-**
1) DNS, 2) Septal perforation 3) Polyps 4) cyst or tumours 5) Congested or Atrophied or Hypertrophied or pale mucosa 6) Watery or mucoid. or mucopurulent or purulent or blood stained, or foul nasal discharge 7) foreign bodies or Rhinoliths. 8) unilateral or bilateral lesions 9) probing should be performed gently for polyps, pedunculated masses, foreign bodies and Rhinoliths. 10) Obstruction of the air way (Rhinomanometry).11) In hyper trophied nasal mucosa for better examination topical decongestant drops are instilled.

**Examination of Oral Cavity in Relation to Nasal Paranasal diseases**
a) Gingio buccal sulcus should be inspected for oro antral fistula (communication between oral cavity and maxillary sinus)

b) Soft palate should be examined for bulging down wards due to mass in the naso pharynx like tumour, antrochoanal polyps.

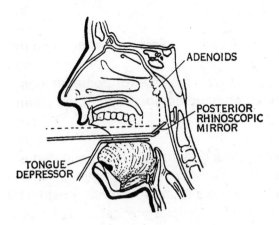

The Posterior Rhinoscopy

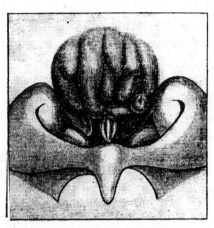

Posterior rhinoscopic view of adenoids and
Eustachian cushion

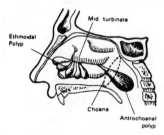

Diagram of nasal polypi

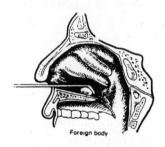

Technique of removing a nasal foreign body

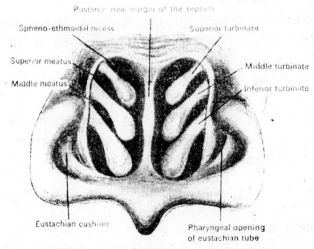

Structures seen by Posterior Rhinoscopy

## Posterior Rhinoscopy :-

Examination of posterior parts of Nasal cavity is known as posterior rhinoscopy .

Posterior rhinoscopy is performed with the help of posterior rhinoscopic mirror, it is slightly difficulty method need co operation of the patient and experience to perform.

**Method :-** The patient is asked to open the mouth, a tongue depressor is used with left hand to depress the anterior 2/3 of the tongue, patient is advised to breath quietly through the nose and relax. A warmed post nasal mirror is held in the right hand and passed into oropharynx between the posterior pharyngeal wall and soft palate without touching (if the mirror touches the soft palate, palatal arches posterior 1/3 of tongue or posterior pharyngeal wall it causes reflex gaging) light is focussed on the mirror then the reflected image of post nasal cavity and nasal pharynx will be seen, the following points can be seen as the reflected image.

1) The Posterior end of free margin of septum.
2) On either sides to septum posterior choanae are seen.
3) Posterior ends of turbinates, superior, middle meati, maxillary, posterior ethmoidal and sphenoidal sinus secretions are seen.
4) Antro choanal polyp may be seen as a greyish pale smooth swelling coming from choanae into Naso pharynx ..
5) Superior surface of soft palate is seen with secretions, newgrowths, polyps ,foreign bodes etc
6) Laterally Eustachian, choanal openings, Pharyngo tympanic tubes with tubal tonsils, the site is behind the posterior end of inferior turbinates on either sides .
7) Fossa Rosen muller is the frequent site of malignancy is seen behind the eustachian tubes.
8) Inflamed adenoids in children may be visualised as a pinkish mass at the junction of roof and posterior pharyngeal wall .
9) Roof of Nasopharynx can be seen.

Children cannot give co-operation for this examination.

## Electrical Nasopharyngoscopy :-

Electrical Nasopharyngoscope is passed through nasal cavity and Nasopharynx and the lesions can be seen directly.

## Digital Palpation of the Post nasal space and Naso Pharynx :-

The cheek of the patient is pressed in between the jaws (after the mouth has been opened) with the left hand of doctor so as to prevent the biting or closure of the jaw the examiner should stand on the right side of the paient then pass the fingers of the right hand behind the soft palate into the Naso pharynx (It is needed in doubtful cases of malignancy of Naso pharynx and in children for adenoids.) to palpate the lesions, if any.

## Examination of Nasopharynx with retracted soft palate :-

Rubber catheter should insert into oropharynx from the nose and the two ends tied togher this retracts the soft palate and thus allows a direct view of the Naso pharynx.

## Trans illumination test  for sinuses :-

It is specially for maxillary and frontal sinuses, It is conducted in a dark room by illuminating the oral cavity with low voltage torch when the mouth is closed thelight transmitted if seen through the walls of sinus, they are normal. if  not diseased . No body is follwing this technique Now a days due to the availablity of X-ray.

## Palpation for tenderness of  the para nasal sinuses :-

a) In maxillary sinusitis tenderness is elicited on the canine fossa at the cheek.

b) In frontal sinusitis tenderness is elicited just above the inner canthus of the eye (medial portion of floor of the sinus)

c) In Anterior ethomoidal sinusitis tenderness is elicited at the midway between inner canthus of eye and Nose.

d) Rest of the sinuses are deeply seated so tenderness cannot be palpated.

## Posture test :-

It is for the differential diagnosis of frontal sinusitis and maxillary sinusitis

Pus should be cleaned at the middle meatus if it reaccumulates quickly that is coming from **frontal sinus**. If the patient's head is turned to the normal side and Kept for some time, if pus accumulates that is from **maxillary sinus**.

Radiograpy - Sinogram sinoscopy confirms the diagnosis.

# NASA ROGA SAMANYA NIDANAM :
## ( Common Aetiology of Nasal diseases )

" Nasahi shiraso dwaram "

Nose is only the gate way for the drug administration or for the elimination of doshas from the head. so only having utmost importance among the all.

Two nostrils are exposed to the atmosphere for smell sensation and respiration so only prone to attacks of bacteria, virus, fungus, allergic reactions, degenerative changes, injuries etc.

The few common aetiolgical factors are here under.

| | | | |
|---|---|---|---|
| 1) | Vegava rodha | - | Suppressing the natural urges. |
| 2) | Ajeerna | - | Indigestion |
| 3) | Rajo sevana | - | Exposing to dust |
| 4) | Ati bhashya | - | more talking |
| 5) | Pralapa | - | Irrelavant talking. |
| 6) | ucchiir bhashana | - | Loud talking. |
| 7) | Krodha | - | Anger |
| 8) | Rutu Viparyaya | - | Seasonal changes or Apatya in the seasons |
| 9) | Shirobhitapa | - | Head Exposing to sun storke. |
| 10) | Nishi jagara | - | Awakening (not sleeping) at night |
| 11) | Diwa swapna | - | Sleeping in the day time. |
| 12) | Sheeta ambu panam | - | Drinking cold water, cold drinks, ice etc. |
| 13) | Avashyaya | - | Exposing to snow or Moisture |
| 14) | Ati miithuna | - | Indulging more sex. |
| 15) | Bhaspa Sevana | - | Exposing to vapours or Fumes |
| 16) | Dhooma sevana | - | Exposing to Vapours or fumer |
| 17) | Ucchitha shira shayana | - | Resting the head in height during sleeping. |
| 18) | Neecha shira shayana | - | Resting the head down wards while sleeping. |
| 19) | Pravasa | - | Change of place or atmosphere by tours |
| 20) | Abhighatha | - | Injury to Nose or head |
| 21) | Krimi | - | worm infestation or infection |
| 22) | Diving in impure water | - | |
| 23) | Inhaling the poisonous flowers | | |
| 24) | Nasal picking. | | |

25) Nasal Foreign bodies
26) Ati vyayama          -          Doing more exercise
27) Shoka          -          Weeping.
28) Systemic infections (TB syphilis leprosy etc.)
29) Peripheral infective lesions like tonsils, Adenoids, Pharyngitis etc.
30) Inhaling teekshna vidaha dravyas
31) Beeja dosha - Heriditory causes
32) Congenital causes 33) Cranial neuralgia 34) Malnutrition and Hypo vitaminosis 35) Indiopathic causes, By above causes vatadi doshas vitiate and accumulate in the head and causes Nasa rogas.

## Common Prepdisposing factors of Nasa rogas in brief :-

1) ill health 2) General debility 3) Chronic systemic diseases like TB syphilis leprosy etc. 4) Head and Nasal injuries 5) Allergic factors like, Dust smoke vapour cold exposures, inhaling poisonous flowers, seasonal changes etc 6) Inflammatory lesions by bacteria or virus or fungus 7) Peripheral infective foccus like tonsilitis Adenoids contageous eye infections 8) Irritative factors other than allergy, like Nasal picking or foreign bodies.

## Classification of Nasal Diseases :-

1) According to sushrutha Nasal diseases are 31
2)          "          Bhavamishra and yogaratnakar 34 diseases.
3)          "          Vagbhata  18 diseases
4)          "          Charak - no specific number is mentioned.

1) Sushrutha's Classification of nasal diseases  = 31
they are,
1) Apeenasa or peenasa (Atrophic rhinitis)
2) Puthi nasya or puthi nasa ( Ozaena Or atrophic rhinitis)
3) Nasa paka or Ghrana paka  (furunculosis or vestibulitis)
4) Shonitha pitta or Raktha Pitta (Epistaxis)
5) Puya shonitha or puya raktha (Lupus in the nose, chronic rhinitis)
6) Kshavathu or kshava (Vasomotor rhinitis or Allergic rhinitis)
7) Bramshathu (Mucoid discharge from the thickened mucosa of sinus.
8) Dheeptha or Deepthi (burning irritation in the nose) .
9) Nasanaha or prathinaha (Deviation of Nasal septum ).
10) Parisrava (rhinorrhoea)
11) Nasa sosha (Atrophic rhinitis or Rhinitis sicca )
12 to 15,  4 types of Nasa arsha (Polyps of the nose)
16 to 19, 4 types of sopha (Oedema in nasalcavity
20 to 26  7, types of arbuda (Tumours or growths of the nose)
27 to 31, 5 types of pratishyaya of the nose (Rhinitis)

**2)According to Bhava mishra and yogaranakar 34 Nasal diseases,**
they are,
Nasa Raktha pitta is 4 types According to these authors - but only one according to sushrutha so 3 diseases more than sushrutha ie - 31 + 3 = 34.

**3) Accordig to Vagbhata 18 diseases.**

| | Bhavamishra | Vagbhata |
|---|---|---|
| 1) | Arsha 4 types | One type so 3 less |
| 2) | Shopha 4 types | Note explained so 4 less |
| 3) | Arbuda 7 types | one type so 6 less |
| 4) | Raktha Pitta 4 type | not explained so 4 less |
| 5) | Bramshathu 1 type | not explained so  1 less. |

Vagbhata reduced = 18 diseases

so,  34 -18=16, then he added
17)     Dusta Pratishyaya
18)     Putaka.
Total List the diseases of nose as per Vagbhata
1)      Apeenasa 2) Puthinasya 3) Nasa Paka 4) Brusha kshava 5) Deepthi 6) Nasanaha 7) Parisrava 8) Puya shoonitha 9) Nasa sosha 10) Nasa arsha 11) Nasa arbuda 12) Dusta Pratishyaya 13) Putaka, (14 to 18,) 5 types of pratishyaya.

**4)      According to Charak**

He has not mentioned the total list of the diseases but explained more than 20 diseases.

# 1 to 5) PRATISHYAYA (Rhinitis)

**Defination :-**
A) 1) " Vatam Prati abhimukham shyayo gamanam Kaphaadeenam yatra sa pratishyayah "

Prathi = Opposite direction (means to out side)
Shyaya = Moment of the doshas.( elmination of dosha)

i.e. - Kaphadi doshas are eliminated out through the nose, is known as pratishyaya.

2) " Prati kshanam shyayathi ithi Pratishyayah "
Kaphadi doshas are Continuously eliminated out through the nose so only called as Pratishyaya.

## B) Importance of Pratishyaya :-

It is explained as the most improtant disease among the nasa roga. charaka explained that if the disease is not treated properly or neglected, causes so many complications of Nose, ear, throat, head, eye and other parts of the body.

**Ex :-** Dusta Pratishyaya, kshavathu, Nasa sosha, Pratinaha, Parisrava, Puthi nasa, apeenasa, Nasa Paka, shotha, arbuda, puyaraktha, Aroomshika, shiro roga, Karna roga, Netraroga, Khalithya, Arjuna, swasa, Kasa, Jwara, Raktha pitta, swarabhedha, sosha, Andhatwa, Bhadirya, agnimandya, Aghranatwam (Anosmia ) etc.,

## C) Nidana (Aetiologoy ) :-

The common aetiological factors of Nasa roga are really explained for pratishyaya only, this shows the importance of pratishyaya among the nasa rogas, once again the aetiological factors are given in brief.

1) Tridosha vitiating factors

ex in take of cold things, exposure to rain, snowfall, swimming in water, taking in-compatible food etc.

2) Mano dosha vitiating factors.

ex Excessive Anger, fear etc.

3) Abhighataj Karana (injuries)

shiro abhighata - nasa abhighata etc.

4) Irritative factors or Allergic factors

ex exposure to dust, smoke, exposure to cold wind or sunstroke etc.

5) Because of other chronic diseases (specific infections)

ex Tuberculois, Leprosy, syphilis etc.

6) Debilitative factors :-

ex ill health, weak personality, loss of immunity, low socio economic status, living in unhygienic surroundings etc.

7) peripheral lesions (due to mucosal continuity) pharyngeal, laryngeal, oral, auricular, blood borne infections etc.

**Note :-**" The Description is given at common aetiological factors (samanya Nidana ) of Nasa roga.

**Poorva roopa of Pratishyaya :-**

1)Shirogurutwam (heavyness of the head)  2)Kshavathu (Sneezing) 3) Angamarda (Body pains) 4)Romaharsha (Horripulations)5) Jwara (Fever) 6) Aruchi (Tastelessness) 7) Shirashoola (Head ache) 8) Ashrusrava (Lacrimation) 9) Netra Kandu (itching sensation at inner canthus especially) 10) Burning or itching sensation in nasal cavity 11) Taludarana (Dryness and crackings in the palate 12) Lala srava (salivation) 13) Dryness of throat etc.

**E) Samprapthi of Pratishyaya :-**

The vitiated vatadi doshas either individually or together accumulates in the shiras, then propogates to the nose and causes the Pratishyaya etc diseases.

**F) Bhedas :-** Types of pratishyaya, 5 types they are :-
1) Vataj Pratishyaya 2) Pittaja Pratishyaya
3) Kaphaj Pratishyaya 4) Raktaj  Pratishyaya
5) Sannipathaj Pratishyaya.

**1) Vataja Pratishyaya (Sub acute Rhinitis)**

**Clinical Features :-**

1) Nasal obstruction 2) Watery ,cold, fresh, nasal discharge 3) Dryness in the throat Lips and Palate 4) Pain and discomfort in the nose 5) Increased sneezing. 6) Pricking pain at teeth, Temporal region and in head 7) Chira Paka (Delayed suppuration of doshas ) 8) Distaste in the mouth 9) Hoarseness of the voice 10) charaka explained these symptoms under vataj peenasa - so according to charak pratishyaya and peenasa are one and same.

**2) Pittaja Pratishyaya (Acute Rhinitis)**

**Clinical features :-**
1)      Yellowish or reddish hot nasal discharge.
2)      The person becomes weak and anaemic
3)      High temparature (Fever) causes severe burning pain in the nose mouth and throughout the body
4)      Thirst
5)      Nasal furunculosis or ulceration
6)      Giddiness
7)      Becomes inactive tired and weak.

## 3) Kaphaj Pratishyaya (Chronic or Hypertrophic rhinitis )
### Clinical Features :-
1) Cool whitish thick nasal discharge comes from nose .
2) Heaviness in themouth and head .
3) Anaemia (Pale or whitish skin)
4) Oedema of eye and its appendages
5) Severe itching sensation in the head throat- Palate and lips.
6) Cough 7) Sweet taste in the mouth 8) Difficulty in respiration
9) Heavyness of the body 10) Vomitings (vomitis the Kapham).

## 4) RAKTAJ PRATISHYAYA
(Acute Rhinitis Or Acute influenza)

### Clinical Features :-
1) Hyperaemia of eye (Conjunctiva)
2) Blood stained nasal discharge or bleeding from the nose.
3) Foul smell through nose and mouth .
4) Loss of smell sensation (Anosmia)
5) Manifestation of small magots in the nose 6) Chest Pain 7) Fever
8) Cough 9) Severe discomfort and itching sensation
10) Signs and symptoms of Krimija shiro roga.

## 5) Sannipathaja Pratishyaya :-
or Tridoshaja Pratishyaya

### Clinical Features :-
1) Frequent attacks of Common cold.
2) Kaphadi doshas some times suppurates and some times doesn't suppurate (Apakwa or Pakwa ).
3) Severe Pain in the Nose and head.
4) The symptoms are like peenasa
5) All the symptoms of three doshas present.
6) It is explained as Asadya (incurable).

## DUSTA PRATISHYAYA

Sushrutha explained it as the complication of pratishyaya so not counted separately But vagbhata expalined it in addition to the 5 types of pratishyaya.

**Clinical Features :-**
1) Some times nasal discharge comes and some times nose get dried.
2) some times nose obstructed and some times normal .
3) Foul smell exhibited while respiration
4) Anosmia loss of smell sensation)
5) Kasta sadya vyadhi (difficult for cure)

Charaka described it in detail, according to him it occurs as a complication of pratishyaya, the clinical features are sneezing, dryness of nose, Nasal obstruction Rhinorrhoea, foulsmell from nose and mouth, Rhinitis, furunculois, oedema of Nasal mucosa, tumours of nose, blood stained mucopurulent discharge, ulcers, shiro roga (diseases of head), ear diseases, eye diseases, Bald head (Khalithya), Grey hair (Phalitha), thirst, Tiredness, cough, fever, Bleeding disorders, Hoarse Voice and Dehydration (sosha) etc.,

Sushrutha also explained that if Pratishyaya is not treated in time leads to Dusta Pratishyaya and assoicated with Deafness, Blindness, Anosmia cough, Loss of appetite and oedema etc.,

So for having so many complications it is said as Kasta sadya (difficult for cure) vyadhi.

### PEENASA - APEENASA - PRATISHYAYA

1) Most of the acharyas said that peenasa and apeenasa are same with wording difference and also said this is the chronic or progressive stage of pratishyaya.

2) Vagbhats said peenasa and apeenasa are different but these two are chronic or progressive stages of pratishyaya.

3) Vagbhata said that Apeenasa contain pain, ghur ghur noises in the nose and sticky nasal discharge more than peenasa.

ie. Symptoms are more complicated with more obstructive lesions in nose as follows.

The order of severity is -- "Appeenasa > Peenasa > Pratishyaya".

1)      Pratishyaya Contain less complications and with running nose (no Sensory loss).

2)      Peenasa contain more complications than pratishyaya with sticky nasal discharge .

3)      Apeenasa contain more complications and more obstructive lesions than peenasa ( Anosmia and other Indria vikara are observed).

But according to sushrutha above peenasa and Apeenasa are one and same and said it is as the complication of pratishyaya (sannipathaja Pratishyaya symptoms are equalant to peenasa).

## 6) APEENASA ACCORDING TO SUSHRUTHA :-

1) Symptoms of pratishyaya present, additionally following points are observed .

2) Vitiated Kapha causes stickynasal discharge .

3) Vitiated Pitta causes dryness, burning sensation and nasal obstruction

4) Vitiated Vata causes lesion of sensory organs (Indriavikar.) Like Anosmia (loss of smell sensation)  and pain.

### Apeenasa According to Vagbhata .

Vitiated Kapha causes nasal obstructon, ghur ghur noises in the nose, difficulty in respiration, yellowish sticky discharge oozes (Singhanakam) continuously and also causes loss of smell sensation, is explained as Apeenasa, the severity is more than peenasa and Pratishyaya.

### Other Authors :-

The Kapha dosha of mastishka get dried or burnt by pitta and produces blood stained nasal discharge with pain itching and burning sensation.

### Kartheek:-

Apeenasa and peenasa are one and same but samprapthi (Aetiopathology) is different.

### Bhavamishra - yogaratnaker :-

Pratishyaya if infected by Krimi produces the similar symptoms  of Krimija shiro roga in Apeenasa.

# APAKWA PEENASA OR NAVA PRATISHYAYA OR AMA PEENASA
### (According to Vruddha sushruth )

**Clinical features :-**

1) Aruchi (taste lessness) 2) Vairasya (Un pleasant taste in the mouth)
3) Nasa srava (Rhinorrhoea)
4) Body Pains 5) Arathi (restless ness)
6) Shiro gurutwam (Heaviness of head) 7) Kshavathu (sneezes) 8) Jwara
(Fever) 9) Amam 10) Symptoms of Nava or Taruna pratishyaya or Acute Rhinitis are present.

11) According to madhavakar- Hoarse or reduced voice, and Nishteevana
(Spitting) Explained additionally to the above.

**Pakwa Peenasa or Pakwa Pratishyaya**

According to **Vruddha sushrutha .**

1)      Tastelessness and un pleasant taste, reduces.
2)      Body pains reduces.
3)      Lightness in the head.
4)      Normal tone of the voice.
5)      Nasal discharge becomes sticky and yellowish .

**Note :-** The knowledge of Ama & Pakwa stages of peenasa is essential for
the treatment.

## PRATISHYAYA SAMANYA CHIKITSA
### (Common treatment principlesof pratishyaya)

While giving treatment for pratishyaya it is very important to know
whether the disease is in Ama stage (nava Pratishyaya ) or in pakwa stage
(jeerna pratishyaya)

## Nava Pratishyaya or Ama pratishayaya Chikitsa

1) Langhana for 3 to 5 days
2) Swedana
3) Administration of Deepan pachan drugs.
4) "      " Amla ushna teekshna drugs or diet.
5) Usage of Hot water for drinking and bathing.
6) Oral usage of milk + Ardraka swarasa
7)      "        shunti + guda or sharkar.

8) Oral usage of Anupamamsa, curd, masha, kulutha, Lavan, katudravya, Amla, mulaka and medicated alcoholic preparations (madya)

9) Dhooma Narya with Ghritha Sakthu

10) Ghritha pana and snehan Nasya is contra indicated.

## Pakwa Pratishyaya or Jeerna Pratishyaya Chikitsa

1) Ghritha pana gives rasayana effect .
2) Swedana with Amla dravyas.
3) Vaman Karma with the yoosha prepared with milk + tila + masha + vamaka drugs.
4) Virechana
5) Teekshna dhooma Pana
6) Kavalagrah or gandoosha
7) Shiro virechan nasya
8) Aasthapan vasti
9) Resting in a perfect room where there is no pollusion of the air, dust and smoke (nivatha sthana)
10) Covering the head with hot and thick clothes .
11) Oral in take of :-

Jangala mamsa, Guda, Goksheera, chanak, Trikatu, Yava, Godhuma, Dadhi, Dadima, Dasha moola Kashaya, Aardraka, shunti, Yastimadu, Hareetaki, Katphala, chitra moola, Vasa, Tulasi, Kantakari, Haridra dwayam tankan and ikshurasa, amla Katu Tikta Kashaya Lavana sneha shrungibhasma, Trijathaka, pancha kola, pancha valkala, vidanga, Abhraka, Talisa patra, Triphala, Ajamoda, pudina, Varthaka, Patola, Masha, Tila, kulutha, mudga, ushnodaka, Ghritha and ksheera etc are beneficial either single remedy or selected drugs are taken for the treatment.

12) Usage of Hareetaki preparations like chitraka hareetaki or agastya hareetaki etc.
13) Usage of guda dadhi and maricha compound (Bhavamishra)
14) Drinking of cool water while going to bed at night (chakradatta)
15) Usage of Katphaladi churna
16) Oral usage of Panchamoola ksheera
17) Oral usage of Sarpi guda.(ghee + guda)
18) Oral usage of shadanga yoosha
19) Oral usage of Vyoshadi churna or vati (Trikatu, Talisa patra, Chavya, Tinthidika, Amla vetas, chitra moola, Jeeraka - each 2 phala; Lavanga, Ela, Japatri each 1 phala; purana guda 50 phala.

20) Usage of

Lakshmi vilas ras, Maha lakshmi vilas ras, Naradeeya Lakshmi vilas ras, Lagusutha sekar ras, Sanjeevani vati, Tribhuvan Keerthi ras, mrut yunjaya ras, Rama bana ras, Godanthi bhasma, Pancha Kola kwatha, chyavan prasha, panchamrutha ras, Talisadi churna, sithophaladi churna, Trijatha Kadi vati, Karpooradi vati, Trikatu churna, Khadhiradivati, Yastimaduchurna, Pushakara moola churna, Tankan bhasma, Kanchanara guggulu, Triphala guggulu, Nimbadi guggulu, Triphala ghritha, vasaghritha, patoladya ghritha, Vasavalehya etc drugs are beneficial, in different types of pratishyaya.

**21) Nasya Yogas :-**

a) Katphala, Apamarga, maricha, piipali, shunthi, vidanga, manashila, vacha, Hingu etc drugs can be used for pradaman Nasya

b) Tulasi, vasa, Kantakari, Trikatu, choraka, Ardraka, Tarkari, vacha, Jeerak, etc drugs can be used for Avapeedan Nasya.

c) Katu Teekshna ghritha, Navana Nasya

d) Bharangyadi taila Nasya

(Bharangi, Madan Phala, Tarkari, Tulasi, gomutra shodhana (should boil in Gomutra) then add sarshapa taila, vacha, Lamba, vidanga, Kusta, pippali, Karanja, ) cha-chi-26

e) Trikatu, saindhava lavan, kutaja, jeerak,should be grinded in Avimutra and used for Nasya .

f) Medicated oil prepared from Bala, Atibala, Bruhathi, vidanga, Kantakari, Vishnukrantha, mudgaparni, Rasna, punarnava, Tila taila,nasya.

g) Chorak, Tarkari, Vacha, Jeerak, Krishna Jeerak, Avapeedan Nasya.

**22) Dhooma Pana :-**

a) Devadaru, Apamarga, Danthee moola, Ingudee, Varthi should be prepared, for dhooma Pana.

b) Shatahwa, Twak, maricha, ela, bala moola, Shyonaka moola, Erenda moola, chitra moola, bilwa, Aragwada.

c) Dhooma pana with Ghritha sakthu .

**23) Contra Indications of pratishyaaya :-**

The following things or restricted for the usag

a) Cool water in take,or Bathing, b) Coitus c) Sleep d) Worries e) Suppression of natural urges f) Fresh alcoholic Preparations g) Oil less items. h) Weeping i) Anger j) Exposure to dust smoke etc k) Fridged items l) Kapha Vruddhi kara Ahara vihara should not take.

# VATAJ PRATISHYAYA VISESHA CHIKITSA
## (Special treatment for Vataj Pratishyaya)

**1) Snehakarma** (Shiro Abhyanga and Sneha pana )
a) If pain present, head massage is advised with Luke warm vata hara oleus medicines .

b) Oral administration of Vata hara ghritas like Rasnadi ghritha, Vidarigandhadi ghritha, pancha lavan ghritha, pancha moola ghritha, Yava kshara + ghritha, mamsa rasa and Luke warm milk etc.,.

**2)     Sweda Karma :-**
a) Pani sweda and upanaha sweda when associated with pain at Tem poral frontal and vertex regions of head .

b) Sneha and Sankara sweda is advised when Nasa Srava Kshavathu and Nasanaha are associated.

**3)     Niruha vasti with Vatahara dravya.**

**4)     Snigda dhuma Pana (dhooma Nasya)**
a) Shatahwaadi dhuma pana ( Shatahwa, Twak, Bala moola shyonaka, Erenda, Bilwa, Aaragwada, Madhushchista, Vasa and ghritha)
b) Dhooma Pana with Ghritha + Sakthu
c)Inhalation of the powders of Rohisha, jaji, vacha,Tarkari,choraka etc
d) Inhalation of the powders of Twak, Patra, maricha,Ela and jeerak.

**5)     a) Sneha Nasya like in Arditha vata :-**
b) Sneha Nasya with the oil prepared with Tila + Aja ksheera + yastimadu churna, Tila oil, Rasna, Yastimadu, saindhava lavana kalka; Dasha moola Kashaya - Oil should be prepared and used for Nasya.

**6)** Taking of Light, Luke warm, oleus, Vata hara diet, Hot water for drinking and for bath, Resting in Hot and perfect room without the polusion of dust and smoke.

**7)** Patient should be free from Tensions, worry, exercise, irrelavant Talking and coitus. etc.

## PITTAJA PRATISHYAYA VISESHA CHIKITSA
(Special treatment for Pittaja Pratishyaya)

1) Treatment of Pittaja and Rakthaja pratishyaya is merely similar.

2) Cool applications (Lepa- Seka) with chandana, usheera, Aamalaki etc drugs.

3) Cool items for eating and for drinking.

4) Oral in take of Tiktha Yoosha, Jangala mamsa, Godhuma , Yava, shali, Ksheera, ghritha and sheetha veerya Aushadha.

5) snigda madhura virechana

6) Gandusha or Kavala with Padmaka, sarja rasa, Chandana, Priyanga Patranga, madhu, sharkara, Draksha, madhulika, Gojee,shreparnee, Yastimadu.

7) a) Oral intake of Kakolyadi ghritha
b) Shunthi + milk + ghee.
c) Madhura and Tiktha ghritha.

**8) Nasya Karma :-**
a) Nasya with the oil prepared with patha, Haridra, Daru haridra moorva, pippali, Jathi pallava, danthi etc.
b) Nasya with the oil prepared from
Tila tail 1 part        Milk 10 parts.
Other Kalka dravyas - Dhava twak, Triphala, Shyama, shree parni, Yasti madu, Bilva, Haridra etc.
c) Nasya with Brungaraj swarasa.

## 3) KAPHAJ PRATISHYAYA VISESHA CHIKITSA
(Special treatment for Kaphaj pratishyaya )

A) If heaviness of head and Anorexia are assoicated.
1) Langhana 2) Ghritha Abhyanga to shiras 3) Mrudu sweda 4) Vaman with Trikatu, Yava Kshara and ghritha 5) Nasya (charaka - chikitsa - 26th Chapter )

**B)   If doshas are Mild :-**
1) Ghritha pana 2) Oral intake of Yavagu prepared with milk Tila and masha and vamaka dravyas for vaman Karma to eliminate the Kapha dosha 3) Langhana (charaka chikitsa 26th Chapter)

**c)    Nasya Yoga :-**
   1) Bharangyadi taila - (Prepared with Bharangi, madan phala, Tarkari tulasi, boiled with Go mutra and add sarshapa taila, vacha, laksha, Lamba, vidanga, Kusta, pippali, Karanja ) (Ch-Chi. 26)

   2) Teekshna nasya (Pradamana Nasya with the powders of manashila Trikatu, Vacha, Vidanga, Hingu, Guggulu etc). (Ch. chi-26)

   3) Nasya with Trikatu, Saindhava lavana, Kutaja, jeerak, vidanga, grinded in Avi mutra and used for Nasya (A.H.U. 20 -13).

   4) Nasya with the oil prepared from Bala, Atibala, Bruhati, Vidanga, Kantakari, vishnu krantha, mudga parni, Rasna, punarnava and Tila Taila.

**D)    Dhooma Pana :-** With the varthi prepared from Nishotha, Apamarga, Danthi, Devadaru, ingudee.
**E)    Swetha Sarshapa Shiro Lepa**
**F)    Hot water usage for drinking and for Bathing etc.**

### 4) SANNI PATHAJ PRATISHYAYA VISESHA CHIKITSA
(Special treatment for Sannipathaja Pratishyaya )

1) Tridosha hara chikitsa.
2) Katu Tiktha ghritha for oral administration.
3) Teekshna dhooma pana.
4) Teekshna Kavala grah.
5) Katu rasa medicines and diet

**6) Nasya :-**
a) Rasanjanadi taila nasya (rasanjana, ativasa, musta, Bhadradaru and Taila).

**b) Shiro Virechan Taila :-**
(Medicated oil prepared from Musta, chavya, patha, Katphala, pippali, Pippali moola, Katuki, sarshapa, vacha, Tuttha, Karanja, saindhava lavana, Bhadradaru, Taila).

   c) Jangala mamsa, ksheera, uthphalaadi pushpha, Vata hara Aushada , Prakshepa dravya, Boiled according to ksheera paka vidhi, Ghree should be prepared from the above medicated milk, it can be used for Nasya in all types of Pratishyaya

   d) Tiktha taila or ghritha can be used for Nasya.

7) **Kavala graha :-**

1) With the Tiktha Kashaya

2) With the decoction of musta, chavya, patha, Katphala,Pippali, Pippali moola, katuki, sarshapa, vacha, tuttha, Karanja, saindhava Lavan, Bhadradaru etc. drugs.

## Dusta Pratishyaya :-

1) All the above treatments

2) Krimi hara treatment

3) Kshaya hara treatment

4) Rasayana therapy

5) It is Yapaya Vyadhi

### 6) Dhooma Nasya With

Trikatu, Erenda beeja, vidanga, Devadaru, Ativ vasa, Kusta, Ingudee, Kantakari, Nishotha, swetha sarshapa, puthi matsya, Agni mantha, peelu, shigru beeja, these should be grinded in Ashwa vit rasa, Ashwa and gaja mutra . dip the kshouma Vastra varthi in above compound and is used for Dhooma Nasya.

7) vidangadi Nasya

8) Gomutra + go Pitta Nasya

9) Surasadi Krimi hara drugs

10) Luke warm water for Nasa and pana in the early morning.

## APEENASA CHIKITSA
### (Treatment of Apeenasa)

1) sneha 2) Sweda 3) Vaman 4) Virechan 4) Laghu Teekshna ushna ahara 5) Hot water in take 6) Dhooma Pana 7) Avapeedan Nasya.

1) Avapeedan Nasya
Hingu, Trikatu, Kutaja, shivati, Laksha, tulasi, Katphala, Vacha, Kusta, sarshapa, vidanga, Karanja, shigru.

2) The Medicated oil prepared from Above drugs + sarshapa taila + Go mutra, Tila taila, used as nasya.

3) Medicated oil prepared from Pathadi taila used as Nasya (patha, haridra dwayam, pippali, moorva, Jaji patra, taila)

4) Shigru taila Nasya.

5) Vyaghree taila Nasya.

6) Shatbindu ghritha Nasya.

7) Dhooma Nasya with Madhuschita + guggulu

8) Shatahwadi dhooma Nasya

9)    Internal administration of
      a) Guda + dadhi + maricha
      b) Chitraka ksheera
      c) Pancha mooli Ksheera
      d) Vidanga Kwatha + Guda + Ghritha.
      e) Vidanga shaskuli or Godhuma Shaskuli,
      f) Katphaladi churna or Kashaya
      g) Vyoshadivati
      h) Pratishyaya chikitsa, especially Kaphaja Pratishyaya Chikitsa.

# EXTERNAL NOSE

**Congenital deformities :-**
    1) Choanal atresia - closure of the anterior nasal apertures and posterior nasal apertures
    2) Congenital deformitiy in size shape of nose as Flattening, Bifid nose etc.
    3) Dermoid cyst :- Occurs in the midline between the alar cartilages on the bridge of the nose.
    4) Nasal glioma :- A solid tumour produce swelling on the bridge of the nose and is connected to meninges by a stalk but the swelling doesnot increase by straining coughing
    5) Encephalocele :- Herniation of meninges and brain tissue through a dehiscence in frontal bone and the swelling increases by straining and coughing.
    6) Cleft lip :- Failure of fusion of maxillary process and median nasal process.
    7) Cleft palate - Failure of palatine process to fuse with each other and with nasal septum.

**Diseases of External Nose :-**
**1) Furunculosis of the nose (Nasa Paka)**

This is an acute infective condition of the root of the hair follicle or sebaceous gland in the nasal vestibule, caused by staphylococcus aureus, pre-disposing factors are nose picking or pulling of hair .

**Clinical Features :-** Localised redness, swelling, pain, tenderness, crust formation and nasal obstruction
**Complications :-** cellutitis of face and upper lip, and cavernous sinus thrombosis
**Treatment ;-**  1) Local and systemic antibiotics.
            2) Analgesics and antiinflammatory drugs.
            3) Anti histamine drugs to relieve nasal irritation.
            4) Local hot-fomentation.

## 2)    Vestibulitis :-

Diffuse infection of the skin of the anterior nares may result from
1) Trauma as in nose picking, this produces ulceration and crust formation
2) Persistent nasal discharge leads to excoriation and infection of the skin
of the nasal vestibule

**Clinical Features :-** Ulceration, crust formation, pain and discomfort in the
nasal vestibule.

**Treatment :-** 1) Local application of antibiotic or Hydrocortisone ointment
2) Treating the pre-disposing factors
3) Systemic antibiotics and Anti inflammatory drugs.

## 3)    Erysipelas :-

Iti is an acute strepto coccal inflammation of the skin and subcutaneous tissue of the nose.

**Clinical Features :-** Redness, vesicles formation on the nose and face,
headache, fever and malaise (no intra nasal signs and symptoms)
**Treatment :-** 1) Pencillin is drug of treatment
2) Symptomatic treatment.

## 4)    Acne Rosacea :-

Enlarged superficial blood vessels in the skin of nose and cheeks,
giving the skin a dusky red and shining appearance (commonly seen in meno
ause women )

## 5)    Lupus erythematosus :-

The skin of the nose and cheeks are affected with the butterfly shaped
erythema patches with scaling followed by atrophic scars.

## Herpes Simplex :-

Vesicular eruption around the nasal vestibule and lips caused by Herpes simplex virus
**Treatment :-** 1) Local antibiotics or Hydro cortisone
2) Symptomatic treatment.

## 6)    Herpes Zoster :-

Vesicular eruptions along the cutaneous nerves of face heals by scaring and causes severe pain

## 7)    Rhino Phyma :-

Hypertrophy of the sebaceous glands of the tip of the nose, produces
bulbous projection called potato nose or Rhino phyma .

**Treatment :-** Surgical excision of the hypertrophy.

**8)    Deformities of External Nose :-**
1) Congenital flat or Bifid nose
2) Developmental improper development of nose and septum along with face.
3) Traumatic lesions.
4) Infections - septal abscess syphilis and Leprosy.
5) Tumours may cause deformity and destruction.
**Treatment :-**  Rhino Plasty.
6) Atresia of Anterior nares occurs congenitally and due to small pox Rhinoscleroma and Young's operation for atrophic Rhinitis.

**9)    Fracture of  Nasal Bones :-** Symptoms are deformity, pain, swelling, Epistaxis and Nasal obstruction.Treatment depends upon the condition.
**Treatment :-**  Anti inflammatory ; correction of deformity or Rhinosepto plasty under general anesthesia.

**10)    Haematoma and abscess of Septum :-**
The trauma may be followed by extravasation of blood and it causes a smooth round swelling on both sides of the septum it may be transformed in to abscess after infection.

**11)    Tumours of the external nose:-** It may be benign or Malignant.

**Benign tumours :-** 1) Papilloma frequently occur in nasal vestibule and require surgical excision
2) Haemangiomas occurs in the skin of the nose and require diathermy coagulation or excision.

**Malignant Tumours :-**
1) Basal cell carcinoma or rodent ulcer occurs in the skin of the nose as a raised pigmented nodule which ulcerates, doesn't heal and destructs the nasal cartilages and adjacent facial tissue.

**2) Squamous Cell Carcinoma :-**
This lesion may occur in the nasal vestibule or on the skin of the external nose with progressive bleeding ulcer along with raised margins.

**Treatment :-** Radiotherapy and surgery.

# RHINITIS (PEENASA OR PRATISHYAYA )

Rhinitis is the inflammation of the nasal mucous membrane owing to infection, Allergy and trauma. It may be classified as follows.

I) **Infective Rhinitis :-**
   A) **Acute Rhinitis :-**
      a) Non specific acute Rhinitis - common cold
      b) specific acute Rhinitis - Diphtheria.

B) **Chronic Rhinitis :-**
   a) Non specific chronic Rhinitis
      1) Simple Chronic Rhinitis.
      2) Hyper trophic Rhinitis.
      3) Atrophic Rhinitis.
      4) Rhinitis Sicca
      5) Rhinitis Caseosa.
      6) Malignant granuloma.

   b) **Specific Chronic Rhinitis :-**
      1) Rhino sporidiosis.
      2) Rhino scleroma.
      3) Syphilis.
      4) Leprosy.
      5) Tuberculosis, Lupus Vulgaris.
      6) Fungus infections like
      Aspergillosis, actinomycosis, moniliasis.

II) **Non Infective Rhinitis :-**
   a) Allergic Rhinitis (Seasonal Perennial)
   b) Vasomotor Rhinitis.

## Infective Acute Non Specific Rhinitis :-
I/A/a) Common Cold (coryza)
Acute inflammation of nasal mucosa is called Acute Rhinitis. Pri mary infection is by virus and secondary infection is by bacteria

**The Causative Organisms :-**
   **Virus :-** Rhino Virus, influenza virus, adeno virus .
   **Bacteria :-** Strepto coccus haemolyticus, micoro coccus.
catarrhalis, pneumo coccus, staphylo coccus, Haemophilus influenzae etc.

**Clinical Features :-**

These are in 4 Stages :-

**1)     Ischaemic stage :-** Burning sensation in the naso pharynx, irritation, dryness in the nose, sneezing paraxysmally, shivering and malaise may develop.

**2)     Hyperaemic Stage :-** Profuse rhinorrhoea (Watery discharge), blocking of nose, anosmia, fever and head ache.

**3)     State of Secondary Infection :-** The watery nasal discharge thickens with yellow or greenish colour due to secondary infection.

**4)     Stage of Resolution :-** It occurs commonly in 5 to 10 days.
     **Complications :-** Naso pharyngitis, pharyngitis, sinusitis, Acute otitis media, Laryngitis, Bronchitis, Pneumonia etc.,

     **Treatment :-** There is no specific treatment but following treatment principles prevent the secondary infection, complications and give relief symptomatically.

**A)     General Treatment :-** (Systemic treatment )
     1) Analgesics and Anti pyretics reduce pain and fever .
     2) Antibiotics controls secondary infection.
     3) decongestants reduce nasal congestion.
     4) Anti histamines reduce nasal irritation.
     5) Vitamines, B,complex, C, etc protects mucosal hygiene.
     6) Warmth and rest restores the health.
     **B) Local Treatment :-**
     1) Menthol steam inhalation.
     2) Decongestant Nasal drops.
     c) Surgical correection of septum, hypertrophic turbinates tonsils and adenoids etc, and contact should be avoided.

# I/A/b) Nasal Diphtheria :-
     It is an infective specific acute Rhinitis usually occurs in children, the causative organism is corynebacterium diptheriae. It may be the primary disease or secondary to faucial diphtheria.

**Clinical Features :-**
1) Blood stained nasal discharge on one or both sides.

2)   Excoriation of the skin around the nose .
3)   Greyish white colour membrane formation on septum or in ferior turbi nates which bleeds on removal .

**Diagnosis :-** By clinical features, and by Bacteriological examination.

**Treatment :-**
   1) Anti toxin  -   10000 units of the serum
   2) Antibiotics like erythromycin and pencillin.
   3) Symptomatic treatment.
   4) Rest.

**B)     Infective Chronic Rhinitis**
**1/B/a) Non Specific chronic Rhinitis.**
   **1) Simple chronic Rhinitis.**

**Aetiology :-**
   a) Recurrent attacks of acute Rhinitis may lead to chronic Rhinitis.
   b) Pre-disposing factors are sinusitis, tonsilitis vasomotor rhinitis, Nasal obstructions, Atmospheric pollution, over usage of nasal drops. smoking, alco holism, general debility and hypothyroidism.

**Clinical Features :-**
   1) Ischaemic stage and Hyperaemic stage of Acute Rhinitis present but less severe .
   2) post Nasal drip and Nasal blockage is more marked.
   3) The Nasal secretions are thick and viscid.

   **Treatment :-** 1) Elimination of predisposing factors
                    2) Alkaline Nasal douchings
                    3) Symptomatic treatment like in acute Rhinitis.

## 2)   CHRONIC HYPERTROPHIC RHINITIS

   It is due to chronic nasal, paranasal infection and due to nasal allergy. The aetiological factors. are like chronic simple Rhinitis. Rhinitis medicamentosa (over usage of Nasal decongestants ) is the often responsible factor for this condition.

**Clinical Features :-**
1)   Hypertrophied, Congested nasal mucosa with enlarged turbinates is the main finding .

2) Nasal obstruction
3) Rhinorrhoea - thick visicid nasal discharge.
4) Development of Polyps in the further aggravation of the symptoms.

**Diagnosis -**
1)Hyper trophied turbinates, congested mucosa
2) Posterior Rhino scopy reveal the mulberrry like posterior ends of inferior turbinates.

**Treatment :-**
1) Topical nasal decongestants gives relief temproarily
2) a) Electro cautery b) Submucous diathermy
c) Cryo surgery d) Partial tubinectomy etc.
are benefical in hypertrophied turbinates.

### 3) ATROPHIC RHINITIS (OZAENA)

This is a chronic inflammatory condition of the nose characterised by atrophic changes of the nasal mucosa and burbinates, expell foul smell from the nose and causes anosmia. It may be primary or secondary to some other diseases.

**a) Primary atrophic Rhinitis :-**
Causative factors :-
1) Cocco bacillus of perez, Klebsiella foctidis ozaenae and diphtheroid organsisms etc.
2) Heriditory, Hormonal, Nutritional deficiencies vitamin deficiencies (A & D), Infection, Broad nasal cavities and due to other factors

**b) Secondary Atrophic Rhinitis :-**
Atrophic changes are produced due to chronic specific infections like syphilis, leprosy, lupus vulgaris, tuberculosis and Rhino scleroma; extensive Nasal surgery and chronic sinusitis etc.

**Pathology :-**
As a result of chronic inflammatory changes the ciliated columnar epithelium of nasal cavity and turbinates atrophies and shows squamous meta placia, blood circulation reduced, secretions stagnated and result in secondary infection and crust formation, due to loss of sensation and foetor attracts the flies (maggots) and patient looses the sense of smell and touch of air.

**Clinical Features :-**

1) Dryness in the nose 2) wide nasal cavities with crust formation. 3) The nose emits foul smell 4) Anosmia (merciful anosmia) - the patient doesnt feel his foul smell which is coming out and he doesnt smell the other things also. 5) Head ache 6) Epistaxis 7) Atrophic changes in the mucosa and turbinates.8) Nasal obstruction 9) Depressed bridge of the nose (due to atrophic changes.)

**Complications :-**

1) sinusitis 2) Middle ear infections.
3) Atrophic pharyngitis 4) Psychological
Complications like depression and may become an introvert.

**Investigations :-**

1) Xray for the detection of sinusitis and tuberculosis etc.
2) VDRL for detecting syphilis.
3) Haemogram for detecting anaemia.
4) Dermotological examination for detecting Leprosy.
5) Nasal smear for detecting leprosy and tuberculosis.
6) Biopsy
7) Clinical findings.

**Treatment :-**

1) The cause should be treated.
2) Improving the nasal hygiene by preventing the crusting by putting antibiotic nasal drops. alkaline douche, ex: nasal drops 25% glucose in glucerine, and by local infiltration of placental extract (Placentrex) etc.
3) Systemic antibiotics, nutrients, vitamines, vasodilators .
4) Surgical treatment.

**4)      Rhinitis Sicca :-**

It is a mild form of atrophic Rhinitis occurs usually in dry hot dusty environment.

The main feature is drying and crusting in the anterior one third of the nasal cavity.

**Clinical Features :-**

1) Drying and crusting of anterior 1/3 of nasal caivty.
2) Nasal irritation.
3) Ulceration in the Nasal mucosa. and leads to epistaxis.
4) Septal performation in deep ulcerations.

**Treatment :-**
1) Lubrication of Nose with vaseline ghee or oil etc.
2) Alkaline nasal douching.
3) Care from dry hot dusty environment.

## 5) Rhinitis Caseosa (Nasal Cholesteatoma )

This is a rare chronic inflammatory condition of the nose assoicated with formation of granulation tissue and a cheesy epithelial debris (caseous material) in the nose, this may result from chronic sinusitis, presence of foreign body or due to dis integration of nasal polyp .

**Treatment :-** 1) Removal of caseous material  2) Improving of Nasal hygiene 3) Should treat the underlying cause.

## 6) Malignant granuloma :-

This is of two types.

**1) Stewarts granuloma :-** is a localised progressive ulceration of the tissues of the nose sinuses and pharynx, produces destructive lesions in the bones, cartilages and soft tissues.

**Treatment :-** Radio therapy

**2) Wegener's granulomatosis :-**

It is a necrotizing granuloma affecting the nose lungs and kidney.

**Treatment : -**
1) Cytotoxic drugs.
2) Steroids.
3) Antimetabolites.

### I/B/b) SPECIFIC CHRONIC RHINITIS

**1) Rhino Sproidiosis :-**

The diseases is caused by the fungus "Rhino sporidium seeberi" or "R. Kinealyi" (Spore-bearing fungus). It is usally limited to coastal states . Like Kerala, Andrapradesh, madras, Karnataka, Maharashtra .

It occurs mostly to farmers and is predisposed by trauma. The mode of infection is thought to be the dust from the dung of infected cattle, the nasal mucosa affects, but lesions are seen in Naso pharynx , pharnx bronchi and skin, clinically characterised by formation of bleeding papillomatous and polypoidal lesions which have a strawbery appearance.

The clincial features are Rhinorrhoea, Nasal blockage epistaxis and, protrusion of extra growths. The disease. spreads to lungs, liver, spleen, eyes and genitalia.

**Treatment :-**
1) Excision of the growth and cauterisation of the base or cryosurgery or laser surgery may be beneficial.

## 2)    Rhino Scleroma :-
It is a progressive granulomatous disease of respiratory tract caused by Klebsiella Rhinoscleromatis (Frisch bacillus) .

It is a chronic infection of the nose characterised by sclerosis and stenosis of the nasal passage.
Clinical features canbe explained. in four stages.
**1) Prodromal stage Or catarrhal stage:-** Rhinorrhoea present.
**2) Atrophic stage :-** Atrophic changes in the nasal mucosa.
**3) Nodular Stage :-** Bluishred nodules appears at the muco cutaneous junction of septum.
4) Stenotic or fibrotic or cicatrising stage - stenosis of nose and na sopharynx develops.

**Diagnosis -** History, - Clinical examination and biopsy confirm the disease.
**Treatment :-**
1) Antibiotics like streptomycin, chloramphenical, rifampcine steroids. tetracyclines may prove helpful.
2) Surgery to re-establish the air way.

## 3)    Syphilis :-
Primary and secondary stages of syphilis are rarely seen in the nose. in the tertiary stage Gummatous ulcer (ulcerative nodule) develops in the bony part of the septum. The associated symptoms are bony septal perfora- tion. depression of the nasal bridge, pain and head ache particuly during night, marked tenderness and offensive nasal discharge.

If the disease aggravates causes complications like stenosis of the nasal cavity collapse of the Nasal bony frame, perforation of the palate and atrophic rhinitis etc

**Treatment :-** 1) Anti Syphilitic treatment
                 2) Symptomatic treatment.

178

## 4) Leprosy :-

The causative organism is mycobacterium leprae. Nasal lesions are commonly seen in lepromatous leprosy, affected part is Antero inferior part of nasal septum. initially a nodule forms which leads to ulceration and perforation of the nasal septum with deformity of nose., Later the palate and the larynx may be involved. The patient complaints of nasal obstruction, crust formation, blood stained nasal discharge, nodular thickening of mucosa of inferior turbinate, atrophic rhinitic changes and stenosis of anterior nares.

**Diagnosis :-** 1) Clinical Picture
2) Nasal smear test for A.F. Bacilli
3) Biopsy of granuloma

## 5) Tuberculosis :-

It is secondary to pulmonary tuberculosis, it rarely affects the nose, it may form a granuloma at the cartilaginous septum resulting in destruction and perforation.

The clinical features are nasal obstruction, discharge, crusting , pain and On examination ulcerative nodular granulomatous lesion with septal perforation is seen.
**Treatment :-** Anti tuberculous treatment .

## 6) Lupus Vulgaris :-

It is a tuberculous infection of low virulence, usually involves the mucocutaneous junction at the vestibule of the nose, with ulceration and apple jelly nodules formation. The nasal septum may perforate and the nose may be deformed . Symptoms of atrophic rhinitis follows, the disease spreads to pharynx larynx and Lungs.
**Treatment :-** Anti tuberculous treatment
**Note :-** Other chronic specific rhinitis are uncommon.

### II ) NON INFECTIVE RHINITIS

#### 1) Allergic Rhinitis :-

It is a common disorder which is usually characterised by spasmodic attacks of severe sneezing and rhinorrhoea, occurs due to altered reactivity, of the nasal mucosa to certain allergens like.

**a) Exogenous allergens :- Inhalants** (dust pollens, animal odour, feathers, moulds, house dust and mites), **ingestants** (food like eggs, fish milk citrus fruits etc),

**Contactants** (cosmetics and powders), **irritants** (fumes and smoke), **drugs** (aspirin, hypotensive drugs, iodides, and nasal drops). **infections** etc.,

**b) Endogenous allergens :-**
Intestinal helminths, tissue proteins, etc.

**Predisposing factors :-** a) Hereditory factors, b) Hormonal effects during puberty or pregnancy, c) climate - change in Humidity and atmospheric pollution d) Emotional factors etc.

**Pathology :-**
Antigen (allergen) + mucosa --- Histamines released, causes vaso dilatation, increased capillary permiability, copious secretions from mucosal glands, leads to congestion oedema and swelling of mucosa, there is cellular infiltrations of mucosa by Eosinophils, plasma cells. and lymphocystes, Because of oedema and swelling secondary bacterial infection occur, as the disease progresses there are chances for polyp formation in the nose and sinuses. other complications are serous otitis media, suppurative otitis media, Bronchial asthma etc.

**Clinical Types ;-** 2 types are
   1) Seasonal - Due to inhalant allergens, climate environmental changes
   2) Perennial - affects through out the year.

**Signs & Symptoms :-**
**1)    Symptoms :-**
   Nasal irritation, paraxysmal sneezing, watery copious rhinorrhoea, nasal obstruction and anosmia.

**2)    Signs :-**
   a) **Acute stage -:-** Pale nasal mucosa with excessive secretions
   b) **Chronic stage :-** Blusih or purplish mucosa due to venous stasis.
   c) **Infection :-** Secondary bacterial infection is added.
   d) **Polyps:-** may be present.

**Concomitant Allergy :-**
   a) **Eyes :-** Itching and watering of eyes is often present.
   b) **Ears :-** Eustachian tube blockage may leads to middle ear
      problems.
   c) Allergic Pharyngitis.
   d) Allergic bronchial asthma.

**Diagnosis :-**
1) Clinical features & History
2) Nasal secretion may contain Eosinophils.
3) Haemogram shows Eosino philia
4) Stools for helminths.
5 Intra dermal skin test,
6) Nasal provacation test.
7) Elimination test for food.
8) RAST (Radio allergo sorbent test)

**Treatment :-** 1) Avoidance of the allergen 2) Desensitization 3) Anti histamines 4) Steroids 5) Nasal decogestants. 6) Symptomatic treatment 7) Surgical correction of the predisposing diseases like deviated nasal septum, hypertrophied turbinates etc.

## 2) Vasmotor Rhinitis :-

It is a non infective condition occurs due to vaso motor disturbances consequent to autonomic disfunction. various factors play a part in its causation like psychogenic instability. emotional conditions, hormonal changes. climate varations antihypertensive drugs Anti depressants and decongestants.

The Aetiological factors are merely similar to allergic Rhinitis. except allergens.

**Clinical Features :-**
1) Sneezing is less than Allergic Rhinitis .
2) Symptoms appear more frequent than Allergic rhinitis.
3) Lacrimation is occasional
4) Nasal obstruction and Rhinorrhoea are more marked.
5) Eosinophilia is less marked.
6) Nasal mucosa is markedly swollen
7) Skin tests for Allergy are negative.
8) Anti histamine response is variably.
9) Vidian neurectomy is helpful.

**Treatment :-** Except desensitization, rest of the treatment is similar to Allergic rhinitis.

# SINUSITIS (Dusta Pratishyaya)

(Shirashoola can be co-related to sinusitis)

The mucosal inflammation of the paranasal sinuses, may be acute or chronic, commonly associate with rhinitis, is known as sinusitis. Commonly one or two sinues affect, if all sinuses are involved resulting in pansinusitis.

**1) Maxillary sinus :-** is most commonly involved due to inadequate drainage of this sinus owing to the position of the ostium which is situated near the roof of its medial wall and due to its relation to the upper premolar and molar teeth which present at the floor of the sinus 2) Frontal sinusitis is very less frequency 3) Ethmoidal sinusitis and 4) Sphenoidal sinusitis are very rare.

## ACUTE SINUSITIS (MAXILLARY)

**Predisposing Factors :-**
**1) Nasal infections :-** common cold, influenja, deviated nasal septum, hypertrophic turbinates, polyps, tumours etc causes stagnation of sinus secretions and infection follows.

**2) Nasal Allergy :-** Leads to nasal obstruction and inadeqate drain age of sinus secretions.
3) Forcible blowing of nose.
4) Swimming and diving, cold exposure .
5) Barotrauma.
6) Dental infection - especially upper premolar and molar teeth.
7) Trauma to the sinus.
8) Blood borne infection
9) Peripheral infections like Tonsilitis adenoids etc.
10) Lowered resistence
11) Atmospheric Pollution
12) General diseases like influenza Measles, whooping cough and other specific diseases like tuberculosis, leprosy etc.
13) Chronic suppurative lung diseases,
14) Virul infections.
15) Bacterial infection by strepto cocci, pneumo cocci, micro coccus catarrhalis, staphylo cocci, Haemophilus- influenzae , Bacillus pyocyaneus, Bacillus coli, Bacillus necrodentalis, Bacillus Pfeiffer, Bacillus friedlanders.

**Pathology :-**

    **a) Catarrhal stage -** Congestion and oedema of mucosa and hyper-trophy of mucous glands.

    **b** Exudation :- Due to increased glandular activity, secretions collect in the sinus which are mucoid initially.

    **c) Purulent Stage :-** Infection Progresses and there is thick mucopu-rulent discharge - some times comes out through the ostium or produce empyema of the sinus.

**4)    Stage of Complication :-**

    Pan-sinusitis , middle ear infections, pharyngitis, laryngitis, tracheo-bronchitis, ophthalmic problems, osteo myelitis of maxilla, Asthma, muco-cele, pyocele and oro antral fistuala .

**5)    Stage of Resolution :-**

    It depends upon the virulence of virus, resistence of the body and antibiotics administered .

**symptoms :-**  1) Discomfort at naso pharyngeal region.

    2) Pain at maxillary region, may radiate to eyes teeth ear and frontal sinus - aggravate on bending down, coughing and sneezing .

    3) Nasal discharge mucoid or purulent or blood stained (foul smelling discharge suggestive of dental origin .

    4) Blocking of Nose due to oedema of mucosa.

    5) Nasal resonance due to blocking of nose

    6) Dry cough due to post nasal drip.

    7) Epistaxis is due to congestion of mucosa.

    8) Fever headache, malaise etc.

**Signs :-**

    1) Slight oedema at the affected area

    2) Tenderness over the cheek and Floor of the sinus.

    3) Anterior rhinoscopy reveals the congestion of Nasal mucosa and turbinates especially at middle turbinate.

    4) Posterior Rhinoscopy may reveal purulent discharge trickling down through the choana .

**Investigations :-**
    1) Posture test

    1) Patient is asked to be in sitting position then discharge in the nose is wiped out if discharge reappears in middle meatus that is from forntal sinus.

    2) Patient is asked to lie down on un effected side if discharge reappears that is from maxillary sinus.

**2)      Transillumination test :-**
    In dark room a lighted bulb is placed in the oral caivty, if the sinus is translucent infra orbital crescent appears if not absent .

3)      Radiography of paranasal sinuses.
4)      Bacteriological examination of Nasal smear for culture and sensitivity.
5)      Endoscopy of nose and para nasal sinuses.

**Treatment :-**
    1) Antibiotics 2) Decongestants 3) Analgesics 4) Antihistamines. 5) Rest 6) Local decongestant drops 7) Steam inhalation. 8) Antral puncture is advised if medical treatment fails (it is conducted either in Local or general anaesthesia, the Procedure consist of inserting of trocar with canula in to the maxillary sinus through inferior meatus to wash the sinus with lukewarm water to irrigate the exudates out.

## 2)    Acute Frontal Sinusitis :-
    It is less common than maxillary sinusitis, aetio-pathology is similar to maxillary sinusitis except the following .

    1) Dental infection cannot cause frontal sinusitis
    2) Maxillary sinusitis may cause secondary frontal sinusitis via fronto nasal dust

    3) Pain in the frontal region and may radiate to the temporal and parietal regions, it is maximum in the morning and gradually subsides during the course of the day.

    4) Tender ness present at the medial part of the floor of sinus above the inner canthus.

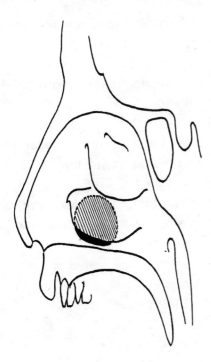

Site of intranasal antrostomy

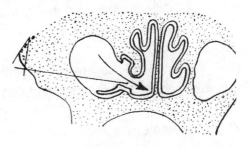

Intranasal Antrostomy (right).

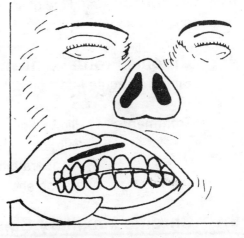

*Sublabial incision for Caldwell-Luc operation*

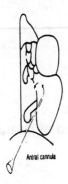

Antral puncture
cannula in the
maxillary antrum
inserted through the
inferior meatus.

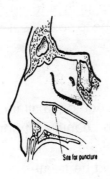

Lateral wall of the
nose with the inferior
turbinate removed to
show the site for
antral puncture

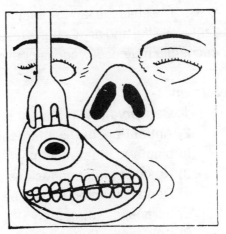

*Opening in anterolateral wall of maxillary sir*

5)    The discharge from the frontal sinus appears in the middle meatus in upright position of the patient.

6)    Complications are ostemyelitis, orbital complications, cavernous sinus thrombosis and intra cranial complications.

7)    Treatment is similar, in addition trephening the floor at the medial end of frontal sinus done for washing the sinus with antibiotic solution.

3)    Ethmoidal and sphenoidal sinusits are rare, ethmoidal sinusitis causes pain in the eyes or behind the eyes, sphenoidal sinusitis may produce occipital or central headache.

## 4)    Chronic Frontal Sinusitis :-
Similar to acute infection but pain and tenderness is less severe.

Treatment :- 1) Elimination of pre-disposing factors
2) Surgical drainage of frontal sinus.
3) An operation of frontal sinus similar to caldwell - luk operation should be performed occasionally.

## 5)    Chronic Maxillary Sinusitis

It is similar to acute infection but pain and tenderness are mild or absent,Hawking and dry Cough present due to post nasal discharge, Hyposmia or cacosmia may occur occasionally.

## Treatment :-
1) Conservatory treatment is like Acute maxillary sinusitis.
2) Antral Puncture with trochor and canula. at anterior end of inferior turbinate to irigate the maxillary sinus.
3) Nasal obstructing lesions should be treated.
4) Dental infection should be treated.
5) Intranasal antrostomy.
6) Cald well - Luk, operation is advisable, if repeated purulent secretion is found during antral wash - in this a sub-labial incision is given through canine fossa.

# NASAL FOREIGN BODIES

Nasal foreign bodies are common in children and infants. The common foreign bodies are buttons, seeds, beads, peas, papers, rubber, plastic materials and maggots (in poor hygienic and suppurative diseases of Nose and Paransal sinuses)

Parents brings the child to the hospital for the following reasons .
1) With the history of insertion of foreign bodies.
2) Foul smell (unilateral) with nasal discharge.
3) Pain, headache, crawling sensation and worms coming out of the nose in the case of Maggots.

**Removal of foreign bodies :-**
Foreign bodies like buttons, sponges, papers etc should remove with forceps. round objects such as peas, beans etc should be removed with hook.

The child should be holded properly by an assistant, the tip of the hook is introduced along the roof of the nose and placed behind the foreign body, the foreign body is lodged in the angle of the hook and brought out . In a non co -operative child General anaesthesia will be necessary .

For Maggots, Nose is irrigated with chloroform water or Packed with gauze soaked in ether, this stupifies the maggots which are washed out in large numbers. Then Nose is packed with turpentine for 24 hours, and Nasal douching is repeated with antibiotics.

**Rhinolith :-** Calcareous mass often found in the nose The deposits of corbonates and phosphates of calcium and magnesium formed around a foreign body, blood clot or mucous and leads to blackish or Brownish calcareous mass formation.
**Cinical features :-** Pain, Nasal obstruction, Nasal discharge and epistaxis.
**Treatment :-** Removal of mass and anti-inflammatory therapy should be given.

## 7) POOTHI NAASA OR POOTHI NASYA
### Atrophic Rhinitis Or Ozaena or Frontal sinusitis

Vitiated pitta Raktha and Kapha Produces vitiation at Gala and Talu moola and expel foul smell (Vitiationof Vata) Through nose and mouth is known as poothi Nasa (Sushrutha. U. 22).

Vitatied doshas by deranging the talu moola expel foul smell with Kapha through Nose and mouth                    (Vagbhata. A.H.U. 19)

It can be corelated to atrophic rhinitis.

**Videha :-** Vitiated pitta Raktha and Kapha accumulates in shiras, get burnt by Pittoshma, causes pain in the eyes and temporal region, expel foul smell, blood stained Yellowish nasal discharge with itching sensation and fever, it is known as poothi nasyam, it can be co-related to frontal sinusitis.

**Treatment :-**
**1)** Like Apeenasa (Su) and Kaphaja peenasa (Vag)
**2)** Sneha, sweda, vaman, mrudu virechan, ,
   dhooma pana. Avapeedan Nasya-sneha nasaya, Langan, teekshna ahara and hot water utility for daily needs.

**3)      Avapeedan Nasya :-**
   Hingu, Trikatu, swetha purarnava, Vatsak, Laksha, shireesha beeja, Katphala, Vacha, Kusta, shigru, vidanga, Karanja - Swarasa Nasya.

**4)      Snehan Nasya :-**
   Medicated oil prepared with the Above drugs, sarshapa taila and gomatra is used for Nasya.

5)      Vyaghree taila Nasya or vyaghree swarasa (The medicated oil pre pared from Vyaghree, danthi beeja, vacha, shigru, trikatu, saindhava lavan and Taila).

6)      Shatbindu ghritha Nasya. (The medicated ghee prepared from Bringaraj, Lavanga, yastimadu, Kusta, shunthi - Ghritha).

7)      Oral in take of guda + Maricha + dadhi.

8)      "   Vidanga churna + godhuma pista, Shaskuli should be prepared.

9)      "   godhuma pista + guda + ghritha.

## 8) NASA PAKA OR NASIKA PAKA
(Nasal furunculosis or Herpes or Dermatitis of the Nasal vestibule.)

a) vitiated Pitta dosha causes acute inflammatory changes by the erup-tion of small piticas (Vesicles) in the nasal cavity, the piticas suppurates and discharges sticky secretion with atrophic changes (Su. u. 22).

b) Vitiated Raktha and pitta produces furuncles in the nose, associ-ated with pain, burning sensation, redness and oedema, is known as Nasa paka (cha- chi - 26 ).

c) Vitiated Pitta dosha causes vitiation in twak and mamsa of nose and leads to eruption of furuncles associated with pain, burning sensation and oedema, is Known as ghrana paka                          (A.H.U. 16)

**Treatment :-**
### 1) Pitta hara Chikitsa

### 2) External :-
a) Application of ghritha or shathadhoutha ghritha
b) Seka with the decoction of ksheeri vruksha (Pancha valkala
c) jalouka Mokshana.

### 3) Internal :-
a) Pitta hara Ahara - Vihar
b) Oral intake of ghritha + ksheera
c)        "        Jangala Mamsa rasa
d)        "        Kiishora guggulu
e)        "        Manjistadi quath, chandanasav.
                  Shadanga paneeya, usheerasav, Tandulodak etc
f)        "        Praval, Muktha, shukti, gyrika etc.,
g) Sneha, mrudu sweda, Lepa, seka, sneha dhooma, mrudu virechan and nasya (Anutaila nasya).

## 9) POOYA SHONITHA OR POOYA RAKTHA
(Frontal sinusitis, Hypertrophic or chronic Rhinitis)

It is of 2 types 1) Doshaj or Nija 2) Aaganthaja or Abhighataja.
**1) Nija or doshaj :-** due to pitta and Rakta vitation
**2) Aaganthuja or abhighataja :-** Due to injury to frontal region.

Either due to pitta Rakta doshas vitation or due to injury to frontal region of head, blood stained pus discharge comes through Nasal cavity is known as pooya Raktha .
**Vagbhata** Added the symptoms like pain and burning sensation in the head.

**Treatment :-**
1) Vaman 2) Avapeedan nasya (Rechan nasyam ) 3) Teekshna dhooma pana 4) In mild case Raktha peenasa chikitsa should be done 5) In severe case Nadi vrana chikitsa should be done.

**Note :-** Nasa arbuda, Kshayarbuda, Abhighata, Phiranga, nasal Paranasal chronic diseases, Nasa arsha etc may lead to pooya Rakta.

189

# 10) KSHAVATHU

( Allergic rhinitis or Vaso motor Rhinitis )

It is of 2 types - 1) Doshaja 2) Aaganthuja

## 1) Doshaja Kshavathu :-

Vitiated vatadi doshas affects the shrungataka marma of Nasal caivty. and so the vitiated vata and kapha dosha forcibly eliminated through nose with sounds frequently. is known as doshaja kshavathu, (sushrutha)

## 2) Aaganthuja Kshavathu.

The Nasal shrungataka Marma is stimulated by the following causes and produces sounds through nose with nasal discharge Frequently . the irritative factors are inhalation of katu Teekshna items like maricha tobacco and chillies. nasal picking with sticks, direct exposure to sun rays etc.,

**Vagbhata :** - Explained above two types as one in the name of Bhrushakshava

**Charaka** - Viatiated Vata by irritating shrungataka marma causes the Kshavathu .

## Treatment :-

1) Ghrita pana 2) ghritha abhyanga 3) Shiro vasti. 4) mrudu Sweda to shiras 5) Snigda dhooma 6) Nasya 7) Pratishyaya chikitsa 8) Avoiding the allergic foctors. 9) Pradaman Nasya with 10) Avapeedan Nasya with Pippali, shunthi, maricha, vidanga, sighru beeja, 11) Shatbindu taila Nasya. 12) Sneha nasya prepared with Shunthi, kusta, pippali, velli, draksha, Tila taila.

13)     Oral intake of agastya hareetaki
14)          "          Chitraka hareetaki
15)          "          Maha Lakshmi vilas ras
16)          "          Sheleshma shiilendra ras
17)          "          Rasayan chikitsa
18)          "          Anti allergic treatment Preventive as wellas curative .
19)     Rest.

# 11) BRAMSHATHU

Hypertrophic or chronic rhinitis , frontal sinusitis

The accumulated Kapha of shiras (Because of repeated sneezes the nasal mucosa becomes inflammed or get hypertrophied ) dissolved, burnt by pittoshma and expels sticky salty mucus discharge through the nasal cavity is known as Bramshathu. It is secondary to the ksavathu and the treatment is as like **Kshavathu.**

# DEEPTHA OR DEEPTHI
## (ACUTE CATARRHAL RHINITIS)

It is due to pitta and Raktha vitiation, associated with Burning sensation in the nose, smoky feeling, un-tolerable pain and tenderness.

**Treatment :-**
1) Pitta Raktha hara chikitsa
2) Cool applications, (Lepa seka ) ex - shatadautha ghritha
3) Modhura Tiktha kashaya (Ahara)sheeta veerya Aushada and sheetala vihara .
4) The following remedies can be given for external and internal usage.

Chandana, usheera, Nagakesara, musta, muktha, ghritha, shunthi, pravala pisti, chandanadi vati, Chandanadi loha, Lagu Sathasekara ras, Triphala guggulu, Nimbadi guggulu, shadanga paneeya, Ksheeri sarpi chandanasav, usheerasav etc. drugs are useful.

5) Brumhana or shamana Nasya should be given
ex 1) Rasanjana Nasya
2) Ksheeri sarpi Nasya.

# 13) GHRANA SRAVA &
# NASA SRAVA OR NASA PARISRAVA
## (Acute or chronic Rhinorrhoea )

The kapha (mucosa) of shrungatak area of the nose is affected and discharges colourless watery secrections from the nose continuously and more severe at nights, is known as nasa srava or parisrava.

**Charak -** Solid, yellowish, pakwa, Nasasrava comes by the vitiation of masthishka.

**Bhavamishra & Yoga ratnakar :-**
Some times solid discharge and some times watery discharge comes through the nose, is known as Nasa srava.

**Treatment :-**
1) Shiro virechan
2) Hingu, Vyoshadi Teekshna Avapeedan Nasya.
3) Teekshna dhooma pana (Devadaru, chitramoola)
4) Aja mamsa sevana
5) Gandak rasayana usage
6) Pratishyaya Chikitsa.

## 14) NASA SOSHA (Atrophic Rhinitis )

Vata and Pitta causes dryness of nasal mucosa, leads to difficulty in olfaction and respiration, is explained as Nasa sosha.

**Charaka :-** Vitiated vata causes dryness of nasal mucosa and shrungataka marma, is explained as Nasa sosha.

**Treatment :-**
1) Ghee + Milk -          for oral intake
2) Kseera Sarpi          "
3) Jangala Mamsa          "
4) Anutaila Nasya
5) Sneha          6) Mrudu sweda
7) Sneha dhooma pana.

## 15) NASA GATHA RAKTHAPITTA (Epistaxis)

Bleeding from and through the nose is calledas Nasagatha Raktha Pitta, it comes under the Classification of urdwagatha Raktha pitta .
1) According to dosha it is 4 types , they are.
a) Vataj b) Pittaja c) Kaphaj d) sannipathaj
(madhavkar explained Dwandaja Ratapitta also)

**2) Dwi Prabhavam :-**
A) a) Yakruth (Liver ) b) Pleeha (spleen )
B) a) Aamashayaja b) Pakwashayaja
C) a) Snigdoshna b) rukshnoshna

**3) Dwi marga**
a) Urdwa gatha b) Adhogatha
(others explained Tiryakgath as 3rd, some body ubhaya gatha as 3rd )

**Samprapthi :-** 1) Doshaj 2) Aaganthuja.
1) The Pitta, Raktha predominent vitiated doshas while propogating in the body moves in 3 drections a) upward b) Downward c) Both or irregular, if doshas passes in upward direction there are chances for nasal bleeding.

(Madhava kara explained that in Kapha Predominence doshas moves in upward direction, vata predominence doshas moves in downward direction and in vata Kapa Predominence doshas moves in Both the direction)

2) Shiro or Nasa Abhighata (Injury ) causes nasal bleeding

# CLINICAL FEATURES OF NASAL BLEEDING

**Based on Doshas :-**

**1) Vataj Raktha Pitta :-** Thin, rough, foamy, black Nasal bleeding.

**2) Pittaja Raktha Pitta :-** The blood is blackish, Decoction like, smoky, and resembles like Agaru and anjana.

**3) Kaphaja Raktha Pitta :-** Blood appears bulk, oily, sticky and in whit colour

**4) Tridoshaja Raktha Pitta :-** All the symptoms of tri-doshas present.

**Treatment :- 1)** Shodhana therapy in strengthy patients

**2)** Shamana or Stambana therapy in weak patients.

**3) Pitta -** Raktha hara treatment should be given.

**4) Sandhanam -** Adjoining the margins or suturing the lesion

**Skandana -** Processing of blood coagulation by dusting medicated powder.

**Pachana -** Medical cauterisation

**Dahana -** Electric Cauterisation.

**5)** Cool applications, drops, and dusting the powders of, ex: musta, usheera, Naga kesara, chandana, doorva etc.**6)** Cause should be treated whether Local or systemic **7)** Nasya with milk and sugar **8)** Nasya with doorva swarasa or ghritha or draksha or ikshurasa or ksheera or dadima puspa swarasa or spatika + sharkara or pancha ksheeri kashaya or Hreeberadi kasaya or palaandu moola swarasa or vasa swarasa or Yasti ghritha or babula patra swrarasa, or Apamarga patra swarasa, or Aamalaki swarasa etc.**9)** Oral administration of Vasa swarara, Avaleha or ghritha.**10)** Oral administration of Chandanasav usheerasava etc drugs.**11)** Ghritha Pichu. **12)** Internal usage of the drugs. Like swarna gyrica, sutasekara ras, Pravala Pisti, mukta pisti, shankha bhasma, chandanadivati, lakshadi guggulu, Kamaduda ras, shubra bhasma, Rakta bandini vati. **13)** Santarpana chikitsa.

# EPISTAXIS

The Bleeding from the nose (unilateral or bilateral) occuring due to local or systemic caues is known as epistaxis .

| I) | 1) Anteror | 2) Posterior |
|----|------------|--------------|
| II) | 1) spontaneous | 2) Induced. |

**Causes of Epistaxis :-**

**A) Local causes -**

**1) Congenital :-** Multiple telangiectasis or Osler's disease.

**2) Traumatic:-** Trauma to the nose, para nasal sinuses or head, nose picking (especially at littles area), surgical trauma, Barotrauma etc.

**3) Inflammatory :-** Nasal diphtheria, Acute vestibulitis, acute Rhinitis, Acute sinusitis, Adenoids, Chronic Rhinitis, chronic sinusitis, Rhinitis sicca, atrophic rhinitis, Rhino sporidiosis, Tuberculosis, syphilis, leprosy, lupus, etc.

**4) Neoplastic :-** Benign and malignant tumours.

5) Idiopathic

**6) Miscellaneous :-** Foregin bodies, maggots, rhinoliths, vicarious menstruation.

**B) General Causes :-** or systemic caues

1) Hypertension. **2)** Bleeding disorders like leukaemia, haemophilia, Purpura, agranulocytosis, Hodgkin's disease, anaemia etc **3)** increased pressure in superiorvenacava due to mitral stenosis, superior mediastinal tumours, whooping cough, pneumonia, Bhronchitis, tumours of mediastinam and neck **4)** drugs - salicylates, quinine, phosphoras etc **5)** Debilitative disorders infective viral fevers, measles, varicella, erysepelas, influenza, Rheumatic fever, endo carditis. **6)** Chronic renal failure, uraemia, Toxaemai **7)** Miscellaneous - Caisson disease, high altitudes. Vicarious menstruation **8)** Idio pathic causes.

**Pathology :-** 1) 90 % of the cases the bleeding point is Little's area or Kiessel bach's plexus for the rich blood supply due to the anastamosis of many vessels like Anterior ethmoidal, sphenopalatine, posterior ethmoidal, greater palatine and superior labial arteries, it is situated about 6 to 8 mm within the vestibule and 6 mm above the floor of the nose.

2) The area above the middle turbinate receives blood supply from anterior ethmoidal artery, Bleeding chances or there

3) Woodruff's plexus - behind the posterior end of the inferior turbinate (venous anastamosis present here ) it is also a site for bleeding per Nose.

**Clinical Features :-**

1) Quantity may vary from Little to profuse, the symptoms depends upon the quantity of blood loss.

2) Bleeding if anterior, can be seen; if post nasal may be swallowed by the patient or he may spit it out or come as Haemoptysis or Haematemesis.And the other symptoms are 3) Anxiety 4) Discomfort 5) general debility 6) shock 7) If cause is systemic the Local symptoms may appear.

**Investigations :-**

    1) Blood pressure    2) Haemogram
    3) Coagulation test    4) Radiography
    5) CT Scan         6) Endoscopy 7) Biopsy.

**Treatment :-**

    1) If there is any specific cause that should be treated.
    2) First aid
    a) ice or cold pack application on the bridge of nose to arrest the bleeding by reflex vasoconstriction
    b) Pinching the nose at Littles area for 2 to 3 minutes.
    3) Anterior nasal packing with a gauze soaked in liquid paraffin or other lubricants.
    4) Posterior nasal packing is advised if bleeding does not stop by anterior nasal packing
    5) If the bleeding is due to Local atrophic causes - Lubricant ointment should apply
    6) If bleeding point is Visible that should be cauterised.
    7) sedation should be given in suitable doses.
    8) Blood transfusion if blood Loss is severe
    9) Calcium vitamines C, K and other haemostate may be given
    10) Antibiotics to prevent the infection following nasal packing.
    11) Ligatin of the external carotid artery distal to lingual artery or Eth moidal arteries in the pterygo maxillary fossa.

### 16) NASA NAHA OR NASA PRATINAHA
### ( Deviated nasal septum)

    The udana vayu is get encircled (Aavrutha) with Kapha and causes vitiation in its own place (swa marga viigunya), leads to Nasal obstruction and difficulty in respiration, is known as Nasaanaha or Nasa Pratinaha

    It canbe co-related to deviated Nasal septum, Nasal polyp or cyst or tumour of Nasal cavity those causes nasal obstruction and dfficulty in respiration.

**Treatment :-**

    1) Intake of Oleus substances after meals
    2) meal with mamsa rasa
    3) Ghritha pana 4) Snigdha dhooma
    5) Shiro vasti 6) Nasya with Anu taila or shatbindu taila For oral, massage nasya and for shiro vasti 7) Usage of bala taila
    8) Nasa sosha chikitsa 9) Brumhana chikitsa.

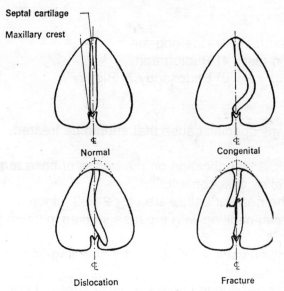

Septal cartilage

Maxillary crest

Normal

Congenital

Dislocation

Fracture

Causes of deviated nasal septum.

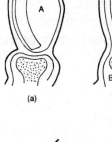
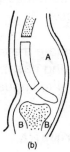
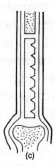

(a)

(b)

(c)

Septoplasy i) Creation of anterior tunnel (A) ii) Creation of inferior tunnels (B) and excision of inferior strip of cartilage iii) Criss-Cross incisions on cartilage to break spring.

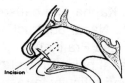

Incision

Incision for the submucosal resection of the nasal septum

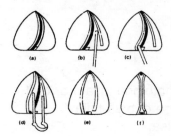

(a)     (b)     (c)

(d)     (e)     (f)

Steps of the SMR operation (a) Incision; (b) Elevation of the mucoperichondrial flap on one side; (c) Elevation of the mucoperichondrial flap on other side; (d) Use of Killian long bladed speculum for separating the mucosal flaps from the nasal skeleton; (e) Excision of the deviated nasal septum leaving behind the framework; (f) The end result.

196

## DEVIATED NASAL SEPTUM (D.N.S.)

Deviated Nasal septum is a common and frequent abnormality, requires the treatment when it produces the symptoms.

**Aetiology ;-**

1) Heriditory causes
2) Congential causes - compression of nose and upper jaw in the intra uterine period due to abnormal posture.
3) Defective development of septum
4) Rapid Growth of septum in relation to face so septum buckled to accommodate it self.
5) High arch of palate may cause buckling of cartilagenous spetum
6) Excessive development of middle and inferior turbinate.
7) D.N.S. is secondary to the nasal tumours polyps and masses.
8) Trauma to the Nose or upper jaw
9) Recurrent Nasal Paranasal infections.
10) general debility and un hygienic condition.

**Clinical features :-**

1) Asymptomatic - there may be no symptoms
2) Blocking of the nose either unilateral or bilateral
3) Headache due to sinusitis, Vacum head ache, Neuralgic head ache etc.
4) Recurrent cold due to stagnation of fluids and infection.
5) epistaxis - due to stimulation of little's area
6) Anosmia 7) Deformity of external nose 8) Dryness of mouth and pharynx 9) On examination of nasal cavity septum appears as deviated either in C shape or S shape or in irregular shape and the turbinates apppears as hypertrophied.

**Complications :-**

1) Recurrent Sinusitis.
2) Middle ear infections.
3) Mouth breathing
4) Asthma
5) Atrophic rhinitis.

**Treatment :-** It is required when patient has persistent or recurrent symptoms due to deviated nasal septum permanent relief is obtained by the submucoous resection of nasal septum (S.M.R. operation) or septoplasty.

In the early stage decongestant drops and antibiotics gives relief but when there is gross deflection surgical correction is only the choice of treatment.

# S.M.R. (SUB MUCOUS RESECTION ) OPERATION

The Nose is Locally anaesthetised by packing the nose (on bothsides) with a solution of 4 % Lignocaine with 1:100000 adrenaline, further anaesthesia is achieved by sabmucosal infiltration of 2% Lignocaine with 1:100000 adrenaline (General anaesthesia is advocated in an un cooperated patient).

Patient is operated in a semi sitting position under Local anaesthesia and in supine position under general anaesthesia.

**Method :-** 1) An incision is made usually in the deviated side through the mucoperichondrium upto the cartilage, just beyond and parallel to the muco cutaneous junction.

2) The mucoperichondrium is then elivated from the deviated portion of the septum by a suitable elvator.

3) Then the cartilage is incised along the first incision this should be carefully done to avoid injury to the muco perichondrium of opposite side, then the opposite mucoperichondrium should be elivated by introducing a suitable elevator.

4) With the long bladed nasal speculum the mucosal flaps are separated from septal cartilage, then with the help of Ballenger swivel knife and luc forceps the deviated cartilaginous and bony parts of septum should be removed but care should be taken to preserve some part at roof and columella to avoid deformity of external nose

5) Suturing of the flaps is usually not necessary but nose is pack with veselline ribbon gauze to prevent the sticking of mucosa and injury.

## Post Operative Care :-

1) Anti biotics Analgesics and Antiinflammatories are given 5 to 7 days
2) Nasal packs are removed after 48 hours then Nasal decongestants should use for few days
3) Application of ointment or oleus things to the nose to loosens crusts or clots.
4) Forcible blowing of nose should be avoided .
5) Rest for a week.

## Complication :-

Haemorrhage 2) Septal haematoma 3) Septal abscess 4) Septal perforation 5) Adhesions of septum with lateral wall 6) Saddle nose 7) flappy septum 8) Neuralgic pain a) Intra cranial complications.

# (17 to 20 ) NASA ARSHA (NASAL POLYP )

The Twak (Skin ), Mamsa (muscle ), medas (fat tissue ) are vitiated by vatadi doshas and produce polyp like growth is called arsha.

It is of 6 types in general (for guda arsha) they are 1) Vataj 2) Pittaj 3) Kaphaj 4) Raktaj 5) Sannipataj 6) Sahaj

But in Nasa rogas Nasa arsha are explained as 4 types they are 1) Vataj 2) Pittaj 3) Kaphaj 4) Sanni pataj.

## Clinical Features :-
1) Difficulty in respiration 2) Sneezing 3) Rhinitis 4) Foul smell from nose 5) headache 6) Nasal Speech.

## Treatment :-
It can be corelated to Nasal Polyps, treatment is excision of the polyps, in shalya tantra 1) Aushada 2) Shastra 3) Kshara 4) Agni Karma are explained for the treatment of Arshas.

# 21-24) NASA SHOPHA :-
It is an oedema like thing that does not contain any sac in side like tumour. it may occur due to infection, Allergy and trauma. .

It is of 4 Types :
1) Vataja 2) Pittaja 3) Kaphaja 4) Sanni pataj

**Symptoms :-** Like arshas.

**Treatment :-** Shotha hara, shoola hara, Vrana ropana, pratishyaya chikitsa should be given.

# 25-31) ARBUDA (TUMOURS )

The Raktha and mamsa are vitaited by vatadi doshas and produces a round hard and deep rooted growth is known as arbuda.

a) Madhava kara explained 6 types.
1) Vataj 2) Pittaja 3) Kaphaj 4) Rakthaj 5) Mamsaja 6) Medoja.

b) According to Shalakya tantra 7 types in the nose.
1) Vataj 2) Pittaja 3) Kaphaj 4) Raktaj 5) Mamsaja 6) Medoja
7) Sannipataj.
It produces obstructive inflammatory irritative symptoms in the nose.
It can be co-related to tumour of the nose.

**Treatment : -** 1) Aushada 2) Shastra 3) Kshara 4) Agni Karma according to the condition of the tumour.

## Nasal Polyp :-

Polyp is a pedunculated hypertrophied oedematous mucosa of Nose or para nasal sinuses. The Nasal polyps are inflammatory in origin but not Neoplastic - polypoidal swellings are shaped like polyp but not polyps.

**Types :-** Usually 2 types.

1) Antrochoanal Polyp it arises from the maxillary antrum, grows towards the back of nose (Posterior nares) and reaches Naso pharynx and oropharynx, commonly single doesnt recur after perfect excision.

2) Ethmoidal polyp, multiple, bilateral, arises from ethmoidal sinus and grows towards anterior nares.

## Pre-disposing factors :-
1) Allergy                        ex:  Ethmoidal polyp
2) Vasomotor          -          Due to imbalance between sympathetic and Para sympathetic nerves of nose
3) Infection          -          Long Standing bacterial and viral infection
4) Mixed causes
5) Bernouilli's phenomenon - (Negative pressure in the sinuses )..
6) Polyp saccharide changes in the ground substance.

## Pathology :-

## Macroscopic Pathology :-
**a) Antra choanal Polyp :-** Prolapsed mucosa hangs from the roof of the antrum, becomes oedematous, through the ostium of maxillary sinus and haitas semilunaris reaches the choana then to the Naso pharynx and oro pharynx.

**b) Ethmoidal Polyps :-** Multiple, Bilateral, the prolapsed mucosa swells and hanged downwards and forwards in the nasal cavity.

## Microscopic Pathology :-
The Nasal polyp consist of Soft smooth bluish white masses. The ciliated columnar epithelial  covering undergo squamous meta plasia due to chronic irritation, the stroma is fibrillar and oedematons, Lympho cytes, Eosino phils and plasma cells are included. The blood vessels and nerves are scanty so only polyp is painless and avascular.

## Clinical Features :-
1) Nasal obstruction which is not relieving with nasal decongestant.

200

2) Sneezing and watery nasal discharge present in Allergic cases. 3) Mucopurulent discharge in infected cases.4) Broadening of nose in Ethmoidal polyp 5) Snoring and mouth breathing.6) Headache epiphora and post nasal drip 7) In anterior Rhinoscopy ethmoidal polyp look like a bunch of grapes, smooth oval pale blue pink or reddish in colour and pain less. 8) in Posterior Rhinoscopy Antro choanal polyp looks rounded smooth greyish bluish in colour.

**Investigations :-** 1) Nasal secretion contain Eosinophils 2) Radiograpy of sinues 3) Biopsy.

**Treatment :-**
1) Removal of the causes
2) Anti histamines - decongestants - Antibiotics.
3) Excision of the polyps.
4) Ethmoidectomy in recurrent ethmoidal polyp
5) Removal with cald well- luc operation, in recurrent Antro choanal polyp.

**Differential Diagnosis of Polyp :-**

**1) Hypertrophied turbinate :-**
It is pink in colour, tender , firm to feel, probe cannot passed around the tubinate and it shrink with decongestant drops.

**2) Rhinosporidiosis :-**
Mass arises from septum , strawberry like in appearance, arises to people of costal area due to fungus infection.

**3) Malignancy :-** Contain granulomatous bleeding poly poidal swelling - Histopathology confirms the disease.
**4)** Angioma of Nasal septum, single red smooth and bleeds readily
**5) Meningo cele :-** Prolongation of meninges into nasal caivty as polyp like swelling. aspiratin of fluid and Histopathology confirm the disease
**6) Hamartoma :-** It is adevelopmental malformation consisting of tumour like growth of tissue - Benign in origin but rarely becomes malignant.
**7) Adenoids -** Radiography of Naso pharynx confirm the adenoids locating at the junction of roof and posterior pharyngeal wall.
**8) Naso pharyngeal malignany :-** In posterior Rhinoscopy irregular growth is seen with lymph node meta stasis .

**Note :-** So after excision of Polyp- Histopathology in necessary to confirm the disease.

# Tumours of the Nose and Paranasal Sinuses :-

The benign tumours are not so common in the nose and para nasal sinuses. the following are rarely observed.

**Benign Tumours :**

1) Papilloma 2) Adenoma 3) Haemangioma 4) Fibroma 5) Osteoma 6) chondroma 7) Osteoclastoma 8) Chordoma 9) Rhinophyma etc.

**1) Papilloma :-** Single or multiple, sessile or pedunculated tumour mostly arises from the skin of vestibule or anterior part of septum - Surgical excision is treatment of choice .

**2)    Adenoma :-** It is rare but may become malignant .

**3)    Fibroma :-** It is rare, commonly arises from septum and turbinates.

**4)    Haemangioma :-** 3 types capillary cavernous and multiple telangiectasees (Osler's disease ). The commonest is capillary types occurs at septum, osler's disease occurs at Little's area and causes bleeding. excision. and cautery is the treatment.

**5)    Osteoma** 3 types .

a) Campact osteoma occurs in frontal sinuses

b) Cancellus osteoma occurs in maxillary and ethmoidal sinuses and

c) Fibrous dysplacia - maxillary and ethmoidal bones are deformed . Excision of the excessive tissue is the choice of treatment for cosmotic purpose.

6) Chondroma 7) Chordoma 8) Osteo clastoma and Rhino phyma are rare.

**Malignant tumours :-**

Malignant tumours of nose and para nasal sinuses occurs 0.2% of the malignancy of total body (Very less when compared to other parts of body). Rare in the nasal cavity, more frequent in maxillary sinus, less frequent in Ethmoidal sinus, Rare in frontal and sphenoid sinus.

a) **Squamous cell carcinoma** is the commonest type involving the nose with eruption of bleeding polypoidal mass- causes Nasal obstruction and bleeding.

**Treatment :-** wide surgical excision and Radio therapy

b) **Adeno carcinoma** occurs in maxillary sinus.

c) **Melanoma :-** Rare blackish mass develops inside the nose.

d) **Chondro sarcoma** & meta static tumours are very rare.

e) **Inverted papilloma** develops in the lateral wall of nose as red or greyish mass, it is known as Ringertz's tumour.

f) Olfactory neuroblastoma develops from sensory olfactory epithelium at cribriform plate of ethmoid bone.

The common clinical features are 1) Nasal obstruction. 2) epistaxis 3) Blood stained nasal discharge 4) Pain and head ache  5) Peripheral lesions like proptosis, epiphora, Toothache swelling of check and palate etc.

**Diagnosis :-**  1) Xray

           2) Biopsy

     **Treatment :-**  Excision, radio therapy  or chemotherapy etc.

# CYSTS OF NOSE AND PARANASAL SINUSES

**Sinuses :-**

Cysts are of different types.

1) Congenital cysts

2) Cystic odontomes

     a) Cyst of eruption - Bluish swelling on unerupted deciduous tooth or permanent tooth .

     **b) Dentigerous Cyst :-**  Arises from the follicle around an unerupted tooth. the tooth is seen in the cyst cavity on xray -Treatment is to remove cyst along with tooth.

     **c) Dental cyst :-**  The infected tooth produces apical granuloma which forms cyst .

     **Treatment :-** Excision along with carious tooth.

     **d) Adamantinoma :-**  A diffuse swelling on mandible with eggshell crackling - treatment is radical excision.

**3) Mucocele :-**  A cystic swelling of sinus (mostly Frontal some times ethmoid) due to blockage of sinus ostium resulting in thinning and expansion of sinus wall.

     **Treatment :-** Excision and re establishment of drainage.

**4) Dermoids :-**  Occurs midline of the nose and extend into septum and inner outer margins of orbit .

**5) Haemorrhagic :-**  Bone cysts found in the mandible may be due to trauma.

# MUKHA ROGA
# (DISEASES OF THE
# ORAL CAVITY & THROAT)

## मुख रोग संख्या

''मुखरोगाः पंचषष्टिर्भवन्ति सप्तस्वायतनेषु। तत्रायतनानि-ओष्ठौ, दन्तमूलानि, दन्ताः, जिह्वा, तालु, कण्ठः, सर्वाणि चेति। तत्राष्टावोष्ठयोः पंचदश दन्तमूलेषु, अष्टौ दन्तषु, पंच जिह्वायां, नव तालुनि, सप्तदश कण्ठे, त्रयः सर्वेष्वायतनेषु॥

(सु॰ नि॰ अ॰ 26)

यथा-ओष्ठे गण्डे द्विजे मूले जिह्वायां तालुके गले॥
वक्त्रे सर्वत्र चेत्युक्ताः पंचसप्ततिरामयाः।
एकादशैको दश च त्रयोदश तथा च षट् ॥
अष्टावष्टादशष्टौ च क्रमात्

(अ॰ हृ॰ उ॰ अ॰ १७)

## मुखस्वरूप

ओष्ठौ च दन्तमूलानि दन्ता जिह्वा च तालू च।
गलो मुखादि सकलं सप्ताङ्ग मुखमुच्यते॥

## मुखरोग-संख्या

स्युरष्टावोष्ठयोर्दन्तमूले तु दश षट् तथा।
दन्तेष्वष्टौ च जिह्वायां पंचस्युर्नवतालुनि॥
कण्ठे त्वष्टादश प्रोक्तास्त्रयः सर्वेषु च स्मृतः।
एवं मुखामयाः सर्वे सप्तंषष्टिमता बुधै॥

(भा॰ चि॰ म॰ ४)

## वग्भट के मत से मुखरोग निदान

मात्स्यमाहिषवाराहपिशितामकमूलकम्।
माषसूपदधिक्षीरशुक्ते क्षुरसफाणितम् ॥
अवाक्शय्यां च भजतो द्विषतो दन्तधावनम्।
धूमच्छर्दनगण्डूषानुचितं च सिराव्यधम्॥
क्रुद्धाः श्लेष्मोल्बणा दोषाः कुर्वन्त्यन्तर्मुखान् गदान्।

(अ॰ हृ॰ उ॰ अ॰ 21)

205

# ANATOMY AND PHYSIOLOGY OF ORAL CAVITY (MUKHA )

The mouth Or the oral cavity consists of Two parts. a smaller anterior vestibule and a bigger posterior mouth proper, these are seperated by teeth and gums and having connection from beyond the last molar teeth when mouth is closed, parotid glands and mucous glands of lips and cheeks are open into the vestibule of mouth. The mouth proper has a floor roof and communicates posteriorly with the pharynx by the Oropharyngeal isthmus. The vestibule of mouth is bounded externally by the lips and Cheeks and internally by the upper and Lower teeth.

## Lips :- (Osta)

Lips are, Two, soft movable structures which surround the oral aperture. . By incisivus superioris and inferioris lips attached to the bone (Maxilla and mandiable ) and also attached by the respective median fold of mucous membrane, known as frenulum. It contains free border, attached border and adjoining angle (Angle of mouth), a shallow median groove present at the centre of upper lip, known as philtrum. It is having two surfaces - cutaneous surface (Externally) and mucosal surface (Internally), The layers of lips from out to inwards are as follows. 1) Cutaneous layer 2) Muscle Layer (Orbicularis Oris) 3) Sub mucous layer (contain labial salivary glands ) 4) Mucosa (Reddish pink transparent layer.)

## Muscle Attachments of the Lips :-

**1)Levator Labii superioris alaeque nasi :-**
Raises and everts the upper lip and dilates the nostrils.
**2) Levator labii Superioris :-**
Elevates the upper lips slignt laterally.
**3) Zygomaticus minor :-** Elevating upper lip.
**4) Levator anguli Oris :-** Raises the angle of lips.
**5) Zygomaticus Major :-** Raises the lips upwards iaterally as in laughing
**6) Mentalis : -** Raises and Protrudes the lower lip.
**7) Depressor Labiii inferioris :-**
Depress the lips downwards little laterally.
**8) Depressor anguli oris :-** Angle of mouth is depressed down wards and Laterally.

**Note :-** The 8 Mucsles are supplied by facial Nerve only.

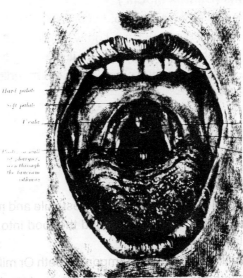

Hard palate
Soft palate
Uvula
Palatopharyngeal arch
Palatoglossal arch
Tonsil
Posterior wall of pharynx, seen through the isthmus faucium

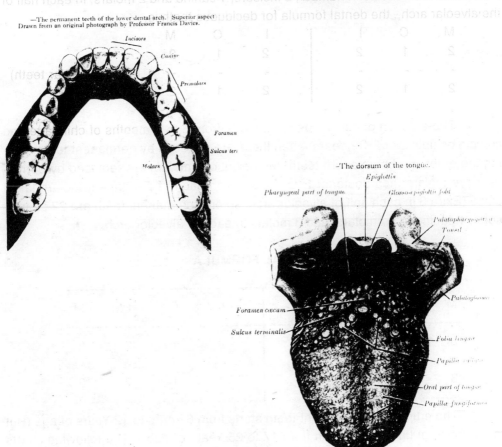

—The permanent teeth of the lower dental arch. Superior aspect
Drawn from an original photograph by Professor Francis Davies.

Incisors
Canine
Premolars
Foramen
Sulcus ter
Molars

—The dorsum of the tongue.
Epiglottis
Pharyngeal part of tongue
Glosso-epiglottic fold
Palatopharyngeal
Tonsil
Palatoglossus
Foramen caecum
Sulcus terminalis
Folia linguae
Papilla vallatae
Oral part of tongue
Papilla fungiformes

**B)     Gums (Dantha Moola ) :-**

Gums Or gingivae is a fold of dense Vascular fibrous tissue, covered by mucous membrane, being lined by lightly keratinised squamous epithelium, which is continuous with the mucosa of cheek - it is having two parts, Attached part is firmly adherent to alveolar process of maxillae and mandible, free part surrounds the neck of teeth like a collar.

**Nerve Supply :-**

Maxillary and mandibular nerves, branches.of Trigeminal Nerve.

**C)     Teeth (Dantha )**

The Oral cavity is divided into vestibule and mouth proper by teeth and gums. Teeth are useful to cut, tear and grind the food into small pieces.
Teeth are classified into.

1) Deciduous teeth Or Temporary teeth Or milk teeth and .2) Permanent teeth. Deciduous teeth are 20 in number, 2 incisors, 1 canine and 2 molars, in each half of the alveolar arch,. the dental formula for deciduous teeth is.

| M | C | I | | I | C | M | |
|---|---|---|---|---|---|---|---|
| 2 | 1 | 2 | | 2 | 1 | 2 | |
| - | - | - | | - | - | - | (No premolar teeth) |
| 2 | 1 | 2 | | 2 | 1 | 2 | |

The eruption of deciduous teeth starts from 6 to 9 months of child age and completes upto 2 or 2 1/2 Years. Then these are replaced by permanent teeth. During the eruption of permanent teeth, the deciduous molars are replaced by permanent pre-molars then posterior to pre-molars eruption of permanent molars takes plase (Extra 3 in each half of alveolor arch, so only permanent teeth are 32 ; 2 incisors , 1 canine, 2 premolars, and 3 molars in each of alveolor arch.

### DENTAL FORMULA

| M | PM | C | I | | I | C | PM | M |
|---|----|----|---|---|---|---|----|---|
| 3 | 2 | 1 | 2 | | 2 | 1 | 2 | 3 |
| - | - | - | - | | - | - | - | - |
| 3 | 2 | 1 | 2 | | 2 | 1 | 2 | 3 |

The eruption of permanent teeth starts from 6 Years to 12 Years of age (But the eruption of Last molar teeth from 17 to 25 Years of age ). The following charts denote the time of eruption of each tooth.

**Eruption of Deciduous Teeth :-**

| Sl.No. | Name of Tooth | Age of the Child. |
|---|---|---|
| 1. | Lower Central incisors | 6 to 9 months of child age |
| 2. | Upper Central incisors | 8 to 10 Months . |
| 3. | Upper Lateral incisors | 15 to 21 Months. |
| 4. | Lower Lateral incisors | 15 to 21 Months. |
| 5. | First Molar | 15 to 21 Months. |
| 6. | Canine | 16 to 20 Months. |
| 7. | Second Molar. | 21 to 24 Months. |

**Eruption of Permanent Teeth :-**

| Sl.No. | Name of Tooth | Age of the Child. |
|---|---|---|
| 1. | Ist Molar | 6 Years. |
| 2. | Medial Incisor | 7 Years. |
| 3. | Lateral incisor | 8 Years. |
| 4. | Ist Pre-molar | 9 Years. |
| 5. | 2nd Pre-molar | 10 Years. |
| 6. | Canine | 11 to 12 Years. |
| 7. | 2nd molar | 12 Years. |
| 8. | 3 rd molar (Wisdom teeth) | 17 to 25 Years. |

## Discription of the Teeth :-

The tooth has root, a crown and a neck, The portion burried within the jaw is called as root, while the portion projecting beyond the gum is called crown, and neck is the constricted portion situated at the junction of above two parts. At the apex of the each root has a pin point aperture known as apical Faramen For the transmission of. the vessels and nerves.

## Structure of the Teeth :-

Each tooth is composed of Enamel, cement Dentine, and pulp.

1) Enamel is white in sensitive substance that covers the crown of the tooth.

2) Cement is bony and covers the roots of the teeth.

3) Dentine is the yellowish basis of the tooth which is Extremely sensitive which covered by Enamel (at crown area) and cement (at root area ).

**4)** **Pulp :-** Dentine contain a cavity within known as pulp cavity that usually opens at the tip of the root through a Foramen known as apical foramen that gives transmission for vessels and nerves.

Each tooth contained in a conical bony socket ; between the root - and bony socket a vascular layer know as peridontal membrane present which is covered by gum and attached by an epithelial Layer which may destructed by age and leads to Exposing of cement.

**Discription of the Structure of Teeth :-**
**Incisors :-** 8 in number , 4 in each jaw. It is chisel shaped with an incising margin, upper incisors are bigger than lower and medial incisors are bigger than Lateral. The two labial tubercles of the crown Form the cutting margin and one lingual tubercle remains rudimentary - The root is single, conical with lateral curvature.

**Canine :-** 4 in number 2 in each jaw, it is longest of all teeth. 2 labal tubercles of the crown are fused to Form a large cone and one lingual tubercle is well defined. the root is single & elongated.

**Premolars :-** 8 in number, 4 in each jaw, 2 labial tubercles of crown and lingual tubercles appear in pyramidal shape (cusp- like) and have single root (The root of first upper pre-molar is bifurcated).

**Molars :-** 12 in number, 6 in each jaw. The crown contain 2 labial and 2 lingual tubercles in upper jaw and 2 labial and 1 Lingual tubercles in lower jaw. 3 roots present in upper molars and 2 roots in Lower molars.

**Blood Supply :-**
**Upper Jaw :-** Molars and premolars - by posterior superior alveolar branches of maxillary Artery.
Incisors and canine - by Anterior superior alveolar branches of inferior orbital artery.

**Lower Jaw :-** All the teeth are supplied by inferior alveolar branches of maxillary artery.

**Nerve Suuply :-**
**Upper Jaw :-** Molars and pre molars by maxillary nerve and canine and incisors by infra orbital nerve, lower jaw by the mandibular nerve.

# TONGUE (JIHWA )

The Tongue is a mobile organ, bulges upwards From the floor of the mouth, it is coverved by straitified squamous epithelium and consists of a mass of straited muscle. Interspersed with little fat and numerous glands. It consists of
a) root of tongue b) Apex or tip of tongue c) Dorsum
d) Inferior surface and e) Right and Left margins Or borders.

**a) Root of Tongue :-**
It is attached to the hyoid bone and mandible and in between the attachments it comes in contact with Genio hyoid muscle and Myelohyoid muscles, it transmits the nerves and vessels which supply it.

210

**b) Apex or tip of Tongue :-** It is free anterior end of tongue, that rests against the incisor teeth.

**c) Dorsum of Tongue :-** The dorsum of tongue extends from the tip of tongue to the anterior suface of the epiglottis. It is separated into Oral part (Palatine Part) and pharyngeal part by a "V" shaped sulcus terminalis, the apex of which points posteriorly and is marked by a pit the formen caecum, A shallow median groove extends from the tip of tongue to the foramen caecum. The mucosa of Oral part is rough and thick due to presence of papillae (Most of papillae contain taste buds) where as pharyngeal part or mucosa is smooth thin and nodular in appearence due to the presence of small lymph follicles (Lingual tonsils ) in sub mucosa. Posteriorly the mucosa is continuous with anterior surface of epiglottis and the glosso epiglottic fold connects the tongue with the epiglottis.

**Inferior surface and sides of Tongue :-**
The inferior surface and sides are covered with thin smooth mucosa, in the middle a raised fold of mucosa joins the inferior suface to the floor of mouth known as frenuium Liguae. on each side of Frenulum Linguae deep Lingual veins present, on lateral sides of Lingual veins there is fringed Fold of mucosa known as plica fimbriata and in the floor the openings of sub mandibular ducts, present on sub lingual papillae .

**Actions of Tongue :-**
1) Organ of Taste.
2) Helps in deglutition.
3) Hels in speech
4) Helps in mastication of food.

**Muscles of Tongue :-**
( Extrinsic Muscles :-)
**1) Genioglossus :-** The anterior fibres of the muscle, depress the tongue to enlarge the Oral cavity and the posterio- inferior fibres help to protrude the tongue, it is supplied by Hypoglossal Nerve.

**2) Hyoglossus :-** It depress the sides of the tongue to enlarge the Oral caivty, it is supplied by Hypoglossal Nerve.

**3) Styloglossus :-** It pulls the tongue postero superiorly as in swallowing, it is supplied by Hypoglossal Nerve.

**4) Palatoglossus :-** It draw the soft palate inferiorly on to the posterior part of the dorsum of the tongue (elevation of tongue ) it is supplied by pharyngeal plexus formed by glossopharyrgeal and vagus complex,

**5) Chondro Glossus :-** It is a part of hypoglossus, it inserts into intrinsic muscles, in between Hyoglossus and genio glossus.

**Intrinsic Muscles :-**
1) Superior longitudinal muscle curls the tip of tongue upwards and roll it posteriorly.

2 ) Inferior longitudinal muscle curls the tip of tongue inferiorly, with superior logitudinal it retract and widen the tongue.

3) Vertical muscle :- Increases the length of tongue for protrusion.

4) Transverse muscle :- Narrow the tongue and increases its height.

**Motor Nerve Supply :-** All the above muscles except palatoglossal are supplied by Hypoglossal nerve.

**Note :-** Actions of the individual muscles is explained above and others also occurs by the complex combinations.

**Sensory Nerve Supply :-**
1) **Lingual nerve,** branch of Trigeminal, for general sensation of Anterior 2/3 of tongue.
2) **Chorda tympani,** branch of facial, for taste sensation of Anterior 2/3 of tongue.
3) **Glosso pharyngeal,** :- Nerve for posterior 1/3 of tongue for general and taste sensation.
4) Superior laryngeal - nerve, branch of vagus, supply to the small area adjacent to epiglottis.

**Vessels of Tongue :-**
1) Lingual and deep artery of tongue, to the anterior 2/3 part.
2) Dorsalis linguae artery, to the posterior.

**Veins :-**
1) Deep vein and Lingual vein follow,the corresponding arteries.

**Physiology of Tongue :-**
The sense of Taste and smell are closely interrelated, sense of taste doesnot evolve solely, in the absence of olfaction (Smell sensation) taste sensation is remarkably altered. Primary taste sensations are 4 - a) Sweet (From the tip of tongue ) b) Sour (From the sides of tongue ) c) Bitter (From the back of tongue ) d) Salt (Dorsum of tongue Anteriorly). and other tastes are e) Metallic f) Alkaline.

Tongue is mainly concerned with taste sensation (Other functions speach, mastication and deglutition) Taste buds are the end organs of taste, located in the mucosa of the epiglottis, pharynx, under surface of palate and lateral walls of papillae which present in the Anterior 2/3 of Tongue.

**Papillae of the Tongue :-** Thickly distributed over the Anterior 2/3 of tongue, these are modifications of mucosa, visible to the naked eye and designed to increase the surface area of mucosa.

**1) Vallate Papillae :-** 8 to 12 in number, large in size present in front and parallel to the sulcus terminalis, theses is are encirded by trench like Furrow(Vallum) so only named as vallate papillae.

**2) Fungi Form Papillae :-** More numberous at sides and apex of tongue, round in shape and appears as bright red spots.

**3) Filiform Papillae :-** Numerous in number, present at Anterior 2/3 of dorsum of Tongue, conical cylindrical in shape, run parrallel to vallate papillae and at the apex run transversely.

**4) Papillae Simplices :-** These cover whole of mucosa of tongue, consist of closely set microscopic elivations of corium.

### Taste Buds (Gustatory Calyculi )

These are modified neuro epithelial cells, arranged in flask shaped groups in the epithelium of tongue, inferior surface of palate, oro pharynx etc., (Taste buds absent in the mid dorsum of tongue). Broad base resting on corium and its neck opening between the cells of epithelium by an orifice known as gustatory pore. 2 types of cells a) Gustatory cells and. b) Supporting cells present. gustatory cells occupy the central portion of taste bud, spindle shaped with sperical nucleus, the peripheral processes (gustatory hair ) ends at the gustatory pore, nerve fibres enter the base of the taste bud, loose their myelin sheath and either invaginate the gustatory cell or lie between them. The substance that should be tasted must be in solution- Normally saliva acts as solvent.

## Factors influence the taste Sensation :-

1) **Area :** If bigger wider area is stimulated, taste sensation perfectly carried out, if not negligible.

2) **Temparature :-** Taste sensation is modified with temparature - at $30^0$ to $40^0$ c maximum Taste sensation is observed.

3) **olfaction :-** Taste sensation have link with olfaction, if olfaction sensation is poor, Taste sensation also poor.

4) **Individual variation:-** Changes person to person as per their taste preferences.

5) **Adaptation :-** Taking Tea after eating of Sweets, sweet sensation of Tea reduces.

6) **Acceptance and rejection of Foods.**

**Ex :-** Sweets mostly accepted, Acid and salts in higher concentration is rejected.

## Pathway of Taste Impulses :-

From Anterior 2/3 of Tongue Taste fibres to Lingual Nerve, to Chorda tympani, to facial Nerve, to Geniculate ganglion, to Dorsal nucleus of facial Nerve (Upper part of nucleus of tractus solitarius) to posterior ventral nucleus of thalamus, to inferior part of post central gyrus of cerebral cortex.

## From Posterior 1/3 of Tongue :-

Taste fibres to glosso pharyngeal Nerve - to petrous ganglion-to Dorsal nucleus of glossopharyngeal Nerve (Lower part of nucleus of Tractus solitarius) - to posterior ventral nucleus of Thalamus. to inferior part of post central gyrus of cerbral cortex.

**Note :-** 1) The General sensation From Anterior 2/3 through lingual Nerve, branch of Trigeminal Nerve.

2) Superior laryngeal Nerve branch of Vagus Nerve supply to the small area adjacent to Epiglottis.

# SOFT PALATE (TALU)

The soft palate is a flexible musular flap which extends postero inferiorly from the posterior edge of the hard palate into the pharyngeal cavity. It Forms an incomplete septum between mouth and pharynx. the Uvula is hanging down From the middle of its free posterior border which is continuous with palato - pharyngeal arches on each side.

**Upper or Dorsal Surface :-**

It is convex and is continuous with the floor of nasal cavity. Lower or Anterior suface is concave and an elivated smooth ridge named median rephe present at its median plane. posterior or inferior surface is free margin and contain Uvula centrally. Superiorly attached to the lower border of hard palate and on each side it is attached to the pharynx with palato pharyngeal arches. The dorsal surface is lined with columnar ciliated epithelium where as ventral surface is lined with satraitified squamous epithelium. The soft palate contain double fold of mucus membrane which contains the following structures in between them.

**A) Palatal Muscles :-**
1) 2 Levator Palatini muscles (elevates the soft Palate)
2) 2 Tensor Palatini Muscles (it make the anterior part of soft palate rigid).

**Note :-** By the action of these 2 muscles soft palate is elivated and drawn posteriorly against posterior pharyngeal wall and shuts off Nasal part of Pharynx thus permits swallowing without regurgitation of Food into Nose. etc.,

2) 2 glosso Palatini Or Palatoglossus muscles (Draw the soft Palate inferiorly on to posterior part of tongue by that it cuts off mouth against pharynx thus permitting respiration to cotinue during sucking Or chewing).

4) Pharyngo palatini muscle Or Palato Pharyngeous muscle (it prevents the soft Palate From being Forced into pharynx while blowing through mouth.)

5) Musculus Uvulae (Shortens and tenses the uvula).
**B) Palatal Aponeurosis :-**
Thin fibrous lamella not only supports the muscles but also strengthens them.
**C) Palatal Glands.**
**D) Arteries :-**
1) Ascending Palatine from facial artery.
2) Palatine branch From ascending pharyngeal, artery.
3) Lesser Palatine, branch of descending palatine, branch of maxillary artery.
4) Dorsal branches of Lingual artery.
**E) Nerves :-**
1) Greater and Lesser Palatine nerves From pterigo palatine ganglian.
2) Pharyngeal plexus (Glossopharyngeal + Vagus Nerves )

# HARD PALATE

Hard palate is formed by the palatine process of two maxillae and Horizontal palates of palatine bones. It s upper surface forms the floor of the nasal cavity and is lined by columnar ciliated epithelium and Lower surface Forms the roof of mouth which is lined by straitfied squamous epithelium, its muco - periosteum is much thicker and contains a large number of mucous glands, greater palatine vessels nerves and naso palatine nerves, posteriorly it is attached to soft palate, on either sides it is continuous with the alveolar arches formed by two maxillae.

# CHEEKS

The cheeks are directly continuous with lips and have 6 (Six) layer they are 1) Skin 2) buccal pad of Fat 3) Bucco pharyngeal Fascia 4) Buccinator muscle. 5) Molar glands 6 ) Mucous membrane.

Buccal pad of Fat is more in infants to increase the rigidity of cheeks and assists in sucking process, parotid duct passes above the buccal pad of fat, pierces buccinator and its facia and enters the mouth opposite to the second upper molar teeth, and molar glands open into mouth at opposite last molar teeth by piercing Buccinator muscle.

Zygomaticus major risorius and platysma muscles also come in the formation of cheek Naso labial sulcus forms a demarcation line between lips and cheeks.Buccinator muscle helps in mastication of Food.

Masseter, Temporalis and medial pterygoid helps to close the mouth and lateral pterigoid to open the mouth.

## PHARYNX (GALA )

Pharynx is a wide muscular tube, 12 to 14 cm long which is lined throughout with mucous membrane, it extends from the base of the skull to the level of the body of the 6th cervical vertebra (Lower border of cricoid cartilage ) where it is continuous with Oesophagus. Widest part of pharynx corresponds to the level of the base of the skull about 3.5cm. and narrowest part is at the Oesophageal Orifice about 10.5 c.m.

Pharynx is divided into 3 compartments they are as follows :1) Naso pharynx 2) Oropharynx 3) Laryngeo pharynx .

**1) Naso Pharynx :-** Extends from the base of skull to the soft palate, it lies posterior to the nasal cavities and septum. pharyngeal busa and pharyngeal tonsils (adenoids) present in the mucosa and sub mucosa at the junction of roof and posterior pharyngeal wall, naso pharyngeal isthmus present at the floor, 2 Posterior nasal apertures present in its anterior surface, and openings of auditory tubes and tubal tonsils present in the lateral wall.

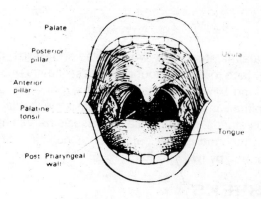

Palate

Posterior pillar

Anterior pillar

Palatine tonsil

Uvula

Tongue

Post Pharyngeal wall

*Structures seen on opening the mouth*

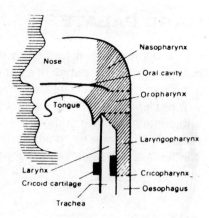

Nose

Tongue

Larynx

Cricoid cartilage

Trachea

Nasopharynx

Oral cavity

Oropharynx

Laryngopharynx

Cricopharynx

Oesophagus

*Three parts of the pharynx.*

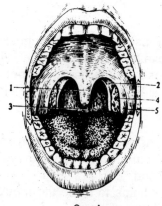

1
3
2
4
5

Oropharynx:
*1*—uvula, *2*—palatopharyngeal arch, *3*—posterior pharyngeal wall, *4*—palatine tonsil, *5*—palatoglossal arch

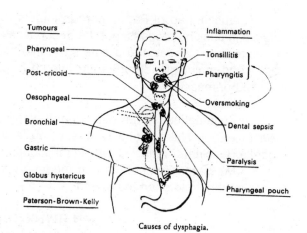

Tumours

Pharyngeal

Post-cricoid

Oesophageal

Bronchial

Gastric

Globus hystericus

Paterson-Brown-Kelly

Inflammation

Tonsillitis

Pharyngitis

Oversmoking

Dental sepsis

Paralysis

Pharyngeal pouch

Causes of dysphagia.

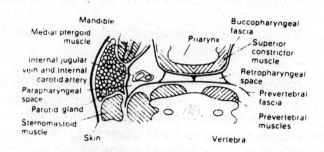

Mandible

Medial ptergoid muscle

Internal jugular vein and internal carotid artery

Parapharyngeal space

Parotid gland

Sternomastoid muscle

Skin

Pharynx

Vertebra

Buccopharyngeal fascia

Superior constrictor muscle

Retropharyngeal space

Prevertebral fascia

Prevertebral muscles

*Retropharyngeal and parapharyngeal spaces.*

216

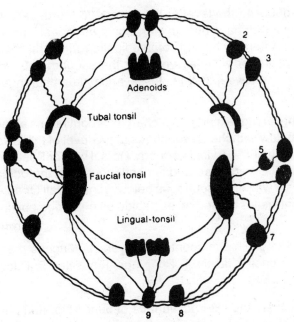

1. Retropharyngeal
2. Styloid
3. Lateral pharyngeal
4. Behind sternomastold
5. Bifurcation of cartold
6. In front of sternomastold
7. Angle of jaw (Jugulo-diagastric)
8. Hyoid
9. Sub-mental

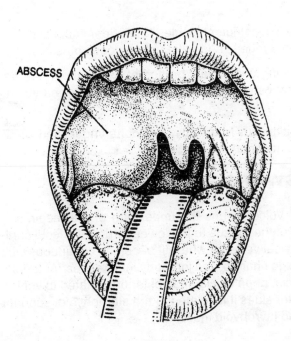

Acute peritonsillar abscess

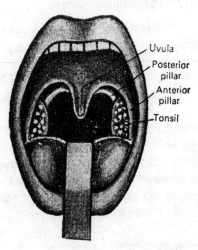

Examinagtion of the tonsils

**2) Oropharynx :-** It lies opposite the level of the second to fourth cervical vertebrae, superiorly it is continuous with naso pharynx through pharyngeal isthmus and inferiorly with laryngopharynx. Anteriorly having communication with Oral cavity through oropharyngeal isthmus, posterior wall lies opposite the second to Fourth cervical vertebrae in the lateral wall in between palato glossal and palato pharyngeal arches palatine tonsils present.

**3) Laryngo Pharynx :-** The laryngeal part of the pharynx is continuous above with Oral part of the pharynx and below with the Oesophagus at the level of the lower border of cricoid cartilage, opposite the 6th cervical vertebra. Dorsal wall or Posterior wall lies opposite 5th and 6th cerrvical vertebrae and is continuous with the dorsal wall of Oropharynx above and dorsal wall of Oesophagus below, ventral wall Or anterior wall is formed by larynx. Lateral wall is formed on each side by pharyngo epiglottic fold and by piriform fossa.

**Pharyngeal Wall :-** The wall of Pharynx contain 5 layers 1) Mucous membrane 2) Sub-mucosa 3) Pharyngo basilar fascia 4) Pharyngeal muscles 5) Bucco pharyngeal fascia.

Bucco pharyngeal fascia covers the external surface of buccinator and pharyngeal muscles and pharyngo basilar fascia covers the internal surface of pharyngeal muscles.

The muslces of pharynx are 3 constrictor muscles (Superior middle and inferior ), stylo pharyngeus, Salpingo pharyngeus and palato pharyngeus muslces.

**Blood Supply ;-** 1) Ascending pharyngeal branch of external corotid, Ascending palatine and Tonsilar branches of facial. greater palatine and pharyngeal braches of maxillary artery.

**Nerve Supply :-** Pharyngeal plexus formed by glossopharyngeal and vagus nerves. External and recurrent laryngeal nerves.

# LARYNX(SWARA - YANTRA)

The larynx is the Organ of Voice, Forms the upper part of the respiratory passage and Extends from the root of the tongue to the lower border of cricoid cartilage - opposite the level of 6th cervical vertebra where it becomes continuous with trachea. Superiorly it open into laryngo pharynx and inferiorly into trachea. Anteriorly it is covered by skin, superficial fascia, deep fascia and posteriorly related to ventral surface of Laryngo pharynx, on either sides it is related to the sternohyoid, superior belly of Omohyoid, sternothyroid and thyrohyoid muscles.

**Measurements :-**

|  | Male | Female |
|---|---|---|
| Length | 44 mm | 36 mm |
| Transverse Dia meter | 43 mm | 41 mm |
| Antero posterior Diameter. | 36 mm | 26 mm. |

The structure of larynx contain 9 cartilages ,3 paired cartilages and 3 single cartilages, they are as follows which are connected with ligaments and membranes.

**Paired cartilages**
1)  Arytenoid Cartilages
2)  Corniculate Cartilages
3)  Cuniform Cartilages

**Single Cartilages**
1) Thyroid Cartilage
2) Cricoid Cartilage
3) Epiglottis.

### i) Epiglottis :-

It is a leaf like thin cartilage present in between the base of tongue and inlet of larynx. It consists of upper Lower and 2 lateral borders and 2 surfaces (Anterior lingual surface and posterior laryngeal surface). Upper border is free and convex, Lpwer border is attached to posterior surface of thyroid cartilage a little below to thyroid notch by **Thyro epiglottic ligament.** Upper part of lateral borders is free but lower part of lateral border is attached to **Ery epiglottic membrane.** Upper part of anterior surface is free but lower part of anterior surface is attached to the Dorsum of tongue by Glosso epiglottic fold, sides by **Pharyngo epiglottic Fold** and to the Hyoid bone by **Hyo epiglottic ligament ,** Posterior surface or laryngeal surface is concave at sides and concavo convex from above down wards. The convex lower surface of epiglottis is known as **Tubercle.**

### Thyroid Cartilage :-

It is the largest of all cartilages, Consists of two lamina which are fused ante-riorly to form an angle and makes a sub cutaneous prominence known as **laryngeal prominence (Adam's apple).** Superiorly two lamina forms V shaped notch known as **Thyroid notch.** The cartilage is convex anteriorly and concave posteriorly. It con-tain superior and inferior horns. Superior horn articulates with Hyoid bone by **Thyro hyoid membrane .** inferior horn articulates with cricoid cartilage. Inferior border gives attachment to **crico thyroid membrane and muscle .** outer surface (lateral) gives insertion to sternothyroid, thyrohyoid and inferior constrictor of pharynx. Inner surface gives attachments to **Vestibular and Vocal ligaments.** Thyro arytenoideus thyro epiglotticus and vocal muscles. The angle gives attachment to **Thyro epiglot-tic ligament.**

### Chicoid Cartilage :- It is situated below the thyroid cartilage. its lower bor-der forms the lowest limit of larynx and becomes continue as trache. It consist of quadri lateral plate posteriorly and an anterior arch by which it resembles signet ring.

In posterior surface a vertical ridge present that gives attachment to longitu-dinal fibres of Oesophagus., on either sides gives Origin to crico arytenoideus poste-rior. Anteriorly on either sides crico thyroideus, posteriorly inferior constrictor of phar-ynx and From the junction of 2 surfaces inferior horn of thyroid articulates . In Upper border towards the anterior surface cricovacal membrane and crico arytenoideus lateralis arises and the lower border is attached to trachea by Crico tracheal liga-ment.

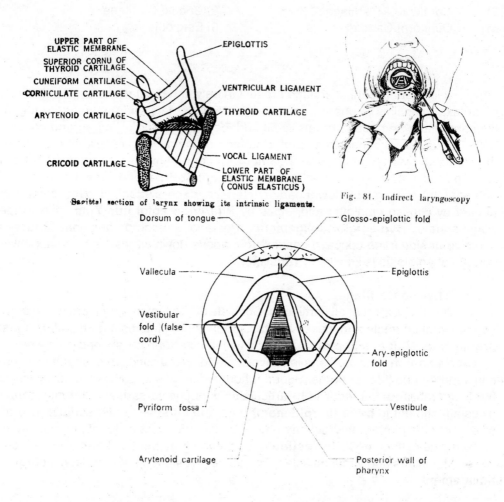

UPPER PART OF ELASTIC MEMBRANE

SUPERIOR CORNU OF THYROID CARTILAGE

CUNEIFORM CARTILAGE

CORNICULATE CARTILAGE

ARYTENOID CARTILAGE

CRICOID CARTILAGE

EPIGLOTTIS

VENTRICULAR LIGAMENT

THYROID CARTILAGE

VOCAL LIGAMENT

LOWER PART OF ELASTIC MEMBRANE ( CONUS ELASTICUS )

Sagittal section of larynx showing its intrinsic ligaments.

Fig. 81. Indirect laryngoscopy

Dorsum of tongue

Glosso-epiglottic fold

Vallecula

Epiglottis

Vestibular fold (false cord)

Ary-epiglottic fold

Pyriform fossa

Vestibule

Arytenoid cartilage

Posterior wall of pharynx

The Larynx on mirror examination (indirect laryngos-

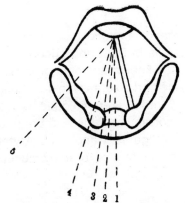

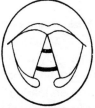

**QUIET RESPIRATION**

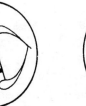

**DEEP INSPIRATION**

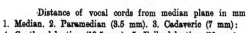
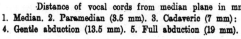

·Distance of vocal cords from median plane in mm
1. Median. 2. Paramedian (3.5 mm). 3. Cadaveric (7 mm):
4. Gentle abduction (13.5 mm). 5. Full abduction (19 mm).

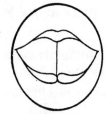

**PHONATION**
*Various positions of vocal cords*

**PARALYSED CORD**

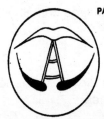

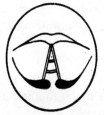

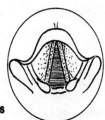

Inflammation

**A. UNILATERAL ABDUCTOR PARALYSIS  B. BILATERAL ABDUCTOR PARALYSIS**

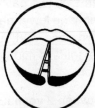

**C. UNILATERAL PARALYSIS
WITH COMPENSATION
BY UN PARALYSED**

*. Positions of paralysed vocal cords:(a) Unilateral abductor paralysis,
(b) Bilateral abductor paralysis, and (c) Unilateral paralysis with
compensation by unparalysed*

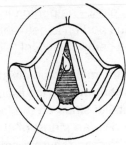

Vocal cord polyp

221

**Arytenoid Cartilage :-**

These are placed at the upper border of lamina of cricoid cartilage on the posterior part of the larynx, pyramidal in shape and consists of 3 surfaces a base and an Apex.

The Base articulates with the upper border of lamina of cricoid, postero laterally gives insertion for crico arytenoideus lateralis in front and crico arytenoideus posterior from behind. Anteriorly a short process known as vocal process present that gives attachment to vocal ligament. The Apex articulates with corniculate cartilage **Posterior Surfaces** is concave and is covered by Arytenoidues transaversus, **Antero Lateral surface** is convex and contain irregular ridges. to the upper area vestibular ligament and to the lower area vocal ligament and crico Arytenoideus lateralis are attached. The **Medial surface** is smooth and covered by mucous membrane.

### 4) Corniculate Cartilages :-

These are two small conical nodulesof Yellow elastic cartilage present within the Ary epiglottic fold being placed at the Apex of arytenoid cartilage.

### 5) Cuniform cartilages :-

These are also two small nodules of Yellow elastic cartilage contain within Ary epiglottic fold, superio lateral to the corniculate cartilages.

### Cavum Laryngis (Cavity of Larynx )

It extends from laryngeal inlet (Communicates with pharynx) to the lower border of the cricod cartilage where it communicates with trachea.

It is incompletely divided into 3 compartments by two pairs of mucous folds, the upper pair of mucous folds are vestibular folds and the lower pair of mucous folds are vocal folds. The portion in between inlet of larynx and vestibular folds is upper division. the portion in between vestibular and vocal folds is middle sub division and the portion below the vocal folds is lower sub division.

In the middle sub division, the fissure in between 2 vestibular folds is known as **Rima Vestibuli** and the fissure in between 2 vocal folds is known as **Rima glottidis,** the packet like sinus on the lateral wall of the larynx between vestibular and vocal folds is known as **sinus of the larynx,** The saccule of larynx present in between vestibular fold and thyroid cartilage that contain numerous glands which pour out secretions by which larynx always kept lubricated.

Rima glottidis is the narrowest part of larynx and fissure changes its shape and form during phonation and respiration. When two vocal folds are adducted high pitch sounds are produced and when two vocal folds are abducted low pitch sounds are produced. (lower range of pitch in the male voice than female due to greater lenght of vocal folds 2.5 cm than female. 1.7 cm.)

## Muscles of Larynx :-

**a) Extrinsic Muscles :-** These concerned with upward and down ward movements of larynx.

1. Supra hyoid for elevating the larynx and trachea.
2. Infra hyoid for depressing the larynx and trachea.

**b) Intrinsic Muscles :-**

Regulates the condition of Rima glottidis.

**1. Adductors of Vocal folds (closure of glottidis )**
A) Crico arytenoideus lateralis.
B) Arytenoideus transversus.
C) Crico thyroid.
d) Thyro arytenoid.

**2) Abductors of Vocal Folds (Opening of glottidis )**
A) Crico arytenoidei posteriores.

**3) Tensors of Vocal Folds.**
A) Crico thyroidei muscles.

**4) Relaxation of Vocal Folds**
Thyro arytenoidei and Vocalis muscles.

**5) Closure of inlet of larynx.**
Oblique arytenoids.

**6) Widening of inlet of larynx.**
Thyro epiglotticus.

**Blood Supply :-**

Superior and inferior laryngeal arteries (Branches of superior thyroid artery and inferior thyroid artery respectively). superior and inferior laryngeal veins opens into superior and inferior thyroid venis respectively.

**Nerve Supply.**
**Motro Nerve Supply :-**

The recurrent laryngeal Nerves supply all the muscles of larynx except crico thyroideus which is supplied by external laryngeal nerve branch of superior laryngeal Nerve. (Arytenoideus having double nerve supply a) Recurrent laryngeal Nerve and internal laryngeal Nerve branch of superior laryngeal Nerve.)

**SENSoRY NERVE SUPPY :-**

**Above the Vocal folds By :-** Internal laryngeal Nerve.
**Below the Vocal Folds By :-** Recurrent laryngeal Nerve.

# MUKHA ROGA VARGEEKARANA
## Classification of diseases of Mukha.

Mukha is formed by the combination of following
7 parts.
1) Osta (Lips) 2) Dantha moola (Gums) 3) Dantha (Teeth) 4) Jihwa
(Tongue) 5) Talu (Palate) 6) Gala (Throat) 7) Mukhadi (the total)

## CLASSIFICATION OF DISEASES OF MUKHA

| | | |
|---|---|---|
| 1) Accroding to sushrutha Mukha Rogas | | 65 |
| 2) " Vegbhata " | | 75 |
| 3) " Bhava Mishra " and yoga ratnakar | | 67 |
| 4) " Charaka " | | 64 |
| 5) " Sarangdhar " | | 74 |

| Sl. No. | Affected part | Sushrutha | Bhava Mishra | Sarang dhar | Vagbhat |
|---------|---------------|-----------|--------------|-------------|---------|
| 1. | Osta roga (diseases of Lips) | 8 | 8 | 11 | 11 |
| 2. | Dantha Moola (diseases of gums) | 15 | 16 | 13 | 13 |
| 3. | Dantha roga (diseases of teeth) | 8 | 8 | 10 | 10 |
| 4. | Jihwa roga (diseases of tongue) | 5 | 5 | 6 | 6 |
| 5. | Talu roga (Diseases of palate) | 9 | 9 | 8 | 8 |
| 6. | Gala roga (diseases of Throat) | 17 | 18 | 18 | 18 |
| 7. | Mukha dhi (Sarvaj) | 3 | 3 | 8 | 8 |
| 8. | Ganda roga (Extra . by Vagbhat) | - | - | - | 1 |
| 9. | Total | 65 | 67 | 74 | 75 |

# 1. वातिक ओष्ठ-प्रकोप

कर्कशौ परुषौ स्तब्धौ कृष्णौ तीव्ररुगन्वितौ ।
दाल्येते परिपाट्येते ह्योष्ठौ मारुतकोपतः ॥

(सु॰ नि॰ अ॰ 16/5)

ओष्ठकोपे तु पवनात् स्तब्धावोष्ठौ महारुजौ ।
दाल्येते परिपाट्येते परुषासितकर्कशौ ॥

(अ॰ हृ॰ उ॰ अ॰ २१)

तत्र खण्डौष्ठ इत्युक्ते वातेनौष्ठौ द्विधाकृतः ॥

(अ॰ हृ॰ उ॰ अ॰ २१)

# 2. पैत्तिक ओष्ठप्रकोप

आचितौ पिटकाभिस्तु सर्षपाकृतिभिर्भृशम् ।
सदाहपाकसंस्रावौ नीलौ पीतौच पित्ततः ॥

(सु॰ नि॰ अ॰ 16/6)

पित्तात्तीक्ष्णसहौ पीतौ सर्षपाकृतिभिश्चितौ ।
पिडिकाभिर्बहुक्लेदावाशुपाकौ

(अ॰ हृ॰ उ॰ अ॰ २१)

# ३. कफज ओष्ठप्रकोप

सवर्णाभिस्तु चीयेते पिडकाभिरवेदनौ ।
कण्डूमन्तौ कफाच्छूनौ पिच्छिलौ शीतलौ गुरू ॥

(सु॰ नि॰ अ॰ 16/7)

शीतासहौ गुरू शूनौ सवर्णपिटिकाचितौ ।

(अ॰ हृ॰ उ॰ अ॰ २१)

# 4. सान्निपातिक ओष्ठप्रकोप

सकृत् कृष्णौ सकृत् पीतौ सकृच्छ्वेतौ तथैव च ।
सन्निपातेन विज्ञेयावनेकपिडकाचितौ ॥

(सु॰ नि॰ अ॰ 16/8)

सन्निपातादनेकाभौ दुर्गन्धास्त्रावपिच्छिलौ ॥
अकस्मान् म्लानसंशूनरुजौ विषमपाकिनौ ।

(अ॰ हृ॰ उ॰ अ॰ २१)

## 5. रक्तदुष्ट ओष्ठप्रकोप

खर्जूरफलवर्णाभि: पिडकाभि: समाचितौ ।
रक्तोपसृष्टौ रुधिरं स्त्रवत: शोणितप्रभौ ॥

(सु॰ नि॰ अ 16/9)

रक्तोपसृष्टौ रुधिरं स्त्रवत: शोणितप्रभौ ॥
शर्जूरसदृशं चात्र क्षीणे रक्तेर्बुदं भवेत् ॥

(अ॰ ह॰ उ॰ अ॰ २१)

## 6. मेद्येदुष्ट ओष्ठप्रकोप

मेदसा घृतमण्डाभौ कण्डूमन्तौ स्थिरौ मृदू ।
अच्छं स्फटिकसङ्काशमास्त्रावं स्त्रवतो गुरू ॥

(सु॰ नि॰ अ 16/11)

तैलाभश्चयशुक्लोदौ सकण्डूवौ मेदसा मृदु ॥

(अ॰ ह॰ उ॰ अ॰ २१)

## 7. मांसदुष्ट ओष्ठप्रकोप

मांसपिण्डौ गुरू स्थूलौ मांसपिण्डवदुद्गतौ ।
जन्तवश्चात्र मूर्च्छन्ति सृक्कस्योभयतो मुखात् ॥

(सु॰ नि॰ अ 16/10)

## 8. क्षतज वा अभिघातज ओष्ठप्रकोप

क्षतजाभौ विदीर्येते पाट्येते चाभिघातत: ।
ग्रथितौ च समाख्यातावोष्ठौ कण्डूसमन्वितौ ॥

(सु॰ नि॰ अ 16/12)

## जलार्बुद

जलबुद्बुदवद् वातकफादोष्ठे जलार्बुदम् ॥

(अ॰ ह॰ उ॰ अ॰ २१)

## गण्डरोग-गण्डालजी

गण्डालजी स्थिर: शोफो गण्डे दाहज्वरान्वित: ॥

(अ॰ ह॰ उ॰ अ॰ २१)

## Osta Rogas (Diseases of Lips )

According to sushrutha Osta rogas are 8 and according to Vagbhata osta rogas are 11, They are as Follows :

### A) Sushrutha's Classification ( 8 Diseases )
1) Vataj Osta Prakopa (cracked Lips)
2) Pittaj Osta Prakopa (herpes labialis - aphthous ulcer)
3) Kaphaj osta Prakopa (Herpes Labialis)
4) Rakthaja Osta Prakopa (Lip granuloma)
5) Sannipathaja Osta Prakopa (aphthous ulcer-carcinoma)
6) Mamsaja Osta Prakopa (Epithelioma of Lips)
7) Medoja Osta Prakopa (Hypertrophy of Lips)
8) Abhighataja Osta Prakopa (Hare - Lip)

### B) Vagbhata's Classification. (11 Diseases)
1 to 8 diseases are same as above, and the additional 3 diseases are.
9) Khandausta (hare-lip)
10) Jalaarbuda (Soft Cyst in lip appearing like water bubble)
11) Grandhi (Cyst in lip)

3, Osta rogas - 1) Sannipathaj 2) Mamsaj 3) Rakthaja osta Prakopa are Asadyam)

## 1) VATAJA OSTA PRAKOPA (CRACKED LIPS)

Vata dosha vitiates and Osta (Lip) becomes stony hard (Karkasha), rough (Parusha), stiff (stabda), blackish (Krishna varna), Painful (Atiruk), and with crackings Or Fissures (Sputanam). This condition also visible in cold wind exposure, infection and injury. " If osta (Lip) is bifurcated by the vitiation of Vata it is named as Khandausta". and " In abhigathaj Osta Prakopa also lips bifurcates but the following differences are there.

| Vataja Osta Prakopa | Abhighataj Osta Prakopa |
|---|---|
| 1) Only vata vitiates | Vata - Kapha and raktha vitiates. |
| 2) No history of injury | History of injury present. |

**Treatment of Vataj Osta Prakopa :-**

1) a) **Abhyanga :-** with chathur snehas + madooschista (wax) and also with Yastimadu + Lodhra + Sariba + Shravani + Neelothphala + Patola +Kakamachi+ tailam.

2) **Nadi Sweda :-** With vata Hara dravya Kashaya.
Ex. ( Erenda Patra + Ksheera - Pakwa Kashaya).

3) **Upanaha sweda :-** (Salavana Swedam ).

4) **Shiro Vasti :-** With Vata hara taila

**Ex :-** Bala taila or Ksheera Bata taila

5) **Nasya :-** with vata hara taila. **Ex :-** 1) Bala taila.

2) Yastimadukadi taila. 3) Kakolyadi taila. etc.

6) **Prathisarana:-** with a) Sarala niryasa + Sarjarasa + Devadaru + guggulu + Yastimadu (for local application.) b) Taila+ + ghritha + Sarja rasa + Rasna + guda + saindhav lavana + gyrica - Pakwa taila+ madooschistam (for local application).

7) **Internal Yogas :-** Ghrithapana, mamsa rasa sevana, shotha hara, shoola hara, Krimighna, vathaghna and vrana ropana yogas should be used.

**Ex :-** 1) Rasnadi guggulu Or Triphala guggulu. 2) Gandak rasayan 3) Maha Rasnadi quatha. etc.

## 2) PITTAJA OSTA ROGA :
### (Herpes Labialis Or simplex, aphthous ulcer).

Pitta dosha vitiates and small papules (Piticas) resembling sarshapa beeja Originates on lips. Lips become bluish Or Yellowish and associate with daha (burning sensation), paka (ulceration), srava (discharge ) and the patient is unable to eat Katu vidaha dravyas (desires cold applications ).

### Treatment :-
" For Pittaja - Rakthaja and Abhighataja Osta Prakopa treatment is similar
1. Pitta dosha hara chikitsa. 2) Like the treatment of pittaja vidradi. 3) Jalaukaavacharara to remove impure blood (blood letting process) 4) Abhyanga (Massage) with ghritha Prepared from Giloya + Yastimadu + Chandan + ghritha 5) Prathisarana - Lodra + sarja rasa + Madhu + Yastimadhu (Local application) 6). Sheetala, vrana ropana, and Raktha pitta hara Chikitsa should be given. 7) Internal Yoga - Daha shamana, shotha hara, Pitta raktha hara, Vrana hara and Krimighna Yogas should be given.

> **Ex : -** 1) Triphala guggulu
> 2) Lagu sootha sekara ras, tabs
> 3) Chandanasav or usheerasav
> 4) Sarivadyarista.

## 3) KAPHAJA OSTA PRAKOPA
### (Herpes labialis)

Kapha vitiates and exhibits same coloured, small papules on the lips, lips become oedematous, heavy, sticky pain less, with itching sensation, cannot bear cool touch and discharges sticky. Cool and thick fluid from the lesion if piticas get suppurate.

**Treatment :-**

1) Kapha hara chikitsa 2) Raktha Mokshan 3) Shiro virechana 4) Kapha hara dhooma pana 5) Swedana 6) Kavala or Gandoosha (with kapha hara decoctions) 7) Pratisaran :- Trikatu + Sarja Kshara + Yava kshara + Vidalavana + madhu. 8) Internal Yogas (Shotha hara, shoola hara, krimighna and Kaphagna ).
  a) Kanchanara guggulu Or Triphala guggulu.
  b) Trijathakadi VatiOr Lavangadi Vati or Kapha hara Vati.
  c) Sariva Or Manjista Or Khadhira Asava Or Arista.

## 4) SANNIPATHAJA OSTA PRAKOPA
**(Aphthous-ulcer Carcinoma of lips ).**

Tridoshas vitiate the lips and lips discoloured into black Or Yellow or white, multiple papules erupt on the lips, discharges sticky foul fluid from the lesion and associate with severe pain. Swelling, ulcer may develop Or may not develop, the signs and symptoms are very irregular and uncertain.

**Treatment :-**
It is Asadya Vyadhi, but can be tried with Tridosha hara Chikitsa.

## 5)    Rakthaja Osta Prakopa :-
**(Lip Granuloma )**
The Raktha dosha vitiates and manifest the papules resembling the colour of Kharjura Phala, the papules bleeds and red tumour develops on lips.
**Treatment :**
Asadya Vyadhi, but can be tried Like Pittaja osta Prakopa.
(Raktha Mokshan - shodhan - Shaman Chikitsa )

## 6) MAMSAJA OSTA PRAKOPA
**(Epithelioma of Lips )**

The flesh of lips vitiates (Mamsa Vikruthi ) and exhibits hard stout inflammed lips and maggots (Krimi) produced from the angles of mouth.

**Treatment :-** It is Asadya vyadhi But According to Modern science : excision and radio therapy. is the choice of treatment.

## 7) MEDOJA OSTA PRAKOPA
**(Macrochelia Or herpes Labialis Or Hypertrophy of Lips )**

It is due to vitiation of medo dhathu in which lips become stout, soft, heavy, sticky, with severe itching sensation and discharges thick fresh fluid resembling Ghritha manda (the upper fresh part of ghee when dissolved) Or spatica.

**Treatment :-** 1) Ruksha swedam 2) Bhedana and Medo nirharana 3) Shodhana 4) Agni Karma 5) Pratisarana - with priyangu + Triphala + Lodra + madhu.

## 8) KSHATHAJA OSTA PRAKOPA
### (Hare lip)

It is due to injury to lips in which cracking Or fissures Or bifurcation of lips takes place. it associates with pain and itching sensation.

**Treatment :-**    1) Like pittaja osta Prakopa.
                        2) If injury is deeper.

Lekhana and Seevana has to do (Osta sandhana by suturing).

## 1) KHANDAUSTA (BY VAGBHATA).
### (Hare lip )

It is due to vata vitiation in which the lips bifurcates.
**Treatment :-** a) Medical treatment b) Surgical treatment.

    **a ) Medical Treatment :-** 1) Vata hara Chikitsa , 2) Vataja osta prakopa chikitsa.
    **b) Surgical treatment :- 1) Sneha 2) Sweda**
    **3) Lekhana :-** The bifurcated surfaces should be scrated with vreehi mukha shastra to have bleeding surfaces for proper healing after suturing.
    **4) Sevana Vidhi :- 5) Pratisaran :-** Application of Shata dautha ghritha Or Yastimadhukadi taila (Yastimadu + Jyothismathi + Lodhra + Mundi + sariba + Kamala + Patola + Kakamachi + Taila).
    **6) Bandhana** (bandaging ) 7) Vata hara shamana taila nasya.

# 2) GRANDHI (CYST)

The Vitiated kaphadi doshas produces a cyst on lips known as grandhi, it associate with itching sensation.

## 3) JALAARBUDA
### (Cyst in the lips)

It is due to the vitiaton of Vata and Kapha in which a cyst resembles water bubble appears on the lips, known as jalaarbuda.
    **Chikitsa :-**
    a) If the cyst or abscess is superficial (utthana) :- Bhedhana -dosha nirharana and prathisarana (Katuki, shunti Kaseesa, Kshara, lavan, Pippali, maricha, + madhu) should be done for. Vrana ropana.
    b) If the cyst Or abscess is deep rooted (Gambheera) Kshara and Agni karma should be done.

## GANDALAJI
### (Cellulitis of the Cheek.)

It is a single disease develops in Ganda sthala in which an immobile cyst Or swelling (Sthira shopha ) developes inthe Cheeks (ganda Sthala), and it assoicates with fever and burning sensation.

    **Treatment :-**
1) Vrana hara Chikitsa. (Vrana shopha Chikitsa should be given.)

## OSTA ROGAS (DISEASES OF LIPS) BY SUSHRUTHA

| Sl. No. | Name of Disease | Vitiated dosha | Signs and Symptoms | Treatment Principle. |
|---------|-----------------|----------------|--------------------|--------------------|
| 1. | Vataj Osta Prakopa (Cracked lips) | Vata | Lips become hard rough stiff painful blackish & with crackings. | 1) Osta abhyanga 2) Sweda 3) Pratisarana 4) Shirovasti 5) Snehan Nasya. |
| 2. | Pittaja Osta Prakopa (Herpes Labialis) | Pitta | Bluish Or Yellowish papules resembling Sarshapa beeja appears on lips, associate with burning sensation, ulcers and patient desires cool applications. | 1) Pitta, or Raktha, or Vidradi Chikitsa has to give 2) Raktha Mokshan 3) Sheeta lepa. |
| 3. | Kaphaj Osta Prakopa (Herpes labialis) | Kapha | Same coloured small papules erupt on Lips and the lips become stout heavy sticky with itching sensation. | 1) kaphahara Chikitsa 2) Raktha mokshan 3)Teekshna Pratisaran 4) Kavala. |
| 4. | Sannipathaja Osta prakopa (Aphthous ulcer, carcinoma) | Tridoshas | Lips are spread with multiple papules appears in black or Yellow Or white. symptoms are irregular and uncertain. | Asadya. |
| 5. | Rakthaj Osta Prokopa (Lip granuloma) | Raktha | Red coloured papules resembling kharjura phale erupts on lips, bleeds and a red tumour develops on lips. | Asadya. |
| 6. | Mamsaja Osta pra-Kopa (Epithelioma of lips) | Mamsa. | Hard stout inflammed lips with maggots at the angles of lips. | Asadya. |

231

| Sl. No. | Name of Disease | Vitiated dosha | Signs and Symptoms | Treatment Principle. |
|---|---|---|---|---|
| 7. | Medoja Osta Prakopa (Hyper trophy of lips) | Medodhathu | Lips become stout soft heavy sticky with itching and discharges fluid resembling ghritha manda. | 1) Ruksha sweda 2) Bhedhan 3) Shodhan 4) Agni Karma 5) Prathi saran. |
| 8. | Kshataja osta Prakopa (Hare lip) | Abhighata | Fissures or cracks appear on lips due to injury and associate with pain burning sensation | 1) Pitta hara chikitsa 2) Lekhana 3) Seevana 4) Pratisarana 5) Bandana. |

## ADDITIONAL 3 DISEASES OF LIPS- BY VAGBHATA

| Sl. No. | Name of Disease | Vitiated dosha | Signs and Symptoms | Treatment Principle. |
|---|---|---|---|---|
| 9. | Khandausta (hare Lip) | Vata | Lips bifurcates - assoicate with pain and burning sensation. | 1) Pitta hara Chikitsa 2) Lekhana-seevana-Bandhana |
| 10) | Jalaarbuda (water bubble like cyst ) | Vata, Kapha | A cyst resembling water bubble appears on lips. | 1) Bhedhan and malanirharan 2) Kshara karma 3) Agni Karma |
| 11. | Grandhi (Cyst) | Kapha | Cyst. erupt on lips due to the vitiation of Kaphadi doshas | 1) Sneha 2) Sweda 3) Chedan 4) Pratisaran. |

232

# दन्तमूल गत रोग

## 1. शीताद

शोणितं दन्तवेष्टेभ्यो यस्याकस्मात् प्रवर्त्तते।
दुर्गन्धीनि सकृष्णानि प्रक्लेदीनि मृदूनि च॥
दन्तमांसानि शीर्यन्ते पचन्ति च परस्परम्।
शीतादो नाम स व्याधि: कफशोणितसम्भव:॥

(सु॰ नि॰ अ॰ 16/14,15)

श्लेष्मरक्ते पूतीनि वहन्त्यस्रमहेतुकम्॥
शीर्यन्ते दन्तमांसानि मृदुक्लिन्नासितानि च।
शीतादोसौ–

(अ॰ हृ॰ उ॰ अ॰ २१)

## 2. दन्तपुप्पुटक या दन्तपुप्पुट

दन्तयोस्त्रिषु वा यस्य श्वयथू: सरुजो महान्।
दन्तपुप्पुटको ज्ञेय: कफरक्तनिमित्तज:॥

(सु॰ नि॰ अ॰ 16/16)

दन्तयोस्त्रिषु वा शोफो बदरास्थनिभो घन:
कफास्रात्तीव्ररुक् शीघ्रं पच्यते दन्तपुप्पुट:।

(अ॰ हृ॰ उ॰ अ॰ २१)

## 3. दन्तवेष्टक

स्रवन्ति पूयरुधिरं चलदन्ता भवन्ति च।
दन्तवेष्ट: स विज्ञेयो दुष्टशोणितसम्भव:॥

(सु॰ चि॰ अ॰ 16)

## 4. उपकुश

वेष्टेषु दाह: पाकश्च तेभ्यो दन्ताश्चलन्ति च॥
आघट्टिता: प्रस्रवन्ति शोणितं मन्दवेदना:।
आध्मायन्ते स्रुते रक्ते मुखं पूति च जायते॥
यस्मिन्नुपकुश: स स्यात् पित्तरक्तकृतो गद:

(सु॰ नि॰ अ॰ 16/21,22)

233

उपकुश: पाक: पित्तासृगुद्भव: ॥

दन्तमांसानि दह्यन्ते रक्तन्युत्सेधवन्त्यत: ।

कण्डूमन्ति स्त्रवन्त्यस्त्रमाध्मायन्तेसृजि स्थिते ॥

चला मन्दरुजो दन्ता: पूतिवक्त्रं च जायते ।

(अ॰ हृ॰ उ॰ अ॰ २१)

## 5. दन्तवैदर्भ

घृष्टेषु दन्तमूलेषु संरम्भो जायते महान् ॥

भवन्ति च चला दन्ता: स वैदर्भोऽभिघातज: ।

(सु॰ चि॰ अ॰ 16/23)

घृष्टेषु दन्तमांसेषु संरम्भो जायते महान् ॥

यस्मिंश्चलन्ति दन्ताश्च स विदर्भोऽभिघातज: ।

(अ॰ हृ॰ उ॰ अ॰ २१)

## 6. वर्धन

मारुतेनाधिकोदन्तो जायते तीव्रवेदन: ।

वर्धन: स मतो व्याधिजिते रुक् च प्रशाम्यति ।

दन्तोधिकोऽधिदन्ताख्य: स चोक्त: खलु वर्धन: ।

जायामानेतिरुग् दन्ते, जाते तत्र तु शाम्यति ॥

(अ॰ हृ॰ उ॰ अ॰ २१)

## 7. अधिमांस

हानव्ये पश्चिमे दन्ते महांछोथो महारुज: ॥

लालास्त्रावी कफकृतो विज्ञेय: सोधिमांसक: ।

दन्तमूलगता: नाड्य: पंच ज्ञेया यथेरिता: ॥

(सु॰ नि॰ अ॰ 16/25,26)

दन्तान्ते कीलवच्छोफो हनुकर्णरुजाकर: ॥

प्रतिहन्त्यभ्यवह्रातिं श्लेष्मणा सोधिमांसक: ।

(अ॰ हृ॰ उ॰ अ॰ २१)

## 8. शौषिर वा सुषिर

श्वयथुर्दन्तमुलेषु रुजावान् कफरक्तज: ।
लालास्त्रावी स विज्ञेय: कण्डूमान् शौषिरो गद: ॥

(सु॰ नि॰ अ॰ 16/18)

श्वयथुर्दन्तमूलेषु रुजावान् पित्तरक्तज: ॥
लालास्त्रावी स सुषिरो दन्तमांसप्रशातन: ।

(अ॰ हृ॰ उ॰ अ॰ २१)

## 9. महाशौषिर

दन्ताश्चलन्ति वेष्टेभ्यस्तालु चाप्यवदीर्यते ।
दन्तमांसानि पच्यन्ते मुखं च परिपीड्यते ॥
यस्मिन् स सर्वजो व्याधिर्महाशौषिरसंज्ञक: ।

(सु॰ नि॰ अ॰ 16/19)

स सन्निपाताज्जवरवान् सपूयरुधिरस्रुति: ॥
महासुषिरमित्युक्ते विशीर्णद्विजबन्धन: ।

(अ॰ हृ॰ उ॰ अ॰ २१)

## 10. परिदर

दन्तमांसानि शीर्यन्ते यस्मिन् ष्ठीवति चाप्यसृक् ॥
पित्तासृक्कफजो व्याधिर्ज्ञेय: परिदरो हि स: ।

(सु॰ उ॰ अ॰ 16/20)

## 11 से 15) दन्तनाड़ी

शोफं न पक्वमिति पक्वमुपेक्षते यो
यो वा व्रणं प्रचुरपूयमसाधुवृत्त: ।
अभ्यन्तरं प्रविशति प्रविदार्य तस्य
स्थानानि पूर्वविहितानि तत: स पूय: ॥
तस्यातिमात्रगमनाद् गतिरित्यतश्च
नाडीव यद् वहति तेन मता तु नाड़ी ।

(सु॰ नि॰ अ॰ 20/9)

# DANTHA MOOLA VYADHIES
## Diseases of Gums.

(A) According to sushrutha 15 diseases.
(B)     "        Bhavamishra 16 diseases.
(B)     "        Saranghadhara 13 diseases.

They are as follows :-

## A) SUSHRUTHA'S CLASSIFICATION - 15 DISEASES.

1) Sheethada (Spongy gums or Bleeding gums )
2) Dantha Pupputaka (Gingivitis - Gumboil-Alveloar abscess)
3) Dantha Vestak (Pyorrhoea alveolaris)
4) Upakusha (Pyorrhoea alveolaris - stomatitis)
5) Dantha Vydarbha (Allergic gums)
6) Vardana (Extra tooth eruption)
7) Adhimamsa (Impacted wisdom tooth)
8) Saushira (Apical abscess or Gingivitis)
9) Maha Saushira (Concrum Oris)
10) Paridhara (Concrum Oris-Gangrenous stomatitis)
11) Vataj Dantha nadi (Sinuses of gums)
12) Pittaj           "      -do-
13) Kaphaj         "      -do-
14) Sannipathaj     "      -do-
15) Abhighataj      "      -do-

**B)**     **Bhavamishra's Classification - 16 Disease.**
1 to 15 - same as sushrutha and the additional 16th disease is **Datha Vidradi.**

**C)**     **Vagbhata's Classification - 13 Diseases.**
3 diseases are not explained by vagbhata from the above classification (16-3=13), The omitted 3 diseases are 1) Dantha Vestak 2) Vardhana.
3) Paridhara
Rest of the Classification is as like above.
Among the diseases of gums.
**2 diseases are asadya, they are**
**1) Sannipathaj Danthanadi 2) Saushira.**

**Note :-** Maha saushira is more complicated than saushira. so maha saushira may also Asadya like saushira - and Bhoja said " maha saushira " is Tridoshaja and causes death within 7 days.

# 1) Sheethaada :-
## Spongy gums Or Bleeding gums.:-
It is a diseases in which Kapha and Raktha doshas vitiate the gums and the following abnormal changes are manifested.

1) Gums become soft 2) bleeding from gums. 3) blackish dis colouration with accumulation of debris on gums 4) foul smell from mouth 5) Severe pain and finally gums are destructed Or emaciated.

This condition is commonly observed due to 1) Vitatmin-C, defficiancy (Scurvey), 2) Injury to gums due to recurrent Oropharyngeal infections, Oral unhygienic conditions, improper brushing of teeth and improper mouth wash etc 3) allergic changes in gums (allergy to tooth paste, very hot or cold liquids.).

**Treatment :-**
**General Principle :-** Swedana, Raktha mokshana, pratisarana, Gandoosha and Nasya
**1) Rakthamokshana :-** Alabu and Gati are commonly used Or jalauka or gums are rubbed with coarse powders (Dantha gharshana choorna). The main idea behind Raktha Mokshana is to remove impure blood from the affected area.

2) Pratisarana yogas (Application of Medicine to the lesion)
a) Priyangau Triphala and musta.b) Musta, Arjuna twacha, Triphala, Priyangu, Shunti, Rasanjan + Madhu.c) Kaseesa Lodra Pippali Manashila Priangu Tejohwa + Madhu (Pratisarana Or Kavala).d) Dadima twacha, Triphala, rasanjan, shunti, saindhava lavana, musta + honey.e) Lavana and Sarshapa taila as tooth powder.

**3) Gandusha Or Kavala Ghaha.**
Gandoosha should do with the decoctions of
a) Musta, Arjuna twacha, Triphala, Priyangu, Rasanjan, and shunti.b) Shunti and parpataka . c) Vataghna taila and ghritha . d) Ksheeri Vruksha Kashaya e) Shunti, Sarshapa, Triphala. Musta. and rasanjan. f) Babbula twak kwatha.

**4)    Nasya :-**
a) If vata is associated snehana nasya. b) If kapha associated madukadi Triphala taila nasya. (yastimadu, utphnala padmaka triphala + taila) c) If Raktha assoicates :- Triphala ghritha Nasya.
**5)    Internal Yogas :-**
Shoola hara, shotha hara, Raktha stambana, vrana ropana yogas should give ex 1) Triphala guggulu, Kanchanara guggulu Lakshadi guggulu etc. Anti inflammatroy analgesic drugs 3) Lagu suthasekara ras, tabs (Anti allergic) 3) Sarivadi vati Or Trijathakadi vati Or Khadhiradi vati (mukha shodhana ) etc ; are very useful to reduce the inflammation of gums.

**Note :-** (Brushing should be avoided and Fine powders of Tiktha Kashaya ras should use for dantha dhavana.)

## 2) DANTHA PUPPUTAKA
(Gingivitis - gum boil- alveolar abscess)

It is a disease in Which the kapha and Raktha dosha vitiate and cause pain and Oedema (hard cystic swelling resmbling Badari Phala ) in 2 or 3 gums (root of teeth) and suppurates quickly.

**Treatment :-**
a)	**According to Sushrutha .**
1) Raktha mokshana then application of Kshara, pancha lavana and Madhu (Pratisarana)
2) Shiro Virechan	3) Kavala	4) Snigda bhojana.

B)	**According to Vagbhata :-**
Sneha, Sweda, Chedan, or Bhedan, or Lekhana, Then application of Yastimadu Sarjakshar shunti and saindhava Lavana to the affected area.

C)	**Modern :-**
If gum is totally infected and root of the tooth also effected, extraction of tooth, incision and drainage to irrigate of pus (Bhedan) and anti inflammatory treatment should be given.

## 3) DANTHA VESTAK
### (Pyorrhoea alveolaris )

It is due to Raktha vitiation in which the root of the tooth is infected impure blood and pus discharges, and leads to destruction of the root of tooth following tooth deay.

(Foul breath, coated tongue, Pigmented teeth, (tartars) and collection of debris at the neck of the tooth, causes infection and leads to above condition.)

**Treatment :-**
1) Raktha mokshana.
**2) Prathisarana :-** Local application of the medicated powder prepared with Lodra Yastimadu,Laksha, Chandan + Honey. **3) Arogya vardini vati with cow milk - Local application . 4) Gandoosha :-** Ksheeri Vruksha Kashaya + Honey + Ghee. **5) Nasya :-** with medicated ghee prepared with Kakolyadi dravya, Dashaguna Ksheera, 6) Swetha manjan & Dashan samskar choorna for brushing 7) Khadhiradi vati for Chewing. 8) Irimedadi taila or sarshapa taila, application to the gums then gargling with Luke warm water 9) Raktha and pitta hara Chikitsa should be given.

## 4) UPAKUSHA
### (Pyorrhoea alveolaris - stomatitis.)

It is pitta Raktha prakopaja Vyadhi, in which Gums ulcerate (Paka), bleeds and bulges again, associated with burning sensation, pain, itching sensation, foul smell (from mouth), and tooth decay.

**General Treatment Principle :-**
1) Vaman 2) Virechan 3) Shiro virechana 4) Raktha mokshan 5) Pratisarana 6) Kavala  7) Nasya. 8) Raktha Pitta hara Chikitsa .

**1) Raktha Mokshana :-** With Gojihwa Patra or madalagrashastra

**2) Pratisaran :-** a) Trikatu, Lavan, + Madu.
b) Laksha, Priyangu, Patanga, Kusta, Saindhava Lavana, Gyrika, Kusta, Shunti, Maricha, Yastimadhu Rasanjan, + Ghrithamanda or Madhu.

3) **Kavala :-**
   A) Pippali, Swetha, Sarshapa Shunthi, Vetasa with Hot water.
   B) Ghritha prepared with Kakolyadi Madhur. dravya.
   C) Ksheeri Vruksha Kashaya + Madhu
   D) Pancha Pallava kashaya + Madhu + Ghritha + Sharkara.
   E) Sahacharadi taila.
   F) Irimedadi taila.

4) **Nasya :-** Ghritha Prepared with kakolyadi madura draya.

## 5) DANTHA VYADARBHA .
### (Allergic gums )

It is a traumatic disease of gums occurs by improper usage of tooth brush Or & Sticks (Dantha Kaasta) while brushing the teeth. The associated symptoms are pain, swelling of gums and tooth decay.

**Treatment :-**
1) Shodhana with Mandalagra shastra and application of Sarja kshara. 2) Cold applications. 3) Sheetha gandoosha. 4) Sheetha Nasya.

## 6) VARDANA (EXTRA TOOTH)

Madhavakara called it as **Khalli vardan** and vagbhata called it as **Adhidantha.**

Extra tooth erupt due to the vitiation of vata, during the eruption severe pain associates and get relief after complete eruption.

**Treatment :-**
1) Extra tooth should be removed and agni karma has to do at the site. 2) Krimi dantha Chikitsa. 3) Vrana Chikitsa.

# 7) ADHI MAMSA

(Impacted Wisdom tooth ) (Tooth ache during the eruption of wisdom tooth).

It is kaphaj vyadhi, The disease occurs at the site of last molar teeth; due to the stricture, oedema of gum, narrow place, tooth eruption becomes late, severe pain swelling of gums, salivation, discomfort and itching sensation present upto the completion of the teeth eruption

**Additional Points By Vagbhata :-** Causes pain in the ear, Maxilla and mandible.

**Treatment :-**

1) Adhimamsa chedan and Prathisarana with Vacha, Chavya, Patha, sarja Kshara, Yava Kshara + madhu. **2) Kavala : -** Pippali + madhu. **3) Mukhadhavana :-** With the decoction of patola, Triphala, Nimbatwak. etc. 4) Shiro Virechana. 5) Virechana dhooma.

## 8) SAUSHIRA OR SUSHIRA
### (Apical abscess Or Chronic gingivitis.)

The Kapha and Raktha doshas vitiate and causes a painful swelling in the gums, associated with salivation and itching sensation, is named as saushira (sushrutha). and according to vagbhata the vitiated Pitta and Raktha doshas causes pain, Oedema and destruction of gums and tooth is explained as saushira.

**Treatment :-**
1) Raktha mokshana (Sushrutha), Su. Chi. 22 chapter)
2) Chedhan and Lekhan (Vagbhata) Ah. Uth. 22 Cahpter)

3)   **a) Pratisarana :-** With Lodra musta Rasanjan + Madhu (Sushrutha )
     **b) Pratisarana :-** With Lodra,musta, shata pushpi,Triphala, Rasanjan, Patang, phalasha pushpa, Katphala + Madhu (Vagbhata)

4)   **a) Gandoosha : -** With the decoction of above drugs (Vagbhata)
     b) Gandoosha with Ksheeri Vruksha Kashaya (Sushrutha)

5)   **Nasya :-** With medicated ghritha prepared with sariva, Neela Kamala, Yastimadhu, Lodra, Agaru, Chandan (for Kalka). 10 times milk, Ghritha.

## 9)   Maha Saushira (Concrum Oris )
The Tridoshas vitiate and causes pain swelling ulceration and destruction of gums, and associate with tooth decay, cleft palate and pain in the oral cavity. (Sushrutha)

**Vagbhata :-** Bleeding pus discharge from the gums with Fever, due to the vitiation of Tridoshas and Raktha dosha .

**Bhoja :-** Herelip, Cleft palate and cracked teeth are also associated and Kills the patient within 7 days.

**Treatment :-**
Like in saushira.

## 10) PARIDHARA
### (Concrum Oris Or Gangrenous stomatitis)

The Pitta Raktha and Kapha doshas vitiate, gums are destructed and bleeds while spitting. (Su. Ni. 16th Chapter).

**Treatment : -**
Like in Sheetada (Su. Chi. 22nd Chapter)

## 11-15) DANTHA NAADI (SINUSES OF GUMS)

It is of 5 types, they are.
1). Vataja Dantha Naadi 2) Pittaja Dantha Naadi. 3) Kaphaja Dantha Naadi 4) Shalyaja Dantha Naadi . 5) Tridoshaja Dantha Naadi.

If gum abscess is not drained in time and is neglected, the pus Or infected fluid propogates into the deeper structures and vitiate the twak Raktha mamsa and asthi of gums and causes sinuses (cavities) which are filled with pus and infected fluids that causes severe complications, even the maxilla and mandible are destructed.

**Treatment :-**
1) Upanaha Swedam (Hot applications) 2) Nadi Vidarana (incision of sinus) 3) Puya nirharana (pus drainage) 4) Prakshalana (Cleaning the gum cavity) 5) Purana Or pratisarana (Application of medicine) (Sushrutha), Su. Chi. 22 chapter) 6) Nadi Vrana Chikitsa. (Ulcer therapy ).

**Special Treatment : -**
1. Dantha Nirharan (Tooth Extraction)  2. Lekhana (Scraping at the site to remove pus and impure blood) 3) Kshara Or Agni Karma. (cauterisation) . 4) Pratisarana. (Applicaton of medicine.)

## COMMON YOGAS

Following tooth powders are helpful in the infammatory conditions of gums.
1. Babbula, Bakula, Jamun Sticks, used for brushing the teeth .
2. Application of Swetha Manjan :- Katika 1kg, Saindhava Lavana 1/2 Kg. spatika 250 grm. Maricha 25 gr. and kapur 12 grm. the fine powder is used as tooth powder.
3. **Jeerakadya Choorna :-** application of fine powder (Tooth powder) of Jeerak, Saindhavalana Hareetaki, shalmali kantak (Yoga ratnakar).
4) **Kanadya Choorna :-** Regular application of fine powder of pippali - saindhava lavana and jeera to the gums (Yoga ratnakar).
5) Dashamoola taila Or ghritha + Madhu (Honey). Gundoosha for treating the chala dantha

6. Sahacharadi taila gandoosha for treating the Chala Dantha.

7. Bhadra mustadi Vati - Kavala to treat the Chala dantha (Yoga Ratnakar) (Badra musta, Hareetak, Trikatu, vidang, Nimbapatra, grinded with gomutra and used for chewing).

8. Fine Powder of Tejobala beeja and Twacha, Haridra dwayam, kusta. Patha, Katuki, Lodra, manjista and Nagar musta, is used as tooth powder.

9) The tablets prepared from Trikatu, Yavakshar, Manahshila Haritala, saindhava lavana, Daruharidra, is used for chewing .

**Pratisarana - Kavala and Gandoosha with the drugs prepared with Kashaya Tiktha Dravya, is very useful in the disorders of gums and teeth.**

# DISEASES OF GUMS (DANTHA MOOLA VYADHEIS )

| Sl.No. | Name of the Disease | Doshas | Signs and symptoms | Treatment Principle. |
|---|---|---|---|---|
| 1. | Sheetada (Bleeding gum) | kapha Raktha | Gums become Painful, soft, black with foul smell, debris Collection on gums, and finally destructed and bleeds. | Swedana, Rakthamokshana Pratisarana Gandoosha and Nasya. |
| 2. | Dantha Pupputa (Gingivitis-gum boil) | Kapha Raktha | Pain and Oedema at the roots of 2 or 3 gums and suppurates quickly. | Raktha mokshana, Kshara Pratisaran, Gandoosha & Nasya. |
| 3. | Dantha Vestak (Pyorrhoea alveolaris) | Raktha | The Root of teeth are infected, accumulation of pus and blood causes destruction of teeth and follows tooth decay. | Raktha mokshan, Pratisaran, Gandoosha, and Kavala. |
| 4. | Upakusha (Stomatitis) | Pitta Raktha. | Gums ulcerates, bleeds and bulges again associated with pain, burning sensation and itching | Shodhan-Raktha mokshan, Prathisaran, gandoosha and Nasya. |
| 5. | Dantha Vydarbha (allergic gums) | Abhighatha | It is a traumatic condition of gums. associated with pain Oedema and Tooth decay. | Shodhan,Kshara, Prathisaran, Cold applications, Sheetha Nasya, and gandoosha. |
| 6. | Vardhan (Extra tooth) | Vata | Extra tooth erupts, during eruption pain, Oedema, itching, associates (Pain subsides after eruption of tooth). | Extra tooth should remove then Agni Karma and Vrana Chikitsa. |

243

| Sl.No. | Name of the Disease | Doshas | Signs and symptoms | Treatment Principel. |
|---|---|---|---|---|
| 7. | Adhimamsa (impacted Wisdom tooth) | Kaphaja | It occurs at the site of last molar tooth, during eruption pain Oedema salivation associates after eruption symptoms get controlled. | Adimamsa Chedan, Prathisarana, Kavala, Vrana Chikitsa. |
| 8. | Saushira (Ch-gingivitis) | Kapha-Raktha Pitta or Raktha | Painful swelling at gums associates with Salivation and itching | Raktamokshana, Gand-oosha,Pratisaranand nasya. |
| 9. | Maha Saushira (Concum Oris) | Tridoshas | Gums inflame and suppurate, associates with tooth decay, cleft palate and stomatitis. | Like Saushira. |
| 10. | Paridhara (Gangrenous stomatitis) | Pitta Raktha Kapha. | Gums destructed and bleeds while spitting | Like Sheetada. |
| 11. | Vataj Dantha nadi | Vata | | |
| 12. | Pittaja Dantha nadi | Pitta | If gum abscess is not treated perfectly in time, the pus propogates into deeper | Incision and drainage of sinus, Prakshalana, |
| 13. | Kaphaj Dantha nadi | Kapha | Structures and vitiate Twak, Raktha, | Pratisaran, gandoosha. |
| 14. | Sannipataj Dantha Nadi | Tridosha | mamsa and asti and causes Severe complications. | |
| 15. | Abhigataj Dantha (Sinus in gums). | Trauma. | | |

244

# दन्त रोग

## 1. दालन

दाल्यन्ते वहुधा दन्ता यस्मिस्तीव्ररुगर्दिताः ।
दालनः स इति ज्ञेयः सदागतिनिमित्तजः ॥

(सु॰ नि॰ अ॰ 16/28)

वातादुष्णंसहा दन्ताः शीतस्पर्शेधिकव्यथाः ॥
दाल्यन्त इव शूलेन शीताख्यो दालनश्च सः ।

(अ॰ हृ॰ उ॰ अ॰ २१)

## 2. दन्तहर्ष

शीतमुष्णं च दशनाः सहन्ते स्पर्शनं न च ।
यस्य तं दन्तहर्षं तु व्याधिं विद्यात् समीरणात् ॥

(सु॰ नि॰ अ॰ 16/30)

दन्तहर्षे प्रवाताम्लशीतभक्षा क्षमाद्विजाः
भवन्त्यम्लाशनेनेव सरुजा श्चलिता इव

(अ॰ हृ॰ उ॰ अ॰ २१)

## 3. दन्तशर्करा

शर्करेव स्थिरीभूतो मलो दन्तेषु यस्य वै ।
स दन्तानां गुणहरी विज्ञेया दन्तशर्करा ॥

(सु॰ नि॰ अ॰ १६/32)

## 4. कपालिका

दलन्ति दन्तवल्कानि यदा शर्करया सह ।
ज्ञेया कपालिका सैव दशनानां विनाशिनी ॥

(सु॰ नि॰ अ॰ 16/33)

साप्युपेक्षिता
शातयत्यणुशौ दन्तात् कपालानि कपालिका ।

(अ॰ हृ॰ उ॰ अ॰ २१)

## 5. भञ्जनक

वक्त्रं वक्रं भवेद्यस्मिन् दन्तभङ्गश्च तीव्ररुक् ।
कफवातकृतो व्याधिः स भञ्जनकसंज्ञितः ॥

(सु॰ नि॰ अ॰ 16/31)

## 6. कृमिदन्तक, कृमिदन्त

कृष्णशिछद्री चल: स्रावी ससंरम्भो महारुज: ।
अनिमित्तरुजो वातात् विज्ञेय: कृमिदन्तक: ॥

सु. नि. अ. 16/29

समूलं दन्तमाश्रित्य दोषैरुल्वणमारुतै: ।
शोषिते मज्जि सुषिरे दन्तेन्नमलपूरिते ॥
पूतित्वात् कृमय: सुक्ष्मा जायन्ते तत: ।
अहेतुतीव्रार्त्तिशम: ससंम्भोसितश्चल: ॥
प्रलून: पूयरक्तस्रुत् स चोक्त: कृमिदन्तक: ।

(अ॰ ह॰ उ॰ अ॰ २१)

## 7. श्यावदन्त

योसृङ्ग्मिश्रेण पित्तेन दग्धो दन्तस्त्वशेषत: ।
श्यावतां नीलतां वापि गत: स श्यावदन्तक: ॥

(सु॰ नि॰ अ॰ 16/34)

## 8. हनुमोक्ष

वातेन तैस्तैर्भावैस्तु हनुसन्धिर्विसंहत: ।
हनुमोक्ष इति ज्ञेयो व्याधिर्दितलक्षण: ॥

(सु॰ नि॰ अ॰ 16/35)

## 1. कराल

करालस्तु करालानां दशनानां समुद्गम: ॥

(अ॰ ह॰ उ॰ अ॰ २१)

## 2. दन्तचाल

चालश्चलद्द्विर्दशनैर्भक्षणादधिकव्यथ: ॥

(अ॰ ह॰ उ॰ अ॰ २१)

## 3. दन्तविद्रधि:

दन्तमांसे मलै: सास्त्रैर्बाह्यान्त: श्रयथुर्गुरु: ।
सरुग्दाह: स्रवेद् भिन्न: पूयास्रं दन्तविद्रधि: ।

(अ॰ ह॰ उ॰ अ॰ २१)

# DANTHA ROGAS
## (Diseases of Teeth)

According to :-

| | |
|---|---|
| Sushrutha | \| |
| Bhavamishra | \|        8 Diseases only |
| Madhava Kara | \| |

Vagbhata       =        10 Diseases

## A) SUSHRUTHA AND BHAVAMISHRA'S CLASSIFICATION OF DANTHA ROGAS.

8 Diseases, they are as follow :-

1) Dalana (Tooth ache or Odontina or Cracked tooth)
2) Krimi Dantha (Caries tooth)
3) Dantha harsha (Sensitivity of tooth due to exposed nerve Filament).
4) Bhanjanka (Broken teeth or falling of Teeth)
5) Dantha sharkara (Tartars)
6) Kaplika (Tooth Enamel separation )
7) Shyava dantha (Black or bluish teeth)
8) Hanu Moksha (mandibular dislocation)

## B) MADHAVA KARA'S CLASSIFICIATION OF DANTHA ROGAS = 8

1 to 7 diseases are same as above; **8)** dantha Vidradi (Alveolar abscess Or gumboll)

## C) VAGBHATA'S CLASSIFICATION OF DANTHA ROGAS (10)

**1 to 7** are same as above (except few wording differences they are as follow.
Dalana (sushrutha) sheetha dantha (Vagbhata)
Bhanjanaka (sushrutha) = Dantha bheda (Vagbhata)
**8)** Karala (ill formed teeth).
**9)** Chala dantha (Loose teeth)
**10)** Adidantha (eruption of extra tooth).

**Note :-  Vagbhata and Madhava Kara were not explained Hanu moksha.**

# 1) DALANA
### (Tooth ache or Odontina or Craecked Tooth )

The Vitiated Vata causes untolerable cutting type of pain in the teeth, is known as dalana.

Vagbhata called it as sheetha dantha why because the patient cannot able to eat or drink cold items. **(Sheetha asahishnutha).**

This condition commonly observed in the Old, caries teeth, cracked teeth - in which the nerve filament of teeth is exposed.

**Treatment :-**

As per sushrutha it is Asadhya Vyadhi. But Vagbhata explained the following treatment principles.

1) Sweda with hot water (Hot water gargling) 2) Dantha pali lekhan (Scraping of external coating on tooth (Lekhana with vreehi mukha shastra) 3) After lekhana, Agni Karma with hot Oils (ushna taila). 4) Dantha Pali Gharshan or pratisarana with, fine powders of Musta, saindhava lavana, dadima twacha, Triphala, Rasanjan, Priyangu, jambuasti, Shunti + Madhu. 5) Kavala with Kseeri Vruksha Kashaya. 6) Nasya with Anutaila.

## 2)    Dantha Harsha :-
(Odontitis due to exposed Nerve filament Or due to caries teeth).

The vitiated vata causes (Vata + Pitta + Other Acharyas) the disease in which the patient cannot able to take hot or cold things (sour things also - Vagbhata) " **Sheetha - Ushna-Amla asahishnutha "**

This condition commonly observed in Krimi dantha or **Dantha kshaya** (caries teeth ) in which due to cracking or perforation of teeth the nerve filament is exposed and causes sensitivity to cold or hot things.

**Treatment :-**

**1) Kavala Or Gandoosha :-**

a) With Lukewaram Oils (Chathur Sneha sarpi - taila vasa and Majja). b) Trivruth ghritha Or with Vataghna Aushadas. c) Yastimadu, Tila and Kseera (ksheera Paka Aushada). d) Sarshapa taila Or Narayan taila Or vishnu taila or prasarini taila.

**2) Nasya :-** Snehan nasya.**3) Dhoma Pana :-** Snehika dhooma pana.**4) Shiro Vasti:-** with vataghna taila. **5) Snigdha bhojan** Like mamsarasa, Kseera - Navaneetha and ghritha . **6) Vatahara Chikitsa.**

## 3)    Dantha Sharkara (Tartars)
It is due to improper cleaning of mouth and teeth by which vitiated vata dry . the Kapha and dantha mala (The waste Precipitations on teeth) and so the teeth appears with yellow or brown coloured precipitations and foul smell. If it is not treated in time leads to tooth decay and other complications..

**Treatment :-**

1) Nidana Parivarjana (Proper brushing and gargling etc). 2) Shareera shodhana (Vamana Virechana etc.,) 3) Dantha mala Lekhana without injuring the enamel and gums(scraping of the Yellow pigment). 4) Pratisarana with Kshara + Madhu. 5) Poorana with Laksha + Madhu (filling). 6) Kavala Or Gandhoosha like in Dantha harsha.

Accoring to modern science also the principle is Lekhana Prakshalana and purana only (Scaling - washing and filling)

## 4)    Dantha Kapalika :-
(Enamel separation due to caries tooth Or injuries)

The disease Dantha Sharkara if not treated in time, causes injury to the enamel of teeth (the outer strong covering of teeth) and fall in small pieces and leads to destruction of teeth, is known as kapalika. Signs and symptoms are pain, burning and sensitivity to hot and cold things.

**Treatment : -** It is Kasta Sadya Vyadhi but advised to treat like Dantha Sharkara and Dantha harsha.

## 5)    Bhanjanaka :-
(Cracked Or fissured teeth).

Vagbhata called it as ' Dantha bhedha ." it is Kapha vataj disease in which teeth fall down or broken due to facial paralisis (mukha vakratha) and associate with severe pain .

**Treatment :-** 1) kapha Vataghna Chikitsa 2) Ardhitha Vata Chikitsa 3) Abhyanga with Narayan taila 4) Swedan 5) Vasti 6) Gandoosha with Yastimadu, tila-Ksheera paka 7) Kavala with Aakara Karavadi Yoga 8) Erenda taila panam.

## 6)    Krimi Dantha :-
(Dental Caries.)

It is Vataj, tooth destructing disease (affecting the teeth due to oral un hygeinic conditons like improper brushing of teeth, improper washing of mouth, bitting the hard items, Taking very hot or very cold items, picking of teeth with needles neglecting the Dantha moola rogas, Dantha sharkara, Kaphalika. Shyava vadantha etc.,) in which tooth becomes black, perforate, become loose, discharges foul fluid and assoicate with pain swelling etc.

**Vagbhata :-** Explained the aetio pathology more discriptively as follows :-

| | | |
|---|---|---|
| Vata Vitiation | —ε | Dantha moola Shotha  —ε |
| Dantha Kshatha | —ε | Sushira (Perforation)  —ε |
| - Dantha Majja sosha | —ε | Production of Krimi -  —ε |
| - Dantha Shoola, Srava | —ε | Chala dantha. -  —ε |
| - Puya Raktha Srava | —ε | Tooth decay.  —ε |

Vaghbata's discription is merely equal to modern dental science.

**Treatment :-**
**A) If tooth is not moving**
1) Swedana 2) Rkatha Mokshan 3) Vataghna Avapeedana nasya 4) Sneha Ganoosha 5) Bhadra daarvyadi Lepam (application) 6) Snigdha bhojan. etc .

**B) If tooth is moving at the site :-** Extraction of tooth and cauterisaton (Agni karma) .

**C) If tooth is perforated :-** a) Filling the gap with Guda Or madhuschista and daha Karma b) Filling the gap with the milk of Sapthacchada or Arka.

**D) For Pain Relieving :-**
1) Dhoopana with the seeds of Kantakari. 2) Keeping the vati in mouth, prepared with - Hingu Katphala, Kaseesa, Sarja Kshara, Kusta and Vidanga. 3) Sariva Kalka, Mukha Dharana (chewing) as Krimighna. 4) Ardhraka + Krishna Lavana, Mukha dharara (chewing) as Krimighna. 5) Vataghna taila, ex :- Narayana taila for Gandoosha 6) Brahatyadi Gandoosha. 7) Medicated oil prepared from Hingu, Katphala, Kaseesa, Sarja Kshara, Kusta, vidanga, oil-gandoosha. 8) Application of Clove Oil at the site. 9) Sarshapa taila Nasya. 10) Medicated oil prepared from Vidari, Yastimadu, Kasheruk, Shrungatak, 10 times of milk-taila, Nasya.
" If pain is not relieved by above treatments, the tooth should be extra-cted "

The tooth should not extract in children, Old, weak vatarogi, If comulsory care should be taken for extraction to prevent complications. (Upper teeth should not remove ) after extraction snigdha sheetha madura Chikitsa should give (A.H.U. 22-26).

**Apathya :-** Dantha rogi should not take sour, cold, Rough hard items.

# 7)    Shyava Dantha (Black Tooth )

It is due to Vata, pitta and Raktha vitiation (Vagbhata); Pitta and Raktha vitiation (Sushrutha). Due to the vitiation of doshas the enamel (Dantha twacha ) is burnt and becomes black or blue, is known as shyava dantha.

**Treatment :-** Asadya Vyadhi.
(It is asymptamatic and so no need of any treatment ).

# 8) Hanu Moksha :-
(Dislocation of Mandible).
It is not related to dantha rogas, but contain dantha shoola so sushrutha added it in dantha rogas. Due to head injury, Loud talking, bitting hard substances, and lifting the heavy weights, Vata dosha vitiates, deranges the Hanu sandhi and causes the disease.
**Treatment :-**
1) Arditha Vata Chikitsa. 2) Shiro Vasti. 3) Nasya 4) Dhooma 5) Upanaha Sweda.

**Additional Diseases of Vagbhata :-**

## I) Karala :- (ill formed teeth)

Irregular shape, size and positioned teeth is explained as Karala.

It may be due to adenoids, chronic naso pharyngeal catarrh, congenital abnormelities, Malnutrition, Oral unhygein, chronic debilitative diseases, recurrent dental disorders and caries. etc.

### Treatment : -
**1) Cause Should Treated :-**

**ex** improving immunity powder, suplementing the required vitamines and minerals, treating the chronic naso pharyngeal and oro pharyngeal infections etc.

" In modern dental medical science different technieques are there to treat irregularities of teeth. "

## 2) Chala Dantha :- (Loose tooth)

Really it is a symptom arises by neglecting caries teeth, cracked tooth, tartars, gum diseases etc.,.

Loose teeth causes pain and discomfort during eating Or drinking it causes so many complications even the healthy teeth and mandible Or maxilla also affected.

### Treatment :-
1) Sneha and Dasha moola quath Gandoosha .2) Gharshana (Rubbing).
with Tutha, Lodra, Pippali, Triphala, Raktha Chandan saindhava lavana. etc.
3) Snigda nasya.4) Snigda Kavala.5) Snigda bhojana

## 3) Adidantha (Explained in Dantha Moola Rogas )

### I) Dantha Vidradi (Alveolar abscess or gum boil )
Explained By :- Madhavakara.

Vitiated Raktha causes burning painful Oedematous gums that discharges blood stained pus when suppurates.

### Treatment :-
**A) In Ama Stage :-** a) shamana Chikitsa b) Katu Teekshna ushna Kavala and Lepa.c) Katuki, Kusta, Punarnava, Mesha Shrungi, Yava- For rubbing at the site.

**B) In Patwa Stage :-**
a) Bhedhan. b) Puya nirharana c) Shothahara Vrana ropana Chikitsa.

**C) If Gambheera (deep rooted) :-** Agni Karma should be done.

## DANTHA SHOOLA .

**Chikitsa :-**
1) Hingu, Katphala, Kaseesa, Sarjakshara, Kusta, Vidanga, Pratisaran.
2) Hingwadi taila gandoosha.
3) Erenda, Bruhati dwaya, mundi, siddha taila gandoosha.
4) Kantakari beeja dhoopana.
5) Clove Oil application.

If pain is not under control and tooth is moving with pus discharge, tooth extraction has to do and then following ,medication should given.
1) Yastimadu + taila has to apply to the site.
2) Vidari, Yastimadu, Shrungataka, Kasheru, Ksheera Siddha taila Nasya.

# DISEASES OF TEETH - (DANTHA ROGA) (BY SUSHRUTHA - 8 DISEASES)

| Sl.No. | Name of the disese | Dosha | Sign - Symptoms | Treatment Principle |
|---|---|---|---|---|
| 1. | Dalan (SU) Sheeta dantha (Vag) (Odontina-Toothache) | Vata | Severe untolerable cutting pain in the teeth and cannot bear the cool things (Sensitivity to cool things - Sheethasahishnutha) | Sushrutha - Asadya Vagbhata :- Swedan - Lekhan Pratisarana -gandoosha |
| 2. | Dantha harsha (Exposed nerve fila ment of tooth) | Vata (Pitta) | Due to vitiated Vata patient cannot take cool or hot things (Sheetha - Ushna Asahishnutha) | 1) Sukoshna gandoosha 2) Nasya 3) Dhooma Panam 4) Vata hara Chikitsa. |
| 3. | Dantha Sharkara (Tartars) | Vata Kapha | Due to improper mouth wash or brushing of teeth Kapha and Ama accumulates on teeth and get dried by vitiated Vata and teeth 3) Gandoosha appears with Yellowish brown precepitations. | 1) Dantha mala Lekhan 2) Kshara + Madhu Pratisaran Gandoosha 4) Nasya. |
| 4. | Kapalika Enamel separation | Vata Abhignata | If dantha sharkara is neglected, the tartars. and enamel spearated in small pieces. | 1) Asadya 2) Like dantha Sharkara. |
| 5. | Bhanja naka (SU) Dantha bheda (Vag) | Kapha Vata. | Teeth fall down or broken due to mukha Ardiktha Vakratha (Facial Paralysis) assoiated with pain. | Ardiktha Vata chikitsa. |
| 6. | Krimi Dantha (Dantal carious) | Vata | Tooth becomes loose, black, perforated and discharges foul fluid, assoicate with pain and oedema- causes tooth decay. | 1) If tooth is strong : Lepa Gandoosha. 2) Moving :- Extraction of Tooth and agni Karma. 3) Perforated :- Filling. |

| No. | Disease | Dosha | Description | Treatment |
|---|---|---|---|---|
| 7. | Shyava Dantha (Blackish tooth) | Vata Pitta Raktha. | Due to Vitiation of doshas the enamel is burnt and tooth become black. | Asadya. |
| 8. | Hanu Moksha (Dis location of Mandible.) | Vata | Due to Loud talking bitting hard things, Lifting heavy weight, Vata, vitiates and deranges the Hanu Sandhi and causes the disease.it causes tooth ache. | Ardhitha Vata Chikitsa. |

## ADDITION 3 DISEASES OF VAGBHATA

| No. | Disease | Dosha | Description | Treatment |
|---|---|---|---|---|
| 1. | Karala | Vata | Irregular size shape position of teeth | Nidana Parivarjana |
| 2. | Chala Dantha (Loose tooth) | Doshaj Aganthaja | Loose tooth causes pain and discomfort during eating and drinking | Prathisarana Gandoosha, if not controlled. extraction of tooth is must. |
| 3. | Adidantha (Extra tooth) | Vata | Extra tooth erruption is called adidantha and during the eruption pain assoicates and after eruption pain subsides. | 1) Dantha Nirharan 2) Agni Karma. 3) Gandoosha. |

**Extradisease of madhavakara**

| No. | Disease | Dosha | Description | Treatment |
|---|---|---|---|---|
| 4. | 1) Dantha vidradi (Alveolar abscess) | Raktha | Gums are vitiated by Raktha and get inflammed with pain and oedema, after suppuration discharges blood stained pus | 1) Shaman Chikitsa. 2) Bhedan 3) Prathisaran. |

# जिह्वागत रोग

## 1. वातिक कण्टक

जिह्वानिलेन स्फुटिता प्रसुप्ता भवेच्च शाकच्छदनप्रकाशा ॥

(सु॰ नि॰ अ॰ 16/37)

शाकपत्रखरा सुप्ता स्फुटिता वातदूषिता ॥

(अ॰ ह॰ उ॰ अ॰ २१)

## 2. पैत्तिक जिह्वाकण्टक

पित्तेन पीता परिदह्याते च चिता सरक्तैरपि कण्टकैश्च ॥

(सु॰ नि॰ अ॰ 16/37)

जिह्वा पित्तात् सदाहोषा रक्तैर्मासांकुरैश्चिता ॥

(अ॰ ह॰ उ॰ अ॰ २२)

## 3. श्लैष्मिक जिह्वाकण्टक

कफेन गुर्वी वहला चिता च मांसोद्गमैः शाल्मलिकण्टकाभैः

(सु॰ नि॰ अ॰ 16/37)

शाल्मलीकण्टकाभैस्तु कफेन वहला गुरुः ॥

(अ॰ ह॰ उ॰ अ॰ २२)

## 4. अलास

जिह्वातले यः श्वयथुः प्रगाढः सोलाससंज्ञः कफरक्तमूर्तिः ।
जिह्वां स तु स्तम्भयति प्रवृद्धो मूले तु जिह्वा भृशमेति पाकम् ॥

(सु॰ नि॰ अ॰ 16/38)

कफपित्तादधः शोफो जिह्वास्तम्भकृदुन्नतः ।
मत्स्यगन्धिर्भवेत् पक्वः सोलसो मांसशातनः ॥

(अ॰ ह॰ उ॰ अ॰ २१)

## 5. उपजिह्वा घा उपजिह्विका

जिह्वाग्ररूपः श्वयथुर्हि जिह्वामुन्नम्य जातः कफरक्तयोनिः ।
प्रसेककण्डूपरिदाहयुक्त प्रकथ्यतेसावुजिह्विकेति ॥

(सु॰ नि॰ अ॰ 16/39)

प्रबन्धनेधो जिह्वायाः शोफो जिह्वाग्रसन्निभः ।
साङ्कुरः कफपित्तास्रैर्लालोषास्तम्भवान् खरः ॥
अधिजिह्वः सरुक्कण्डूर्वक्याहारविधातकृत् ।
तादृगेवोपजिह्वस्तु जिह्वाया उपरिस्थितः ॥

254

(अ॰ ह॰ उ॰ अ॰ २१)

# JIHWA GATHA ROGAS
## (Diseases of Tongue)

A) According ot sushrutha Jihwa rogas are 5, they are
       1) Vataja Jihwa kantaka (Chronic glossitis)
       2) Pittaja Jihwa kantaka (Acute glossitis)
       3) Kaphaja Jihwa Kantaka (Chronic glossitis - Leuco Plakia)
       4) Alasa (Sub lingual cyst or abscess)
       5) Upajihwak (Ranula or Cystic swelling)

B)     According to vagbhata Jihwa rogas are Six (6) they are.
       1 to 5 are same as sushrutha - and 6) Adhijihwaka.

## I) Vataja Jihwa Kataka.
## (Chronic glossitis)

The Vata vitiation changes the smooth regular suface of tongue into rough dry thorny and cracked with loss of taste perception, loss and sensation, discomfort, pain and burning sensation.

### Treatment :-
Like Vataja Osta Prakopa.

1) Abhyanga with (Chatur snehas) 2) NadiOr Upanaha sweda. 3) Sneha Pratisarana. 4) Snehan Nasya. (Vata hara, Vrana ropana, Shothahara, Chikitsa has to give.)

## 2) Pittaja Jihwa Kantaka (Acute Glossitis).

Vitiated Pitta causes inflammatory changes in tongue, the tongue appears in red or Yellow colour with, red thorny buds. The symptoms - pain, burning sensation discomfort and loss of taste perception.

### Treatment :-
**1) Raktha Mokshana :-** By rubhing the surface of tongue with the leaves of Gojihwa or shephalika. (impure blood is removed.) 2) Sira Vyadana. 3) Pratisarana with Kakolyadi Madhura sheetha dravyas. 4) Kakolyadi dravya Kwatha Gandoosha. 5) Kakolyadi dravya Milk + Sneha Siddha, Sneha Nasyam. 6) Pitta hara ahara and vihara.

## 3) Kaphaj Jihwa kantaka.
## (Chronic glossitis - Leukoplakia)
Vitiated kapha causes the Jihwa as heavy, thick, wide and is scattered with thorny buds resembling shalmali Kantaka and assoicated with pain discomfort itching sensation and sticky salivation.

**Treatment :-**

1) Lekhana Or Gharshana with the leaves of Gojihwa Or Shephalika to remove impure blood. 2) Raktha mokshana. **3) Pratisarana :-** Trikatu Sarshapa and Saindhava lavana + Madhu = for lepa gandoosha and Nasya. 4) Kavala grah with Swetha Sarshapa + Saindhava lavana **5) Yusha Sevana :-** Food + Yusha prepared with patola Nimba twak, Varthaka, Yava Kshara etc.,

**4)     Alasa :-**
**(Sub lingual cyst Or abscess).**

Tridoshas (Kapha Raktha Or Pitta predominently ) Vitiate and causes a dread ful swelling underneath the tongue by which immobilasation of tongue and suppuration of root of tongue occurs, it is known as Alasa, after suppuration it causes destruction of muscles of tongue and Expels Matsya gandam.

**Treatment :-**

Asadhyam. But can try with the following treatment Principles.
1) Virechan 2) Raktha mokshan 3) Kavala 4) Shiro Virechan 5) Dhooma 6) Vaman. 7) Nasya.

The disease with short duration is sadyam. chronic Or with long duration is Asadhyam.

**5)     Upa Jihwa :-**
**(Ranula Or Cystic swelling of tongue :-**

Vitiated Kapha and Raktha doshas causes a cystic swelling resembling tip of tongue (jihwaagra), and pushes the tongue upwards, assoicated with itching sensation salivation and burning sensation. (Vagbhata called it as adhi jihwaka).

**Treatment ;-**

A) Raktha Mokshana Lekhana - Pratisarana - Nasya - Gandoosha and Dhooma Panam.
B) Chedan and Teekshana dravya Pratisaran (Vagbhata)
**Pratisarana dravyas :-** Katuki, Pippali - Nimba etc

**6)     Adijihwa :-**

Sushrutha explained it in Kantha rogas, the discription of Adhijihwaka is equal to the sushruta's Upajihwaka and Vagbhata said the cyst arises below the tongue and pushes it upwards. (According to vagbhata Upajihwaka arises above the tongue and adhijiwaka arises below the tongue )

**Treatment :-**
Chdan Lekhan Pratisarana.

**Note :-** Among the jihwa roga Alasa is only Asadya.

# DISEASES OF TONGUE (JIHWA ROGAS).

| Sl. No. | Name of the Disease | Dosha | Signs and symptoms | Treatment Princiiple. |
|---------|---------------------|-------|---------------------|------------------------|
| 1, | Vataj-Jihwa Kantak (Chronic glossitis) | Vata | Dry rough thorny appearence of tongue with Crackings and loss of Sensation | 1) Abhyanga 2) Sweda 3) Sneha Pratisaran 4) sneha gandoosha 5) Sneha Nasya. |
| 2. | Pittaja Jihwa Kantak (Acute glossitis) | Pitta | Inflamed tongue (Red Or Yellow colour) ulceration, thorny appearence of mucosa with pain and burning sansation. | 1) Raktha Mokshan 2) Sheetha Pratisaran 3) Sheetha Kavala Nasya. |
| 3. | Kaphaj Jihwa Kantak (Chronic Leucoplakia) | Kaphaj | Thicky bulky heavy tongue with thorny appearence of mucosa of tongue (like shalmali Kantaka) assoicated with itching and salivation | 1) Raktha Mokshan 2) Teekshna Pratisaran 3) Shodhan Nasya 4) Teekshan Gandoosha. |
| 4. | Alasa (Sublingual abscess Or Carcinoma) | Tridosha and Raktha | A dreadful swelling underneath the tongue that causes immobilisation and suppuration of tongue. | Asadya. |
| 5. | Upajihwaka (Cystic Swelling) | Kapha Raktha | A Cystic swelling resembling the tip of the tongue, puspes the tongue upwards (Vagbhata called it as adijihwa) 3) Gandoosha 4) Nasya | 1) Lekhan 2) Pratisarana |
| 6. | Adijihwk (Cystic swelling | Kapha Raktha | A cyst arises on the dorsum of the tongue (Vagbhata called it as upajihwaka) | 1) Lekhan 2) Pratisaran 3) Gandoosha 4) Nasya. |

257

# तालुगत रोग

## 1. गलशुण्डिका या कण्ठशुण्डी

श्लेष्मासृग्भ्यां तालुमूलात् प्रवृद्धो दीर्घः शोफोध्मातवस्तिप्रकाशः ।
तृष्णाकासश्वासकृत् सम्प्रदिष्टो व्याधिवैद्यैः कण्ठशुण्डीतिनाम्ना ॥

तालुमूले कफात् साक्षात् मत्स्यवस्तिनिभो मृदुः ।
प्रलम्बः पिच्छिलः शोफो नासयाहारमीरयन् ॥
कण्ठोपरोधतृट्कासवामिकृद् गलशुण्डिका ।

(अ॰ ह॰ उ॰ अ॰ २१)

## 2. तुण्डिकेरी

शोफः स्थूलस्तोददाहप्रपाकी प्रागुक्ताभ्यां तुण्डिकेरी मता तु ॥

(सु॰ नि॰ अ॰ 16/42)

## 3. अध्रुष

शोफः स्तब्धो लोहितस्तालुर्देशे रक्तज्ज्ञेयः सोध्रुषो रुग्ज्वराढ्यः ॥

(सु॰ नि॰ अ॰ १६)

## 4. कच्छप वा तालुकच्छप

कूर्मोत्सन्नो अवेदनोशीघ्रजन्मारक्तज्ञेयः कच्छपः श्लेष्मणा स्यात् ॥

(सु॰ नि॰ अ॰ 16/43)

कच्छपः कच्छपाकारश्चिरवृद्धिः काफादरुक् ॥

(अ॰ ह॰ उ॰ अ॰ २१)

## 5. अर्बुद

पद्माकारं तालुमध्ये तु शोफं विद्याद्रक्तादबुंदं प्रोक्तलिङ्गम् ॥

(सु॰ नि॰ अ॰ 16/43)

पद्माकृतिस्तालुमध्येरक्तच्छृवयथुरर्बुदम् ॥

(अ॰ ह॰ उ॰ अ॰ २१)

## 6. मांससंघात

दुष्टं मांसं श्लेष्मणा नीरुजं च तान्वन्तःस्थं मांससङ्घातमाहुः ॥

(सु॰ नि॰ अ॰ 16/44)

दृष्टं मांसं निरुजं तालुमध्ये कफाच्छूनं मांससङ्घातमाहुः ॥

(मा॰ नि॰)

## 7. तालुपुप्पुट

निरुक् स्थायी कोलमात्रः कफात् स्यात् मेदोयुक्तत् पुप्पुटस्तालुदेशे ॥

(सु॰ नि॰ अ॰ 16/44)

कोलाभः श्लेष्ममेदोभ्यां पुप्पुटो निरुजः स्थिरः ॥

(अ॰ हृ॰ उ॰ अ॰ २१)

## 8. तालुशोष

शोषोत्यर्थं दीर्यते चापि तालुः श्वासो वातात्तालुशोषः सपित्तात् ॥

(सु॰ नि॰ अ॰ 16/45)

वातपित्तज्वरायासैस्तालुशोषस्तदाह्वयः ॥

(अ॰ हृ॰ उ॰ अ॰ २१)

## 9. तालुपाक

पित्तं कुर्यात् पाकमत्यन्तघोरं तालुन्येनं तालुपाकं वदन्ति ॥

(सु॰ नि॰ अ॰ 16/45)

पित्तेन पाकः पाकाख्यः पूयास्रावी महारुजः ॥

(अ॰ हृ॰ उ॰ अ॰ २१)

# TALU ROGAS
## Diseases of Palate

    A) 9 diseases according to sushrutha
    B) 8 diseases according to Vagbhata.

## A) Sushrutha's Classification ( 9 diseases)

    1) Gala Shundi (Elongated Uvula Or Uvulitis)
    2) Tundikeri (Tonsilitis)
    3) Adhrusha (Palatitis)
    4) Kacchapa (Adenoma of Palate)
    5) Talu arbuda (Epithelioma or Carcinoma of Palate)
    6) Mamsa Sanghatha (Adenoma or fibroma of Palate)
    7) Talu Pupputa (Epulis or fibroma or Cyst of Palate)
    8) Talu sosha ( Atrophy of Palate)
    9) Talu Paka (ulceration of palate)

## B)    Vagbhata's classification (8 diseases )
He has not explained tundikeri in Talu rogas but explained it in Kantha roags. So only 8 diseases according to him. he added Talu pitica in Place of Adhrusha.

**Note :-** Among 9 diseases Talu Arbuda is only Asadya - Talu sosha aushada Sadya, remaing chedan sadya Vyadhies (chedan and Bhedan for tundikeri and Talu Pupputa)

# 1) Gala Shundi (Kantha Shundi)
( Elogated Uvula Or Uvulitis)

    The vitatied Kapha and Raktha doshas produces soft lengthy bulk swelling in palate (Talu moola ), Resembles swollen bladder (Admaatha Vasti Prakasham- Matsya Vasti nibham) and manifest the symptoms like, Obstruction while swallowing the food, irritation in the throat, dry cough, dyspnosa, thirst, Vomiting through nose and fever.

**Treatment :-**
    **1) shaman Chikitsa :-**
    1) Kavala Gandusha Nasya and Dhooma panam 2) If the disease is not controlled chedan karma is advised.

    **2) Chedan Karma :-**
    Gala shundi has to firmly handled with samdamsha Yantra and with mandalagra shastra the lower 1/3rd part should cut by leaving the upper 2/3. Excessive cutting causes bleeding complications. and improper cutting causes complications like salivation Insomnia and aggravation of the disease.

**Pashchyath Karma (Post chedan therapy regimen):-**
    1) Prathisarana with maricha, Ateesa patha, Vacha, kusta Shyonak, rasna, saindhava lavana + madhu.

2)      **Kavala:-**With the decoction of Vacha, ativisha, patha, Rasna, Katuki, and nimba.

3)      **Dhooma Pana :-** With Panchangee Varthi prepared by Ingudi, Kinihe, danthi, Trivruth and Devadaru.

4)      Kshara Siddha mugda Yoosha bhojan

**Uvulitis :-**

It is an inflammatory condition of Uvula (the free central posterior border of soft palate). The disease occurs due to

1) Recurrent or Chronic Oropharyngeal Or Upper respiratory tract infections
2) Dust smoke and cold allergy (cold wind Or cold items allergy)

elongated Uvula causes irritation at Posterior dorsum of tongue, Oro pharynx and produces irritative dry cough thirst, pain during deglutition, fever and pharyngitis etc.

**Treatment :-**

1) Broad spectrum antibiotics.
(Ex. Erythromycetin)
2) Anti inflammatories and Analgesics.
Ex. Ibuprofen Or Diclophenac sodium .
3) Anti histamines and cortisones
(Betamthasone and Dexamethosone, Pheneramine maleate and chore phenaramine maleate).
4) Lukewarm salt water gargling .

If the disease is not controlled the lower 1/3 parts should excise under local anaestheia.

## 2) Tundikeri (Tonsilitis)

The Vitiated Kapha and Raktha doshas causes a bigcystic swelling resembling the fruit of Vana Karpasa, the assoicated symptoms are Burning sensation, Pricking pain in the throat and with suppurative cyst.

(Note :- Vagbhata explained it in gala rogas)

**Treatment :-**

**A) Shamana Chikitsa**

Kavala Gandusha Dhooma and Nasya.

B) If the disease is not controlled by shamana chikitsa, Shastra Chikitsa like galashundi has to do (chedan)

" According to modern also it is Chedana sadya Vyadhi (Tonsilectomy) But Dalhana explained it as Bhedan sadya vyadhi.

**Pratisarana :-** with Gruha dhooma + Katu Varga dravyas.

**Nasya :-** Taila Prepared with Apamarga beeja, Vishnukrantha, danthi, Vidanga, Saindhava lavana and Tila Kalka.

**Note :-** Shoola, shotha, grandhi hara, Aushada's should give **Ex : -** Kanchanara guggulu Or Triphalaguggulu, Gandak rasayan, Chopa chenyadi churna . Khadhiradi vati, Sarivadivati etc., are helpful to reduce the inflammation of the tonsils.

# TONSILITIS

The palatine tonsils are subepithelial lymphiod collections situated in between faucial pillars. These help in Protecting the respiratory and alimentary tracts from bacterial invasion and are thus prove to frequent attacks of infection.

" The inflammation of tonsils, is known as Tonsilitis. "

## A) Acute Tonsilitis :-

**Aetiology :-** It may occur as a Primary infection of tonsil, Or secondary to upper respiratory tract viral infections, The causative Organisms are, Haemolytic strepto coccus, staphylo coccus, haemophilus influenzae, and pneumo coccus. Poor Orodental hygiene, Poor nutrition and congested surroundings are important predisposing factors.

## Pathology :-

1) Tonsils are inflammed and lymphoid follicles convert into small abscesses which discharge into crypts known as **catarrhal tonsilitis**.

2) Multiple white spots of exudative collections in crypts on an inflamed tonsilar surface is known as **Folllicular Tonsilitis**

3) Some times exudation from crypts Form a membrane over the surface of Tonsil, is known as **membranous tonsilitis.**

4) Whole tonsil if uniformly congested is known as . **Parenchymatous tonsilitis.**

### Clinical Features :-

**Symptoms :-** Sore throat 2) Fever 3) Painful deglutition 4 Malaise 5) Headache, 6) Anorexia 7) Body pains. 8) Earache, 9) Constipation 10) Tachycardia.

**Signs :-** 1) Enlarged congested tonsils 2) Raise of temparature 3) Tonsils are stubbed with yellowish spot 4) Surrounding part of Pharynx are often inflammed (Soft palate and uvula) 6) Enlarged Tonsilar lymph nodes with tenderness (Jugulo digastric lymph nodes).

**Treatment : -** 1) Bed rest 2) Giving plenty of fluids. 3) Administration of Broad spectrum antibiotics (Erythromycetine Ampicilline pencillin etc.,) Analgesics Antiphyretics and Anti inflammatory drugs 4) Salt Water (Lukwarm) gargling.

**Complicatios :-** 1) Chronic Tonsilitis 2) Peri tonsilar abscess (Quinsy) 3) Parapharyngeal abscess 4) Acute otitis media 5) Acute nephritis 6) Rheumatic fever.

## Chronic Tonsilitis :-

Chronic inflammatory changes in the tonsils are usually the result of recurrent acute infections treated inadquately. It is of two varieties 1) Chronic Parenchymatous tonsilitis 2) Chronic fibrotic tonsilitis.

### Clinical Features :-

**Symptoms :-** 1) Recurrent sore thorat 2) Difficulty in deglutition 3) Discomfrot in throat 4) Un pleasent taste (cacagus) and bad smell in mouth (Halitosis ) 5) Change of Voice.

**Signs :-** 1) Hypertrophic tonsils and protruding out of the pillars 2) Congested tonsils, crypts appear open from which epithelial debris may be squeezed on pressure 3) Enlargement of jugulo digastric lymph nodes.

**Treatment :-** 1) Treatment should give to control the infection of Tonsils Nasal and para Nasal sinuses

2)      Broad spectrum antibiotics.

3)      Analgesics and anti-inflammatories.

4)      Anti histamines.

5)      Surgery of Nasal and Paranasal abnormalities
        Ex septal deviation (DNS), Adenoids, Nasal Polyps etc.,

6)      If the disease is not responding to medical treatment, surgical excision of Tonsils is must (tonsilectomy).

**Complication :-**

1)      Peritonsilar abscess 2) Para Pharyngeal abscess

3)      Intra tonsilar abscess 4) Tonsilolyths.

5)      Rheumatic fever 6) Acute nephritis.

**Tonsilectomy :-** Excision of tonsils, is known as tonsilectomy.

**Indications :-** 1) Failure of conservative treatment 2) Chronic tonsilitis 3) Repeated attacks of acute follicular tonsilitis 4) After the attach of peritonsilar abscess (Quinsy) 5) Huge enlargment of tonsils causing mechanical obstruction for swallowing and respiration. 6) Chronic enlargement of regional lymph nodes with sore throat 7) weight loss 8) Persistent carrier to strepto coccus haemolyticus and Diphtheria bacilli . 9) Carcinoma of tonsil 10) Benign tumours of tonsils.

11)     Tonsilitis if causes secondary effects in other organas ex Rheumatic fever, Acute glomerulo nephiritis, chronic suppurative otitis media. etc.,

**Contra Indications :-**
        1) Severe diabetes 2) Gross Hypertension 3) blood dyscrasias (Bleeding Coagulation defects, aplastic anaemias and Purpura) 4) Allergy - asthama 5) During epidemic of polio 6) Systemic infections 7) Debilitative diseases 8) presence of acute local infection 9) During menstruation 10) During pregnacy.

**Investigation Needed :-**
        1) C.B.P. 2) Hb% 3) Bleeding and coagulation time 4) Blood sugar - Cholesterol, uric acid levels etc., 5) Urine examination to know kidney damage and other metabolic disorders 6) Blood pressure 7) General examination of Heart & ECG
8) Enquiry about menstruation, pregnancy, Allergy and other past medical history.

## 3)      Adrusha (Palatitis)

The Vitiated Raktha dosha causes red coloured hard Oedema in Talu, associated symptoms are pain and fever.

" Vagbhata not explained this diseases. "

**Treatment :-** 1) Shamana chikitsa :

Abhyanga, pratisarana, kavala, gandusha, dhooma pana, nasya and sweda (Rakta dosha hara chikitsa should be given.

" Now a days for palatitis only shamana chikitsa (Anti inflammatory treatment) is practicing. "

2) If the disease not responds to shamana chikitsa, shastra chikitsa (Like gala shundhi) is advised i.e. sneha - sweda - chedan and prathisarana.

## 4) Talu kacchapa (Adenoma of Palate) :-
The vitiated Kapha dosha causes a painless, slowly developing and slowly suppurating whitish or pale coloured oedema (Arakta vruddhi ) which resembles kacchapa (Dorsum of Tortoise) originates in Talu.

**Treatment :-**
1) Shamana Chikitsa :-
Abhyanga, Sweda, Pratisarana, Kavala Gandoosha, Dhooma and Nasya.
2) Shastra Chikitsa - Chedana, if Shamana Chikitsa get failure Chedana is advised like Galashundi.

## 5)    Talu Arbuda :-
### Epithelioma Or Cancer of Palate

The Vitiated Raktha doshas causes Red coloured Arbuda in middle part of Talu, resembles Raktha padma (Red lotus)

**Treatment :- Asadhya Vyadhi. (Rejected for treatment )**
**Note :** (If Arbuda is newly developed, can try with the following treatment principle. ) 1) Chedana and 2) Pratisarana with sarjakshara, shunti + Honey 3) Taila + Mmadhu - Gandoosha 4) Teekshna taila nasya.

## 6)    Mamsa Sanghatha (Fibroma of Palate)
The Vitiated Kapha dosha causes painless Oedema in the Talu Mamsa. (Sushrutha).
**Vagbhata :-** Kapha + Raktha, doshas Produces painless swelling in the middele part of talu is known as talu samhati.
**Treatment :-** 1) Shaman Chikitsa 2) Chedan Chikitsa like Galashundi

## 7)    Talu Pupputa
### (Epulis Or Fibroma Or Cystic Swelling )

The vitiated Kapha dosha and Medo dhathu causes painless fixed swelling at Talu, resembles kola phala (Badari phala ), is known as Talu pupputa.
(It is a non specific cystic swelling (Fibroma) commonly arises due to trauma).

**Treatment :- Sushrutha :-** Like Galashundi (Chedan - Pratisaran)
**Vagbhata :-** Lekhana, Prathisarana, Kavala and nasya.

## 8) Talu Sosha .
### (Atrophy of Palate - Cleft Palate.)

It arises Due to 1) vata and Pitta vitiation 2) Pipasa nigraha (suppressing the thirst urge ) 3) Vata Pitta Jwara 4) Parishrama (Exersion ), The talu get dried, some times bifurcates and associates with swasa (Dyspnoea).

**Treatment : -**
1) Nidana Parivarjanam (Treat the cause) 2) Vata Pitta hara Chikitsa. 3) Ghee should take after meals. 4) Pippali shunti - Pakwa jala panam (boiled water with pippali, shunthi) 5) Pippali shunti - Pakwa ghritha panam (ghee prepared with pippali, shunthi)6) Amla dravya Or Sneha drava Gandoosha 7) Snigda Jangala mamsa rasa sevana. 8) Ksheeri sarpi Nasya (Nasya with Ghee prepared from milk)  (ghritha or snehapanam is contra indicated in Thirst).

## 9) Talu Paka
### (Palatitis Or ulceration of Palate ).

The vitiated pitta causes severe dreadful ulceration (Talu Paka ) in Talu- (painful pus discharging ulcer in Talu) (vagbhata).

Ulceration of palate may be classified as follows :-
1) Simple ulceration 2) Syphilitic ulceration (phirangaja) 3) Lupoidal ulceration (Charmakeelaja) 4) Epithelioma (malignant carcinoma - Ghatakaarbuda).

**Treatment :-**
1) Nidana Parivarjanam 2) Pitta - Visarpa hara Chikitsa 3) If Talu is not suppurated (Apakwa) a) Kaseesa Madhu and rasanjan - should be applied at the site  b) Kavala with sheetha Kashaya, and Madhura dravyas like Kakolyadi etc., 4) If Talu get suppurated (Pakwa) a) Asta Pada Vatha Bhedan (eight limbed incision) b) Teekshna Ushna Pratisarana c) Kavala with Vasa, Nimba twak, and patola etc., dravyas.

**Talu Pitika : -** Explained by only vagbhata in which vata dosha vitiates and produces painful, rough, hard and exudating piticas (Polyps) in Talu, known as Talu pitica

**Treatment : -** 1) Shaman Chikitsa
        2) Shastra Chikitsa.

# DISEASES OF PALATE (TALU ROGAS )

| Sl. No. | Name of the Disease | Dosha | Signs and Symptoms | Treatment . |
|---|---|---|---|---|
| 1. | Gala shundi (Elongated Uvula) | Kapha Raktha | Doshas vitiate the root of Talu and Produces a soft lengthy bulky swelling resembling vasti of matsya, it obstructs the throat and causes irritation thirst cough and dyspnoea. | 1) Shaman Chikitsa, if get failure 2) Chedan, Pratisaran. |
| 2. | Tundikeri (Tonsilitis) | Tridosha | A swelling resembling the fruit of Vana Karpasa develops at Talu, that causes pain burning and obstruction of throat | 1) Shaman Chikitsa if get failure.2) Chedan /bhedan & Pratisaran. |
| 3. | Adhrusha (Palatitis) | Raktha | Red Coloured hard Oedema develops in talu, assoicated with pain and fever | 1) Shaman if get failure 2) Chedan, Pratisaran |
| 4. | Kacchapa (Adenoma of Palate) | Kaphaj | Painless slowly growing Oedema develops resembling the dorsum of tortoice, in talu | 1) Shaman chikitsa, if get failure. 2) Chedan, Pratisaran. |
| 5. | Talu arbuda (Epithelioma Or (Carcinoma of Palate) | Rakthaj | Red Coloured arbuda resembling padma Karnika, develops in Talu | Asadya (Rejected for treatment) |
| 6. | Talu Pupputa (Cystic swelling) | Kapha, Medo dhathu | Vitiated doshas causes painless swelling resembling Kola Phala develops in talu | 1) shaman Chikitsa 2) Bhedan/Chedan 3) Pratisaran 4) Kavala. |

266

| SI. No. | Name of the Disease | Dosha | Signs and Symptoms | Treatment |
|---|---|---|---|---|
| 7. | Talu Sosha (Atrophy of Palate) | Vata Pitta | Talu get dried, bifurcates and associate with dyspnoea, due to suppressing the urge of thirst, Exertion and fever etc. | 1) Nidana Parivarjan  2) Vata Pitta hara. Brumhana Chikitsa. |
| 8. | Mamsa Samghatha (fibroma of Palate) | Kapha Raktha | Painles Oedema in Palate | 1) Chedan 2) Pratisaran. |
| 9. | Talu Paka (Ulceration of Palate) | Pitta | Vitiated Doshas causes ulcer in Palate | 1) Pitta hara Chikitsa 2) Asta pada Bhedan 3) Pratisaran |
| 10. | Talu Pitica (Polyp) | Vataj | Painful rough hard exudating piticas (Polyp Or follicles ) erupts in Talu | 1) Shastra Chedan Pratisaran. |

267

# कण्ठगत रोग

## 1. रोहिणी

गलेनिल: पित्तकफौ च मूर्च्छितौ पृथक्समस्ताश्च तथैव शोणितम्।
प्रदूष्य मांसं गलरोधिनोङ्कुरान् सृजन्ति यान् सासुहरा हि रोहिणी॥
जिह्वां समन्ताद् भृशवेदना ये मांसाङ्कुरा: कण्ठरोधिन: स्यु:।
तां रोहिणी वातकृतां वदन्ति वातात्मकोपद्रवगाढ़युक्ताम्॥

(सु॰ नि॰ अ॰ 16/48)

जिह्वाप्रबन्धजा: कण्ठे दारुणामार्गरोधिन:॥
मांसाङ्कुरा: शीघ्रचया रोहिणी शीघ्रकारिणी।

(अ॰ हृ॰ उ॰ अ॰ २१)

## 2. पित्तज रोहिणी

क्षिप्रोद्गमाक्षिप्रविदाहपाका तीव्रज्वरा पित्तनिमित्तजा स्यत्।
स्रोतोनिरोधिन्यपि मन्दपाका गुर्वी स्थिरा सा कफसम्भवा वै॥

(सु॰ नि॰ अ॰ 16/49)

पित्ताज्वरोषातृण्मोहकण्ठधुमायनान्विता।
क्षिप्रजा क्षिप्रपाकातिरागिणी स्पर्शनासहा॥

(अ॰ हृ॰ उ॰ अ॰ २१)

## 3. कफज रोहिणी

स्रोतोरोधिन्यपि मन्दपाका गुर्वी स्थिरा सा कफसम्भवा वै॥

(सु॰ नि॰ अ॰ 16/49)

कर्फन पिच्छिला पाण्डु:

(अ॰ हृ॰ उ॰ अ॰ २१)

## 4. त्रिदोषजा रोहिणी

गम्भीरपाकाप्रतिवारवीर्या त्रिदोफलिङ्ग त्रयसम्भवा स्यात्।

(सु॰ नि॰ अ॰ १६)

गम्भीरपाका निचयात् सर्वलिङ्गसमन्विता।

(अ॰ हृ॰ उ॰ अ॰ २१)

## 5. रक्तज रोहिणी

स्फोटाचिता पित्तसमानलिङ्गासाध्या प्रदिष्टा रुधिरात्मिकेयम्॥

(सु० नि० अ 16/50)

असृजा स्फोटकाचिता।

तप्ताङ्गारनिभा कर्णरुक्करी पित्तजाकृतिः॥

(अ० हृ० उ० अ० २१)

## 6. कण्ठशालुक

कोलास्थिमात्रः कफसंभवो यो ग्रन्थिर्गले कण्टकशूकभूतः।

खरः स्थिरः शस्त्रनिपातसाध्यस्तं कण्ठशालूकमिति ब्रुवन्ति॥

(सु० नि० अ 16/51)

दोषैः कफोल्बणैः शोफः कोलवद् ग्रथितोन्नतः॥

शूककण्टकवत् कण्ठे शालूको मार्गरोधनः।

(अ० हृ० उ० अ० २१)

## 7. अधिजिह्विका

जिह्वाग्ररुपः श्वयथुः कफातु जिह्वाप्रबन्धोपरि रक्तमिश्रात्।

ज्ञेयोधिजिह्वः खलु रोग एष विवर्जयेदागतपाकमेनमे॥

(सु० नि० अ 16/52)

प्रबन्धनोधो जिह्वायाः शोफो जिह्वाग्रसन्निभः।

सांकुरः कफपित्तास्त्रैर्लालोषास्तम्भवान् खरः॥

अधिजिह्वः सरुक्कण्डूर्वाक्याहारविधातकृत्।

तादृगेवोपजिह्वास्तु जिह्वाया उपरिस्थितः॥

(अ० हृ० उ० अ० २१)

## 8. वलय

बलास एवायतमुन्नतं च शोफं करोत्यनगतिं निवार्य।

तं सर्वथैवाप्रतिवारवीर्य विवर्जनीयं वलयं वदन्ति॥

(सु० नि० अ 16/53)

वलयोनातिरुक्शोफस्तद्द्वेवायतोन्नतः॥

(अ० हृ० उ० अ० २१)

## 9. वलास

गले तु शोफं कुरुतः प्रवृद्धौ श्लेष्मानिलौ श्वासरुजोपपन्नम् ।
मर्मच्छिदं दुस्तरमेतमाहुर्वलाससंज्ञं निपुणा विकारम् ॥

(सु॰ नि॰ अ॰ 16/54)

## 10. एकवृन्द

वृत्तोन्नतो यः श्वयथुः सदाहः कण्ड्वन्वितोपाक्यमृदुगुरुश्च ।
नाम्नैकवृन्दः परिकीर्तितोसौ व्याधिर्वलासक्षतजप्रसूतः ॥

(सु॰ नि॰ अ॰ 16/55)

## 11. वृन्द

समुन्नतं वृत्तममन्ददाहं तीव्रज्वरं वृन्दमुदाहरन्ति ।
तं चापि पित्तक्षतजप्रकोपाद् विद्यात् सतोद पवनासृजं तु ॥

(सु॰ नि॰ अ॰ 16/56)

वृन्दो वृत्तोन्नती दाहज्वरकृद् गलपार्श्वगः ॥

## 12. गिलायु

ग्रन्थिर्गले त्वामलकास्थिमात्रः स्थिररोल्परुक् स्यात् कफरक्तमूर्तिः ।
संलक्ष्यते सक्तमिवाशनं च स शस्त्रसाध्यस्तु गिलायुसंज्ञः ॥

(सु॰ नि॰ अ॰ 16/58)

मांसकीलोगले दोषै रेकोनेकोथवाल्परुक्
कृच्छ्रोच्छ्वासाम्यवहतिः पृथुमूलो गिलायुकः

(अ॰ हृ॰ उ॰ अ॰ २३)

## 13. गलविद्रधि

सर्वं गलं व्याप्य समुत्थितो यः शोफो रुजो यत्र च सन्ति सर्वाः ।
स सर्वदोषो गलविद्रधिस्तु तस्यैव तुल्यः खलु सर्वजस्य ॥

(सु॰ नि॰ अ॰ 16/59)

व्याप्तसर्वगलः शीघ्रजन्मपाको महारुजः ॥
पूतिपूयनिभस्त्रावी श्वयथुर्गलविद्रधिः ।

(अ॰ हृ॰ उ॰ अ॰ २३)

## 14. गलौघ

शोफो महानन्नजलावरोधी तीव्रज्वरो वातगतोर्निहन्ता ।
कर्फन जातो रुधिरन्वितेन गले गलौघः परिकीर्त्तयतेसौ ॥

(सु॰ नि॰ अ॰ 16)

बाह्यान्तः श्वयथुपर्घोरो गलमार्गार्गलोपमः ।
गलौधो मूर्धगुरुतातन्द्रालालाज्वरप्रदः ॥

(अ॰ हृ॰ उ॰ अ॰ २३)

## 15. स्वरघ्न

योतिप्रताभ्यन् श्वसिति प्रसक्तभिन्नस्वरः शुष्कविमुक्तक्रण्ठः ।
कफोपदिग्धेष्वनिलायनेषु ज्ञेयः स रोगः श्वसनात् स्वरघ्नः ॥

(सु॰ नि॰ अ॰ 16/61)

श्लेष्मरुद्धानिलगतिः शुष्ककण्ठो हतस्वरः ।
ताभ्यन् प्रसक्तं श्वसिति येन स स्वरहानिलात् ॥

(अ॰ हृ॰ उ॰ अ॰ २१)

## 16. मांसतान

प्रतानवान् यः श्वयथुः सुकष्टो गलोपरोधं कुरुते क्रमेण ।
स मांसतानः कथितोवलम्बी प्राणप्रणुत् सर्वकृतो विकारः ॥

(सु॰ नि॰ अ॰ 16/62)

## 17. विदारी

सदाहतोदं श्वयथुं सरक्तमन्तर्गले पूतिविशीर्णमांसम् ।
पित्तेन विद्याद् वदने विदारीं पार्श्वेविशेषात् स तु येन शेते ॥

(सु॰ नि॰ अ॰ 16/63)

## गलाबुंद

जिह्वावसाने कण्ठादावपाकं श्वयथुं मलाः ।
जनयन्ति स्थिरं रक्तं नीरुजं तद् गलाबुर्दम

(अ॰ हृ॰ उ॰ अ॰ 21)

## गलगण्ड के सामान्य लक्षण

वातः कफश्चैव गले प्रवुद्धौ मन्ये च संसृत्य तथैव मेदः ।
कुर्वन्ति गण्डं क्रमशः स्वलिङ्गैः समन्वितं तं गलगाण्डमाहुः ॥

(सु॰ नि॰ अ॰ 11/22)

पवनश्लेष्ममेदोभिर्गलगण्डो भवेद् बहि: ।
वर्धमान: स कालेन मुष्कवल्लम्बते नीरुक् ॥

(अ॰ ह॰ उ॰ अ॰ २१)

निबद्ध: श्वयथुर्यस्य मुष्कवल्लम्बते गले ।
महान् वा यदि ह्रस्वो गलगण्डं तमादिशेत् ॥

(सु॰ नि॰ अ॰ 11/29)

## वातज गलगण्ड

तोदान्वित: कृष्णसिरावनद्ध: कृष्णोरुणो वा पवनात्मकस्तु ।
मेदोन्वितश्चोपचितश्च कालाद्द्रवेदतिस्निग्धतरोरुजश्च ॥

(सु॰ नि॰ अ॰ 11/23)

पारुष्ययुक्तश्चिरवृद्ध्ययपाकौ यदृच्छया पाकमियात् कदाचित् ।
वैरस्यामास्यस्य च तस्य जन्तोर्भवेत्तथा तालुगलप्रशोष: ॥

(सु॰ नि॰ अ॰ 11/24)

कृष्णोरुणो वा तोदाद्य: स वातात् कृष्णराजिमान् ।
वृद्धस्तालुगले शोषं कुर्याच्च विरसास्यताम् ॥

## कफज गलगण्ड

स्थिर: सवर्णोल्परुगुरुकण्डू: शीतो महांश्चापि कफात्मकस्तु ।
चयाभिवृद्धिं कुरुते चिराच्च प्रपच्यते मन्दरुज: कदाचित् ॥

(सु. नि. 11/25)

स्थिर: सवर्ण: कण्डुमां शीतस्पर्शो गुरु: कफात् ।
वृद्धस्तालुगले लेपं कुर्याच्च मधुरास्यताम् ॥

(अ॰ ह॰ उ॰ अ॰ 21)

माधुर्यमास्यस्य च तस्य जन्तोर्भवेत्तथा तालुगलप्रलेप: ॥

(सु. नि. अ. 11)

## मेदोजगलगण्ड

स्निग्धो मृदु: पाण्डुरनिष्टगन्धो मेद:कृतो नीरुगथातिकण्डू:
प्रलम्बतेलावुवदल्पमूलो देहानुरुपक्षयवृद्धियुक्त: ।
स्निग्धास्यता तस्य भवेच्च जन्तोर्गलेनुशब्दं कुरुते च नित्यम् ॥

(सु. नि. अ. 11/26,27)

# DISEASES OF THROAT
## (Gala Or Kantha Rogas.)

| |  | | | |
|---|---|---|---|---|
| 1) | According to | Sushrutha | 17 | Diseases. |
| 2) | " | Bhava mishra | 18 | " |
| 3) | " | Vagbhata | 18 | " |
| 4) | " | Sarangdhara | 18 | " |

They are as follows :-

| Sl.No. | Name of the Disease | Modern Name. |
|---|---|---|
| 1. | Vataj Rohini | ⎤ |
| 2. | Pittaj Rohini | ⎥ |
| 3. | Kaphaj Rohini | ⎬ Diphtheria |
| 4. | Rakthaj Rohini | ⎥ |
| 5. | Sannipathaj Rohini | ⎦ |
| 6. | Kantha Snaaluka | Adenoida |
| 7. | Adijihwa | Epiglottitis |
| 8. | Valaya | Tumour in throat |
| 9. | Balasa | Benign tumour |
| 10. | Ekavrunda, Vrunda | Benign tumour |
| 11. | Gilaya | Benign tumour |
| 12. | Shathaghnee | Retropharyngeal abscess |
| 13. | Gala Vidradi | Retropharyngeal abscess |
| 14. | Gala ugha | Retropharyngeal abscess |
| 15. | Swaraghna | Paralysis of larynx |
| 16. | Mamsatana | Malignant tumour |
| 17. | Vidari | Malignant tumour. |

**Note :-**

1) Shushrutha counted Eka Vrunda and Vrunda as a single disease because of similarity, So only according to him Gala rogas are only 17

| Sl.No. | Vagbhata not explained | Vagbhata Explained. Additionally |
|---|---|---|
| 1. | Adijihwa | 1. Vataj Gala ganda |
| 2. | Eka Vrunda | 2. Kaphaj Galaganda |
| 3. | Balasa | 3. Medoja Galaganda |
| 4. | Mamsa Tana | 4. Galaarbuda |
| 5. | Vidari | 5. Tundikeri. |

Among 18 diseases vagbhata not explained the 5 diseases of Sushrutha and added extra five diseases which are given in above chart.

273

**Note :-**

Sushrutha explained Tundikeri in Talurogas (Diseases of Palate) and Adijihwak in Galarogas (Dieseases of Throat). But Vagbhata explained Tundikeri in Galarogas and Adijihwa in jihwa rogas (Diseases of Tongue).

# ROHINI
## (Diphtheria)

It is a complicated, trouble some and poor prognostic disease of throat. The Tridoshas (Vata, Pitta Kapha) and Raktha either separately or togetherly vitiate and produces a hard quickly spreading, dreadful and throat obstructing swelling (Single or multiple) that causes difficulty in Respiration and food in take, is known as ROHINI.

It is of 5 types
1) Vataja Rohini 2) Pittaj Rohini 3) Kaphaj Rohini
4) Rakthaj Rohini 5) Sanni pathaj Rohini

| Sl. No. | Name of the Disease | Fatal time. |
|---|---|---|
| 1. | Vataj Rohini | Causes death in 7 days |
| 2. | Pittaj Rohini | Causes death in 5 days |
| 3. | Kaphaj Rohini | Causes death in 3 days |
| 4. | Rakthaj Rohini | Causes death immediately (Asadya) |
| 5. | Sannipathaj Rohini | Asadya. |

**Note :-**

The prognosis of the disease is very poor, Rakthaj and Tridoshaj Rohini are Asadya So treatment should be tried for the rest of the diseases (Vataj, Pittaj and Kaphaj ) only

## 1) VATAJ ROHINI

The vitiated Vata dosha causes a painful throat obstructing swelling at the root of Tongue. The symptoms are Dryness of mouth and throat, pain in jaws and ears, obstruction for respiration and food intake and other general complications of Vata are also associated It is known as VATAJA ROHINI a very complicated disease that causes death in 7 days if proper treatment is not given in time.

**Treatment :-**

1) Bahya Abhyanga (massage) with Lukewarm Vatahara Oils (Chatur Sneha).

2) Oral intake of luke warm medicated Oils (Chatur snehas - Sarpi taila - Vasa - Majja). 3) Light fomentation (Mrudu Swedam) in General aswellas Local. 4) Vamana Karma (emesis therapy ). 5) Raktha Mokshana :- with anguli shastra or Nakha (Nails), Lekhana has to do at the lesion. 6) Application of saindhava lavana (Prathisarana) to the lesion where Lekhana has conducted. 7) Lukewarm gargles (Gandoosha) with Chatur Snehas. 8) Lukewarm gargles (Gandoosha) with the decoction of Hareetaki with Madhu.

9)    Lukewarm garlges (Gandoosha ) with the decoction of panchamoola. 10) Gandoosha and Nasya, with the medicated Oil prepared form Ela, punarnava, Kantakari, Khapitta, Godugda and tila taila. 11) Nasya Karma with Tila taila. 12) Dhoomapanam with Vatahara Aushada. 13) Shotha hara shoola hara, krimighna Jwarahara medicines, Local aswellas systemic can be given.

## 2) PITTAJA ROHINI

The vitiated pitta dosha causes quickly originating, spreading and suppurating swelling at the root of tongue. it is an unbearable, very painful, disease with severe burning and fever thirst vertigo drowsiness unconsciousness other complications of pitta dosha are also associated. It is known as PITTAJA ROHINI , a very complicated disease that causes death in 5 days if proper treatment is not given intime.

**Treatment :-**
1) Abhyanga (massage) with cold oils. 2) Sneha panam (Ghritha etc.,). 3) Light fomentation(Mrudu Sweda) General and Local. 4) Vaman Karma (Emesis therapy). 5) Raktha Mokshan with anguli shastra Or Nakha (Nails ) Lekhana Karma has to do, at the lesion. 6) Application of the paste (Pratisaran) Prepared from Raktha Chandan, Lodra, Priyangu, sugar and Honey to the lesion where Lekhana has conducted. 7) Gargles (Kavala- Gandoosha) with the cold decoctions prepared from chandan, Lodhra, Priyangu Sharkara and Honey. 8) Gargles (Gandoosha ) with the decoctions of Draksha and parooshak. 9) A medicine for Gargling, Nasya and for Oral intake of Ghritha Prepared From Triphala Lodra Sariva.Kashmari Yastimadu Milk and Ghee (Ghrita Paka Vidhi)

## 3) RAKTHAJ ROHINI

The vitiated Raktha Dosha causes a dreadful, Red coloured swelling in the throat with severe burning pain and earache (pain in ears). All the symptoms of pittaja Rohini are also associated.

**Treatment :-**
It is an incurable and highly complicated, disease that causes death immediately. But treatment can be given as like pittaja Rohini for suppressing the symptoms temporarly.

## 4) KAPHAJ ROHINI

The vitiated kapha dosha produces a whitish, immobile, sticky, bulk, throat obstructing and slowly suppurating swelling in the throat, associated with atropic changes pain and dyspnoea. If it is neglected kills the person within 3 days.

**Treatment :-**
1) Lekhan and Raktha Mokshan 2) Prathisaran with Ghruhadhooma + Katuki Powder. 3) Nasya and Gandusha with the Oil prepared from apamarga, aparajitha Vidanga danthi saindhavalavana and taila.

## 5) SANNIPATHAJ ROHINI

The Tridoshas vitiate and produces a dreadful, most complicated, deep rooted, Incurable, quickly suppurative disease in the throat, all the symptoms of Tri-dosha appears in this variety.

**Treatment :-** Asadya. (Rejected for the treatment )

## COMMON TREATMENT PRINCIPLES OF THROAT DISEASES.

1) Lekhan and Raktha Mokshan. 2) Prathisaran Or Lepa
3) Kavala Or Gandoosha. 4) Nasya Karma. 5) Dhooma Panam.

1)    Oral intake of decoction prepared with Daru Haridra, Nimba patra, Rasanjan, and indrayava.
2)    Decoction of Hareetaki with Honey.
3)    Gandoosha & Pratisaran with Triphala Trikatu Yavakshara Daruharidra Chitraka Rasanjan Patha Tejobala and Nimba with shuktha Or gomutra.
4)    Local application of Amlavetas Malkangini musta devadaru Shunthi. Vacha Danthi and Moorva.
5)    The yogas explained is Sarva Sara mukha rogas are also useful in gala rogas.

## DIPHTHERIA

It is a dreadful contageous disease caused by Coryne bacterium diphtheria, a gram positive Organism, usually spread by droplet infection and its incubation period is 2 to 4 days.

It commonly occur in 5 to 12 Years of age group. It is mostly eradicated but still a problem in developing countries like India. The disease commonly occurs in the mucosa of Nose, Nasopharynx oralcavity, Oropharynx and larynx, etc., but rarely affects the conjunctiva and genital tract.

**Clinical Features :-**
Clinical features depends upon the site of infection

**A) Nasal diphtheria :-** The clinical features are, fibrinous rhinitis, chronic rhinitis, excoriation of anterior nares, blood stained mucopurulent nasal discharge, inflamed nasal mucosa, formation of greyish white thick layer on nasal mucosa which is not separatable and bleeds when try to separate it, finally it causes nasal nasopharyngeal obstruction and systemic toxaemia (infection also spread to other mucous membranes of body and vital organs .

**B)    Faucial diphtheria - Clinical Feature :-**
Faucial diphtheria may be primary disease Or secondary to Nasal diphtheria, infection spreads to oral cavity and oropharynx.

276

The greyish white layer develops on tonsils Uvula soft palate and posterior pharyngeal wall. pain in the throat, difficulty in deglutition, mild Fever, head ache, Tachycardia, cervical lymphadenopathy (bull's neck appearence), Throat Obstruction and systemic toxaemia are associated.

**C)     Laryngeal Diphtheria :-** Clinical features . Diphtherial infection spreads to larynx and produces Greyish white layer on vocal cords, laryngeal vestibule, subglottis and trachea. Due to inflammatory changes in larynx, causes dyspnoea and Asphyxia.

**Complications :-**
        1) Throat Obstruction (Difficulty in deglutition of food and water ). 2) Nose and Larynx if affected causes dyspnoea and Asphyxia. 3) Myocarditis and peripheral Vascular problems. 4) Neuritis. 5) Kedney and Liver Problems.

**Treatment of Diphtheria.**
1)      Identification of the disease by clinical (features ) findings.
2)      Deep intra muscular injection of Anti diphtheric. Serum 10000,I.U. to 50.000, I.U. should give to neutralise the toxins.
3)      Administration of suitable antibiotics (By culture/Sensitivity).
4)      Bed rest.
5)      Symptomatic treatment.
6)      The main complication of the disease is Breathing problem for that " Trache Ostomy " Operation is only the alternative, in which an artificial hole is done in tracha, in between 3rd and 4th rings, and tracheostomy tubes are inserted. So antiinfective precautions should take tosave from pulmonary complications.

# 6) KANTA SHAALUKA (ADENOIDS )
(Noso Paryngeal Tonsil)

It is Kaphaj, Shastra sadya Vyadhi, vitiated, Kapha produces an immobile rough and hard cyst resembling the seed of Kola Phala (Badari Phala ) in the throat, causes throat obstruction dis comfort pricking pain (Like pricking with thorn and hook ) and sounds during respiration.

**Treatment :-**
        1) It is Shastra Sadyam (only surgical treatment is needed). 2) Similar surgey is explained for " Kanta Shaaluka Tundikari Gilay and Vrunda, i.e. - Bhedan Or Lekhan. 3) Raktha Mokshana. 4) Ghee + Yavanna. 5) Kaphaj Rohini Treatment. 6) Shodhan Chikitsa. 7) Breathing exercises etc.,

**Adenoids**
**Naso Pharyngeal Tonsils.**

Hypertrophied Naso pharyngeal tonsils are called as adenoids.
        As the child grows the size of naso pharyngeal tonsils diminishes and dis appears by pubety, But due to recurrent upper respiratory tract infections ( in 3 to 10 Years of age group) instead of atrophic changes, the nasopharyngeal tonsils get hypertrophied and causes nasal and aural complications.

**Signs and Symptoms :-**
   Frequent attachs of Cold, persistent Mucopurulent nasal discharge, nasal obstruction, snoring, nocturnal cough (due to post nasal discharge), infection of paranasal Sinuses (Sinusitis) headache, enlarged mass of adenoids on posterio superior wall of nasopharynx, pinched nostrils, dull look, mental instability, retracted upper lip, protruding teeth, obstruction to nasal breathing, opened mouth (for respiration) , earache deafness, tinnitus, otorrhoea, loss of appetite and on palapation of Naso pharynx adenoids have a feel like bag of worms.

**Diagnostic Criteria :-**
   1) Nasal obstruction and Open mouth. 2) Apearence of adenoid facies. 3) Posterior Rhinos copic Examination . 4) Palpation of Naso pharynx. 5) Lateral view Xray of Naso pharynx.

**Complications :-**
   1) Recurrent attaches of Otitis media. 2) Sinusitis 3) Speech problems. 4) chronic nasal changes (Prinched Nose etc.,) 5) Adenoid Cysts.

**Treatment**
**Conservatory Treatment :-**
   1) Antibiotics (Erythromycetin etc.,) 2) Analgesics and anti inflammatory drugs. 3) Anti allergic drugs. 4) Nasal decongestants (Nasal drops and systemic drugs).

   If the disease is not controlled by above treatment. surgical excision of adenoids, (Adenoidectomy), is only the next alternative treatment. Commonly adenoidectomy is done along with tonsilectomy under general anaesthecia. St clair Thomson adenoid curette with a guard is the instrument more commonly used for adenoidectomy.

   The adenoid curette is held in the right hand and passed behind the soft palate to the end of the nasal septum. it is pressed against the roof of Naso pharynx to engage the adenoid mass, then with downward and forward movement the adenoids are curetted out and are help up in the guard of curette. a second stoke may need to clear the roof, post nasal cavity is packed for few minutes to arrest bleedng, then Antibiotics, anti inflammatories analgesics and anti histamines are prescribed.

# ADIJIHWAK
## (Epiglottitis)

   The vitiated Kapha and Raktha doshas produces a swelling above the tongue resembling the tip of tongue, is named as Adijihwa. It becomes incurable (Asadya) when suppurated.

**Note : -** According to Vagbhata Adijihwa and Upajihwa are the diseases of tongue. in which
   Swelling above the tongue is " **Upajihwa**"
   Swelling below the tongue is " **Adijihwa**"

**Treatment :-**
1) Lekhana and Pratisaran with Yavakshara. 2) Shiro Virechan Nasya. 3) Kapha and Raktha dosha hara Gandoosha. 4) Kapha Raktha hara dhooma panam.

It can be correleted to Epiglottitis (Inflammation of epiglottis), it is a rare condition. If it is not severe can be controlled with Antibiotics Analgesics, Anti inflammatories and Anti histamine drugs.

## 8) VALAYA
### (Tumour in throat either benign Or Malignant)

" Charaka Called it as Bidalika.

The vitiated Kapha produces a lengthy, bulk complicative, round and throat Obstructing. Swelling that causes difficulty for food intake, it is named as Valaya.

It is Asadya (incurable) and said to be rejected for treatment.

**Treatment :-** Incurable disease.

## 9) BALASA .
### (Benign Or malignant tumour of Throat )

The vitiated Kapha and Vata dosha produces a dreadful swelling that causes pain breathlessness and injury to vital parts (Marmaabhighatha), it is known as Balasa.

**Treatment : -** Incurable disease (Asadya Vyadhi)

## 10) EKA VRUNDA

Vagbhata not explained this disease.

The vitiated Kapha and Raktha doshas Produce a round bulk, hard, non suppurative cyst in the throat that causes pain, itching sensation burning sensation and throat obstruction, it is known as Eka Vrunda.

**Treatment :-**
1) Shodhan (**Raktha Mokshan** Nasya etc.,) 2) Prathisaran (Local Application of the medicine ) with Yava Kshara. 3) Gandoosha. 4) Dhooma Panam. 5) Kaphaj Rohini Chikitsa.

## 11 VRUNDA

The vitiated pitta and Raktha or vata and rakta. produce a bigger, painful, swelling in the throat (in the lateral side of throat by vagbhata ) with fever and burning sensation, it is known as Vrunda.

**Note :-** (vedana Daha Jwara are more severe than Eka Vrunda)

279

**Note :-** According to sushrutha and Dalhana - Vrunda and Ekavrunda are similar diseases, So only explained seperately but counted as one and they expained that the severity of pain, burning sensation and fever are more in Vrunda than Ekavrunda.
**Treatment :-** Same as Ekavrunda.

## 12 GILAYU
### (Benign Cyst of Throat )

The vitiated kapha and Raktha doshas produces a hard, immobile, painful cyst (Cysts- Vagbhata ), resembling the seed of Aamalaki Fruit, in the throat that causes difficulty in deglutition of food ( and have a feel that food bolus is obstructed in the throat ) an breathing, it is known as Gilayu, need surgical treatment.

**Treatment -**
1) Surgical Treatment like Kantha shaaluka Tundikeri and Vrunda.
2) Kaphaj Rohini Treatment.
3) For Oral intake and for Gargling usag of Musta, Trikatu Ativisha, Devadaru, Go Mutra, Tikthaushadhas.

## 13) GALA VIDRADI.
### (Retropharyngeal abscess )

The Tridoshas vitiate and produces a painful, quickly originating spreading and suppurating abscess with foul pus discharge that completely obstructs the throat and teases by manifesting the symptoms of vitiated Tridoshas, like pain, burning sensation, oedema, itiching sensation and discomfort etc.

**Treatment :-**
1) If the abscess is not at vital prats (marma sthana ) Bhedhan, pooya nirharan, Shodhan, Ropana has to do (Incision and drainage).
2) Raktha mokshan- then prathisarana and Gandoosha.
**With :-**
Triphala Haridra, Rasanjan, Gyrika, Lodra, saindhava lavan, Raktha chandan and pippali.
Powder is for prathisaran and the decoction is for Gandoosha.

## 14 GALAUGHA
### ( Retropharyngeal Abscess )

The vitiated kapha and Raktha doshas produces biggger oedema Or Cyst in the throat (oedema not only in throat but also externally Vagbhata ), assoicated with fever and obstructs the respiration and food intake, other symptoms are salivation drowsiness heavyness of head and discomfort in throat.

**Treatment :-** Asadya Vyadhi (incurable disease ) but can try as Rohini.

## 15) SWARAGHNA
( Carcinoma Or Paralysis of Larynx. )

The vitiated Vata (Vata + Kapha - Vagbhata ) by affecting shabdavaha srotas Or swara Yantra (Pharynx and larynx ) deranges the function of Vata and produces the symptoms like breathlessness in ability to talk, dryness of throat and giddiness, it is known as Swaraghna which is incurable.

**Treatment :-**
Asadya Vyadhi (Incurable disease.)

### 16) MAMSA TANA
### (Cellutitis Or Carcinoma of Throat )

The vitiated Tridoshas produce an abnormal, spreading, throat obstructing, hanging, Cyst Or Polyp in the throat, it is known as mamsatana which is incurable and rejected for the treatment.

**Treatment :-**
Asadya Vyadhi.

## 17) VIDARI
(Gangrenous Stomatitis Or Retro pharyngeal absess).

The Vitiated pitta and Raktha produce a painful, burning type of red growth (Abscess ) in the throat, the tissue of the abscess gradually get necrosed and exfoliated, it is known as Vidari which is incurable and rejected for the treatment.
**Treatment :-** Asadya (incurable)

## 18) SHATHAGHNEE

The Tridoshas vitiate and produce multiple cysts or Polyps in the throat, that causes throat obstruction, severe pain, burning sensation, head ache, fever and said to be more dangerous and so it should be rejected for the treatment.

**Treatment :**
Asadya (Incurable)

### ADDITIONAL DISEASES OF THROAT, EXPLAINED BY VAGBHATA.

5 Diseases.
1) Galaarbuda 2) Tundikeri 3) Kaphaj Galaganda 4) Medoja Galaganda. 5) Vataj Galaganda.

**1)     Galaarbuda (benign Tumour in Throat )**
The vitiated Vatadi doshas produces a hard, immobile, painless, non suppurative, reddish tumour in the throat. It is known Galaarbuda.

281

**Treatment :-**
1) If the growth is smaller Chedan & Pratisarana should be done (Excision and application of Sarja Kshara shunthi and Honey).
2) Gargling (Gandooshan -With Giloya, Nimba Kashaya + Honey + Tila taila.
3) Nasya and abhyanga
   **With :-** 1) Concentrated Sarshapa Taila.
4) Usage of Yava as food (Yavanna Sevena )

## 2) 3) 4) , GALAGANDA (GOITRE)

A) Sushrutha expalined it in the chapter " Grandhi "
B) Charaka           "           " Shopa "
C) Vagbhata          "           " Gala roga.

It occurs by the vitiation of vata, Kapha and medas So only on the basis of Vitiation it is of 3 types.
1) Vataj Gala ganda
2) Kaphaj Galganada.
3) Medoja Galganda.

Common Features of Galaganda :-

A painless slowly progressive movable (Hangs like scrotum,) cyst develops on the neck, the size of cyst is not unform (changes time to time)

**1)      Vataj Galaganda :-**
A slowly developing blackish red cyst develops on neck, it assoicates with pain and is encircled with black capillary net, some times suppurate and some times not. The other symptoms are Talu sosha, Gala Sosha and Viirasya.

**Treatment :-**
1) Nadi Swedam with Vata hara drugs. 2) Raktha Mokshana 3) Upanah Swedam. 4) If Cyst suppuratives Vrana chikitsa should do with following external applications.

a) Shigru Tilwaka Tarkari (Arani), Gaja Pippali, Swetha punarnava, Neeli, Amrutha, Arka Moola, Trivruth and padmak should be grinded with sura Or Kanji and used as External application.

b) **Guduchi Taila :-** Oil prepared with Guduchi Nimba Kutaja Hamsapadi Pippali Devadaru and Baladwayam.

## 2) KAPHAJ GALAGANDA.

The vitiated Kapha dosha causes, a hard, painless, skin coloured, bigger cyst develops on the Neck with itching sensation, Coldness, formation of Sticky layer on palate and throat and with unpleasant sweetness of mouth.

**Treatment :-**

Like Vataj Galaganda But with more potent drugs.
1) Sweda 2) Vimlapana, 3) Upanaha. 4) Raktha Mokshan 5) Vamana 6) Shodhan Nasya 7) Rechana Dhoomapana. 8) If the cyst suppurates Vrana Chikitsa with the following external applications.
a) Ajaganda, Ativisha, vishalya, Gunja, Karkatata Shrungi, Alabu and Phalasha kshara - grinded with sura or Kanji and applied to the lesion.

**9) Oral Adiministriation of :-**

1) Taila Prepared with the drugs of Vatsakadi group.
2) Jala Kumbhee Kshar + Gomutra
3) Taking of Kodrava diet.

## 3) MEDOJA GALAGANDA .

The signs and symptoms of Kaphaj Galaganda present, additionally abnormal noises in throat, abnormal (obstructed) Voice, Foul smell, and severe itching sensation assciated. The size of the cyst increases and decreases along with body built (if the body build is perfect, cyst increases in size and if the body is emaciated cyst reduces in size ).

**Treatment :-**
1) Like Kaphaj Galaganda Chikitsa.
2) Sira Vyadana.
3) The powder of the drugs of Aasanadi Group + Gomutra, for Oral intake.

4) Daha Karma with Vasa ghritha and madhu, then application of Gorochan + kaseesa + Tutta + Ropana taila (if the disease is not controlled ; incision, should be given to remove the fat, suturing then Healing therapy should be followed as an alternative method )

# ADDITIONAL DISEASES OF THROAT, BY VAGBHATA.

| Sl. No. | Name of the Disease | Modern Name | Vitiation of Dosha | Lakshanas | Treatment. |
|---------|--------------------|-----------| -------------------|-----------|------------|
| 1. | Galarbuda | Benign Tumour in Throat | Vatadi Doshas Sadya | Hard, Painless, fixed non suppurative, red tumour develops in throat. | Chedan. Pratisaran. |
| 2. | Tundikeri | Tonsilitis | Kapha Rakthaja Sadya | Red, bigger, painful swelling develops at Talumoola resembling Karpasa phala . | Bhedhan/Chedan Pratisaran. |
| 3. | Vataj Galaganda | Goitre | Vataj/Sadya | Painful reddish black cyst with black vessels develops on neck. | Sweda, Raktha Mokshana, vrana Chikitsa. |
| 4. | Kaphaj Galaganda | " | Kaphaj/Sadya | Hard painless big cyst develops on neck with itching sensation. | -do- |
| 5, | Medoja Galaganda | " | Medoja /Sadya | Kapha features, Swara Vikruthi, foul smell with itching sensation. | -do- |

284

# DISEASES OF THROAT
## GALAROGAS

| Sl. No. | Name of the Disease | Modern Name | Vitiation of Dosha Sadya-asadhya | Lakshanas | Treatment |
|---------|--------------------|-------------|--------------------------------|-----------|-----------|
| 1. | Vataja Rohini | Diphtheria | Vathaj Kasta Sadya Vyadhi | Painful, throat obstructing Swelling develops in the throat with dryness of oralcavity, obstruct the food and . airway | Sneha -Sweda, Vamana. Raktha Mokshana, Pratisarana, Kavala. it kills the person in 7 days if neglected. |
| 2. | Pittaja Rohini | " | Pittaj/Kasta Sadya | Spreading type of swelling develops in throat with burning pain, fever, thirst, vertigo and unconsciousness. | Treatment principles same as above and kills the person in 5 Days if neglected |
| 3. | Kaphaj Rohini | " | Kaphaj/Kasta Sadya | Fixed, bulk sticky, throat obstructing swelling develops, with atrophic changes in throat | Treatment principles same as above and kills the person in 3 days if neglected. |
| 4. | Rakthaj Rohini | " | Rakthaj/Kasta Sadya | Red swelling develops in throat with burning pain-and symptoms of pitta also present. | Treatment principles same as above and kills the person immediately. |
| 5. | SanniPathaj Rohini | " | Tridoshaj/Asadya | Most complicated swelling with all the above symptoms develops in throat. | Asadya. |

285

| No. | Name | English | Description | Dosha / Sadya | Treatment |
|---|---|---|---|---|---|
| 6. | Kantha Shaaluka | Adenoids | Fixed, hard cyst resembling Badari Phala Develops in throat with pricking pain and discomfort. | Kapha-Shastra Sadya | Bhedan/Lekhana and Prathisaran. |
| 7. | Adijihwa | Epiglottitis | A Swelling develops above the tongue resembling the tip of tongue | Kapha-Raktha sadya | Lekhan-Pratisarana Nasya-Kavala, & dhoomapana. |
| 8. | Valaya | Tumour of Throat | Lengthy bulk, complicative throat obstructing swelling causes obstrution of air and Food way. | Kaphaja Asadya | Asadya. |
| 9. | Balasa | " | Dreadful, painful, throat obstructing swelling that causes injury to vital parts develops in throat. | Vata Kaphaj Asadya | Asadya. |
| 10) | Ekavrunda | " | Round fixed, bulk, hard, non Suppurative cyst with pain, burning anditching sensation develops in throat. | Kapha Rakthaj Sadya | Raktha mokshan Pratisaran Kavala dhoom panam. |
| 11) | Vrunda | " | Bigger, painful burning swelling develops in throat, more complicated than ekavrunda. | Pitta Raktha Or Vata Raktha Sadya. | Asadya. |

| No. | Name | Dosha / Sadya | Symptoms | Treatment |
|---|---|---|---|---|
| 12. | Gilayu | " Kapha Raktha Shastra Sadya | Hard, fixed, painful swelling like Amalaki Seed develops in throat end and obstructs the air and food way | Bhedan/Lekhan Pratisaran Kavala-Dhoomapan |
| 13. | Gala Vidradi Retro Pharyngeal abscess | Tridoshaj Asadya | Painful, suppurating and throat obstructing swelling with features of Tridosha. | Bhedan Shodhan Ropana. |
| 14. | Galaugha | " Kapha Raktha Asadya | Bigger, painful, throat obstructing Swelling with fever, drowsiness and heavyness of head, develops in thorat. | Asadya. |
| 15. | Swaraghna Paralysis of Larynx | Vata Asadya | Shabdavaha srotas is deranged and causes breathlessness, inability or to talk, Dryness of throat and giddiness | Asadya. |
| 16. | Mamsatana Carcinoma of Throat | Tridoshaj Asadya | Abnormally spreading, throat obstructing swelling or polyp develops in throat | Asadya. |
| 17. | Vidari Gangrenous stomatitis | Pitta Raktha Asadya | Painful, burning type of red growth with necrotic Or atrophic changes, develops in Throat. | Asadya |
| 18. | Shataghnee Tumour of throat | Tridoshaj Asadya | Multiple cysts obstructs the throat with burning pain, fever and headache. | Asadya. |

# सर्वसर मुखरोग या सर्वसर मुखपाक

त्रय: सर्वेष्वायतनेषु ॥

सर्वसरास्तु वातपित्त कफ शोणितनिमित्ता

(सु. नि. अ. १६)

स्फोटै: सतोदैर्वदनं समन्ताद्यस्याचितं सर्वसर: स वातात् ।
रक्तै: सदाहैस्तनुभि: सपीतैर्यस्याचितं चापि स पित्तकोपात् ॥
कण्डूयुतैरल्परुजै: सवर्णैर्यस्याचितं चापि स वै कफेन ।
रक्तेन पित्तोदित एक एव कैश्चित् प्रदिष्टो मुखपाकसंज्ञ: ॥

(सु. नि. अ. १६)

करोति वदनस्यान्तर्व्रणान् सर्वसरोनिल: ।
संचारिणोरुणान् रुक्षानोष्ठौ ताम्रौ चलत्वचौ ॥
जिह्वा शीतासहा गुर्वी स्फुटिता कण्टकाचिता ।
विवृणोति च कृच्छ्रेण मुखं पाको मुखस्य च ॥

(अ॰ हृ॰ उ॰ अ॰ 21)

# पित्तज मुखपाक

मुखस्य पित्तजे पाके दाहोषे तिक्तवक्रता ।
क्षारोक्षितक्षतसमा व्रणा:, तद्वच्च रक्तजे ॥

(अ॰ हृ॰ उ॰ अ॰ 21)

# कफज मुखपाक

कफजे मधुरास्यत्वं कण्डूमत्पिच्छिला व्रणा: ।
अन्त:कपोलमाश्रित्य श्यावपाण्डुकफोर्बुदम् ॥
कुर्यात्तद् घट्टितं छिन्नं मृदितं च विवर्धते ।
मुखपाको भवेत् सास्त्रै:, सर्वै: सर्वाकृतिर्मलै: ॥

# ऊर्ध्वगुद के लक्षण

अध: प्रतिहतो वायुरर्शोगुल्मकफादिभि: ।
यात्यूर्ध्वं वक्त्रदौर्गन्ध्यं कुर्वन्नूर्ध्वगुदस्तु स: ॥

(अ॰ हृ॰ उ॰ अ॰ 21)

## पूतिवक्त्रता के लक्षण

पूत्यास्यतां तैरेव दन्तकाष्ठादिविद्विषः ॥

(अ॰ हृ॰ उ॰ अ॰ २१)

## असाध्य मुखरोग

रोगाणां मुखजातानां साध्यानां कर्म कीर्तितम् ।
असाध्या अपि वक्ष्यन्ते रोगा ये तत्र कीर्तिताः ॥
ओष्ठप्रकोपे वर्ज्याः स्युर्मांसरक्त त्रिदोषजाः ।
दन्तमूलेषु वर्ज्यौ तु त्रिलिङ्गयतिसौषिरौ ॥
दन्तेषु च न सिध्यन्ति श्यावदालनभञ्जनाः ।
जिह्वागतेष्वलासस्तु तालव्येष्वर्बुदं तथा ॥
स्वरघ्नो वलयो वृन्दो विदार्यलस एव च ।
गलौघो मांसतानश्च शताघ्नी रोहिणी च या ॥
असाध्याः कीर्तिता ह्येते रोगा नव दशैव च ।
तेषाँ चापि क्रियां वैद्यः प्रत्याख्याय समाचरेत् ॥

(सु. चि. अ. 22/77 से 81)

# SARVA SARA MUKHA ROGAS ( MUKHA PAKA )

| | | |
|---|---|---|
| According to Sushrutha | | 3 Diseases |
| " Sarangdhara | | 5 " |
| " Vagbhata | | 8 " |

## CLASSIFICATION OF THE DISEASES OF MUKHA.

| Sl. No. | Sushrutha | Sarangdhara | Vagbhata |
|---|---|---|---|
| 1. | Vataj Mukha Paka | Vataj Mukha Paka | Vataj Mukha Paka |
| 2. | Pittaj Mukha Paka | Pittaj Mukha Paka | Pittaj Mukha Paka |
| 3. | Kaphaj Mukha Paka | Kaphaj Mukha Paka | Kaphaj Mukha Paka |
| 4. | | Rakthaj Mukha Paka | Rakthaj Mukha Paka |
| 5. | | Sanni Pathaja Mukha paka | Sanni Pathaj Mukha Paka. |
| 6. | | | Urdwa guda |
| 7. | | | Mukhaarbuda |
| 8. | | | Puthi Mukha. |

Sarvasara Mukha rogas are named as " Mukha Paka". occur by spreading competely in the Mukha so only named as Sarvasara mukha rogas.

## NIDANA SAMPRAPTHI OF MUKHA ROGAS.

**Aetio pathology of mukha roga :-**

Lose of appetite, Indigestion, constipation, eating of very hard, hot, cold items; improper cleaning of teeth and mouth Intestinal worms, caries teeth, general weakness, Hypovitaminosis (defficiency of B. Complex, Vit C) Allergy to Tooth powder or paste, physical and chemical traumatic injuries to oral mucosa; pitta and Raktha, vitiating food intake. Due to above causative factors, vatadi doshas vitiate the oral mucosa and causes mukha paka.

### Common Signs Symptoms of Mukha Paka.

1) Inflammation of Oral mucosa. 2) Ulceration in the mouth. 3) Altered taste. 4) Pain Burning Sensation and itching sensation in mouth. 5) Difficulty in mastication and deglutition 6) Headache and discomfort.

### Common Treatment Principles of Mukha Roagas.

1) Sneha - Sweda (Oleation and Fomentation) 2) Shodhan (Vaman, Virechana Nasya, Rkatha Mokshana) 3) Lekhana Or Bhedhana Or Chedan. therapies. 4) Prathisarana (application of medicine ) 5) Kavala Or Gandoosha (Gargling) 6) Dhooma pana (medicated smoking. 7) Nasya (nasal drops) 8) Nidana Parivarjan. (Avoiding the causative factor) 9) Dosha shamana chikitsa. 10) Samyak mukha prakshalana. (Perfect mouth wash).

# COMMON YOGAS FOR MUKHAPAKA

After shareera shodhan, Local treatments should give, among the Local treatments Kavala Gandoosha and prathisaran are having utmost importance in the management of Mukha rogas.

## Medicines for Gargling and for Oral Intake. :-

I) a)   Triphala Kashaya Or Aaragwadadi Kashaya
Or Pancha Pallava Kashaya Or panchakola Kashaya
Or Dashamoola Kashaya Or Pancha Valkala Kasahaya
Or Pancha tiktha Kashaya Or udumbara Kashaya.
Or Shigru Kashaya Or jathi Patra Kashaya.
Or Mutra Or Ksheera Or Madhu Or ghritha Or

Yastimadu Kashaya Or Pancha Lavanas + Water Or shubra Bhasma + Water or Tankan Bhasma + Water.

B)    **1) Patoladi quath :-** Decoction prepared with Patola shunti Triphala Vishala, Karanja, Katuki, Haridra, Daruharidra, Guduchi + honey.

**2) Khadhiradi Kashaya :-** Decoction prepared with Khadhira Agaru Triphala, Arjunatwak, malathi, Babbula twak.

**3) Kshudradi Kashaya :-** Decoction Prepared with kantakari, Guduchi Jathipatra, Daruharidra, Triphala + Honey..

**4) Jathyadi Kashaya :-** Decoction prepared with Jathipatra, Daru-Haridra, Triphala, Dadimapatra, Babbula twak, Badari moola twak - and add Tankan bhasma - shubra bhasma and use for Gargling.

**5) Sapthacchadadi Kashaya :-** Decoction prepared with Sapthacchada, usheera, patola, Musta, Kiratha tiktha, Katuki, Yastimadu, amlavetas, chandan.

**6) Tiladi Kashaya :-** Decoction prepared with Tila, Neelothphala, Ghritha, Sugar, Milk and Lodra.

**7) Dhaarvee Kashaya** + Honey

**8) Jathipatra kashaya** + Honey .

**9) Dhaarree Ghana Kwatha** + Gyrika + Honey

**10) Patoladi ghana Kwatha** + Gyrika + Honey.

(Patola, Nimba , Yastimadu, Vasa, Jathipatra, Babbula, Khadhira sara, Triphala ).

**11)** Go mutra, Hareetaki + Sadapa, Kusta and usheera Kashaya.

C)    Haridradi Taila,      Tila Taila
      Irimedadi Taila,      Arimedadi Taila
      Khadhiradi Taila etc., are used for gargling.

## d)    Tablets and powders for chewing.

1) Triphala, Dweepi, Kiratatiktha, Yastimadu Sarshapa, Trikatu, Musta, Haridra dwayam. Yava Kshara, Vrukshamla, Amlavetas Ashwattha twak, Jambu twak, Amra Twak, Arjuna twak, Dhananjaya twak, khadira sara, the fine powder, is prepared, half (1/2) medicine should be prepared for decoction, then remaining half should be added, heat it and prepared concentrated medicine, tabets are prepared and used for chewing.

2) a) Khadhiradi Vati    b) Lavangadivati c) Trijatha Kadi Vati) Eladi churna e) Krishnajeera + Kusta + Indrayana should  be used for chewing

3) Triphala small pieces or Powder, Yastimadu small pieces Or powder , Amla small pieces Or powder, jathi Patra, Tamala patra + Khadira + Pudeena + Lavanga + Karpoora, for chewing.

## E) Dantha Manjan ;- (Prathisaran)

**1) Pathadi Manjan** :- Patha, Daruharidra, Kusta, Musta Manjista, Katuki, Haridra, Lodra, Tejobala + Honey.

**2) Kaalak churna manjan :-** Gruhadhooma, Rasanjan, Patha, Trikatu Triphala, Yavakshara, Loha bhasama, Tejobala, chiktrak + Honey.

**3) Peetak Churna Manjan :-** Daru haridra, Saindhava lavan, Manashila, Yavakshara, haritala, Ghee and Honey

**4)** Tankan bhasma + Honey Pratisaran

**5)** Shubra bhasma + Honey pratisaran.

**6)** Saindhava Lavana + Honey Pratisaran.

## II)    Nasya Karma :-

Medicated ghee or oil or powder or liquid should be selected according to vitiation of doshas and used as nasal drops.

Ex :-    1) Yastimadwadi Taila  2) Ksheera bala taila etc.

## II)    Dhooma Pana:- Medicine should select According to the vitiation of doshas and use for dhooma pana.

## IV)    If the disease is not controlled by medical treatment, surgical methods like LEKHANA BHEDHANA and CHEDANA has to do in assoication with Pratisarana.

## V)    Same remedies useful in Mukha rogas.

Lakshmivilasras, Maha Lakshmivilas ras, maha lakshmivilas ras with Gold, Naradeeya Lakshmivilas ras, Lagusuthasekara ras, Arogyavardini vati, sarivadi vati, Gandak rasayan tab, Lavangadi Vati Trijathakadi vati, G. 32 tabs, Kanchanara guggulu, Triphala guggulu, Sapthamrutha Loha, khadhiradivati,

Haridra Khanda, Chopacheenyadi  Churna, Yastimadu Churna, Triphala Churna, Panchanimba churna, Trikatu churna, Tankanbhasma, shubra bhasma Rasmanikyaras, vyadhiharan rasayan.Panchatiktha-gugglu-ghritha, Khadhirarista, Sarivadyarista, mahamangistadi quath, Maha Rasnadi quatha, Bhasmas like muktha Pravala, Akeeka, Jaharmohra, shankha etc., are more beneficial in the management of mukha rogas.

# 1) VATAJ MUKHA PAKA
## (Stomatitis )

The vitiated vata dosha causes a single Or multiple ulcers in the Oral mucosa with acute inflammatory changes. The disease is progressive in nature, very painful, mucosa becomes dry and rough. The associated symptoms are inflamed lips tongue and palate, difficulty in opening the mouth and sensitivity to cold items. etc.

## Treatment :-
1) Sneha, sweda (Oleation and Fomentation ) 2) Shodhan Karma (Vaman, virechan, Nasya, Raktha Mokshan) 3) Kavalagraha or Gandoosha (gargles) 4) Snehika dhooma pana (medicated smoking) 5) Snehana Nasya (Vata hara Nasal drops) 6) Nidana Parivarjan (Avoiding causative factors ) 7) Lekhana and prathisarana.

## Some Yoga of Gandoosha (Gargling)
A)      1) Triphala Kashaya 2) Dashamoola Kashaya.3) Rasnadi Kashaya 4) Pancha Pallava Kashaya 5) The decoction of Triphala, patha, Mrudweeka, jathi patra, the decotion + Honey 6) Vata hara taila or ghritha.

B)      **Nasya :-** With Vata hara taila or Ghrita.
C)      **Dhooma Pana :-** Snehika dhooma pana with shalaphaladi drugs. Sarja rasa Khadhiradi vati etc., drugs.
D)      **Pratisaran :-** Local application of medicine  1) Pippali + Lavan + Ela + Honey.2) Pancha lavana + Honey

# 2) PITTAJA MUKHA PAKA
## (Acute Stomatitis )

The vitiated pitta dosha causes inflammation and ulceration of oral mucosa. Smaller reddish yellow papules develop throughout the mouth. causes severe burning pain. altered taste (Bitter mouth), difficulty in mastication and deglutition.

## Treatment :-
1) Sneha, sweda (oleation and Fomentation ) 2) Shodhan Karma (Vaman, virechan, Nasya, Raktha Mokshan etc ) 3) Kavala graha Or Gandoosha (Gargling) 4) Shaman Nasaya 5) Shaman Dhooma Pana 6) Nidana Parivarjana 7) Lekhana and Prathisarana.

A)      **Some Yoga of Gandoosha :-**
1) Triphala Kashaya 2) Pancha valkala Kashaya 3) Vidari gandhadi or kakolyadi Kashaya 4) Pancha Tiktha Kashaya 5) Yastimadu Kashaya 6) Chandana, Usheera, mustadi Kashaya 7) Gargling with Milk Or Sugar cane juice Or Ghee.

B)      **Nasya and Gandoosha :-**
With sheeta Veerya, Pitta hara taila, ghritha Or Kashaya.

293

C) Pratisaran Yoga (Local application of the Medicine with the following drugs
1) Shunti Choorna + Ghritha 2) Amalaki Churna + Water 3) Haridra Chandanadi Lepam 4) Nimba Pallava Kalka 5) Jathi Pallava Kalka etc.,

# 3) KAPHAJ MUKHA PAKA.
## (Sub acute Or Chronic, Stomatitis )

The vitiatied Kapha dosha produces inflammation and ulceration in the oral mucosa, The mouth become sweet sticky with itching sensation and negligible pain. Small cysts Or tumours develop and become more severe by compression and excision.

**Treatment :-**

1) Sneha sweda (Oleation and Fomentatin ) 2) Shodhan Karma (Vaman Virechan Nasya Raktha Mokshan) 3) Kavalagraha and Gandoosha 4) Shodhana Nasya 5) Virechanika Dhooma Pana. 6) Lekhana / Bhedhan / Chedan and Prathisaran 7) Nidana Parivarjana.

**Some Yoga of (gargling) Gandoosha :-**

A) Ghritha Or taila or madhu Or Ksheera
B) Triphala Kashaya Or pancha valkala Kashaya Or Panchakola Kashaya Or Aaragwadadi Kashaya Or Trikatu Kashaya.

C) Haridradi taila Or khadiradi taila.
D) Khadiradi vati Or Trijathakadi Vati Or
Lavangadi vati for chewing.
E) Oral in take of
Ativisha, patha, musta, Devadaru, Katuki, Indrayava, with Gomutra.
F) Oral intake of
Trikatu Or pancha Kola Kashaya.

# 4) SANNIPATHAJ MUKHA PAKAM.

All the symptoms of Tridosha and Raktha dosha are present in this disease.

**Treatment :-** Tridosha hara Chikitsa should be given.

Pratisaran with Haridra, Kaseesa, Kamkshi, Rasanjan, mocha ras + Madhu.

# 5) RAKTHAJA MUKHA PAKA.

Signs symptoms and treatment is like pittaja mukha paka

## 6) URDWA GCDA
### (Intestinal Obstruction)

The Annavaha srotas is obstructed due to Gulma Arsha and Kapha by which the **Apana vayu** is obstructed and propogates upwards and emits foul smell through the mouth

**Treatment :-**　　1) Asadya

　　　　　　　　2) Symptomatic treatment.

## 7) (PUTHI VAKTRATHA)
### (Puthi Mukha )

The Vitiated dosha produces Foul smell in mouth due to improper cleaning of teeth (with dantha Kaasta) and mouth

**Treatment :-**

1) Sneha - Sweda

2) Vaman

3) Teekshna nasya

4) Teekshana Dhooma Pana

5) Brushing of teeth and gargling with manjista, Dhataki, Lodra, priyang, and Padmaka.

6) Sheetada Upakusha Chikitsa (these two are Dantha moola Vyadhies)

7) Gandoosha, with the decoction of Triphala, Jathi Patra., haridra Daruharidra, Guduchi, Nimba and patola etc.,.

8) Irimededi taila Gandoosha.

9) Chewing of Khadhiradi Vati Or Lavangadi vati.

## 8) MUKHA ARBUDA .
### (Tumours in oral cavity)

The Vitiated Kapha dosha produces **blackish white colour tumour** in the oral cavity (in the internal surface of Kapola i.e. cheeks.). By compression incision and excision the disease recurs and aggravates.

**Treatment :-**

1) If tumour is smaller

Chedhan and prathisarana with Kshara + Shunthi + Madhu.

2) Gandoosha with the decoction of Guduchi + nimba + Tila taila + Honey.

3) Teekshna Nasya, Dhooma pana and abhyanga.

4) In take of food prepared with yava.

5) Kapha hara Picchu at Vrana. (Ulcer or lesion)

# ASADYA MUKHA ROGA

| Sl. No. | Name of the Group | Asadya Vyadhies. |
|---------|-------------------|------------------|
| 1. | Osta Rogas | 1) Mamsaja Osta prakopa<br>2) Rakthaja osta prakopa<br>3) Sannipathaja Osta Prakopa. |
| 2. | Dantha Moola Vyadhies | 1) Saushira<br>2) Sannipathaja Danthanadi |
| 3. | Dantha Vyadhies | 1) Shyava Dantha<br>2) Dhalana<br>3) Bhanjanaka |
| 4. | Jihwa Roga | 1) Alasa. |
| 5. | Talu Rogas | 1) Talu arbuda. |
| 6, | Gala Rogas | 1) Swaraghna<br>2) Valaya<br>3) Vrunda<br>4) Vidari<br>5) Balasa<br>6) Galaugha<br>7) Mamsatana<br>8) Shathaghnee<br>9) Rohini (Tridoshaj) |

(In total 19 Disease are Asadya. in mukha roga)

# SARVA SARA MUKHA ROGA.

| Sl.No. | Name of the Disease | Modern Name | Vitiation of Dosha Sadya Asdya | Lakshana | Chikitsa. |
|---|---|---|---|---|---|
| 1. | Vataja Mukha Paka | Stomatitis | Vataja Sadya | Dry - rough progressive Ulceration & inflammation of Oral mucosa associated with pain and sensitivity | Vata hara Chikitsa. Sneha, sweda, Sneha, Gandoosha Snehika dhooma. |
| 2. | Pittaja Mukha Paka | Acute Stomatitis | Pittaja Sadya | Ulceration and inflammation of oral mucosa with severe burning pain and bitter taste | Pitta hara Chikitsa Sneha, Sweda, Gandoosha, (Tiktha Kashaya) Shamana dhooma and nasya. |
| 3. | Kaphaja Mukha Paka | Chronic Stomatitis | Kaphaja Sadya | Ulceration and inflammation of oral mucosa with negligible pain, itching sensation and with unpleasent sweet taste | Kapha hara Chikitsa Sneha, sweda, Teekshna Nasya, Gandoosha, Dhooma, Lekhan and Pratisaran. |
| 4. | Sanni Pathaj mukha paka | Acute Stomatitis | Tridoshaja Sadya. | All the symptoms of Tridosha present | Tridosha hara Chikitsa. |

297

| Sl. No | Name of the Disease | Modern Name | Vitiation of Dosha | Sadya Asadya | Lakshana | Chikitsa. |
|---|---|---|---|---|---|---|
| 5. | Rakthaja Mukah paka | Acute Stomatitis | Rakthaja | Sadya. | All the Symptoms of Vitiated Pitta present | Like pittaja muka paka. |
| 6. | Urdwa guda | Intestinal Obstruction | Kaphaja | Asadya | Apana Vayu is obstructed by kapha - gulma Arsha and emits foul smell thorugh the mouth | Asadya. |
| 7. | Puthi Mukha | Oral unhygienic Condition. | Vatadi | Sadya | Foul smell comes from mouth due to improper brushing of teeth. | Sneha - sweda Kavala, Nasya, dhooma Mukha Prakshalana. |
| 8. | Mukhaarbuda | Tumour in Oral cavity | Kaphaj Shastra | Sadya | White tumour develops in mouth aggravates by excision | Chedan Kshara Pratisaran. |

298

# COMMON SIGNS AND SYMPTOMS OF PHARYNGEAL DISORDERS.

**Symptoms :-**
1)  Pain (Odynophagia) :- Pain on Swallowing and may referred to ear.
2)  Salivation :- it may increase due to infrequent swallowing due to pain, it may be blood stained and with foul smell in malignanay and dental sepsis.
3)  Irritation or Foreign body Sensation in throat due to allergy Or post nasal discharge, foreign bodies inflamed mucosa and malignancy.
4)  Nasal regurgitation due to improper functioning of soft Palate, cleftpalate, short palate and palatal perforation.
5)  Dysphagia :- Due to laryngopharyngeal or Oesophageal diseases.
6)  Swellings of neck :- Lymphadenitis Or metastatic lymph nodes.

**Signs :-** The signs of the diseases depends upon the nature of the disease, but the common signs. are.
1)  Congestion Or oedema Or inflammation of Pharyngeal mucosa,
2)  Mucoid Or mucopurulent Or purulent secretions.
3)  Inflamed glands, development of cysts Or tumours Or abscess or membrane formation Or lymphadenitis are observed.

**Treatment - Principle.**
1)  Cause should be removed.
2)  Culture and sensitivity of throat swab and using Broad spectrum antibiotics accordingly.3) Anti inflammatories analgesics anti pyretics. and anti histamines. etc., drugs. should use.4)Medicated hot gargles Or steam inhalations. 5)Supplementation of Vitamines -Nutrients (Vit-B.C.) 6) Excision of malignant tumours, Radiation, and usage of cytotoxic drugs. 7) Stoping the irritants. 8) Symptomatic treatments.

# DISEASES OF BUCCAL CAVITY ( ORAL CAVITY)

**STOMATITIS :**
Diffuse inflammation of the oral mucosa caused by the following local and systemic diseases.

**Local Causes :-**
**1) Traumatic Stomatitis :-**
It is due to ill fitting of dentures, incorrect brushing of teeth, hot and spiced food, medicaments, fumes, smoke and radio therapy, The epithelium of the palate cheeks and gums becomes eroded, producing painful shallow ulcers, sloughy base and with surrounding hyperaemia.

**Treatment :-**   1) Removal of primary cause 2) Orodental hygiene
3) Antiseptic gargles 4) Supplementation of vitamines (especially
B.Complex) 5) Antibiotics anti inflammatories and analgesics.

**2) Infective Stomatitis :-**
Inflammation of the oral mucosa with bacteria virus Or fungi.

### a) Viral Infective stomatitis :-

Herpes simplex, herpes Zoster etc., involve the mucosa of lips, buccal mucosa and palate and produces small painful vesicles which later ulcerates..

### b) Bacterial stomatitis :-

Acute ulcerative stomatitis commonly caused by the staphy lococcus, streptococcus Or Gonococci infection.

### c) Fungal Stomatitis :-

Stomatitis caused by candida albicans, etc. it is known as thrush Or Moniliasis.

**Treatment :-** 1) Removal of causes 2) Antibiotics 3) Antiseptic Gargles 4) Orodental hypiene 5) Vitamine supplementation 6) Application of 1% Gentian Voilet Or nystatine in glucerine etc.,

## 3) RECURRENT ULCERATIVE STOMATITIS - APHTHOUS ULCERS.

Aetiology is un known but various factors like viruses, endocrine disturbances, psychosomatic factors, habitual constipation, autoimmune reactions, and vitamine deficiencies etc. are suggested.

Single Or multiple small vesicles appear in Oropharyngeal mucosa, the vesicles soon ulcerate and surrounded by erythema. they are very painful and usually occur in gingiobuccal groove tongue. or buccal mucosa.

**Treatment :-** 1) Cause should be ruled out 2) Vitamines and nutrients supplementation, 3) maintainance of Orodental hygiene. 4) Local hydro cortisone usage. 5) Antibiotics - Anti inflammatories and analgesics. 6) Antiseptic gargles.

## 4) ANGULAR STOMATITIS

It is due to ill fitting of dentures and avitaminosis (Riboflavin deficienency) ulceration and cracking of the angles of the mouth is observed as the main sign of th disease.

**Treatment :-** 1) Supplementation of nutriets and Vitamines. 2) Orodental hygiene 3) Removal of the cause 4) Local applications of 1% Gention voilet 5) Symptomatic treatment.

## 5) BEHCETS SYNDROME

This is a disease of un known aetiology characterised by ulceration of the Oral cavity, External genitalia (Some times neurological problems like encephalitis and blindness) and conjunctivitis.

**Treatment :-**
1) Administration of Steroids. 2) symptomatic treatment.

## 6) LICHEN PLANUS

it is a pre malignant condition of unknown aetiology, the mucosal lesions are dull white, milky dots, appears like lacy striae, circular Or anular. Skin lesions usually co exist.

**Treatment :-** Symptomatic treatment

## 7) PEMPHIGUS

Bullus lesions without erythema on oral mucosa and skin, the bullae when repture leaves a raw surface it is also with unknown aetiology.

**Treatment :-**

Administration of steroids and symptomatic treatment.

## 8) STOMATITIS DUE TO DRUGS.

Excessive doses of Bismuth lead iodides and mercury etc., causes the stomatitis.

## 9) STOMATITIS DUE TO SYSTEMIC CAUSES.

Stomatitis occur due to vitamine B. Complex, deficiency, pernicious anaemia, mal- absorption syndrome and haemotalogical lesions (Agranulocytosis - leukemias, poly cythemia, mononucleosis etc.,)

## 10) LEUKOPLAKIA

It occurs as white patches in oropharyngeal mucosa, usually arises by heavy smoking, alcohol, spices, dental sepsis, syphilis and vitamin deficiency, it is a pre malignant lesion.

**Treatment :-**

Avoiding the irritating Factors and Biopsy to rule out malignancy .

## 11) ERYTHROPLAKIA

Red patches on oral mucosa, it is also a premalignant lesion.

## 12) SUBMUCUS FIBROSIS.

It is characterised by diffuse dense white patches on oral and pharyngeal mucosa, due to deposition of Fibrous tissue in submucosa, often associated with Trismus.

**Predisposing Factors.**

Exact cause is unknown but following factors may cause the disease.

1) Irritants- Chewing of paan, Tobacco, Betal nuts, and intake of Chillies and spicy foods. 2) Trauma _ Repeated mechanical and thermal trauma. 3) Nutrition :- Poor Nutrition and Vitamine deficiency. 4) Poor Oro dental hygiene. 5) Achlorhydria and hyperacidity.

**Clinical Features :-**

Trismus, Burning sensation in Oral cavity, recurrent ulcers in mouth, lymphadenitis, (submandibular) involvement of cheeks, leads to failure in blowing whistling and sucking etc., White patches are seen in the Oral cavity on the cheeks, retromolar area, hard palate and soft palate, it leads to difficulty in mastication and swallowing, poor oro dental hygiene, deafness and malignancy may supervene in some cases.

**Treatment :-**

1) Avoiding the irritants 2) Correction of dental hygiene . 3) Local injections of Hydro Cortisonse Or Hyaluronidase. Once a week submucously. 4) Surgery. 5) Physio therapy 6) Symptomatic therapy.

# TUMOURS OF THE ORAL CAVITY.

## A) Benign Tumours.

**1) Cyst -** Usually retention cysts develop in the Floor of the mouth or in tongue (Mucous cysts).

**2) Ranula :-** A cystic swelling develops in the Floor of mouth and under surface of tongue, commonly associate with sublingual salivary gland, appears bluish in colour and require surgical excision.

**3) Haemangioma :-**
It occurs usually on the tongue Or in the inner surface of cheek, it requires surgical excision.

**4) Papilloma ;-**
It usually occurs on the tongue and other parts os oral mucosa, requires surgical excision.

**5) Pleomorphic adenoma-**
It Usually occur on the palate.

**6) Epulis.**
A swelling on gums, having different types a) Fibrous epulis b) Gaint cell epulis c) Malignant epulis It is benign as well as malignant, require surgical excision and radio therapy.

**7) Ludwig's angina :-**
This is an acute inflammatory condition producing cellulitis of Floor of mouth. The patient appears toxic with swelling and Oedema of floor of the mouth and brawny induration of the sub-mandibular and submental region, causes difficulty in swallowing and breathing, the oedema may spread to larynx.
**Treatment :-** 1) Heavy doses of pencillin. 2) Symptomatic treatment.3) may require tracheostomy.

**8) Ameloblastoma :-**
The tumour arises frequently from mandible - benign in nature and need surgical excision.

## B) Premalignant Lesions.
Ex :- Leukoplakia and syphylitic ulcer.

## C) Malignant Tumours :-
Squamous cell carcinoma is the commonest malignancy of tongue and inner aspect of cheek etc., the aetiology is uncertain but factors like tobacco, betel nut chewing, smoking, poor orodental hygiene, thought to play a part for the origination of disease.

The lesions present as a slough covered ulcerated mass with raised margins which bleeds easily on touch, it also involve the adjacent areas and lymph node metastasis is common.

**Treatment:-** Surgery and Radio therapy

# PHARYNGITIS

Inflammation of Pharynx is known as Pharyngitis.

## A) Naso Pharyngitis :-
1) Acute Naso Pharyngitis.
2) Chronic Naso pharyngitis     a) Simple
                                          b) Atrophic.

## 1) Acute Naso Pharyngitis :-
It may be Bacterial Or viral and it follows nasal Or sinus infection.

### Clinical Features :-
Dry ness, burning sensation in naso pharynx, pain while swallowing, Fever, headache and body ache. etc.,

### Treatment :-
Like acute Rhinitis and acute sinusitis.

## 2) a) Chronic Simple Naso Pharyngitis :-
Chronic Nasal Or Sinus Infections may extend and cause the disease.

### Clinical Features :-
Post nasal irritation, inspiratory snoring and mucopurulent sticky discharge with granular pharyngitis.

### Treatment :- 1) Cause should be treated. 2) Alkaline douches and gargles.

## 2) b) Chronic Atrophic Pharyngitis.
Similar to atrophic Rhinitis.

## B) OROPHARYNGEAL AND LARYNGO PHARYNGEAL INFECTIONS.
It is of Two Types-
Acute and Chronic pharyngitis, again they are divided into two, specific and non specific

### Pharyngitis :-

| Acute | Chronic |
|---|---|
| Specific - Non specific | Specific - Non specific. |

## Acute Pharyngitis :-
Acute Inflammation of pharyngeal mucosa is known as Acute pharyngitis.

## 1) Acute Simple Pharyngitis :-
It may occur because of so many Local and systemic causes. Common cold, dental sepsis, mouth breathing, after administration of certain drugs. like potassium lodide, mercury, Arsenic etc., It  is common in other infections like measles Chicken pox, influenza, typhoid etc., inflammatory lesions may also occur after trauma by a Foreign body or after instrumentation.

### Clinical Features :-
Sore throat, mild fever, head ache, body ache, cough dysphagia, slight hoarsness of voice. Examination reveals diffuse congestion of pharyngeal mucosa, tonsils with its pillars, palate, uvula may  be swollen and Resolution usually occurs. in 3 to 7 days (it depends on the seviority of the infection)

**Treatment :-** 1) Bed rest 2) Plenty of fluids 3) Alkaline gargles 4) Giving of suitable Antibiotics, anti inflammatories and analgesics 5) Symptomatic treatment.

## 2) Acute Septic Pharyngitis :-

It is more acute nature than simple pharyngitis, Bacterial in Origion, organisms are strepto coccus haemolyticus, staphylo coccus aureus, pneumo coccus etc.,

### Predisposing Factors :-
1) Low body resistence 2) unhygienic condition. 3) Poverty (malnutrition) 4) Epedemic form in schools and hospitals.

### Clinical Features :-
High Fever, rigor, dysphagia, sore throat, congested pharyngeal mucosa, tonsils and epiglottis, Uvula is swollen and elongated, mucopurulent discharge is sticked to the posterior pharyngeal wall palate, tonsils and pillars, pulse is full and rapid at First then weak and thready, Features of toxaemia and enlarged and tender cervical lymph nodes are Visualised.

### Complications. :-
1) )Oedema of Larynx 2) Ludwigs angina.
### Treatment :-
1) Bed rest 2) C/s of throat swab to detect the infective organism then administration of broad spectum antibiotics accordingly. 3) nutritious soft liquid diet. 4) Analgesics, Antipyretics, Anti inflammatories. 5) Tracheostomy in laryngeal Oedema.

## 3) Ludwig's Angina :-

This is cellulitis and eventually abscess formation in the floor of the oral cavity extending on to the neck, a brawny indurated swelling forms under the chin, there is acute dysphagia and sore throat.
### Treatment :-
1) Incision and drainage of abscess if needed. 2) Broad spectrum antibiotics. 3) Symptomatic treatment.

## 4) Vincent's Angina :-

This is an acute ulcerative lesion of one or both tonsils due to fusiform bacilli and spirochaete. it spreeds to soft palate and gums also

### Predisposing factors :-
Carious teeth, pyorrhoea, - Malnutrition.

**Clinical Features** :- Acute pain in throat, high fever, dysphagia, greyish ulcero membranous patch on one or both tonsils, bleeds easily from mouth, patient appears toxic and with cervical lymphadenitis.

**Treatment :-**
1) High dose of pencillin injections. 2) Antiseptic mouth wash 3) Symptomatic treatment.

## 5) Acute Diphtheretic Pharyngitis :-

Diphtheria is an acute infection due to specific organism Corynebacterium diphtheriae, usually occur in the first decade of age, occurs by airborne or by direct contact.

## Clinical Features :-

Child complains of sore throat, fever and discomfort in throat. There is raised pulse rate, that is disproportionate to the rise of temparature.

The characteristic feature is the greyish white membrane formation on faucial tonsils and extends to Uvula and soft palate. it cannot be easily removed and on removal leaves a raw bleeding surface. The child is often toxic, cervical glands are often englarged and tender due to secondary infection. In advance cases the membrane formation may extend to the larynx causing respiratory obstruction. Neurological and cardiological complications like neuritis myocarditis etc., can occur.

**Diagnosis :-** Swab culture is confirmmatory (Growth of C. diphtheariae or K.L.B.)

**Treatment :-**

1) Anti toxin :- Early administration of anti diphtheric serum (A.D.S.) is always advisable without waiting for bacteriological confirmation. usual dose is 20000 to 100000 Units. 2) Systemic antibiotics (Pencillin is drug of Choice). 3) Nutritious soft liquid diet, 4) Bed Rest. 5) Tracheostomy may be necessary in diphtheretic laryngitis.

## 6) Agranulocytosis Or agaranulocytic Angina :-

This condition is characterised by polymorpho nuclear Leukopenia (marked reduction of neutrophils) associated with Oro-pharyngeal ulceration, pyrexia and severe prostration.

**Actiology :-** Sensitivity to drugs like chloramphenical sulphonamides, cytotoxic drugs and amidopyrine- These causes bone marrow destruction and non formation of neutrophils.

## Clinical Features :-

Head ache, pyrexia, sore throat and malaise Pharyngeal ulcers develop on tonsils, pillars, palate, posterior pharyngeal wall and throughout The gastro intestinal tract. W.B.C. count falls below 3000 per C.M.M. and neutrophils are rarely seen.

## Treatment :-

1) With drawal of the concerned sensitive drugs. 2) heavy doses of pencillin.3) Pentnucleotide is the drug of Choice by injection to stimulate bone marrow. 4) Blood transfusion.

## 7) INFECTIUS MONONUCLEOSIS OR GLANDULAR FEVER :-

It is a viral disease, Some times associated with oral lesions. The causative agent is Epstein-Barr-virus, where there is increase of large mononuclear cells.

**Clinical Features :-**

Sore throat, malaise, weakness, nausea, Vomiting, fever, generalised lymphadenopathy and spleenomegaly.

**Diagnosis :-**

1) **Paul** - bunnell test positive, differential count of W.B.C.

**Treatment :-** Symptomatic

## 8) Moniliasis (Thrush) :-

It is a fungal infection of mouth due to candida albicans, The lesions appear as white Or greyish white patches on Oropharyngeal mucosa surrounded by erythema. The membrane can be removed easily by leaving a raw area, it commonly occurs in the debilitative children.

**Treatment :-**

1)Local application of 1% gention Voilet Or Nystatin inglycerine Or Silver nitrate. 2) Good Nutrition Supplementation.

## 9) Leucaemia :-

Acute lymphocytic leaucaemia some times associate with Oropharyngeal ulcerations with membrane formation.

## 10) Herpes Simplex :-

It is a viral infection causes small vesicles in themouth and Oropharynx, painful ulcers form after rupture of the vesicles.

**Treatment :-**

1) Antiseptic mouth wash. 2) Lignocaine 2% appplication to reduce pain 3) Antiviral drugs like acyclovir. 4) Symptomatic treatment.

## 11) Herpes Zoster :-

Vesicles occur unilaterally in a row on the pharynx Or palate. pain is severe and may referred to the ear.
**Treatment :-** Same as obove.

## CHRONIC PHARYNGITIS

Chronic inflammation of pharynx, may be due to specific Or non specific lesions.

### 1) CHRONIC NON SPECIFIC PHARYINGITIS.

Various aetiological factors (Exogenous endogenous etc) influence and causes the disease, those, predisposing factors are as follows.
1)recurent nasal paranasal infections causes nasal block due to deviated nasal septum, hyper trophied turbinates, nasal polyps, cysts, tumours adenoids etc. So that the patient takes mouth breathing leads to dryness and inflammation of pharynx. 2) Allergic rhinitis 3) Allergic sinustitis 4) Chronic tonsilitis 5) chronic Orodental diseases.

6) Bronchitis 7) Eosinophilia 8) intestinal parasites, 9) Tobacco betelnut chewing, 10) Smoking 11) in take of severe irritants like alcohol 12) atmosphere pollution and 13) emotional factors,causes prolonged irritation to the pharynx and caues diseases.

## Clinical Features :-

Irritation and foreign body sensation in throat, dry cough, pain, Vocal Fatigue and blood stained spit.

## Signs:-
### 1) chronic catarrhal pharyngitis :-

Diffuse congestion of pharyngeal mucosa,

### 2) Chronic Granular Pharyngitis :-

posterior pharyngeal wall appeares to be stubbed with granules - pinkishred in colour (hypertorphy of lymph nodules).

### 3) Follicular pharyngitis :-

Single Or multiple Yellowish cysts develop in pharyngeal wall due to chronic inflammatory changes (mucous glands).

### 4) Lateral band pharyngitis :-

Manifest at the lateral portion of the pharyngeal wall along the track of post nasal discharge.

### 5) Atrophic pharyngitis :-

Atrphic changes in pharyngeal mucosa as a result of extension of atrophic Rhinitis.Examination reveals a dry thin glazed mucosa with wrinkles and crusts.

### Treatment ;-
1) Cause should be treated 2) Hawking should be avoided. 3) Medicated steam inhalation 4) Local alkaline gargles. 5) Chemical Or electric Cautery. 6) Symptomatic treatment.

## Keratosis Pharyngitis :-

It is a condition of unknown aetiology which is characterised by whitish horny out growths on faucial tonsils, base of the tongue and posterior pharyngeal wall. It results from hypertrophy and keratinisation of superficial epithelium, The lesions are hard with no erythema peripherally.

No specific treatment require, subside within few months.

## CHRONIC SPECIFIC PHARYNGITIS

### 1) Tuberculosis Of Pharynx :-

It is secondary to chronic pulmonary tuberculosis. Mucosal ulceration surrounded by area of congestion in Oro pharyngeal region. The Chief complaint is pain and dysphagia, anti tubercular Treatment should be given.

### 2) Lupus of Pharynx:-

It is secondary to Lupus of nose, tubercles appear on pharyngeal mucosa. The nodules break down, ulcerate and heal by cicatrisation.
Anti tubercular treatment should be given.

### 3) Syphilis of Pharynx :-

Pharynx is usually involved in the secondary stage of syphilis , with diffuse congestion, mucosal patches, snail track ulcers and lymphadenitis.

In tertiary syphilis the gummatous ulcer involve hard palate, soft palate and pharynx.

Biopsy and serological tests confirm the diagnosis and pencillin is used as the drug of choice for the treatment.

### 4) Leprosy of Pharynx :-

The pharyngeal involvement is Secondary to nasal and skin lesions. Leprous nodules ulcerate, destruct and perforate the palate and heals with cicatrisation.

# PHARYNGEAL ABSCESSES .

### 1) QUINSY (PERITONSILLAR ABSCESS).

In Quinsy Or peritonsillar abscess  collection of pus outside the tonsilar capsule and medial to superior constrictor muscle, it originates in the peritonsillar tissue as peritonsilitis and culminates into peritonsillar abscess, it is usually unilateral,
**Aetiology :-** Recurrent Tonsilitis, Foreign Body  embedded in tonsil, tonsilar tag left while tonsilectomy and recurrent Oropharyngeal infections, leads to Quinsy.

### Clinical Features :-

1) Pain in throat which refer to ear and aggravate during swallowing 2) Trismus 3) Salivation 4) Rattling sound of saliva while speech. 5) Fever 6) Bodyache. on examination. Anterior pillar of tonsil and uvula becomes inflamed, tonsil is congested, pushed medially and downwards by the abscess.

### Treatment :

1) Antibiotics, anti inflammatories and analgesics to get relieve from pain inflammation and infection. 2) Oral hygiene. 3) Incision and drainage of the abscess, after 4 to 6 weeks tonsilectomy should also perform to prevent recurrence of quinsy.

## 2) Retropharyngeal Abscess.

It is of two types a) Acute b) Chronic.

### a) Acute Retropharyngeal Abscess :-

It occurs due to suppuration of the retropharyngeal lymph nodes, usually affect the children.it is secondary to Oropharyngeal nasopharyngeal, traumatic and exanthematic lesions. etc.

### Clinical Features :-

Fever, malaise, dysphagia. dyspnoea, cough, stiffneck, Oro naso pharyngeal infections, Acute lymphadenitis of jugulo digastric lymph nodes and nodes of upper part of posterior triangle.
**Diagnosis :-** soft tissue X ray of neck lateral view confirm the diagnosis.

### Treatment :-

1) Broad spectrum antibiotics, steroids and symptomatic treatment 2) incision and drainage of abscess transorally.

**b) Chronic retropharyngeal abscess:-** It is due to tuberculosis of cervical spine Treatment consist incision and Drainage and Tubercular treatment.

## 3) PARA PHARYNGEAL ABSCESS :-

The infection spreads to para pharyngeal space From infected tonsil, teeth, Oropharynx, parotid lesions and sub mandibular glands.

**Clinical Features :-**

Patient looks ill, toxic, Febrile, difficulty in swallowing and Trismus. Examination of neck shows a diffuse tender swelling below the angle of mandible on affected side.

**Treatment :-**

1) Broad spectrum antibiotics. 2) Incision and drainage. 3) Symptomatic treatment.

## TUMOURS OF PHARYNX

**A) Tumours of Nasopharynx :-**

1) Benign tumours2) maligant tumours.

**1) Benign Tumours .**

a) Nasopharyngeal Fibroma :- it is smooth lobulated red Or pink tumour, usually, arises from theroot of the naso pharynx, causes nasal obstruction, epistaxis, nasal Voice (rhinolalia clausa ), blocking of eustachian tubes, conductive deafness and by the extension of disease causes broadening of nose (Frog face deformity) proptosis, swelling of cheeks, neuralgic pain and intracranial extension.

**Investigations :-** 1) X ray of Naso pharynx, Base of skull and sinuses. 2) Biopsy.
**Treatment :-**Surgery Or radio therapy.

## OTHER BENIGN TUMOURS ARE.

b) Adenoma c) Papilloma d) salivary tumour e) Enchondroma. f) Angioma. etc.,

**2) MALIGNANT TUMOURS OF NASOPHARYNX .**

The commonest (60 to 75%) malignant tumour of Naso pharynx is squamous cell carcinoma. The commonest site of origin is fossa of Rosen muller.

**Clinical Features :-**

Metastasis in neck glands, conductive deafness, immobility of homolateral soft palate, Trigeminal neuralgia : 2,3,4,6,9, 10, 11, cranial nerves may involve, nasal obstruction. epistaxis. etc.

**Diagnosis ;-** 1) X ray 2) Cytology and biopsy posterior rhinoscopy.
**Treatment :-** 1) Cytotoxic drugs. 2) Radiotherapy
The other malignant tumours of naso Pharynx are
1) Sarcoma 2) Lympho Epithelioma 3) Adeno Carcinoma 4) Chondroma etc.,,

**B) Tumours of Oropharynx.:-**
1) Benign 2) premalignant 3) Malignant tumours.

## 1) Benign Tumours ;-

Benign tumours of Oropharynx are not so common, Papilloma fibroma adenoma, angioma, neurilemma and lipoma are rarely found. Large tumours produce difficulty in breathing, deglutition and have a sensation of lump in the throat.
**Treatment ;-** Excision.

## 2) Premalignant Tumours :-

Leucoplakia is a condition potentially malignant, occurs due to chronic irritation by smoking, chewing of pan and bettlenut. Biopsy should be done to exclude malignancy and irritating factors should be forbidden.

## 3) Malignant Tumours :-

Commonest malignant tumour is **squamous cell carcinoma** the site of Origin is Tonsilo Lingual sulcus and may also originate in tonsils Uvula Palate and lower part of posterior pharyngeal wall. The other malignant Oro pharyngeal tumours are **sarcoma. lympho epithelioma, and adeno carcinoma.**

The common clinical features are sorethoroat dysphagia, difficulty in tongue movements, otalgia, altered speech and upper cervical metastasis.
The cytology and biopsy confirms the diagnosis.
**Treatment ;-** 1) Cytotoxic drugs. 2) Radio therapy

# C) Tumours of Hypo Pharynx Or Laryngo Pharynx :-

This part lies posterior to the larynx extends from the lower limit of the Oropharynx upto the upper end of oesophagus, it includes two pyriform fossae the post cricoid region and the lateral and posterior pharyngeal wall.

Malignant tumours are common than benign. Commonly affects the males of elderly age (except post cricoid cancer that occur in females ) the commonest cauase may be betalnut chewing and smoking. Pyriform fossa, is commonest site for cancer, spread of the disease is vast even upto lungs and other viscera.

## Clinical Features :-

Early symptoms are vague and the patient may complain discomfort in throat Or Pain on swallowing. In the late stages progressive dysphagia is themain symptom along with refered pain in the ear.
**Diagnosis ;-** 1) Indirect laryngo scopy 2) neck examination for lymphnodes 3) X ray of soft tissues of neck 4) Hypo pharyngo scopy 5) Direct laryngo scopy 6) Biopsy 7) X ray chest.
**Treatment :-** Surgery and radio therapy.

## COMMON SIGNS AND SYMPTOMS OF LARYNGEAL, & OESOPHAGEAL DISORDERS.

1) Pain - may radiate to ear. 2) Dysphagia - difficulty in swallowing due to larnygo pharyngeal Or oesophageal lesions. 3) Hoarsness of Voice - with 2 weeks history which is not responding to conservatory treatment. 4) Cough - Irritative cough with expectoration, purulent blood stained foul sputum comes in malignant cases. 5) Dyspnoea with stridor Or Wheezing.

6) Cervical or peripheral lymphadenitis Or metastatic lymphnodes . 8) Congestion or oedema Or inflammation of laryngeal mucosa alongwith pharyngeal mucosa. 9) Mucoid Or mucopurulent Or purulent secretions From throat. 10) Polyps Or cysts Or tumours or paralytic changes are seen in larynx.

## THE TREATMENT PRINCIPLE :-

1) Cause should be removed. 2) Culture and sensitivity of throat swab and using broad spectrum antibiotics accordingly. 3) Anti inflammatory drugs Or analgesics Or antihistamines. 4). Hot gargles. 5) medicated steam inhalations. 6) Vocal rest and Bed rest. 7) Steroids and cough linctus. 8) Avoiding irritants. 9) Endo tracheal intubation Or tracheostomy if needed. 10) Surgery (Laryngectomy) Or radio therapy Or Chemotherapy. for malignant. tumours.

### LARYNGITIS

Inflammation of larynx is known as laryngitis it is of two types.
I) Acute laryngitis A) Specific B) Non specific
II) Chronic laryngitis  A) Specific B) Non specific.

## I/A) Acute Non specific Laryngitis :-
   a) Acute non specific laryngitis.
   b) Acute laryngo tracheo bronchitis.
   c) Acute epiglottitis.

## I/B) Acute Specific Laryngitis.
   a) Diphtheric laryngitis.

## II) A) Chronic Non specific Laryngitis
   a) Chronic non specific laryngitis.
   b) Hyper karatosis (leucoplakia).
   c) Vocal nodule.
   d) Vocal polyps.
   e) Reinka's Oedema.
   f) Atropic laryngitis etc.,

## II/B) Chronic specific laryngitis :-
   a) Tuberculosis
   b) Syphilis.
   c) Lupus,
   d) Leprosy
   e) Scleroma etc.,

## I/A/a) ACUTE NON SPECIFIC LARYNGITIS :
It is the commonest cause of temporary hoarseness of voice.

## Aetiology :-
The infection (bacterial Or viral Or Exanthemata) Common cold, seasonal changes, recurrent attack of infections like tonsilitis, adenoids, sinusitis, rhinitis, pharyngitis, Bronchitis etc., habits or irritative factors like smoking, alcohol. tobacco chewing etc., improper instrumentation during intubation, endo laryngeal surgery and mis use of Voice.

**Clinical Features :-**

Hoarseness of Voice, Rawness feeling in throat, irritative cough, pain, stridor, and constitutional symptoms.

signs observed by indirect laryngoscopy are, congestion of Vocal cords, and other parts of larynx into pinkish red colour, Oedema, exudation, (mucoid initially and purulent in severe cases) white plaques in influanza like infections and restricted movements of vocal cord.

**Complications:-** Infection spreads to Tracheo bronchial tree 2) Dyspnoea 3) Perichondritis.

**Treatment :-**

1) Bed rest 2) Vocal rest (Restrict speaking) 3) Medicated steam inhalation (menthol Or Eucalyptus Oil in Hot water). 4) Hot gargles and neck Fomentation. 5) endo tracheal intubation Or Tracheostomy for Children in stridor. 6) antibiotics antiinflammatories and antihistamines. 7) Steroids and cough linctus. 8) Avoiding irritants. 9) Symptomatic Treatment.

## I/A/b) ACUTE EPIGLOTTITIS.

The epiglottis get inflamed and becomes markedly swollen.

**Clinical Features :-**

Dyspnoea, pain especially during swallowing, Fever and discomfort in throat.

**Treatment :-**

1) Vocal rest 2) Steam inhalation 3) Antibiotics 4) Steroids 5) Tracheostomy may be needed in Children, with stridor.

## I/A/C) ACUTE LARYNGO TRACHEO BRONCHITIS.

It is a severe condition in which larynx and tracheo bronchial tree entirely involved, the child appears toxic, it commonly occur to the people with low resistence power and with virulent infection. It is more complicated than diphtheria.

The common infective organisms are virus, H. influenzae. streptococcus haemolyticus, It causes oedema, congestion and crusting of entire tracheo bronchial tree.

**Clincal Features :-**

High Fever, Cough, hoarsenes of Voice, dysphagia, discomfort in throat and severe dyspnoea. in examination Congestion and Oedema of entire tracheo bronchial tree with membrane formation. rales and Rhonchi of lungs and acute follicular Or ulcerative tonsilitis are seen.

**Treatment :-**

1) Broad spectrum antibiotics. 2) Steriods. 3) Endo tracheal intubation 4) Bronchoscopy to suck the secretions. 5) Tracheostomy may needed in children with stridor.

## I/B/a) LARYNGEAL DIPHTHERIA.

It is due to extention of faucial diphtheria. It may lead to serious complications like laryngeal obstruction.

Coryne bacterium diphthriae is the causative agent, a membrane is formed on larynx and causes laryngeal obstruction.

**Clinical features :-** Mild fever, tachycardia with weak pulse, cough hoarseness of voice breathing problem and greyish white membrane formation on tonsils larynx etc., and chest is clear.

**Investigations :-** 1) C/S of laryngeal swab for coryne bacterium dephtheriae.

**Treatment :-** 1) Antitoxin 40000 to 100000Units. 2) Antibiotics (pencillin or Erythromycetin) 3) Steroids. 4) Oxygen may be needed. 5) Endo tracheal intubation to overcome laryngeal obstruction. 6) Tracheostomy for persistent stridor 7) Fluid intake.

# II) CHRONIC LARYNGITIS.

Chronic inflammation of larynx is known as chronic laryngitis it may occur by specific and nonspecific aetiological factors.

### II/A/a )      Chronic Nonspecific Laryngitis :-

Predisposing factors.:-

Chronic inflammatory focus of tonsils adenoids, teeath, gums, nasal, paransas infections, misuse or over use of voice (Teachers actors singers etc), irritative habits like smoking tobacco chewing alcohol etc., atmospheric pollution with dust fumes etc., repeated attack of acute laryngitis with incomplete treatment leads to chronic laryngitis.

**Clinical Features ;-**

Hoarseness of Voice, dry irritative cough, raw sensation or forgeign body sensation in throat, and patient develops a tendency to clear the secretions of throat (hawking - Choking).

O/E Hyperaemia, hyperplasia, atrophy, oedema, viscid secretions etc,signs are visualised in larynx according to the vitiation.

**Treatment :-**

1) Rest and Vocal rest. 2) Avoid irritative factors those causing the disease, like smoking tobacco chewing, alcohol etc., 3) Inhalation of medicated steams, 4) Traeating the infective sources like tonsils adenoids etc., 5) Change of environment or place of work. 6) Antibiotics expectorent, Anti allergic anti inflammatory and other symptomatic treatments. 7) surgical corrections by Microlaryngoscopy etc.,

### II) A/b) Vocal Nodules (Singer's nodes)

Chronic nodular hypertrophy of free edge of vocal cords (approx - at the junction of anterior 1/3 and middle part) it commonly occurs in the female and those who misues Or over use their Voice continuously for a long time.Ex:-Actors, singers teachere etc., Hoarseness of Voice, strain in Voice, pain in the neck and On examination the nodules appear in pinkish or pearly white and rarely exceeds 1.5 mm of size.

Treatment principles are same but when the nodules are big those should be excised under operative micro laryngoscope.

## II/ A/c ) Vocal Cord Polyp :-

If is a pedunculated lesion arising form the vocal cord usually form anterior commissure and sometimes form both the cords. The polyp may hang down into the sub glottic region and become visible on coughing or phonation.

Clinical features and Treatment is like vocal nodules.

## II/A/d) Laryngeal hyperkeratosis (Leucoplakia)

It is considered to be a pre malignant lesion in which white patches develop on the vocal cords, the exact cause is not known but hyperplasia and hyperkeratosis of epithelium of vocal cords davelops due to chronic irritation to laryngeal mucosa by excessive smoking. tobacco chewing, or due to syphilic infection. etc. The clinical features are hoarseness of Voice and white raised patches on vocal cords Bipsy rules out the malignancy but the patient must remain under continous supervision.

**Treatment :-**
1) Voice rest 2) Biopsy 3) Avoiding irritants like smoking et., 4) Steam inhalation 5) Vit - A supplementation 6) Excision of vocal cords or striping of surface Or Radio therapy

## II/A/e) Reinke's Oedema.

It is Bilateral Polypoidal degenerationand Oedema of membranous Vocal cords in Reinke's space, Indirect laryngoscopy reveals bilateral pale spindle shaped swellings of vocal cords.

**Treatment ;-**Micro surgical excision of stripes of mucosa from membranous cords.

## II/A/f) Atrophic Laryngitis :-

It occurs in association with atropic rhinitis Or atropic pharyngitis, the mucosal glands disappear and there is crusting dryness of throat irritative cough blood stained mucoid secretions and hoarse Vice.

**Treatment :-** Voicerest, controlling the infective focus.

## II/B/a} Tuberculosis of Larynx.

It is usually secondary to pulmonary tuberculosis, mode of infection is by infected sputum blood or lymphatics.

The posterior part of larynx (inter arytenoids region, vocal cords, arytenoids, false cords, epiglottis) is involved.

**Clinical Features :-**

Hoarseness of voice, aphonia, cough, fever, pain on swallowing (refers to the ear) and the movements of vocal cords also affected. The vocal cords initially pale then congested ulcerated in posterior 1/3, the ulceration produces the mouse nibbled appearance, Oedema and perichondritis of larynx develops in later stages (Tuberculoma - ulceration - perichondritis - Cold abscess Formation) It is comfirmed a) Clinical features b) X-ray chest c) Sputum for A.F.B. d) Mantoux test e) Biopsy & hitopathology of granulation.

**Treatment ;-**1) Tuberculosis treatment. 2) Vocal rest. 3) nutritious diet. 4) Symptomatic treatment. 5) Tracheostomy if needed.

## II/B/b) Syphilis of Larynx:-

it is rare now a days. In primary secondary stages of syphilis it doesn't affect the larynx But gumma may occur on epiglottis and anterior 1/3 of Vocal cords in the tertiary stage of syphilis.

**Clinical Features ;-**

hoarseness of voice, difficulty in breathing, anterior part of laryngeal mucosa is deeply ulcerated, perichondritis and laryngeal stenosis occur in late stage.

**Diagnosis :-** 1) VDRL test. 2) Biopay.

**Treatment :-**

1) Anti Syphilis treatment 2) Tracheostomy and laryngoplasty if needed.

## II/B/c  Leprosy of Larynx :-

It is rare diffuse nodular infiltration of epiglottis, arytenoids, false cords and deformity and stenosis of larynx in late stages may result.

## II) /B/d)  Laryngeal Scleroma.

Rhino scleroma of the nose causes the disease but affecting subglottic region of larynx and causes stenosis of larynx.

**Treatment :-** 1) Streptomycin 2) Steroids 3) Tracheostomy 4) Laryngial dilatation.

## II/B/e)  Laryngeal Lupus :-

It is secondary to Lupus vulgaris of nose, The epiglottis, Eryepiglottic folds, arytenoids are involved, destructive lesions, ulceration and cicatrical changes occurs.

**Treatment :-** Anti Tubercular treatment.

## II/B/f) Perichondritis of Larynx :-

Inflammation of laryngeal cartilages due to trauma, infection (T.B. syphilis etc.,) and malignancy.

**Clinical Features :-**

Pain, Hoarseness, inspiratory dyspnoea, Abscess formation and stenosis of larynx.

**Treatment ;-**

1)      Antibiotics 2) Steroids 3) Tracheostomy.

4)      laryngeal dilatation 5) Laryngectomy.

# TUMOURS OF LARYNX

Tumours of larynx classified into 1) Benign tumours 2) Malignant tumours.

## 1) Benign Tumours of Larynx :-

a) Papilloma b) haemangioma c) Fibroma d) Chondroma e) Adenoma f) Myoma g)Lipoma h) Granuloma i) Retention cysts j) Dermoid cyst k) Laryngocele l) Vocal nodules m) Polyp of vocal cord.

Benign tumours are Frequently seen than malignant, among the benign tumours papilomas and Fibroma are common, rest of the diseases are rare.

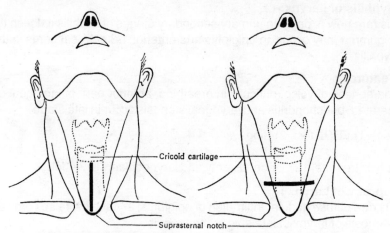

Cricoid cartilage

Suprasternal notch

Vertical incision; for beginners,
and in emergency

Horizontal incision; in elective
operations, for cosmetic reasons.

Tracheostomy incisions.

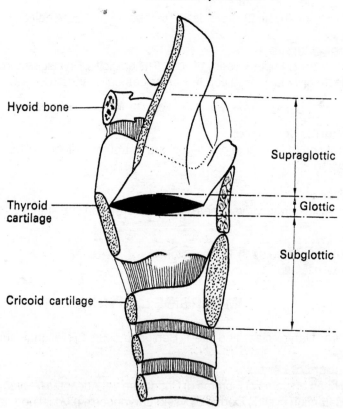

Hyoid bone

Supraglottic

Thyroid
cartilage

Glottic

Subglottic

Cricoid cartilage

Divisions of Larynx for tumour classification.

316

**I) Papilloma :-** a) Single B) Multiple.

## a) Single Papilomas :-
Common in adult male, it usually come from the edge of the vocal cord anteriorly and may be pedunculated. The common clinical features are hoarseness of voice and cough.

**Treatment :-**
Excision by Laryngeal micro surgery and the excised mass is send for histopathological exmination for the conformation of condtion of the disease.

## b) Multiple Papillomas ;-
Common in children and infants, most probably it is viral Origin, originates on vocal cords and ventricular bands but may extend to epiglottis and tracheobronchial tree.

**Clinical Features :-**
Hoarseness of Voice, difficulty in breathing, multiple papillomas fill the larynngeal cavity and spreads completely. if excised like single papilloma,have tendency to recur.

**Treatment :-**
1) Antibiotics Steroids etc., has no use. 2) Repeated surgical excision 3) cryo and laser surgery are also used.

## 2) Fibroma :-
It is usually arises from the Vocal cords and others parts of larynx, it is either new formation of fibrous tissues element or Organisation of sub mucosal haematoma Or inflammatory Origin. It appears as reddish mass with smooth surface. produces hoarseness of Voice.

**Treatment :-**
Excision by Direct micro laryngoscopy.
**Note :-** other benign tumours are not common.

## MALIGNANT TUMOURS OF THE LARYNX.

**Classification :-**
1) Krishaber's (1879) Isambert (1876 ) Classification.
     a)     Intrinsic B) Extrinsic.
2) Lederman's classification.
     a)     Supra glottic carcinoma- 24% - arising in Infrahyoid portion of epiglottis, ventricu lar bands, ventricles and marginal zone (Supra hyoid portion of epiglottis ary epiglottic folds and arytenoids).
     b)     Glottic carcinoma = 66% commonest, arises in vocal cords anterior commissure and posterior commissure.
     c)     Subglottic carcinoma = 10%

It arises in the walls of subglottis (under surface of true cords. )

3) T.N.M. classification is the latest widely accepted classification for malignant tumours.
     T= Tumour, N= lymph nodes.
     M= Metastasis.

Among the malignant (Carcinoma) tumours, squamous all carcinoma is the commonest type of laryngeal carcinoma (adenocarcinoma, basal cell carcinoma Or sarcomas are rare).

**Aetiology :-**

The Exact aetiology is not known but following factors play a part in the pathogenisis, they are.

Chronic irritation by smoking, alcohol, chewing of tobaco and betal nut, prolonged vocal strain, air pollution, Keratosis or leucoeplakia, dietary deficiencies, virus infection etc

## 1) GLOTTIC CARCINOMA OR CARCINOMA OF VOCAL CORDS.

It is the commonest type among the all, common site is free upper surface or margin of the Vocal cord in its anterior 2/3, lymph node involvement is rare, metastasis is only 4%, so prognosis is good if tumour is treated early.

(The spread Occurs locally along the cord to the anterior commissure and may involve the other cord)

## 2) SUPRAGLOTTIC CARCINOMA.

The Growth arises from infrahyoid, epiglottis, ventricular band and ventricles. The tumours are detected in late stages, due to rich lymphatic drainage of this area metastasis to the deep cervical nodes on both side of neck (40%), So only prognosis is very poor. The cauli flower like growth prognosis is better than ulcerative growth.

## SUB GLOTTIC CARCINOMA

It is not common, early detection is difficult. Affecting site is subglottic surface of vocal cord or below the anterior commissure. Lymphatic spread is moderate (17%) to the lower deep cervical and paratracheal pretracheal mediastinal glands.

## CLINICAL FEATURES :-

1) Among 3 types of carcinoma symptoms appear earlier in glottic cancer than others

2) Metastasis also poor 4%, so only prognosis is good in glottic carcinoma.

3) Hoarseness of Voice also earlier symptom in glottic carcinoma.

4) Irritative cough and feeling of discomfort in throat appears early in supra glottic carcinoma.

5) Other common symptoms are pain, dysphagia, dyspnoea, blood stained sputum, cervical lymphadenitis.

# DIAGNOSIS

a) Clinical Features.
b) Histopathology of tumour.
c) Indirect and Direct laryngo scopy
d) Soft tissue X Ray of neck.
e) X ray chest.
f) Biopsy.

**Treatment :-**
The Choice of treatment depends on the extent site, histology of tumour, presence Or absence of neck nodes and distance of metastasis.

1) Surgery- Partial or total laryngectomy with or without neck dissection.
2) Radio therepy.
3) Chemo therapy.

# PARALYSIS OF THE LARYNX AND SPEECH DISDRDERS.

1) Functional paralysis (Bilateral adductor paralysis )
2) Organic paralysis.     A) Motor Paralysis :
                          (B) Sensory Paralysis

**A) MOTOR PARALYSIS.**  (a) Unilaterel     (a1)   In complete
                                             (a2)   Complete
                         b) Bilateral       (b1)   Incomplete
                                             (b2)   Complete.

| | | |
|---|---|---|
| Unilateral | = | Either Right Or Left side |
| Bilateral | = | Both sides. |
| Incomplete | = | Either abductors or adductors. |
| Complete | = | Abductors and adductors. |

**NOTE :-** Unilateral paralysis is only for abductors, adductors commonly Bilaterally paralysed.

**AETIOLOGY :-** Most of the intrinsic muscles of larynx having motor nerve supply of by recurrent laryngeal nerve of vagus except cricothyroid (by superior laryngeal nerve of vagus)

The causes of recurrent laryngeal nerve paralysis are.
1) Central ( Bulbar lesions Or Cortical lesions Or Corticobulbar lesions)
2) Peripheral -Lesions of recurrent laryngeal nerve proper

**1) LEFT RECURRENT LARYNGEAL NERVE PARALYSIS:-**
It is more common.

**CAUSES IN CHEST:-** Carcinoma bronchus, mediastinal growth, carcinoma Oesophagus, mitral stenosis, Aortic aneurism, following patent ductus arteriosis operation, and pulmonary tuberculosis  Or Fibrosis etc.

**CAUSES IN NECK :-** are, carcinoma thyroid, following thyroid surgery, penetrating wounds Malignant metastasis etc.,

## 2) RIGHT RECURRENT LARYNGEAL NERVE PARALYSIS :-

Causes only in neck are - same as on left and right side commonly involved in thyroid surgery, Apical tuberculosis and tumours Aneurism of subclavian artery.

## 3) GENERAL CAUSES :- LIKE DIABETES, SYPHILIS, DIPHTERIA
ENTERIC FEVER, STREPTOCOCAL INFECTIONS.
## 4) INDIOPATHIC CAUSES.

## BILATERAL PARALYSIS.

1) Abductor paralysis causes Idiopathic, malignancy of thyroid, thyroid surgery, carcinoma of Oesophagus, cut throat injury and peripheral neuritis etc.,

## 2) Adductor paralysis:-

It is functional or commonly seen in girls and women with psychological back ground.

## 3) Total Paralysis :-

Viral neuritis, peripheral neuritis etc.,

# c) Superior laryngeal nerve paralysis causes :-

Rarely seen alone, usually involved with recurrent laryngeal nerve

## CLINICAL FEATURES :-

Voice respiration swallowing and position of vocal cords are affected by the vocal cord palsy.

## 1) IN UNILATERAL RECURRENT LARYNGEAL PARALYSIS :-

Raspiration is not usually affected but there is dyspnoea on exertion.
**a) In complete** ( only abductors are paralysed ) Vocal cord occupies median position, voice is unaffected, patient is asymptamatic.
**b) Complete** ( Abductors aswellas adductors are paralysed ). Vocal cords occupies paramedian position and produces hoarse voice.

## 2) BILATERAL RECURENT LARYNGEAL NERVE PALSY.

**a) Incomplete** (abductor palsy) Vocal cords occupies median Or paramedian position, voice unchanged but severe dyspnoea stridor and cyanosis of larynx occurs.
**b) Complete ( Abductor and adductor palsy)**
Cords remain fixed in paramedian position during phonation, respiration unaffected at rest but get dyspnoea on exertion.

## 3) SUPERIOR LARYNGEAL NERVE PALSY

It usually occur along with recurrent laryngeal nerve palsy vocal cords lies in cadaveric position of abduction due to paralysis of cricothyroid muscle. This produces hoarse and feeble voice, inhalation of Food in to larynx due to sensary paralysis.

## INVESTIGATIONS

a) Radiography of Chest to detect malignancy Or enlargment of heart etc.,
b) Radiography of Barium swallow to detect malignancy of Oesophagus.
c) Direct laryngoscopy Or Bronchoscopy or Oesophagoscopy.
d) Blood sugar estimation for diabetes.
e) V.D.R.L estimation for syphilis.
f) E.S.R estimation for Tuberculosis etc.,
g) Neurological investigations.
h) Cardio Vascular investigations.
i) C.T. Scan.

## Treatment

### 1) UNILATERAL PARALYSIS :-

a) Specific cause should be treated.
b) If hoarse Voice present that should be corrected by speech therapy, Taflon paste inj into vocal cords, implantation of cartilage and Arytenoidopexy in mid line (This procedure requires, if paralysis persist for more than 9 to 12 months.)
c) If a symptomatic require no treatment.

### 2) BILATERAL ABDUCTOR PALSY:-

a) Specific treatment for the cause.
b) Intubation Or Tracheostomy for severe stridor and dyspnoea.
c) Arytenoidectomy for the dyspnoea patients.

### 3) SUPERIOR LARYNGEAL NERVE PALSY :-

a) Specific treatment for cause.
b) Ryle tube feeding.
c) Tracheostomy

### 4) BILATERAL ADDUCTOR PALSY.

a) Speech therapy.
b) Psychotherapy.
c) Shock treatment.

## SPEECH AND VOICE DISORDERS.

### Speech disorders.

1) Aphasia - loss of speech due to lesion of cortical speech centre of brain.
2) Dysphasia - Speech disorder due to lesion of cortical speech centre of brain.
3) Dysarthria - speech disorder due to lessions of cranial nerves responsible for production of speech.
4) Stammering - Functional speech disorder where there is break in the flow of speech.

## SPEECH DISORDERS ALSO SEEN DUE TO FOLLOWING.

5) In mentally retarded children.
6) In the cerebral palsy.
7) In Partially deaf child.
8) Cleft palate and palatal palsy.

## VOICE DISORDERS :-

1) Rhinolalia (R. Clausa - R. Aperta) change of Voice due to Nasal paranesal problems.
2) Dysphonia- Hoarseness of Voice (Phonation by ventricular band instead of vocal cords or due to over tensed Vocal cords.)
3) Pubophonia - Cracking of Voice in males at puberty due to emotional as well as hor monal disturbance.
4) Weakness of Voice due to pulmonary insufficiency.
5) Aphonia :- loss of voice due to Bilateral vocal cords paralysis.
6) Vocal asthenia :- Weak Vocie defect due to weakness of Intrinsic muscles of larynx.
7) Stridor - Noisy respiration.

## Treatment :-

1)      Cause should be treated.
2)      Speech therapy is recommended
3)      Auditory and speech therapy for defective speech due to deafness.
4)      Correction of emotional instability.

## HOARSENESS OF VOICE.

A hoarse Voice is rough and unpleasant it results from the lesions of Vocal cords. Causes of hoarse Voice may range from simple laryngitis to malignancy. If hoarse Voice is more than 2 weeks inspite of conservative treatment, laryngeal examination and diagnosis should carried. out

It is due to interference with movements of vocal cords, mass of Vocal cords, Tension of Vocal cords and approximation of edges of Vocal cords.

## CAUSES

## I) LARYNGEAL - LARYNGO PHARYNGEAL

A) Congenital Causes.

1) Laryngeal web at anterior commissure  2) Cyst and tumours of larynx.
B) Traumatic causes.
1) Mis use and over use of Vocie Ex.singers teachers
2) External injuries like strangulation at throat causes haematoma of vocal cord.
3) Internal injuries-inhalation of hot acids, irritant acid, fumes etc.causes laryngitis.
4) Irradiation cauase damage to Vocal cords.
5) Intubation trauma.

C)      Infective Causes :-

Bacteria virus fungus and specific Organism of Tuberculosis syphilis leprosy lupus and scleroma may cause Acute and chronic laryngitis (with hoarse voice)
D)      1) Benign and Malignant tumours of larynx causes Hoarse Voice etc.,

E)      Miscellaneous Causes.

Singer's nodes, Laryngeal Oedema, Laryngeal Polyp, laryngeal stenosis paralysis of recurrent laryngeal nerve of Vagus, Functionalaphonia, laryngocele, prolapse of the ventricle of larynx, and Arthritis of crico arytenoid joints etc.,

II.      Oesophageal Causes :- Cervical - mediastinal malignancy etc.,
causes recurrent laryngeal nerve palsy and hoarseness.
III.      General Causes.

Myxoedema, cardiac Oedema, renal Oedema, diabetes, Syphilis, and lead poisoning may cause recurrent laryngeal nerve palsy.

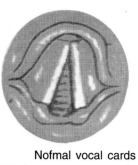

Nofmal vocal cards

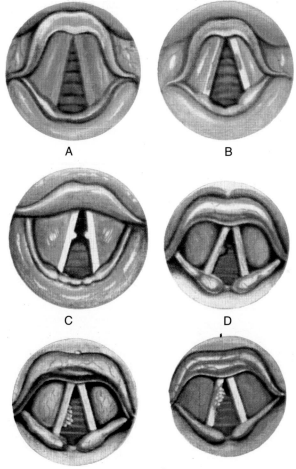

A. Acute simple laryngitis.          B. Submucuous haemorrhage of the vocal cords
C. Singer's nodules               D. Fibroma of right vocal cord.
E. Subglottic (right) carcinoma     F. Carcinoma of right vocal cord.

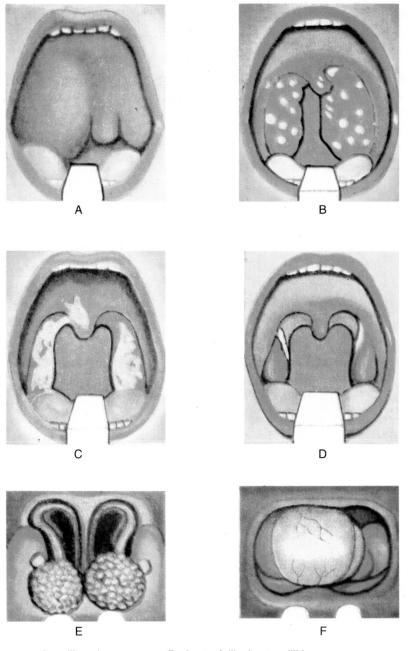

A. Acute peritonsillar absess
B. Acute follicular tonsillitis.
C. Faucial disphtheria.
D. Vincent's angina.
E. Papillary hypertrophy of the
   posterior ends of inferior
   turbinates
F. Antro-choanal polyp (right) as seen by
   posterior rhinoscopy.

**Treatment :-**
1) Cause should be treated.   2) Steam inhalation. 3) Voice rest. 4) Antibiotics to control infection.  5) Anti inflammatories to control Oedema.   6) Speech therapy and congestion.7) Direct laryngoscopy, permits Examination and surgery.

## CONGENITAL ANOMALIES OF OESOPHAGUS

1) Oesophageal atresia 2) Tracheo Oesophageal Fistuala, 3) Congenital Stenosis of oesophagus   4) Webs and diverticula 5) Dysphagia Lusoria.

## SYMPTOMATOLOGY AND DISEASES OF OESOPHAGUS.

1) Dysphagia :- Diffculty in Swallowing.  2) Loss of Weight and lossof appetite. 3) Hyper acidity and heart burn. 4) Regurgitation of Food. 5) Heamatemesis and malena.6) Pulmonary symptoms like cough, hoarse voice and dysponea etc. 7) Spread of malignancy with metastatic lymph nodes.

## DYSPHAGIA.

The word dysphagia means diffuculty in swallowing  the food (painful swallowing is Odynophagia).  It is a symptom of various diseases of mouth, tongue, pharynx,  larynx, Oesophagus and due to pressure on the above parts. So thorough investigations are needed to find out the cause.

**Aetiology :-**    (A) Oesophageal lesions    B) Other than Oesophagial  Lesions.

## (I) OESOPHAGIAL LESIONS.

a) In the lumen - Foreign body Or large bolus.

## b) In the Wall.

Congenital :- Tracheo Oesophageal fistula - stricture.

Traumatic :- Corrosive Food drinks Or poisons.

Inflammatory :- Hiatus hernia after exanthemata and corosive poisoining.

Neoplasma :- Leiomyoma - Carcinoma of Oesophagus.

Neurological :- Paralytic lesions, spasm of cricopharynx and Oesophagus , tetanus myasthenia gravis

Miscellaneous :- Paterson - Brown - Kelly syndrome In female Achalasia (Cardio spasm). etc.,

## (C) Pressure on Oesophagus by :-

Malignancy of thyriod gland, lymph nodes.  Cervical spondylosis Aneurism of aorta, mediastinal tumours, cardiac enlargment, pericardial effusion, Retrosternal goitre, Hepatomegaly etc.,

## (ii) OTHER THAN OESOPHAGEAL LESIONS.

1)      Nose-Nasal obstruction  due adenoids and tumours.
2)      Oral cavity - Trismus, Ludwings angina, stomatitis, glossitis
caroinomatous ulcers on tongue, T.B. of tongue, cleft plate paralysis of soft palate, inflammation of floor of mouth, dental lesions etc.,

3)        Pharynx - Acute tonsilititis, Follicular tonsilitis, quinsy, carcinoma of  pharynx, lesions of pharynx by specific organisms, Retropharyngeal and parapharyngeal abscess, paralytic lesion of pharynx, spastic lesions of pharynx.
4)        Larynx - Carcinoma of larynx, paralytic lesions of larynx, Laryngeal Oedema and spastic lesions of larynx.

III)    **FUNCTIONAL**
        Globus hystericus- painful conditions like glossitis and tonsilitis cause oynophagia.

**Clinical Features :-**
1)      Age 20 to 40 Year suggest cardio Spasm.  50 to 70 Year suggest  carcinoma. Menopause age suggests paterson kelly syndrome.

2)      **Past History :-**
        Anaemia, smoking, alocoholism, Tobaco chewing etc., are contributtory factors for dysphasia.
        Poliomyelitis, diabetes dipththeria may cause neurological lesions.
        History of corrosive poisining suggest stricture of Oesophagus
        History of ingestion of Foreign bodies contribute Obstructive Lesions.
        hysterical patient may have globus hystericus (Lump in throat without any  positive findings, in Female).

3)      **Symptoms.**
1)      Acute dysphagia due to Acute Oesophagitis or due to to Foreign    bodies.
2)      Diffculty in swallowing of solid especially due to malignancy  and stricure and in swallowing of liquids in cardio spasm.
3)      Glossitis, angular stomatitis  and anaemia, Chronic cricopharyngeal, dysphagia occurs in paterson Brown kelly syndrome, in  Menopause ladies.
4)      Regurgitation of Food especially liquids in cario spasm.
5)      Feeling of lump in throat Hysterically in feamle (Globus Hystericus).
6)      Weight  loss, neck glands, Hapatomegaly or Ascites, suggests carcinoma Oesophaus.
7)      Stationary dysphagia suggest Benign condition, progressive dysphagia suggest malignancy.
8)      Slow on set of disease in  malignacy  but rapid onset suggest inflmmatory lesions.
9)      Dysphagia in children suggest congenital lesions and dysphagia  in elders suggest malignancy.
10)     An elderly person with the history of dysphagia for more than 2 weeks and not responding to conservatory treatment suggest malignancy.
11)     There are other so many factors those cause dysphagia are given in the list of aetiology

**INVESTIGATIONS**
1) Clinical Findings 2) Readio logical Examintion for the detection of foreign bodies, Cardio spasm, Oespheged Varices, Stricture, malignancy.   adenoid,  polyps - tumours, retropheryngeal abscesses cardio megaly - media stinal tumours, aortic aneurisms etc., (by plane - Barium and soft tissue X ray )

3)      Heamogram for Hypochromic anaemia, ESR, Hb%, TC & DC etc., to find out specific infections.

4)      V.D.R.L- for syphilis to rule out neurological dysphagia.
5)      Blood sugar for Diabetes to rule out neurological dysphagia.
6)      Tomograms and CT Scan.
7)      Neurological, cardio vascular examination
8)      Endoscopy.
9)      Indirect laryngo scopy - Posterior Rhinoscopy.
10)     neck examination of lymph nodes.
11)     Throat swab for bacteriological Examination.
12)     Routene examination of oral cavity and Oesophagus.

Nose pharynx larynx to detect abnormalities those causing dysphagia.

**Treatment : -**
1)      The cause should be detected and treat accordingly.

**DYSPHAGIA LUSORIA :-**
        It is a congenital abnormality of Dysphagia due to vascular anomalies of chest Ex:- Right aoritic arch, sub clavian artery and patent ductus arteriosus (Diagnosis by Aortography).

**STRICTURE OF OESOPHAGUS :-**
        It is due to congenital, traumatic, inflammatory and malignant. Corrosive poisons etc., causes severe burns and ulcerations that causes stricture depending upon the nature of the cause.

**PLUMMER VINSO SYNDROME:-**
        Progressive dysphagia to solids with hypochromic microcytic anaemia and chronic superficial pharyngo Oesophagitis is known as plummer vinson syndrome.

**OESOPHAGEAL VARIX :-**
        Haemoptesis due to portal obstruction cirrhosis of liver. The condition is found at the cardiac end.

**ACHALASIA CARDIA (CARDIOSPASM)**
        This is a condition characterised by failure of relaxation of the lower Oesophageal sphincter for the passage of food (Oesophgoscopy and Barium meal X Ray confirm the diagnosis).

**CARCINOMA OF OESOPHAGUS.**
        Squamous cell Carcinoma is the commonest type of malignant tumour of Oesophagus, affects in between 40 to 70 Yrs. age group at the middle third of Oesophagus. The growth may be ulcerative proliferative Or infliltrating in nature. The common symptoms are dyscomfort, dysphagia, weight loss, cough and supra clavicular lymphnodes enlargment, it is confirmed by Barium meal X ray, oesophagoscopy, Biopsy.

# KRIYA KALPA (TREATMENT PROCEDURES )

Ayurveda is the life saving science, aimed to preserve the health and to treat the diseases (swasthasyaujaskarm-Aarthasya roganuth).

In Ayurveda to preserve the normal health different methods are explained, they are - Regular practice of Dantha dhavan, mukha Prakshalan, kavala, Gandoosha, Abhyanga, Vyayama, Pratimarsha nasya, Dhooma Paana, Anjana, Pathya Apathya, Rasayan Vidhi, Nidra, Brahmacharya, elimination of Adhaaraneeyavega, and suppression of dharaneeya Vega. in seasonal doshic variation relavant ahar, vihar, Aushada Vidhi, and for special doshic variations-Vaman (for Kapha), Virechana (forPitta) Vasti (for Vata) Raktha mokshan (for Raktha) and Nasya (Shiro-Virechan) are explained to save the body from doshic complications etc.,

In addition to above, a person by indulging Asaatmya Indriaartha Samyoga, Pragyaaparaada, Parinama and other factors, dosha dhatu and malas are affected, becomes abnormal and produce diseases in the body and mind. So it is the aim of the doctor to treat the diseases by different treatment procedures, selection of the procedures should be decided by the doctor by his professional experience. Some of the treatment procedures are exaplained as follows :-

I.      1. Swasthasyaujaskaram (Preventive treatment ) preservation and
           promotion of health.
        2) Artasya roga nuth (curative treatment ) cure of the diseases.
II.     Curative treatment can be grouped as
        1) Diiva Vyapashraya Chikitsa (devine therapy) 2) Yukthi Vyapashraya Chikitsa
        (Rational therapy with drugs diet excercise etc.,3) Satwaavajaya (Psycho
        therapy).

III)    Yukthi Vyapashraya Chikitsa can be grouped as
        1) Antar parimarjana (internal purification) Ex. Shodhan Karma.
        2) Bahir parimarjana (External purification) abhyanga, seka, sweda and
        psychotherapy. 3) Shastra Pranidaana (Surgical treatment) Ex. Chedan,
        Bhedan, Lekhan, Vyadan, Seevan Eshan etc.,

IV.     Shat upakramas (Bahir and Antar Parimarjan )
        A) 1) Langhan (karshan) Catabolic therapy 2) Brumhan (Tarpan) Anabolic
therapy.3) Rukshan (Dehydration therapy). 4) Snehan (Oleation therapy).5) Swedan
(Sudation)6) Stambana (Retaining).

A)      LANGHAN GROUP = Langan, Rukshan and Swedan
B)      BRUMHAN GROUP = Brumhan, snehan and stamban

**LANGHAN.**
   a) Shodan (Elimination ) of doshas Ex:- Pancha karmas.
   b) Shaman (Palliation)

   **Ex.** 1) Deepan (Appetisers) 2) Pachana (digestives Capability) 3) Upavasa (Fasting) 4) Pipasa (Thirst ) 5) marutha (Air bath) 6) Aatapa (Sun bath) and 7) Vyayama (Exercise)

**V.**   1) In Kshaya (Depleted) Restoration (Brumhan)
   2) In Kupitha (Vitiated) - Prashaman (Palliation).
      in chaya prakopa - shodhana therapy and
      in Achaya Prakopa - Shamana therapy.

3)   In vruddhi (Aggravation) - Nirharan (Elimination). (samhatrupa Vruddhi Samshaman therapy and in Vilayana rupa Vrudhi Shodhan therapy.)

4)   In equilibrium of the dosha paripalya (maintenance) etc are advised to maintain normal health.(preservation of condition.)
**VI.**   1) Nidana Parivarjan (Avoiding the causes) 2)Aushada Chikitsa (Drug therapy) 3) Shastra Chikitsa (Surgical therapies.) 4) Kshara karma. 5) Agni karma.

**VIII.**   1) Local treatment (Sthanika Chikitsa) 2) Systemic treatment s (Sarva dehika chikitsa. )
**Note :-** In Shalakya tantra II, ear diseases Nose diseases Throat diseases and Diseases of Shiras are present, in these diseases. common treatment procedures Are as follows:- **1)** Karna Prakshalan (Ear Wash) **2)** karna pramarjana (Dry mopping) **3)** Karna Avadhoolan (Dusting of Fine Powders) **4)** Karna Dhoopan (Fumigation) **5)** Karna Pooran (Filling the ear with medicine drops) **6)** Nasya karma (nasal drops) **7)** Nasa pichu (nasal plug) **8)** Kavala. **9)** Gandhooshan (medicated gargles) **10)** Shirolepa (Application of medicine to shiras) **11)** Shiro Abhyanga (head massage) **12)** Shiro pichu (Putting of medicated varthi at Brahma randra) **13)** Shiro Vasti (Keeping Oleus substances on the head by special Procedure). **14)** Pratisaran (Applying the medicine to the affected site.)

**Note :-** In the treatment principles of most of the diseases first shodhan karma are explained to eliminate deep rooted systemic doshic vitiation then only local treatments are explained - So only here poorva Karma and panchakarma procedures are explained briefly along with E.N.T. Kriya Kalpas.

# A) SNEHA KARMA ) (OLEATION THERAPY)
   It is a process used to induce Oleusness in the body with the help of Sneha Dravyas by " Snehan - Vishyandana and kledana" properties. It is not only Poorva karma (Pre therapy) to panchakarma procedures to mobilise the vitiatted doshas from their sites but also Pradhana Karma (main therapy - One among shat upakaramas - Rukshana Chikitsa) to Vata Vyadhi like diseases. Among the 5 Basic elements (pancha maha Bhuta) Pruthwi and jala are the predominent elements of Sneha dravyas.

### Properties Snehana Drugs :-

1) Snigda (unctuousness) 2) Guru (heavy Or Weight gaining property ) 3) Sheeta (Coolness) 4) Mrudu (Softness) 5) Drava (liquidity) 6) Pischila (Stickyness) 7) Sara (Spreading nature ) 8) Manda (Slow activity ) 9) Sukshma (easily penetrating capacity in to the tissue channels of the body.

### Classifications of Snehas Dravyas.

### 1) According ot Yonibheda (uthpathi) 2 types by Charaka.

a) sthaavara (collected from plants) :- Ex - Tila taila, Erenda taila sarshapa taila etc.,b) Jaangama (Animal products) :- Ex - Milk, Curd, Ghee, animal Fat, Bone marrow etc.

### 2) According to action of drugs - by Sushrutha.

a) Virechanopayogi (Causes motions Or Elimination of doshas through rectum.) Ex. Erenda taila etc., b) Vamanopa yogi (Causes Vomitings Or Elimination of doshas through mouth.) Ex:- madan Phala etc.,. c) Shiro Virechanopayogi (useful to eliminate doshas from Shiras through nose.). Ex. Vidanga, Sarshapa Sneha etc., d) Dusta Vranopayogi (ulcer healing). ex - Karanja, Puthikaranja Sneha etc., e) maha Vyadyupogi (useful in major diseases like Kusta) Ex. Tuvarak taila etc.,f) Mutra Sanga upayogi (Useful in retention of urine). Ex. Eravaaru taila Kushmand taila etc., g) Ashmari upayoga (useful in Urinary Stones), Ex. Bakuchi, Haritaki taila Taila etc., h) Pramehopayogi (Useful in diabetes). Ex. Sarshapa - Nimba Taila etc., i) Pitta Samsrusta Vata (Vata Pitta Vitiation). Ex:- Taal, narikel taila ., j) Krishneekaran Upayogi (Useful in white patches) vibheetaki bhallataka taila k) Pandukaram Upayogi (useful in depigmentation). Ex. Shyonaka Priyang taila etc., l) Kusta upayogi (useful in Skin lesions). Ex:- Devadaru, Agaru taila etc., m) Snehopaga group by Charak. Ex :- Drakshya, Yastimadu, madhu Parni, Meda, Vidarigandha, Kakoli, ksheera kakoli, jeevak, jeevanthi, shala Parni (10 drugs)

### 3) Classificationof sneha drugs according to therapy.

a) Shodhan sneha :- Causes Elimination of doshas by mouth, nose, Rectum by Teekshna Veerya Sneha Aushadas (Ex. Oily drugs used for Vaman - Virechan - Nasya and Vasti).

b) Shaman Sneha :- Causes suppression of doshas in the body by moderate potent Oily drugs- (Ex- Oily drugs used to control Kusta etc., diseases).

C) Brumhan Sneha ;- The oily drugs that gives nourishment to the body (ex:- Ghee).

### 4) CLASSIFICATION OF SNEHA DRAVYA ACCORDING TO IT'S USAGE :-

a) Bahya Sneha :- (External applications) Abhyanga, Lepa, mardan, udavarthan Samvahan, Padaghath, Moordha Taila, Gandoosha, Karna Pooran, Akshitarpan, pariseka, Pichu.

b) Abhyantar Sneha :- (Internal usage )
For food preparations, Drinks, nasal drops and for medicated enema (Vasti).

### 5) Classsification of sneha dravyas accoording to combination of drugs.

a) Yamala sneha - Combinationof 2 Snehas  b) Trivruth Sneha - Combination of 3 snehas c) maha sneha - Combination of 4 Or more snehas.

## 6) Classification of Sneha Dravya according to dosage.

a) Hruseeyasi Matra (test dose ) b) Hraswa matra (minimal dose c) Madyama matra (moderate dose). d) Uttama matra (perfect dose).

## 7) Classification of Sneha dravyas, according ot sneha paka.

a) Mruda paka b) madyama c) Khara paka.

## 8) Classification of Sneha dravyas according ot good quality (uttama Snehas)

a) Sarpi (Ghee) B) Taila (Tila Taila) c) Vasa (Fats) d) Majja (Bone marrow)

# INDICATIONS OF SNEHA KARMA (OLEATION) (SNEHAN YOGYA)

1) Before Fomentation therapy (Sweda Karma) 2) Before Shodhan therapy like Vaman virechan etc., 3) To induce Oleusness in the body or to treat Rough and dry condition cf body. 4) To treat Vata Vyadhi etc., diseases. 5) The people who are having the daily habit of excercise 6) Alcoholic people. 7) Debiliated or Weak persons. 8) Old people 9) Ladies 10) who indulge more sex ( Shukra dhathu Kshaya) 11) Raktha dhathu kshaya (Blood loss Or Anaemic) 12) Anxiety 13) Abhishyandi 14) Timira (Dim Vision or immature cataract) 5) for the improvement of intellect and memory capacity. 16) Improper Opening and closing of eye lids. 17) The persons who have mental tiredness, ministers, Financiers etc., 18) To improve the stamina Or immunity, to face or to prevent the diseases. 19) Before Exercise Or Fighting Or to build the body.

# CONTRA INDICATIONS OF SNEHA KARMA (SNEHAN AYOGYA)

1) Rukshanarha (Those eligible for Rukshana Chikitsta. 2) kapha & medo Vruddhi (fatty persons) 3) Excessive salivation and secretions From Bahirmukha srotas.4) Poor digestive Capacity (Mandaagni) 5) Indigestion(Ajeerna) 6) Thirst (trushna) 7) Un consciousness (moorcha) 8) Pregnancy (Garbinei) 9) Anorexia (Aruchi) 10) Dryness Or atropy of palate (Talu sosha ) 11) Vomitings (Chardi) 12) Ama Dosha 13) Posioning (Visha dosha) 14) More debiliated conditions. 15) After shodhan karma. (After Vaman - Virechan Vasti, Nasaya etc.,)

16) udara rogi (Liver spleen and Ascitic like disorders) 17) Ati sthula (who contian more Fluids and Fat) 18) Unctuous patient (Oily Sticky person) 19) Acute Fever (Taruna jwara) 20) Chronic Alcoholic patient (weakperson) 21) Premature delivered patient (Akaala Prasutha) 22) Gala rogi (The patient who have neck diseases.) 23) Urustamba (Rigid heavy thigh) 24) Dirarrhoea or Dysentry patient 25) Ati Teekshna gni (Who contain severe digestive capacity) 26) Contra indicated Before nasya Vasti and Rakthamokshana.

## RELATION OF SNEHA PAKA WITH THE USAGE ACCORDING TO DIFFERENT AUTHORS :

The medicated Snehas are prepared according to sneha paka vidhi, they are of 3 types 1) Mruda paka 2) Madhyama Paka 3) Khara Paka (Additionally dagdha Paka is explained by Sushrutha and Ama paka by Sarangdhar).

According to the nature of processing of the medicine the usage is depending on, that is as follows According to differenet acharyas.

| Sl. No. | Usage | Charak | Sushrutha | Vagbhat | Sarangdhar. |
|---|---|---|---|---|---|
| 1. | Abhyanga (Massage) | Khara Paka | Madyama paka | Kara paka. | Madyama paka. |
| 2. | Pana (Oral) | Madyama | Mruda | Madyama | Madyama |
| 3. | Nasya (Nasal drops) | Mruda | Madyama | Mrudu | Mrudu |
| 4. | Vasti (Medicated enema) | madyama | khara | madyama | Madyama |
| 5. | Karna Pooran (ear drop) | - | Khara | - | Madyama. |

**Note :-** By above description it is clear that 1) Khara and madyama sneha Paka is used for Abhyanga Vasti and karna Pooran But not the mrudu Paka. 2) Mrudu and madyama paka are used for oral and for nasya - But not the Khara Paka.

## OLEATION THERAPY- SNEHA VIDHI (STEPS OF OLEATION THERAPY )

1) Examination of the patient 2) Determination of duration for Oleation. 3) Determination of dosage for Oleation. 4) Dietetic Management prior to Oleation 5) Collection of materials useful for the therapy. 6) Procedure of sneha Pana 7) Observation of the patient for adequate Oleation or inadequate oleation or excessive Oleation. 8) Complications of the Oleation. 9) Post Snehan Regimen.

1) Examination of the patient is to work out the strength of the patient, diseases and to know whether indicated for Oleation Or not, The strenght of the patient , dosha, dushya prakruthi, Vikruthi are assessed by Dasha Vidha - Asta Vidha, Trividha, Pancha Vidha, shatvidha Etc., Pareekshas.

2) Determination of Duration for Oleation.
a) Determination of Duration for Oleation.
4 to 6 days in   madyama Kosta patients.
and 7 days in   krura Kosta Patients.
b) Vagbhata emphasises that, snehan should continue upto the appearance of symptoms of adequate Oleation, there is no specific time limit.

**Note :-** if Oleation therapy continued longer time it becomes saatmya and doesnot produce shodhana effect in the body .

# 3) DETERMINATION OF DOSAGE FOR OLEATION THERAPY.

The dosage is fixed on the time required for the digestion of Sneha which is taken (Oil digesting capacity).

| Sl. No. | Dosage of drug | Definition | Indications. |
|---------|----------------|------------|--------------|
| 1. | Hriseeyasi Matra | Test dose | Testing dose to know the nature of Kostha. |
| 2. | Hraswa matra | Digestible with 6 hours | Children, Old, Weak. Slight vitiation of dosha, less digestive capacity and in Mrudu Kostha. |
| 3. | Madyama Matra | Digestible with 12 hours | Moderate Strength of body and digestive capacity, moderate vitiation of doshas and in Madyama Kostha. |
| 4. | Uttama Matra | Digestible within 18to 24 hours | Strengthy, good digestive capacity, more vitiation of doshas and in Krura Kostha. |

**Note :-** In Hruseeyasi matra less dosage of Sneha is given for the test dose.

**Dosage is**    1) 2-4-6- Phala    (According to Kosta )
2) 2 1/2 Tolas    (Accepted by the Majority)

## 4)    DIETETIC MANAGEMENT PRIOR TO OLEATION.

Tasty, easily digestible, appetisers, easily absorbable and light Food should be given before the day of Oleation and the Food should contain the follwing qualitities. 1) Liquid diet 2) hot, 3) Regulated Quantiy 4) Incompatible 5) Non sticky 6) Non Oleus 7) and Light food should give to prevent the complications, (on theday of Oleation the previous Food should be perfectly digested).

## 5)    COLLECTION OF MATERIALS NEEDED FOR THE OLEATION

The medicines requried fo the therapy and to treat the complications should be collected.

## 6)    PROCEDURE OF SNEHA PANA (OLEATION METHOD)

1) Mangalaacharan (prayer) 2) Intake of Oleus drug (Sneha Aushada) 3) Waiting for symptoms of adequate or inadequate Oleation 4) Complications - Treatment.

**1) Mangalaacharan (Prayer) :-** Gives mental strength and satisfaction to face the therapy.

**2) Sneha Pana :-** Should give immediately after 15 to 30 minutes of sunrise, shodhan matra should not give in mrudu kosta, the dosage of medicine of oleationis as follows. :-

| | | |
|---|---|---|
| Test day | 2.5 | Tolas |
| Ist day | 5 | Tolas |
| 2nd day | 7.5 | Tolas |
| 3rd day | 10 | Tolas |
| 4th day | 15.0 | Tolas |
| 5th day | 20.0 | Tolas |
| 6th day | 25 | Tolas |
| 7th day | 30 | Tolas. |

**Note :-** 1) dosage should increase gradually by observing th digestive capacity of the patient. 2) If diarrhoea occurs, shodhan matra should stop and Brumhana Or shaman sneha should give. 3) Assurance should be given while the oleation 4) Anupana is Suggested as follows a) Ghritha with Lukewarm water b) Taila with yoosha c) Vasa majja with manda (Boiled Rice Water) 5) Bhallata Sneha panam with Cool water 6) In Vata predominence ghee+ lavana 7) Pitta predomience only ghee 8) Kapha predominence with kshara And Trikatu

## 7) COMPLICATIONS OF OLEATION.
### (Sneha Vyapath)

Complications arises due to the mistakes done during the therapy. These are of two types.
1) Acute complications with the requirment of immediate treatment. 2) Chronic complications without requirement of immediate treatment.

## 1) ACUTE COMPLICATION :

**a)** Indigestion (Ajeerna) **b)** Thirst (Trushna)c) Un consciousnes (Sangyanaash) **d)** Dullness (Tandra) **e)** Nausea (Uthklesha) **f)** Fever (jwara) **g)** Stiffness of body (Stamban) h) Aanaaha. **i)** Anorexia (Aruchi) **j)** Abdominal pain(shoola) k) Aama dosha (Complications of chronic indigestion)

## 2) CHRONIC COMPLICATIONS :

**a)** Kusta (Skin Lesions) **b)** Kandu (itching sensation) **c)** Pandu (Anaemia) **d)** Shotha (Oedema) **e)** Udara roga (G.I.T. diseases) **g)** Arsha (Haemorrhoides) **h)** Stiimitya (Numbness) **i)** Vaaknigraha (difficulty in Speeech)

## 8) OBSERVATIONOF PATIENT FOR
## ADEQUATE OR IN ADEQUATE OLEATION

## FEATURES OF ADEQUATE (SAMYAK SNEHANA).

**A)** **a)** Accelerated digestive capacity (Agni deepthi) **b)** Introlerance ot snehas **c)** Normal motions without discomfort (Oilystools) **d)** Lightness in the body (Laghutwa) **e)** Softness in the body (Mrudutwa) **f)** Oleus Skin (Roughness of skin is removed and Oily shining comes) **g)** Vataanuloman (normal movement of Vayu) **h)** Klama (Feeling of tiredness) **i)** Debility in the body tissues **j)** Thirst (Trushna) **k)** Fresh eructations (shuddha udgar)

## B) FEATURE OF, IN - ADEQUATE OLEATION )
### (Asmyak Sneha Karma )

a) Painful dry Oilless stools (graditha Pureesha) b) Weak digestive capacity (Agni mandya) c) Vata pratiloma (Improper movements of Vayu ) d) Body becomes rough and dry (Rukshaand Khara) e) Burning Sensation in the chest (Uro vidaha) f) Gneral debility and Weakness in the body g) All the Opposite features of Samyak Sneha present

## C) FEATURE OF EXCESSIVE OLEATION.

a) Anaemic (Panduta) b) Heavyness of the body (Gurutwa) c) Rigidity Or stiffness in the body (Stamba) d) Un digested Foodparticles inStools (Apakwa Pureesha) e) Dullness Or Sleepy mood (Tandra) f) Nausea (Uthklesha) h) Salivation (mukha Srava) i) Diarrhoea Dysentry Or Anal Secretions (Guda Srava) k) Burning sensation in Rectum (Guda daha)

# 9) Post Oleation Regimen. (Sneha pashchat Karma)

After Oleation therapy the patient should follow the Following principles upto 7 days.
1) Bed rest, Brahmacharya, Night Sleeping, Warm water intake, Resting in suitable postures and should take easily digestible food.

2) a) The patient should not suppress natural urges. b) Should not expose to hot. Cold, dust, fume and open air. c) Should avoid coarse constipated food, Night arousal, day sleeping, exercise, hard work, journey, anger, loud speaking and anxiety.

## SHAMANA SNEHA VIDHI :-
1) Shaman sneha is used to supress the doshas and to treat the disease.
2) It is given while the patient is hungry (at 9 to 10 AM Or 5 to 6 PM ) for proper digestion of Sneha, for quick spread and to control the vitiated doshas.
3) The dosage of th Sneha is Madyama matra that is 4 tolas to 8 Tolas approximately.

## BRUMHANA SNEHA
Sneha dravyas are given along with food items for the proper nourishment of the body.

Ex :- 1) mamsa rasa. 2) Ksheera 3) Yoosha 4) Bread 5) Food (Rice) 6) Curries.
Snehas are used to prepare the above preparations, the dosage of snehas is approximately 1 to 2 tolas.

## Acchapeya ;-
It is a pure Sneha therapy with out other preparations and so explained as the best for Adequate results.

## Sneha Vicharanas :-

Sneha preparations with food etc., items 24 in number they are as follows :-
1) Odana 2) Vilepi 3) Rasa 4) mamsa 5) Ksheera 6) Dadhi 7) Yavagu 8) Soopa 9) Shaka 10) Yoosha 11) Kambalika 12) Khada 13) Sakthu 14) Tila Pista 15) Madya 16) Leha 17) Bhakshya 18) Abhyanga 19) Gandoosha 20) Karna Puran 21) Nasa Tarpana 22) Akshi Tarpan 23) Basti 24) Uttharabasti.

## Sadyah Sneha :-

It is an Emergency type of sudden Oleation therapy given for a single day without following the general principles.
Ex :- 1) medicated mamsa rasa 2) Ghee + Milk+ Medicines.

## SEASIONAL INDICATIONS OF OLEATION THERAPY.

1) A Good, non cloudy day, after sun rise only oleation should be given.
2) In the Kapha vitiation Or Vata kapha vitiation Oleation should give in day time 3) In the Vata vitiation Or Vata pitta Vitiation Oleation should give at nights, (in Rainy Season with Tila Taila, sharath ruth with ghritha, vasanth ruthu with vasa and majja oleation. should be given.

|  | sneha | Sweda | Vaman | Virecha. |
|---|---|---|---|---|
| Avara | 1to 3 day. | 4th Day | 5th day | 7th day. |
| madyama | 5th days | 6th day | 7th day | 9th day |
| Pravara | 7th days | 8th day | 9th day | 11th day. |

**Note :-** After snehapana - Vasti, Raktha mokshan and Nasya are contra indicated.

## Bhaya Sneha :-

14 Types are explained they are.
1) Abhyang (massage) 2) Lepa (External applications) 3) udwarthan (Rubbing with Oils in Pratiloma direction) 4) mardan (massage with pressure ) 5) Pariseka - (Pouring medicated liquids on body ) 7) Samvahan (Gentle Oil massage) 8) Gandoosha (Gargling the medicated fluids) 9) Shiro tarpan Or moordha taila (medicated Oil applications. etc., on head). 10) Akshi Tarpan (Keeping of medicated sneha on eye ball by special method) 11) Nasa tarpan (Sneha Tarpana nasya) 12) Karna Poorana (instillation of eardrops) 13) maasthishkya (Medicated Oils + paste application to head)

## Shiras Tarpana (Moordha Tailam) :-

It is a special therapy in which the medicated (Snehas) Oils are kept on or poured on the head for a specific time, it is known as moordha taila Or shiras tarpana, It is more beneficial in thediseases of Shalakya tantra (Especially in Shiro roga) then other diseases. it is used for preventive as well as curative aspects.

According to Vagbhata it is of 4 types they are 1) Shiro abhyanga 2) Shiro Seka Or shiro dhara 3) Shiro pichu 4) Shiro Vasti, in these 4 therapies Shiro Vasti is the best then pichu, dhara, Abhyanga and the every method is having it's own importance. (Ref. A.h. SU. 2 - 23 )

# A) Shiro Abhyanga. (Head Massage)

It is a process in which the head is gently massaged with medicated Oils etc., for aspecific period. it is preventive as well as curative therapy. Sushrutha suggested applications of Cool Chakra taila for Shiro abhyanga. The medicine should be selected according to the condition of the disease.

**Use of Shiro Abhyanga :-**
**By Vagbhata.**

It is beneficial in Roughness, itching sensation, dirty collections of scalp and in the diseases of the hair (Ref.A.H. SU. 22 - 24 )

**By Charak.**

By regular shiro Abhyanga a person may get relief from Shira shoola (Head-ache) phalitha (dis colouration of hair), khalitwa (Baldness), Kesha paata (falling of hair), Kesha vikar (Abnormal hairs ), Twak vikar (Abnormalities of Skin of sclap, Indria Vikar (lesions of Sensory organs) and gives strength to head and Scalp. (Ref. Ch.Su. 5-81, 83)

**By Sushrutha .**

Shiro Abhyanga gives relief from Shira shoola, gives colour, complexion to face, proper nourishment to Indrias and head, the hair becomes blackish
(Ref. SU. Chi. 24 -25, 22)

## B) SHIRA SEKA -SHIRO PARISEKA - SHIRO DHARA .

It is a process in which the medicated Oil, ghee, Honey, Butter Milk, Milk, medicated decoctions, Breast milk, Boiled rice water (Kanji) etc., fluids are poured or droped on the head from 4" height by special process for a specific period is known as shiro seka Or shiro pariseka or Shiro dhara . it is mostly useful in Shiro roga than ear, nose, throat, eye and other general diseases.

According to the medicine used for the therapy it is named as follows :-

| 1. | Taila dhara | (Pouring of medicated Oils | ) |
|----|-------------|---------------------------|---|
| 2. | Ghritha dhara | ( " Ghee | ) |
| 3. | Madu Dhara | ( " Honey | ) |
| 4. | Takra Dhara | ( " Butter Milk | ) |
| 5. | Kwatha Dhara | ( ' Decoctions | ) |
| 6. | Ksheera Dhara | ( " Milk | ) |
| 7. | Kanji Dhara | ( " Boiled Rice Water | ) |

**Note :-** 1) Dhara has to do in the mornings in between 7 and 10 AM, and contra indicated in after noon and nights .

2) Leukwarm dhara in Vata and Kapha disorders and Cool dhara in Pitta and Raktha disorders.

## Drug Selection.

The Choice of the drug depends upon the diseases But in general the following sneha are used.

1) In vata and Kapha disorders Leukwarm Tila Taila is used for Shirodhara. 2) In vata and raktha vitiation cool ghritha 3) In Pitta and Raktha Vitiation and Vata + Pitta + Rakta Vitiation Taila and ghritha in equally quantiy is used. 4) In Vata + Kapha disorders Taila one part and Ghritha 1/2 part is used for dhara.

**DURATION OF SHIRO DHARA:-** is 1 to 1 1/2 hours, it is also depending upon the strength of the patient and the disease.

## Time Schedule for Shiro Dhara .

Shiro dhara has to do 14 days Or 21 days.

### A)      14 Days Schedule .

Ist day 1 hour duration.
2nd day to 7th day (duration is increased daily 5 minutes)
7th day1 1/2 hour duration.
8th to 14 day (duration is decreased daily 5 minutes)
14 th day 1 hour duration.

### B)      21 Days Schedule.

Ist day 1 hour
2nd to 7 day (duration increases daily 5 minutes)
8th day to 14th day 1 1/2 hour.
15 to 21 days (Duration decreases daily 5 minutes)
21 st day 1 hour.

## Uses of Shiro Dhara :-
### Vagbhata :-

1) He said Shiro dhara is useful in Arumshika (multiple pustules on scalp), Shiras toda (Pricking pain on scalp), Daha (Burning sensation of scalp and head), paka (inflammatory changes on scalp),Vrana (Ulcers on scalp).(Ref. A.H.SU.22-24) 2) He explained Dashamoola Ksheera shiro Seka in Shira shoola.(Ref.A.H.U. 24 -3)

### Charak.

1) Shira Seka with Ghee Or Milk in Pittaj Shira Shoola. (Ref. Ch. chi. 26-176)
2) Shiro Seka in Shankhaka Shiro Vyadhi (Ref. : ch. si. 9-73)

### Sushrutha :-

1)      Leukwarm shiro dhara with Vataghna milk in Vatik Shira shoola.
       (Ref.su. chi. 26 - 5)
2)      Cool ghee shiro dhara in Pittaj and Rakthaj Shiro roga.
       (Ref. : su U. 26-12, 13)

**Note :-** Kerala people called shiro seka as Shiro dhara, it is mostly useful not only in shalakya vyadhies but alsoin general diseases like psychosis, epilepsy, Neurosis, alcoholism, coma, In somnia, fainting, confusion, excessive purspiration and tiredness etc., disorders.

## The Common Requirements for Dhara.

1) CleanVentilated room. 2) Dhara table or Droni 3) 2 to 5 Attenders and Massagists. 4) Dhara patra (Vessel to hold medicine) 5) Pillows. 6) Furniture (Chairs, Tables, Stools etc.,) 7) Gas Stove 8) Hot water 9) medicines for shiro dhara and to face complications if any 10) Thick cloth for shiro bandan (to prevent the medicine from entering in to the eyes. 11) Eye bandage material 12) Containers to collect the medicine. 13) Stand to hold the dharaa patra.

**1)      Dharaa Patra.** ( Vessel or pot used t o hold the medicine for dhara). It should have wide mouth, 5 to 6" depth with central perforation at the bottom in the size of little finger which is fitted with cotton varthi to allow uniform flow during dhara. The container should have 2 litres capacity to hold the medicated fluid (2 prasta or 1 Aadaka that is approximately 2 litres). The borders of themouth should have been folded outwards so that the neck of the vessel may be tied with rope for handling. The contianer should prepare with Gold, silver, copper etc.,

**2)      Droni or Dharaa Table .**
1) Length of the table 6 feet. 2) Width " 2Feet. 3) height from the ground 1 1/2 to 2 feet 4) depth of the table 4 1/2 to 9 inches.

The surface should be smooth even comfortable to the patient and massagist, it should prepare with Vataghna wood, with head resting and Oil collecting arraangements.

**3) Common Medicines :-**
In Vataj disorders Tila taila, Bala taila, Dashamoola taila; In Kaphaj disroders with honey, nagar, musta. etc; in Pitaja disordes usheera chandan coconut water and ghee etc.

**4) Attenders :-**
2 Attenders are needed for shiro seka, one for pouring the medicine properly and another to collect the oil which is irrigated. after shiro seka, sneha and sweda for total body is advised, for that 5 attenders are needed.

**Shiro Dhaara Therapy.**
A clean Droni is placed in a clean appropriately ventillated room, necessary materials and accessaries are procured and are placed in the therapy room systematically. Dhara patra is fixed at about 4 inches height from the head of the patient in SHUBHA MUHURTHA by SWASTIVACHAN and MANGALACHARAN. Eyes should be bandaged with cotton pads to prevent the entry of Fluids into the eyes. Hair of the patient should cut into small to allow proper absorption of medicine, Shiro bandan has to apply around the head, above the eyebrows with thick cloth to prevent the entry of medicine in to the eyes. head should rest on the pillow properly. The medicine has to pour from 4 inches height on the head with constant speed neither quick nor slow, the medicine should irrigate in different postures of head, Irrigated medicine should be collected time to time from the bottom of the Droni, should be cleaned warmed and should replaced it in the Dhara Patra and Simultaneously the head and limbs of the patient should be given intermittent massage. After the specific time - Sarvanga sneha, sweda are advised to prevent the complications

## C) Shiro Pichu.

Shiro pichu means application of cotton piece or cloth piece by dipping in medicated Oil or ghee on the shiras at Brahma randra (Anterior fontanellae). It is more effective than shiro abhyanga and Shiro dhara. Pichu gives scope for gradual and slow absorption of the medicine, so only said as more effective.

It gives nourishment to the scalp, head, indria, and other organs of the body, it is useful in Kesha Paatha (Falling of hair), Kesha Vikruthi (abnormalities of hair), kesha sputanam (hair fall), Vrana (ulcers ), netra stambana (rigid and ristricted movements of eye ball) and in Shiro rogas etc.,

In addition to shiro pichu some other pichu are also explained like .
Yoni Pichu (pichu is inserted in Vagina)
Guda Pichu (Pcihu is inserted in rectum),
Nasa Pichu (Pichu is inserted in Nasa guha ) etc.,

Note :- if Bigger cloth piece or gauze piece is used by dipping in medicated Oil or ghee that is named as **Plotha.** Ref :- AH. Su. 22-25.

## D) Shiro Vasti.

Vagbhata explained it as the best among 4 types tof moordha taila. It is process in which medicated sneha (Oil Or ghee) are kept on the head, 2 inches above the level of hair with the help of vasti Yantra (leather cap like structure open on both sides ) for a specific period is known as Shiro Vasti. Shiro Vasti Should conduct in the afternoons or in the evenings.

**Shiro Vasti Yantra :-**
It is a leather cap like structure with open base (2 sides of cap is open), it is 12 to 16 inches in length, width should be according to the size of the head of the patient. It is fixed to the head to keep the medicated Oil or ghee on the head for a specific time.

**Shiro Vasti Therapy :-**
1) Sneha, Sweda, Shodhana has to do before shiro Vasti.
2) Hair has to remove (Mundana) Or should cut into small for proper absorption of the medicine.
3) Patient is asked to sit in a chair comfortabely with out any tension.
4) Patient isadvised not to move the head during the therapy.
5) Shiro vastiYantra (leather Cap) has to fix to the head, at the junction of head and cap masha Kalka or godhuma kalka has to apply to prevent the leakage of medicine, then Leukwarm medicated sneha has to pour into vasti Yantra upto 2 inches height above the level of hair. if the medicine become cool that has to exchage with Leukwaram Oil, like that the medicine should kept for a specific time.

When reduction of pain, arrivalof lacrimation (Ashru srava), nasa srava (Nasal discharge), mukha srava (Salivation), appears then Oil should be removed carefully. Then the same oil is used for massage of the shoulders, neck, chest and Back etc., The patient is advised to have bath with hot water and follow the pathya vidhi to avoid complications.

**Note :-** Shiro Vasti is advised for 7 days.

### Duration of Shiro Vasti.

| | | |
|---|---|---|
| 1) In Vata diseases | 10000 Matra Kala | Approx 53 Minuts. |
| 2) In Pitta Diseaes | 8000 Matraakala | Approx 43 Minutes. |
| 3) Kapha diseases | 6000 Matraakala | Approx 31 Minutes. |
| 4) Healthy Person | 1000 Matraakala | Approx 5 to 6 Minutes. |

### Indications ;-

Shiro Vasti is beneficial in the following diseases.

1) Prasupthi (Numbness of scalp ) 2) Arditha Vata (Facial paraysis) 3) Nidraalpatha (Sleeplessness) 4) manya Stamba (neck rigidity) 5) hanugraha and Hanu shoola (Lookjaw ) 6) Arthava Bhedak (migraine, half headache) 7) Shiro roga 8) Daarunaka (Dandruff) 9) Timira (dim vision) 10) Aasya sosha (Dryness of oral cavity ) 11) Nasa sosha (Atrophic Changes in nasal caivty )

## KARNA POORANA.

Putting of medicated Leukwarm Swarasa (Liquid extract of medicine), Taila (Oil), ghritha (Ghee), mutra (Goats urine etc) in to external auditory canal is known as karna Poorana. It is more effective not only in karna rogas but also in other diseases.

Vagbhata and sushrutha advised that a person who practices the karna poorana regularly should get stamina against deafness, neck reigidity (manya shoola) pain in the Jaw (Hanu shoola ) etc., used for karna pooran.

It is indicated in different types of ear diseases (like karna Shoola, karna nada, Badirya, Karna gootha, Karna Srava, karna kandu etc.,) hanu Shoola (pain in the jaws), manya Shoola (pain in neck ) and Shira shoola. (head ache.).

**Note :-** The common Oils are nirgundi taila, Kshara taila, Apamarge taila, Bilvadi tailam, Ksheera bala taila etc.,

### Duration.

100 Matra Kalas in ear disease.
500 Matra kalas in Throat diseases.
and 1000 matra kalas in Shiro rogas.
1) Swaras etc., Before meals. 2) Oil at night .

## Shiro Lepa. :-

It is named as pothicchil according to kerala Therapy. medicated paste is applied on the head in 1/4 1/3 inch thickness, should keep for 1/2 to 1 hour and advised to continue the therapy for 7 days.

It is indicated in Shiro rogas, Arditha Vata, Pakshaghata, Khalithya, Palithya and most of the Neurological problems.

(Hot applications named as upanaha and cool applications named as Lepa).

" The qualities of Shiro Lepa are merely equalant to Takra dhara."
1) Vataghna Aushadha Siddha payasa lepam in Vataja Shira shoola. 2) medicated paste prepared with nala, veteas, Shiivala, Raktha kamala, Chandan, uthphala, padmaka, vamshi, Yastimadu, Musta + Ghee application, in Pittaja shira shoola. 3) Hot application of Flesh of Fish in Kaphaj Shira Shoola. 4) 1Kudava (16Tolas) Amalaki, 2 Kudava (32 Tolas ) Butter Milk prepared from cow milk, 32 Tolas water, heat it upto water evapouration then the paste should be applied on the head it is useful in most of the Shiro rogas.

## Method of Shiro Lepa Therapy.

1) Shiro mundan (hair should remove ) for proper absorptionof medicine. 2) Shiro Abhyanga (head massage) 3) Application of paste to the head which is prepared according to the diseases. 4) Paste should apply in 1/4 Or 1/3 inch thickness only on the scalp not on fore head - and head should be wrapped with banana leaves. 5) Then the medicine should be kept for 1/2 to 1 hour. 6) Then the medicine should be removed and cleaned. 7) Again Oil massage is advised. 8) Patient is advised to have hot water bath 9) Advised to follow pathya vidhi 10) Like this shiro lepa therapy is advised for 7 days.

# GANDOOSHA - KAVALAGRAH.

Charaka explained only Kavala grah But sushruth and Vagbhata explained Gandoosha and kavalagrah. According ot them the difference is, only in the dosage of the drug.

## Gandoosha.

Holding of medicated fluids in the mouth in full quantity for a specific time and then asked to spit it out (Because of full quanitiy, the fluid cannot able to rotate in the mouth.)

## Kabalgrah :-

Medicated Fluids are kept in themouth incompletely and asked to rotate in the mouth for a specific time and then asked to spit it out

**Su. Chi. - 40 -58.**

Note : - According to Sarangadhara, Kalka (Medicated bolus) drugs are used in kavala and Liquids are used in Gandoosha.

Sharangdhar. 4th 10-4.

# CLASSIFICATION OF KAVALA OR GANDOOSHA.

| According to Sushrutha | According ot Vagbhata. |
|---|---|
| 1) Snehan Gandoosha | 1) Snigda Gandoosha |
| 2) Prasadan    " | 2) Shaman         " |
| 3) Shodhan    " | 3) Shodhan     " |
| 4) Ropan      " | 4) Ropan         " |

## 1) Snehan Or Snigda Gandoosha :-

The Drugs should be snigda - Ushna, Madura, Amala, lavana - used in Vata prakopa. The medicine should mix with other Vata hara sneha, mamsaras etc., items.

## 2) Shaman Gandoosha :-

Drugs should be prepared with Tiktha, Kashya and Madura rasa for pitta shaman, But in prasadan gandoosha of sushruth the drugs should be prepared with Madura ,Sheetha for pitta shaman. The both are one and same but explained by different authors for pitta shaman.

## 3) Shodhan Gandoosha :-

Drugs should be prepared with Tekshna, ushna ,Ruksha ,Katu ,Amla ,Lavan rasa for kapha Shaman. The Gomutra, madya, shuktha, madu ,Dhanyamala etc., should be used along with medicines.

## 4) Ropan Gandoosha :-

Durgs should be prepared with ushna, kashaya, Katu, madura, Rasa,for.Vrana ropana (ulcer healing). The Ghritha, ksheera, sneha dravya are used along with the drugs.

## Gandoosha Vidhi.

It is a process having utmost importance in the management of mukha rogas.
It is a Special process as well as pashcyath karma to nasya karma, Vaman
Karma etc., to save the body from the complications of Kapha dosha.

　　　1) Preparationof the patient for Gandoosha
　　　2) Preparation of the medicine according to the condtion of the patient.

**a) Example :-** Triphala - Trikatu, pancha Valkala, Dashamoola, vacha, Yastimadu, etc., drugs should be grinded to prepare kalka (Bolus Or Paste ). to keep in the mouth or to rotate in the mouth.

## b) Liquid Medicines :-

Like Grhitha, Taila, madu, water, madhya, Mamsa rasa, Gomutra, decoctions of medicines, shuktha, kanji etc., drugs.
**c)** According to the vitiation of doshas either kalka Or Kashaya Or mixed  should be selected for the therapy)
3) Gentle massage
4) Light Fomentation|at neck, Cheeck, face, head, shoulders, etc.,
5) Patient is asked to sit in a chair with comfort then the medicine is given to hold in the mouth or to rotate upto the specific time(upto the collection of Kapha in mouth, Nasa Srava etc then the medicine should be spit it out. Pashcyath karma Or other gandoosha should be given.
6) Again Gentle massage and light Fomentation at Neck, face, Cheecks, shoulders head etc.,

## Indication of Gandoosha ;-

　　　1) manya Stamb (neck rigidity ) 2) Shira shoola (Head ache) 3) Karna shoola (otalgia ) 4) Mukha roga (Diseases of Osta, dantha moola, Dantha, jihwa, Talu, Gala) 5) Netra roga (eye diseases) 6) Lala srava (Salivation ) 7) Mukha sosha (Vataj disorders of mouth) 8) Hrullasa (Nausea ) 9) Tandra (Sleeping mood ) 10) Aruchi (Tastelessness ) 11) Peenasa (Rhinitis ) 12) Siro roga.

343

Regular Gandoosha vidhi achieves the following benefits 1) Swara balam (Strength to voice ) 2) Hanubalam (Strenght to Jaws) 3) Strength to face 4) Ruchyam (Better Taste perception 5) Druda dantha (Strong and healthy teeth ) 6) Stamina against Doshaja or Aaganthuja mukha rogas - Shiro rogas, Karna rogas. Nasa roga and Netra roga.

## Time Schedule For Gandoosha :-
The medicated fluids should kept in the mouth upto the manfestation of following symptoms.
1) Collection of Kapham in the mouth 2) Nasa Srava 3) Karna Srava 4) Netra Srava.

Then the drug should spit it out. Then New drug should be kept in the mouth or pashchyath Karma has to do according to the condition of the patient.

## Samyak Yoga Lakshanas of Gandoosha (Symptoms of Adequate Gandoosha):-
1) Relief from the disease or symptoms. 2) Freshness of all Indrias, Face and mind. 3) Lightness of Body 4) Sound sleep 5) Normal taste, appetite, digestion capacity and general health.

## Atiyoga Lakshanas of Gandoosha . (Symptoms of Excessive gandoosha):-
1) Shosha (Dryness of mukha etc., srotas) 2)Daha (Burning sensation)3) Paka (ulceration ) 4) Trushna (Thirst) 5) Aruchi (loss of Taste) 6) Klam (Debility).

## Asamyak Yoga Lakshanas of Gandoosha
## (Symptoms of Inadequate gandoosha):-
1) Alastwa (Lazyness) 2) Agravation of the disease 3) Kapha vitiation 4) Aruchi (Tastelessness) 5) Hrullasa (nausea) 6) Tandra (inactive state Or sleepy mood.)

## Some Important Yogas of Gandosha.
1) Hot water gandoosha in general Kapha disorders of mukha 2) Gandoosha with Kanji Or Dhanyamla in Aruchi 3) Daruharidra - rasa Kriya Or Triphala Kashaya Gandoosha in Mukhapak. 4) Trikatu Sarshapa hareetaki Kalkam + ksharajala Gandoosha in Kaphaj Mukha roga. 5) Tila Kalka + Water gandoosha in Dantha harsha. 6) Ghritha Or Ksheera gandoosha in Pittaja mukha rogas. 7) Ksheeri Vruksha Kashaya gandoosham in Bleeding gums. 8) Decoction of Kaseesa, Lodra, Pippali, manahshlla, priyang, Tejohwa + Honey, Gandoosha in Pyorrhoea (pus discharge from gums) 9) Pancha pallava kashaya + Ghritha + madu + Sugar Gandoosha in (Gingivitis) Upakusha. 10) Gandoosha with Irimedadi, Taila Or sahacharadi taila Or sarshapa taila Or narayan taila Or prasarini taila in gum disorders (Dantha moola vyadhies).11) The decoction of Lodra, musta, jatamamsi, rasanjan, Patranga+ Honey, gandoosha in saushira (Dantha moola Vyadhi). 12) Patola - Nimba, Triphala Kashaya gandoosha in gum disorders 13) Dasha moola Kashaya + Tila Taila gandoosha in Dantha rogas. 14) Trikatu, Sarshapa, Saindhava Lavana, gandoosha in Kaphaja jihwa roga. 15) Kshara jala gandoosha in Kaphaja mukha roga. 16) Tila taila gandoosha is better to do daily to prevent mukharoga 17) Yastimadu Kashaya gandoosha in Mukha paka. 18) Kakolyadi or Vidarigandhadi ghritha gandoosha in Pittaj mukha rogas.

# B) SWEDANA KARMA

Sweating is the physiological process But over sweating or Absence of Sweating is patholgical, Inducing the sweating by heat application is known as swedan Karma. it is beneficial in vata kapha disorders and harmful in pitta, Raktha disorders.

Swedana is a major poorva Karma procedure conducted after sneha Karma and proceedes Vaman karma. it is a process in wihich by the application of the heat Liquification of doshas occurs that relieves stiffness, heavyness, cold and induces sweating. Being the principal poorva karma procedure, swedana is also a specific treatment procedure for number of diseases like vata vyadhi (It is also a main therapy that is one among shat upakramas and quite opposite to stambana therapy).

## Qualities of swedan dravyas.

1) Ushna (Hot) 2) Teekshna (Quickly spreading) 3) Sara (Spreading nature in the all directions) 4) Snidga (oleus- unctuous) 5) Rooksha (Rough - opposite to snigda 6) Sukshma (penetrating into minute channels.) 7) Drava (liquidity ) 8) Sthira (Fixed) 9) Guru (Heavy or bulkness)

### Classification of Swedan Karma .
I) According to Charak
    a) Agni Sweda 13 types. b) Anagni Sweda - 10 types.

II)     a) Snigda Sweda in Vata disorders. b) Ruksha Sweda in Kapha disorders.

III)    a) Ekanga Sweda (Swedan only at the affected part ) b) Sarvanga Sweda (Swedan to thecomplete body)

IV)    a) Mrudu Sweda - in weak persons, less vitiation of doshas and at Heart scrotum eyes etc., b) Madyama Sweda :- moderate Strength of the patient disease and at groins. c) Maha Sweda :- Strengthy people with high vitiation of doshas.

V)     According to Sushrutha and Vagbhata
     a) Tapa Sweda b) ushma Sweda c) Upanaha Sweda d) Drava Sweda.

VI)    a) Shaman Sweda (Remission of the diseases) b) Shodhan Sweda (elimination of doshas )

VII) a) Bahya Sweda (External) b) Abhyanthar Sweda (Internal)

## Swedana Karma - Indications.

1) Pratishyaya (Rhinitis) 2) Kasa (Cough) 3) Hiccah (hiccough) 4) Swasa (Dyspnoea) 5) heaviness of body 6) Karna Shoola (otalgia) 7) manya shoola (Pain at neck region) 8) Shira shoola (headache) 9) Swara bheda (hoarseness of Voice ) 10) Gala grah (neck rigidity) 11) Paarshwa graha (rigid flanks ) 12) prusta grah (rigidity in the dorsum of trunk ) 13) kati graha (rigid Lumbo sacral region) 14) Kukshigrah (rigid abdomen) 15) hanu grah (rigid jaws) 16) Pada - jaanu- janga-uru graha (Rigidity in all parts of Lower limbs) 17) Padaarthi- jaanurathi Jangaarthi Uru arthi (Pain in all parts of Lower Limbs ) 18) Arditha Vata (Facial palsy) 19) Ekaanga Vata (Monoplegia) 20) Sarvaanga Vata (total paralysis) 21) Pakshaghaata (hemi Plegia Or paraplegia)

22) Angamarda (Body pains 23) Aadya Vata 24) Vata kantaka 25) Ghrudrasi Vata 26) Supthi (loss of Sensation) 27) Stamba - Sankocha (Spastic pains) 28) Aanaha 29) Vibandha (Constipation ) 30) Aama Vata 31) Shotha (Oedema) 32) Jrumba 33) Shukraghaath (Retention of Semen ) 34) Mutra kruchra (Dysuria) 35) Muska Vruddi (Orchitis) 36) Moodha garbha (malpresentations during delivary ) 37) Arsha (haemorrhoids) 38) Bhagandar (Fistila in ano ) 39) Arbuda (Tumours) 40) Grandhi (Cysts) 41) kampaVata 42) Shalyaapahrut (after removal of foreign bodies) 43) Samyak Prajatha (after normal delivary) 44) Ashmari (Urinary caliculus 45) Most of vata and Kapha disorders.

## CONTRA INDICATIONS OF SWEDAN KARMA.

1) Raktha and Pitta Disorders 2) Alcoholism 3) Pregnancy 4) jaundice (kamala) 5) Atisara (Diarrhoea) 6) Raktha Pitta (Bleeding disorders) 7) udara roga Spleeno megaly - hepatomegely, Ascites etc. disorders) 8) urakshata (chest injury) 9) Burns 10) Pitta Prakruthi 11) Tired 12) Poisoning 13) unconscious 14) Sthoola (fat) 15) Thirsty 16) Angry 17) Weeping due to mental illness 18) Urustamba 19) Debilitative persons 20) Shukra kshaya 21) Ojo kshaya 22) Timira (Dimvision) 23) Pandu (Anaemia) 24) Visarpa (Skin rashes) 25) Sosha (Dehydrated) 26) Kusta 27) Guda bramsha (prolapse of rectum) 28) Rajaswala (menstruation period) 29) After intake of milk, alcohol, curd, oil etc., 30) Indigestion 31) Madu Meha 32) Pittaja Prameha 33) Ruksha - Shuska deha - (dehydrated) 34) After Virechan 35) Stambana Arha (Those indicated for stambana therapy)

## CLASSIFICATION OF SWEDA ACCORDING TO CHARAK.

a) Agni Sweda  - 13 types b) Anagni Sweda     - 10 types.

### a) Agni SWedas 13 :-
Inducing sweda by heat applicatons they are
1) Sankara sweda, 2) Prastara sweda 3) nadi Sweda 4) pariseka Sweda 5) Avagaha Sweda 6) jenthaaka Sweda 7) Asmaghna Sweda 8) karshoo Sweda 9) kutee sweda 10) Bhoo sweda 11) kumbhi Sweda 12) Koopa Sweda 13) holak Sweda.

### b) Anagni Sweda 10 types .
Inducing sweda by other than heat applications, they are.
1) Vyayama - indulging more exercise 2) ushna Sadan - Residing in hot non Ventillated room 3) Guru praavaran - By covering thick blankets etc., 4) Kshudha - Supressing the hungry 5) Bahupaanam - in take of more alcoholic drinks. 6) Bhaya - By inducing Fear complexion. 7) Krodha - By anger 8) Upanaha - Application of ushna Veerya Aushada 9) Aayath - Fighting 10) Aatap - Sun Bath

### 1) Sankara Sweda - Or Pinda Sweda :-
It is of two types.
a) Snigda Pinda Sweda b) Ruksha pinda Sweda.

## a) Snigda Pinda Sweda :-

The medicated Kalkam (Semi solid paste) which is prepared with coocked rice, Tila, Masha, Kuluttha, Amladravya, Taila, ghritha, Ksheera, payasa and other required medicines should keep in a Fresh, thin white cloth and should prepare poulties or bolus or pinda 4 to 6 according to the requirement, these poulties should dip in hot medicated decoctions and apply to the affected areas for specific time, It is especially indicated in Vata predominent disease.

## b) Ruksha Pinda Sweda :-

Metalic particles, stone pieces, sand and dried faecal material of animals- is heated and applied to the affected area directly or by keeping them in the fresh, thin white cloth like above.

It is especially indicated in Kapha predominent diseases.

Kerala people are practicing this therapy (snigda pinda Sweda) in the name of Shastika shali pinda Sweda Or NAVARAKIZI with advanced techniques.

Time 1/2 to 1 hour - Once or Twice a day.

## 2) Prasthara Sweda :-

Prasthara means stone. In astanga sangraha it is explained as samsthara sweda.

Shali dhanya, Yava, godhuma, masha, Kuluttha, mudga, Kodrava, Tila, mamsa, Payasa etc., are coocked and kept on the 6 feet x 21/2 feet stone uniformly and should cover with medicated leaves Or thin cloth and the massaged patient is asked to lie down on the stone for a specific time. It is meant for sarvanga sweda.

## 3) Nadi Sweda Or Bhaspa Sweda.

a) Bhaspa yantra b) Bhaspa Nalika c) Medicated decoction are required.

The medicated decocotion prepared with Rasna, Erenda, devadaru, Nirgundi, Bala, Shigru, Punarnava, Varuna, guduchi, Amla dravya, Lavana, mutra, Ksheera, Mamsa, or other needed medicines according to the disease should collect in a Big wide vessel. The mouth of the vessel is sealed and 6 feet tube (Bhaspa nalika) is connected to the lateral part of the Bhaspa Yantra. Bhaspa Yantra is kept on the stone for boiling the medicine. The medicated vapour will come through the tube that should be exposed to the massaged part which is affected or to the entire body.

Time :- 1/2 to 1 hours, 7 to 21 days according to the vitiation.

## 4) PARISEKA SWEDA - SNEHA DHARA SWEDA.
## PIZICHIL - PISHIMCHIL.

Droni is a special table used for abhyanga and Sweda in which there is a facility to collect the Oil which is used for the therapy.

Patient is asked to lie down on the droni, Shiro Abhyanga and Kaya Abhyanga has to do before pariseka. Lukewarm medicated decoctions, Oils, ghee, milk, butter milk etc., is poured on the body with the help of dhara patra from 9" height for specific time, kerala people call it as pizichil Or pishimchil. 5 Attenders are required for the therapy, 2- 2 attenders on either sides for giving dhaara and 5th attenders is to collect the medicine from the bottom of droni.

**Note : -** 1) Daily if medicine is changed it is perfect.
2) Milk has to change daily
3) Dhanyamla should change once in 3 daily
4) Taila, after 3 days freshmedicine should add to theold medicine and should change competely after 7 days.
Time :- 1/2 to 1 1/2 Hour daily, for needed duration according to thedisease.

## 5) Avagaaha (Medicated tub Bath)

Medicated decoctions, Oils, milk, ghee, mamsa rasa etc., should be filled in the tub, the patient is asked to dip upto neck for 1/2 to 1 hour, then asked to have hot water tub bath
measure ments of tub :-
Lenght 4 to 6 feet
Width 2 feet
height - 11/2 to 2 feet.

## 6) Jenthaka Sweda :-

A special equidimensional round room is arranged for this therapy. in side the room centrally Angarakosti is arrnanged, peripherally all around the room seating arrangement is done for the patient . A patient after masssage is send in to the room and asked to sit - on the place arranged peripherally - upto specific time (up to the appearance of adequate symptoms of fomentation.

## 7) Ashma ghana sweda :-

It is a type of prasthara sweda in this variety medicines are burnt on on 6 x 2 1/2 feet stone, medicines are removed, Water is sprinkled thin cloth is covered on the stone and the massaged patient is asked to lie down on the stone by covering his bodywith cloth upto the ncek the vapour coming from the stone gives fomentation effect to the patient.

## 8) Karshoo sweda :-

A pit has to dig on the ground in which the bottom should be wide and mouth should be narrow (approximately 4x21/2 feet dimentions) medicines should be burnt in the pit and massaged patient is asked to lie down on a cot which is kept on the pit, for fomentation.

## 9) Kutee seda :-

Massaged patient is covered with thick cloth and asked to sit in a non ventillated room with Angaara kosti, due to absence of air, thick covering, and heat, sweating is produced.

## 10) Bhoo Swedam :-

It is like Ashmaghana sweda but medicines are burnt on earth instead of stone, medicated burnt particles are removed, water is sprinkled, covered with cloth and massaged patient is asked to lie down upto the specific time.

## 11) Kumbhee sweda :-

A pot with medicated decocotion is burried in the earth, a cot Or stool is kept on the site, then hot iron balls are dropped into the decoction then medicated vapours are released those should be exposed to the affected site.

## 12) Koopa Sweda :-

It is like Karshoo sweda but more hot because themouth surface of pit is more wider than the cot dried faecal material is burnt in the pit (medicinal parts are burnt is Karshoo sweda )

## 13) Holaaka Sweda :-

It is also like Koopa sweda but dried faecal material is burnt and is kept underneath the cot instead of pit.

# SWEDA CLASSIFICATION ACCORDING TO SUSHRUTHA AND VAGBHATA.

## 1) Tape Seda :-

Swedana is done with the direct touch of hot or heated objects like metalic things, salt,sand, cloth or hand etc.,

## 2) Ushma Sweda :-

It is indirect Formentation in which swedana is carried out with the touch of vapour liberating from medicated hot items.

## 3) Upanaaha Sweda :-

Swedan by the application of ushna lepa, Sankara Sweda and ushna dravya bandana (Saalavana sweda).

## 4) Drava Sweda :-

Swedan with hot medicated liquids like in pariseka Or Avagaha.

## Sweda Vidhi
### I) Poorva Karma.

1) Collection of requirments like Vessels, medicines for the therapy and to treat complications.

2) Assessment a) About the Common principles like indications, b) Which type of Sweda is required, c) Seasonal indications (maha Sweda in sheeta rutu and mrudu sweda in ushna rutu etc.,) d) Strength of the patient (for more strengthy maha sweda, moderate strengthy madyama sweda and for weak person mrudu sweda ) e) economincal status, estimation of money to purchase the medicines for sweda f) Desha or site of the disease also gives the idea about the sweda (like Aamashaygatha vata - Ruksha Sweda Pakwashaya gatha kapha snigda sweda, vrushan Hrudaya netra mrudu sweda etc.) g) Age consideration is important todice the type of sweda and for treatment

## II) Pradhana Karma :-

1)    Swedavacharan - performing Swedan karma.
2)    Nireckshan :-
Time - Duration, waiting for the features of adequate or inadequate or excess sweda, Taking care about complications.

**Note :-** Method depends upon the type of Sweda which is selected etc.,

## Features of Adequate (Samyaka ) Sweda.

1) Disappearance of cold 2) Relief from pain 3) Relief from stiffness 4) Relief from heaviness 5) Getting smoothness in the body 6) Adequate Sweating 7) Remission of the disease 8) Desire for the cold items.

## Features of Inadequate Sweda (Asamyaka Sweda)

1) Less Sweating 2) No relief from pain, stiffness, heaviness and cold.

## Features of Excess sweda (Ati Sweda)

1) Pitta prakopa 2) Burning Sensation in the body 3) Fainting 4) Heaviness of the body 5) Lethorgy 6) Joint pains 7) Eruption of depigmented papules on Skin 8) Vertigo 9) Thirst 10) Tiredness 110 Fever 120 Vomitings 13) Raktha prakopa.

If above excess symptoms are observed the following measures should be adopted 1) Rakta - pitta shaman, Lepa, Aahara, Aushada has to give.
**Ex :-** Cool applications, cool air, residing in air conditioned room, intake of Sheeta Veerya madhura Tikta Kashaya rasa Aahara, avoiding of katu Amla Lavana rasa and symptomatic treatment.

## Post Swedana Regimen :-

( Sweda Pashchyat Karma)
1) Do not expose to cold Or open air directly. 2) Avoid Cold water 3) Warm water sponging 4) Rest 5) Warm water bath 6) Sleeping after taking light liquid and non sticky food.

## Note :-

1) Swedan then next day vaman
2) Swedan then After 3 days- virechan
3) Nasya, Vasti, Rakta mokshon, should do immediately after swedan.

## FUNCTIONS OF SWEDA.

1) Removes rigidity 2) Reduce heaviness 3) Reduce Coldness 4) Induce Sweating 5) Liquifies the doshas 6) Normally maintenance of Vata dosha 7) Brings softness in the organs 8) Appetiser 9) Brings normal pigmentation and softness to skin 10) Increases desire to take food 11) All the minute channels of the body are purified. 12) Removes unwanted sleep and drowsyness 13) Activates the Joints 14) Eliminates the doshas.

# VAMANA KARMA. (EMESIS THERAPY)

Vamana Karma is one among the panchakarma therapy, especially mentioned to eliminate vitiated Kapha dosha through the oral route, the expelled meterial consist of indigested food, vitiated kapha and pitta.

The aggravated doshas can be expelled out either through oral route or through rectum, for the both virechana word is used but particularly vamana is termed as Urdwa Virechan, it is indicated for elimination of dosha not only in diseased condition but also in healthy condition for the preservation of health.

Sneha and Sweda Karma causes softening mobilisation and liquification of doshas, then brings them from Shakha to Kostha, from here, by Vamana, doshas are expelled out through the mouth.

## PROPERTIES OF VAMAKA DRAVYA.
1) Ushna  2) Teekshna  3) Sukshma 4) Vyavayi  5)Vikasi 6)Prabhava.

**NOTE:-** (a) The drugs those induce vomiting are called as vamaka dravya.
(b) The drugs those helps or enhance the qualities of vomiting are known as Vamanopaka dravya.

## INDICATIONS OF VAMANA KARMA.
1) Peenasa 2) Kusta 3) Navajwara 4) Rajayakshma 5) Kasa 6) Swasa 7) Gala-grah 8) Sleepad  9) Galagand 10) Prameha  11) Mandaagni  12) Vishuchika 13) Alasak 14) Visha Peetha  15) Viddha  16) Adho rakthapitta 17) Mukha praseka 18) Arsha  19) Hrullasa 20) Aruchi 21) Apachi  22) Grandhi 23) Apasmara  24) Unmada 25) Atisara 26) Shopha 27) Pandu 28) Mukha Paka 29) Stanya dysti 30) Arbuda 31) Vidarika 32) Medo roga 33) Grudroga 34) Chitta Vibrama 35) Visarpa 36) Vidradhi 37) Poothi nasa 38) Kantha paka 39) Karna Srava 40) Adhi Jihwak 41) Gala Shundika 42) Kapha Vikar.

## CONTRA INDICATIONS OF VAMANA KARMA.
1) Kshatha Ksheena 2) Ati sthula 3) Ati Krusha 4) Baala 5) Vruddha 6) Durbala 7) Shrantha 8) Pipasitha 9) Kshudhita 10) Karmahatha 11) Bhaarahatha 12) Aadhwahata 13) upavasitha 14) Miithuna prasaktha 15) Adhyayan prasaktha 16) Vyayama Prasakta 17) Chita Prasaktha 18) Kshaama 19) Garbini 20) Sukumara. 21) Vibanda 22) Krumi Kostha 23) Dushchardan 24) Urdwa rakthapitta25) Prasakta Chardi 26) Urdwa Vata 27) Aasthapitha  28) Hrudroga 29) Anuvasitha 30) Udaavartha 31) Mootraa ghaatha 32) Pleeha roga 33) Gulma 34) Udara 35) Ashtheetla  36) Swaropaghaatha 37) Timira 38) Shankhaka 39) Karna Shoola  40) Arsha 41) Akshi Shoola 42) Dukha 43) Brama 44) Paarshwa ruk 45) Vata Vyadhi.

## DRUGS LIST USED FOR VAMANA KARMA.
(a) ACCORDING TO SUSHRUTHA :- Madanphal, Jeemotak, Ikshwaku, Dhamargav, Krutavedana, Sarshapa, Pippali, Karanja, Chakramard, kovidara, Ashwagand Vidul, Shanapushpi, Bimbi, Chitra, Swethavacha etc.

## 4) ACCORDING TO BHAVAMISHRA AND SARANGADHAR.

| Decoction, | Perfect dose | 9 Prasta | = | 576 Tola |
|---|---|---|---|---|
| | Moderate dose | 6 Prasta | = | 384 Tola |
| | Minimum dose | 3 Prasta | = | 192 Tola |
| Kalka | Perfect dose | 12 Tola | | |
| and | Moderate dose | 8 Tola | | |
| Churna | Minimum dose | 4 Tola. | | |

## 5) IDEAL OR PRACTICALLY USING DOSAGE BY MOST OF THE DOCTORS, IS.

| Decoction | 10 to 20 Tolas |
|---|---|
| Powder | 1/2 To 1 Tola. |

## PREPARATION OF THE PATIENT :-

Suitable diet, Snehana, swedana, suggestions and assurances etc., should give before Vaman Karma.

## 1) DIET REGIMEN DURING SNEAHA KARMA.

Light, hot, Non sticky food should give, during the rest day Abhishyandi Kaphoth Klesha (Nausea) food like Anupamamasa, dadhi, Ksheera, Masha, Tila, Drava etc., should give.

**During the day of Vaman :-** Ksheera, Yavagu, ghritha should give, Vaman is conducted after intake of liquid diet only - not in empty stomach.

## 2) SNEHA SWEDA :-

| Abhyantar Sneha | 3 to 7 Days. |
|---|---|
| Abhyanga and Sweda - | 3 Times, in the |
| 1) Last day of Sneha Pana | 2) Rest day 3) During the day of Vamana. |

So, Sneha Pana, Abhyanga, Bashpa Sweda liquifies the doshas and brings them to the Kosta, that should be expelled out by Vaman Karma.

## 3) MAANASOPACHAR:-

Patient should be explained about the therapy and its advantages, tension fear anxiety should be removed; head bath, application of Cented Flavours, wearing of new dress and garlands, taking blessings from God, Brahmins, elders and Friends should be done.

After these preparations, ina a good day vamana karma has to conduct.

## II.    PRADHANA KARMA.

a)    Induction of vamaka Dravya
b)    Service to the Patient and waiting for Vamana.
c)    Waiting for Vamana, Vega -
d)    Determination of Samyak Or Asmyak Vega.
e)    Complications and its Management.

## (a) INDUCTION OF MEDICINE,

Patient is asked to sit in a Chair comfortablely, after examination, the patient is given Vamanopaga dravya like Ksheera, Ikshurasa, madya, mamsarasa etc., to provoke Kapha for proper emesis.

The quantity of milk Or Sugar cane juice shouldbe measured before administration, commonly patient get satifaction after intake to 40 to 64 Lbs (Auns) juice, then madana phala compound (4 parts madana phala + 2 Parts Vacha + 1 Part saindhava lavana with Honey) should be given.

## (b) SERVICE TO THE PATIENT :-

Lukewarm sweda should be done at face chest flankes and back and should wait for 1 muhartha (48 minutes) for Vaman Vega.

Sweating on frontal region, horripulations, balooming of abdomen, salivation, nausea are the Signs of Provokation of dosha to cause proper emesis commonly in one muhurtha 2-3 Vega has to come if not with sticks or madhana phala compound throat should be irritated, and repeatedly salt water Or Yastimadhu kwatha should be given for proper emesis, 10 to 20 Lbs (Auns) Yastimadu Phanta 5 to 8 times should be given that cause 4 to 10 Vamana Vega, than Samples should be collected for analysis.

(c) Vamana Vega Nireekshan.
Waiting for Vamana Vega.

Number of Vamana vegas expelled matter, its quantity, features etc., should be observed carefully to assess the adquate or inadequate emesis.

1st vega after induction of medicine should be Omitted.

| Sl. No. | Emesis grades | Vega Sankya | Dosha | Quantity of Vomited matter. |
|---------|---------------|-------------|-------|------------------------------|
| 1. | Best emesis (Pravara) | 8 | Pitta antha | 2 Prasta = 108 Tola |
| 2. | Moderate Emesis (Madyama) | 6 | Kapha antha | 1 1/2 Prasta=81 Tola |
| 3. | Minimal Emesis Avara | 4 | Kapha antha | 1 Prasta = 54 Tola. |

**(b) VAGBHATA CLASSFICATION :-** Lavana, vacha, Ela, Sarshapa, Karanja, Pipaali, chitrak, Vidanga, Murva, Devadali, Kutaj, Trapusha, Vishala, Bimbi, nimba, madhuka, madanphala.

### (c) ACCORDING TO CHARAKA

| Madanaphala | Yogas | 133, |
|---|---|---|
| Jeemutaka | Yogas | 39, |
| Ikshwaku | Yogas | 45, |
| Dhamargav | Yogas | 60, |
| Kutaj | Yogas | 18, |
| Krutavedan | Yogas | 60, |
| and in Total | | 355 |

He explained moolini, phalini, Pushapa, patra, lavana, Vaman-opaga, Kashya, drugs, and in Kapha pitta Amaashaya Vyadhies he explained madanphala yastimadu, nimbu, jeemuta, Krutavedan, pippali, kutaj, Ikshwaku, Ela, dhamargav etc., drugs.

## VAMANA KALPANAS.

Churna, Vati, kalka, Varti, Kashaya, Leha, sneha, Mamsa ras yavagu, yoosha, Ksheer, dadhi, Takra, Ikshuras, asava, Arista, and with different food items.

## I) VAMAN KARMA PROCEDURE.

I)      Poorva Karma. Essential pre requisites for Vamana

**a) Collection of necessary facilites such as :-** Equipped room, utensils, furniture, spittons, assisting staff and drugs for inducing vamana and to treat the complications.

**(b) Examination of the Patient :-**

Regarding his suitability for vamana, this assessment is done by Asta Vidha, Dasha Vidha Pareeksha etc.

## (c) DETERMINATION OF THE DOSAGE OF VAMANA.

References from classics.

1)      Sushrutha suggests vaman dosage for Decoctions = 16 Tola. Powder and paste = 1 Tola, The other deciding factors are, strength of the patient, disease and digestive capacity.

## 2) CHARAK.

Minimum dosage of drug should eliminate doshas, should be pleasent without producing any complications.

## 3) VAGBHATA.

He said dosage should be fixed basing upon severity of desease, age, Climate, Weather and strength of the patient etc.,

## d) FEATURES OF ADEQUATE EMESIS (SAMYAK VAMAN LAKSHAN)

1)        Proper elimination of doshas first Kapha then pitta.
2)        Lightness in hrudaya moordha, Kantha, Paarshwa, Srotas, indria and body.
3)        Weakness and general debility.
4)        Should not have complications.
5)        Starting and stoping of Vamana Vega should be natural without any stimulations.

## FEATURE OF INADEQUATE EMESIS ( ASAMYAK VAMAN)

1) Improper elimination of doshas  2) Only medicine is expelled out 3) Delayed emesis. 4) uneasyness in hrudaya, Kantha and Srotas 5) Erruption of Spotha, Kotha, Kandu 6) Sticky Salivation. 7) Fever.

### Features of Excessive emesis.

1) Frothy Vomiting. 2) Blood stained vomiting. 3) Pain in the Chest heart and throat. 4) Thirst 5) Delirium 6) Vertigo 7) Un consciousness 8) Burning sensation 9) Insomnia 10) Weakness 11) Death.

### e) Complications of Vamana. (Vamana Vyapath.)

1) Aadmana 2) Parikarthika 3) Hruthgraha 4) Gatragrah 5) Stamba 6) Klama 7) Srava 8) Raktha Pitta 9) Vibramsha 10) Vibanda 11) Atisara 120 Pravahika 13) Vata Shoola 14) Symptoms of Heena Yoga and Atiyoga of Vamana.

### PASHCHATA KARMA. (Post Vaman Regimen.)

1) Rest for 1 Muhurtha (48 Minutes) 2) Dhooma Paana for sroto shuddhi 3) Following the suitable suggestions (Pariharya Vishaya) 4) Samasarjana krama to activate agni 5) Santarpana - nourishing therapy 6) Preparation for proceeding shodhana therapy.

### Suitable Suggestions after Vamana Karma :-

The Patient should avoid. Loud talking, excassive eating, constant sitting, excessive walking, travelling, Anger, Anxiety, heat, Cold,Open air, coitus, night arousal, day sleeping, suppressing of natural urges etc.

# SAMSARJANA KRAMA :-

The Vamana Karma Temporarily diminishes the agni, it has to be revived with th help of appropriate diet schedule for 7 days, itis here under.

| No. of Anna kala. (diets) | No. of the day | Pravara Shuddhi | madyama Shuddhi | Avara Shuddhi |
|---|---|---|---|---|
| | Ist day Morning. | - | - | - |
| 1st | " Night | Peya | Peya | Peya |
| 2nd | 2nd day Morning | Peya | Peya | Vilepi |
| 3rd | " Night | Peya | Vilepi | Yusha |
| 4th | 3rd Day Morning | Vilepi | Vilepi | Mamsarasa |
| 5th | " Night | Vilepi | Akrutha Yusha | Normal diet |
| 6th | 4th Morrning | Vilepi | Krutha Yusha | |
| 7th | " Night | Akrutha Yusha | Akrutha mamsaras | |
| 8th | 5th morrning | Krutha Yusha | Krutha mamsaras | |
| 9th | " Night | Krutha Yusha | Normal diet. | |
| 10th | 6th Morning | Akrutha mamsa rasa | | |
| 11th | " Night | krutha Mamsa rasa | | |
| 12th | 7th Morning | Krutha Mamsa rasa | | |
| 13th | " Night | Normal diet. | | |

Note :-  a) For pravara shuddhi, at 7th day evening normal diet should be given.
b) For Madyama Shuddhi at 5th day evening normal diet should be given.
c) For avara shuddhi at 3rd day evening normal diet should be given.

**Preparation for Proceeding Shodhana karma.**

Vamana pathya vidhi completes upto 7th day then 8th day rest day, 9th 10th, 11th day snehana, 12th 13th, 14th, Rest days and 15th day Swedan and Virechana should be given.

# VIRECHANA KARMA.

It is also one among the pancha karma procedures, commonly proceed after Vamana karma. it is aimed to expell out the pitta predominent doshas through the anal passage, it is safest, and less complicative than Vaman Karma.

## Qualities of Virechana Drugs.

1) Ushna 2) Teekshna 3) Sukshma 4) Vyavayi 5) Vikaasi 6) Predominent basic elements are pruthiwi and Jala. 7) having the effect (Prabhava) of expelling dosas through anal Canal.

**Note :-** Vamana and Virechana drugs are having mostly Similar qualities but oppposite effect is due to the prabhava of the drugs.

## INTRODUCTION OF VIRECHANA DRUGS .
### A) According to Charaka.
1) Best drug of Sukha virechan is Trivruth root
2)      "      mrudu Virechana is Aragwada
3)      "      Teekshna Virechana is Snuhi Ksheera.

**Charaka** - explained in detail about Virechana drugs in Kalpa stana From 7th to 12th chapter ( 6 chapters) and explained 24 5 Virechana Yogas, they are.
a) Shyama Trivruth Yogas 110, b) Snuhi yogas  20, c) Aragwada Yogas 12, d) Tilwaka Yogas 16, e) Sapthala & Shankhini Yogas 39, f) Danthi & Dravanthi yogas 48, in addition to above description Charaka Also given the classification of Virechan drugs as below :-
1) Moolini drugs 2) Phalini drugs 3) Lavan Varga 4) Ksheera Varga 5) Pakwashaya dosha haran dravyas 6) Bhedinee drugs 7) Virechanopaga Varga 8) Pureesha Viraajaneeya 9) Sresta dravyas 10) Virechana dravya sangraha.

## B) ACCORDING OT SUSHRUTHA :-
The Best drug of :
1) Moola Virechan, - Shyama Trivruth  2) Twak Virechan  - Tilwaka 3) Phala Virechana  - hareetaki 4) Taila Virechan -  Erenda Tail  5) Swarasa Virechan - Karavellaka 6) Ksheera Virechan  - Shuni Ksheera.

**Virechan drugs list - by sushrutha & Charaka**.:- Trivruth, Danthi, Dravanthi, Sapthala, Vishanika, Gavaakshi, Snuhi, Swarna ksheeri, Chitrak, Kinihi, Kusha, Kaasha, Tilwaka kampillaka, Ramyak, Patala, Pooga, hareetaki, vibheetaki, Aamalaki, Neelinee, Aaragwada, Erenda, Poothika, Maha Vruksha, Sapthacchada, Jyotismati, Arka, Aavartaki, Vidanga, Lavan, Vacha, Katuki, Drakshna, Yastimadu, Mutra, Ksheera, Karavellaka.

**Important Drugs Commonly used :-**
1) Trivruth 2) Aaragwada 3) tilwaka 4) Snuhi 5) Sapthala 6) shankhni 7) Danthi 8) Dravanthi 9) Erenda Taila 10) hareetaki 11) Yastimadu 12) kakuki 13) Draksha etc.,

**Indications of Virechana.**
1) Jwara 2) Kusta 3) Prameha 4) urdwa Raktha Pitta 5) Bhagandar 6) Arsha 7) Bradhna 8) Pleeha roga 9) Gulma 10) Arbuda 11) Galaganda 12) Grandi 13) Gara Visha 14) Vishoochika 15) Aalasaka 16) Mootra ghata 17) Krimi Kosta 18) Visarpa 19) Pandu 20) Vyanga 21) Shirah Shoola 22) Parshwa shoola 23) udaavartha 24) netra daha 25) Aasya daha 26) hrud roga 27) Neelika 28) Aruchi 29) Netra Srava 30) Nasa srava 31) Haleemaka 32) Swasa 33) kasa 34) Kamala 35) Apachi 36) Apasmara 37) Unmada 38) Vata raktha 39) Yoni dosha 40) Aarthava dosha 41) Timira 42) Udara 43) Avipaka 44) Chardi 45) Visphota 46) Pakwashaya ruja 47) vibanda 48) Vidradhi 49) Shotha 50) Kshatha 51) Dagda Vrana 52) Guda daha 56) Medhra daha 57) Nasa daha 58) Karna daha 59) Aanaha 60) Shleepada 61) Stanya dosha 62) Hrullasa.

**Contra Indications of Virechana.**
1) Kshata guda 2) Guda bramsha 3) Adho Raktha Pitta 4) Langhana 5) Durbala Indria 6) Mandagni 7) Niruha 8) Ajeerna 9) Nava jwara 10) Madatyaya 11) Aadmana 12) Shalyaarditha 13) Abhigatha 14) Ati snigda 15) Ati ruksha 16) Daruna Kosta 17) Kshata Ksheena 18) Ati sthula 19) Ati Krusha 20) Bala 21) Vruddha 22) Shraantha 23) Pippasitha 24) Adwaha 25) Upavasitha 26) Miithuna Prasaktha 27) Adayaan Prasakta 28) Vyayama Praskta 29) Chinta Prasakta 30) Kshaama 31) Garbini 32) Nava prasoota 33) Raja Yakshma 34) Atisar 35) kshuditha 36) Dukhitha 37) Hrudrogi 38) Bhaya bheet.

## DIFFERENT WORDS RELATED TO VIRECHAN BY SARANGADHAR

**1) Anuloman :-**
　　Pureesha, perfectly formed (Pakwa) disintigrated and eliminated out through the anal canal. ex :- hareetaki

**2) Sramsana.**
　　Puresha, imperfectly formed (Apakwa) but forcibly send out side through the anal canal. ex : - Aaragwada

**3) Bhedana.**
　　Acumulated pureesha whether perfectly formed or not, get disintigrated and send out side through the anal canal. ex :- katuki

**4) Rechan.**
　　Pureesha is send out side through the anal canal in fluid form Ex:- Trivruth.

**Virechana Kalpanas :-**
　　The virechan drug can be used in so many forms as follows :-

1) Churna 2) Vati 3) Modak 4) Varti 5) Avaleha 6) Aasava 7) Arista 8) Kwatha 9) Yoosha 10) Yavagu 11) Madya 12) Panak 13) Kseera 14) Takra 15) Dadhi 16) Taila 17) Ghritha 18) Mamsarasa 19) Food preparations 20) Water.

## Virechan - Poorva Karma Procedure.

1) Collectionof requirèd material. 2) Examination of the patient. 3) Preparation of the patient. 4) Fixation of the dosage.

### 1) Collection of Required Material :-

A special well equipped room with furniture, utensils, spittons, bed pans, medicines for Virechana Karma and to treat complicatios, should be collected.

### 2) Examinationof the patient.

Patient should be perfectly examined whether indicated for the therapy or not, the strength of the patient and disease should assess by Asthastana and dashavidha pareeksha etc., suitable drug and dosage for rechana should fix basing on the above factors.

### 3) Preparation of the patient.

Vaman & Samsarjan Krama for 7 days then 8th day rest period, 9-10-11th days again sneha paana, 12-13 14th days for abhyanga and sweda in these day Anabhishyandi pitta vruddhi kara, snigda, drava, ushna, mamsarasa, Amlarasa etc., food items should give, then on 15th day in empty stomach, Virechana therapy should be conducted.

### 4) Fixation of the dosage .

Dosage should be fixed according to the strength of the patient, disease, and digestive capacity etc.,

### According to Sarangdhar.

|                             |                      |
| --------------------------- | -------------------- |
| Decoction perfect dose      | 2 Phala (8 Tola)     |
| Maderate dose               | 1 Phala (4 Tola)     |
| Minimal dose                | 1/2 Phala (2 Tola)   |
| Powder & Paste-perfect dose | 4 Tola               |
| Moderate dose               | 2 Tola               |
| Minimal dose                | 1 Tola.              |

| Sl. No. | Drugs         | Mrudu Kosta   | madyama Kosta    | krura kosta.    |
| ------- | ------------- | ------------- | ---------------- | --------------- |
| 1.      | Erenda sneha  | 1/2 to 2 Tola | 2 to 5 Tola      | 5 to 10 Tola    |
| 2.      | Trivruth      | 1 to 3 Masha  | 3 to 6 Masha     | 1/2 To 1 Tola   |
| 3.      | Draksha       | 1 To 2 Tola   | 2 1/2 To 5 Tola  | 5 To 10 Tola    |
|         | Aragwada      | -do-          | -do-             | -do-            |
|         | Hareetaki     | -do-          | -do-             | -do-            |
| 4.      | Mayaphala     | 1/2 To 1 Rati | 1 To 2 Rati      | 4 to 8 Rati.    |
|         | Snuhi         | -do-          | -do-             | -do-            |
| 5.      | isabgola      | 3 Masha       | 3 To 6 masha     | 1 Tola.         |

**Usage of drugs according to dosha :-**

       1) Vata predominent doshas - Trivruth, Saindhava Lavana, Shuntichurna with Kaanji, 2) Pitta predominent doshas - Trivruth churna and Draksha Kwath. 3) Kapha predominent doshas - Triphala kwatha, Gomutra and Trikatu.

# Virechana - pradhaaana Karma Procedure. (Virechan Therapy)

       1) Induction of Rechana medicine . 2) Service to the patient. 3) Determination of Virechan Vega. 4) Waiting for Adequate, inadequate Or Excessive rechana 5) Complications - Management.

## 1) Induction of Medicine :-

       After perfect preparations when the patient is well prepared physically and mentally, in a good day after worshipping the god, elders, Brahmins etc., in betwween 7 and 8 AM, medicine should be given.

       According to thecondition medicine should be selected for the therapy. Commonly Trivruth churna or.

| Draksha | - | 1 Tola | |
|---|---|---|---|
| Aragwada | - | 1 Tola | + 16 Tola Water |
| hareetaki | - | 1 Tola | Boil it and reduce to |
| Katuki 1/2 | - | 1/2 tola | 1/4, so 4 Tolas decoction is prepared. |

       4 Tolas above compound + 21/2 tola erenda taila
+ 4 Rati Icchabhedhi rasa - is given orally to the patient.

## 2) Service to the Patient.

       After intake of medicine, due to its taste odour and effect there is every possibility of Vomitings so only patient should be advised to Wash the face with Cold water, hot water gargling and intake, chewing and application of Flavoured items and Wearing Or inhaling Flowers etc.,

## 3) Determination of Virechan Vega.

       After drug administartion Virechana vega will start if not repeatedly hot water should be given and mrudu sweda at abdomin should do for the activation of the therapy.

1)      If Virechana doesnt occur on the day, medicine should not give again and in the evening normal diet should give.
2)      The next day medicine should give again.
3)      If Second day also Virehan doesn't occur, by giving 10 days gap Virechana should conduct with sneha ,sweda, vaman etc., procedures.
4)      Care should be taken to collect the expelled matter spearately for the assessment.
5)      For the adequate Virechana therapy pureesha pitta and kapha has to come gradually (Kaphaantha).
6)      While counting the number of vegas the first 2-3 vegas should be avoided.

7) Number of Virechan Vegas for perfect moderate and minimal should be 30-20 and 10 Respectively.

8) Quantity of rechana for perfect moderate andminimal should be 4 Prasta 3 prasta and 2 praste respectively.

9) The vegas should start and stop naturally, after the appearance of adequate symptoms, if drug residue present that should be Vomited by Giving madanphala + Vacha + Saindhava lavana compound.

### 4) Obseravation of Symptoms.

### a) Adequate symptoms of Virechana.

Srotoshuddhi, Indria prasannata, Laghutwa, Vatanulomana, Agni deepana, niramatwa, Kaphaantha Virechana 30-20-10- times of Vega (Pravara - madyama aavara), 4,3,2, prasta pureesha (pravara, madyama, Avara), Absence or Ayoga Or Atiyoga Lakshana, and elimination of doshas in time.

### b) In Adequate symptoms of Virechana.

Vata pitta Kapha prakopa, Agnimandya, Gourava, pratishyaya, Tandra, Chardi, Aruchi, Vata Pratilomana, Daha, kukshi hrudaya Ashuddhi, kandu, Vibanda, mutrasanga, Piticha.

### c) Excessive Symptoms of Virechana.

Vata Pitta Kapha Kshaya, Supti, Angamarda, Klama, Vepadu, Nidra, Dourabalya, Tama Pravesha, unmada, apasmara, hiccough, murcha, Gudabramsha, shoola, Trushna, Brama, Rakta Kshaya and medokshaya.

### 5) Complication .

Aadmana, parikarthika, Srava, hrudgraha, Gatragraha, Raktha pitta, Vibramsha, Stambha, Klama, upadrava.

# Pashchyat karma.
# Post Virechan Regiment.

Except Dhoomapana rest of the method is as like Vamana.

### Virechanottaa karma.
If vasti has togive.

7 days samsarjankram. 8th day rest 9th day Anuvasan Vasti, 3 days food with Jaangala mamsa then Niruha Vasti has to give.

# VASTI KARMA

Vasti Karma is themost important therapy in pancha Karma Procedures, with vivid scope of applicability, It is said as the special treatment for Vata dosha (for pitta Kapha and Rakta also ) it is having the effect of Samshodha, Samshaman, Anabolic, catabolic, restoration of semen etc., dhatus, improves vision, lustre, strength and health, So only given utmost importance in pancha karma procedures and said it is the HALF of the or WHOLE of the treatment.

The word vasti is derived From the vasti Tantra (animal urinary bladder) which is used to introduce the medicated materials through rectum, urethra and Vagina etc.,

## Classification of Vasti Karma.

1) Anatomical classification (adhistana bhed)
a) Pakwashaya gath (Through rectum into Pakwashaya) b) Garbhashaya gath (through Vagina into uterus) c) Mutra Shaya gath (Urethro Vesical) d) Vrana gath (tor wound Or abscess).

2) Pharmaceutical Classification (Dravya bhed)
a) Niruha Vasti Or Aastapan Vasti Or kashaya vasti b) Anuvasan Vasti Or Sneha Vasti.

3) Pharmacological classification (Karma bhed)

I) According to Sushrutha
a) Shodhana Vasti  - It is used to expell the doshas Forcibly.
b) Snehan Vasti :- It is used for Oleation effect - ( Anuvasan Vasti).
c) Lekhan Vasti :- It is used to scrape out medho dhathu Or Kapha dosha.
d) Brumhan Vasti :- It is used to nourish the saptha dhathu (Anabolic activity).

II) According to Vagbhata.
a) Uthkleshan Vasti - It increases the quantity of dosha Or mala.
b) Dosha hara Vasti. :- It is like shodhan Vasti in which doshas are expelled out.
c) Shaman Vasti. :- It suppressess the propogated Or vitated doshas.

III) According to Sarangdhar.
a) Uthkleshan Vasti - it increases the quantity of dosha Or mala. b) Dosha hara Vasti - it is  shodhan Vasti in which doshas are expelled out. c) Shaman Vasti- it suppress the vitated Or propogated doshas. d) Shodhan Vasti- Doshas expelled out Forcibly. e) Lekhan Vasti - it is used to scrape out medo dhathu or Kapha. f) Brumhan Vasti.- Nourishes the dhatus g) Pischila Vasti - Vasti given with sticky items to control Atisara like disorders. h) Deepan Vasti - it is used to regularise the intensity of jatharagni.

IV) According ot Charak.
a) Vataghna Vasti - Controls Vitated Vata dosha b) Bala Varna Kruth- Gives strength and Colour complexion c) Snehan Vasti _ like anuvasan Vasti. d) Shukrakruth - Increases semen. e) Krimighna Vasti - Destructs Krimi. f) Vrushatwa kruth - Increases sex potency.

## 4) Classification of Vasti Based on Number of Vasti.
a) Karma Vasti - 30 Vasti b) Kala Vasti 16 Vasti given. c) Yoga Vasti 8 Vasti should be given.

## 5) Different words used for Vasti.
1) Shodhana Vasti 2) Shaman Vasti 3) Lekhana Vasti 4) Uthkleshan Vasti 5) Brumhana Vasti 6) Karshan Vasti. 7) Rasayan Vasti 8) Vaji Karan Vasti 9) Snehan Vasti 10) Chakshushya Vasti 11) Sangraahi Vasti 12) Varna Prasadan Vasti 13) Karma Vasti 14) Kala Vasti 15) Yoga Vasti 16) Aastapan Vasti 17) Anuvasan Vasti 18) Matra Vasti 19) Yapan Vasti 20) Siddha Vasti 21) Prasrutha Yougika Vasti 22) Dwadash Prasruth vasti 23) Madhu tailkika Vasti 24) Pada heena Vasti 25) Mrudu Vasti 26) Pischila Vasti 27) Teekshna Vasti 28) Raktha Vasti 29) Ksheera Vasti 3)) yuktha ratha Vasti 31) Deepan Vasti 32) Krimighna Vasti 33) Dosha hara vasti.

# I) Aastaapan Vasti Or Niruha Vasti Or Kashaya Vasti :-

Niraha Vasti - Treat the diseases.
Aastaapan Vasti - Restores aging process
kashaya Vasti - Decoction predominent medicines used in this type.

## Example :-

a)  Madhu tailika vasti - Honey Oil are Basic elements of the medicine (honey 2 prasruthi, taila 3 prasruthi, Kwatha 4 prasruth, Kalka 1 prasruthi,
b)  Yaapan Vasti- restores aging and causes Aayur Vruddhi - (ch.Si. 12-5)
c)  Siddha Vasti -Gives strength colour complexion and treats thedisease - (Ch. si -10-3
d)  Yukta ratha vasti -given even in journeys
e)  prasruth yougika Vasti -8 Tolas (1 Prasruthi) medicine is given  (Ch. SI 8-2)
    Ex. Ksheera Vasti, Taila Prasanna vasti.
    Patoladi Vasti - Vidangadi Vasti.
f)  Dwadasha Prasruthi Vasti (Su. Chi 37-30)
    12 Prasruthi (96 Tolas) Medicine is used Ex madhu tailika Vasti.
g)  Pada heena Vasti - 9 Prasruti (72 Tolas) medicine is used (Su. chi. 38-118
h)  Teekshna Vasti (su. Chi. 35 -10 )
i)  Mrudu vasti            "      "
j)  Pischila (sangrahi ) Vasti - (Cha. Chi. 19-64 to 68)
k)  Pischila (Sangrahi ) Vasti - (Cha.Si. 8 to 26 )
                                6 to 83

**Note :-** The dosage of Aastapana Vasti is 12 Prasruthi = 96 Tolas (in general)

## II) Anuvasan Vasti Or sneha Vasti.

It can be given daily and dosen't cause any complications if retained in thebody so only named as Anuvasan Vasti, in the combination of medicines Oily drugs are predominently used so also named as sneha Vasti.

It can be named as follows according to dosage.

a)  Sneha Vasti Dosage
    1/4th of Niruha Vasti  $= \dfrac{12 \text{ prasruthi}}{4}$    =    3 prasruthi
                                                 =    24 Tolas.

B)  Anuvasan Vasti dosage
    1/2 of Sneha Vasti  $= \dfrac{3 \text{ Prasruthi}}{2}$    =    1 1/2 Prasruti
                                             =    12 Tolas.

c)  Matra Vasti dosage
    1/2 of Anuvasn Vasti $= 1 \dfrac{1/2 \text{ Prasruthi}}{2}$   =    6 tolas

## III) Karma Vasti.

Total 30 Vasties are given
among them 18 Anuvasan Vasti and 12 Niruha Vasti.

First anuvasan Vasti is given then Niruha Vasti, like this 12 Anuvasan and 12 Niruha Vasti should give and at last 6 anuvasan vasti should be given.

## IV) Kala Vasti :-

Total 16 Vasties are given among them 10 Anuvasan Vasti and 6 Niruha Vasti

First Anuvasan Vasti is given then Niruha Vasti, like this 6 Anuvasan and 6 Niruha Vasti should be given and at last 4 anuvasan vasti should be given.

## v) Yoga Vasti.

Total 8 Vasties are given, among them 5 anuvasan Vasti and 3 Niruha Vasti
First Anuvasan Vasti then Niruha Vasti like this 3 Anuvasan 3 Niruha Vati should give, at last 2 Anuvasan Vasti should be given.

## Indications of Niruha Vasti.:-

1) Ekanga and Sarvanga roga 2) Kukshi roga 3) Vata, mutra, Pureesha and shukra, Sanga (Retention) 4) Bala Mamsa Shukra and dosha Kshaya 5) Aadmana 6) Anga Supthi 7) Krumi Kosta. 8) Udaavartha 9) Atisara 10) Paarshwa bhed 11) Abhitapa 12) Pleeha dosha 13 Gulma 14) Shoola 15) hrudroga 16) Bhagandara 17) unmada 18) Jwara 19) Bradhna 20) Shirah, Karna, hrudaya, Paarshwa, prushta and Kati shoola 21) Kampa 22) Aakshepa 23) Anga gourava 24) Laghutwa 25) Kshaya 26) Vishamaagni 27) Spik janu Jangha Uru Gulpha Paarshwa Prapada Yoni Bahu Anguli stana Nakha and dantha shoola. 28) Sopha 29) Stambha 30) Antra Koojana 31) Parikartika 32) Vata Vyadhi 33) Jwara 34) Timir 35) Pratishaya 36) Adhimantha 37) Arditha 38) Pakshaghaatha 39) Ashmari 40) Upadamsha 41) Vata Raktha 42) Arsha 43) Stanya Kshaya 44) Manya Graha 45) Hanu graha 46) Moodha garbha 47) Mutra Kruchra.

## Contra Indications of Niruha Vasti.

1) Ajeerna 2) Atisneha 3) Peeta sneha 4) uthklista doshas 5) Alpagni 6) Klama 7) Durbala 8) Kshudhitha 9) Trushnartha 10) Shramaartha 11) Krusha 12) Bhukthaabhaktha 13) Peetodaka 14) Vaamitha 15) Viriktha 16) Krutha Nasya 17) Kruddha 18) Bheetha 19) Mattha 20) Morrchtha 21) chardi Praskta 22) Nishteevana Prasakta 23) Swasa prasakta 24) Kasa Prasakta 25) Hikka Prasakta 26) Baddha gudodara 27) Chidro daru 28) Jalodars 29) Aadmaana 30) Alasaka 31) Vishuchika 32) Aamadosha 33) Aama Atisara 34) prameha 35) Kusta 36) Arsha 37) Paandu 38) Brama 39) arochak 40) Unmada 41) Shoka grasta 42) Sthoulya 43) Kantha sosha 44) Kshatha Ksheena 45) Garbini 46) Bala 47) Vruddha 48) Guda sotha 49) Shopha 50) Alpa Varcha.

## Indications of anuvasan Vasti.

All the indications of Niruha are also indicated for anuvasan, additionally
1) Ati ruksha 2) Vata vyadhi 3) Teekshnagni

## Contra Indications of Anuvasan Vasti.

1) All Contra indications of Niruha Vasti 2) Abhukta bhaktha 3) Nava jwara 4) Pandu 5) Kamala 6) Prameha 7) Arsha 8) Pratishyaya 9) Arochaka 10) Mandaagni 11) Durbala 12) Pleehodara 13) Kaphodara 14) urustamba 15) Atisara 16) Visha Peetha 17) Gara peetha 18) Vishyandi 19) Guru Kostha 20) Shleepada 21) Gala ganda 22) Apachi 23) Krimi Kosta 24) Prameha 25) Kusta 26) Sthoulya 27) Peenasa 28) Krusha.

## Vasti Yantra :-

It is the instrument used to introduce the medicine in to Rectum or urethra or Vagina, it contain 2 parts 1) Vasti Netra 2) Vasti Putaka.

## Vasti Netra :-

It is the metalic tube (Prepared with gold, Silver Copper lead, Tin, Brooze, long, bones, horn, elephant teeth,stainless steel etc.,) Root is bigger and apex is smaller in diameter. to which vasti putaka (Bladder) is attahced, the size depends upon the age and method, vasti netra should be perfect without errors like hraswa, deergha, Tanu, sthula jeerna, shithila, paarshwa Chidra, Vakra etc.,

## Vasti Putak :-

It is an elastic bag used to collect the drug and pressed while the therapy to introduce the medicine into rectum or uterus etc., through vasti Netra, in Olden days perfectly purified urinary bladder is used, but now adays Rubber bladders are available for the usage vasti putaka should be without the errors like Vishama, Mamsala, Chidrayuktha, sthoola, Jalayuktha, vatala, Snigda and Klinna. (Anema cans, bigger syrenges also used.)

# VASTI KARMA PROCEDURE

## 1) Poorva Karma.

The following factors should be considered in Poorva Karma, they are.
1) Dosha (Humors) 2) Aushadhi (Medicine)
3) Desha (climate) 4) Kala (season) 5) Saatmya (Adaptability) 6) Agni (Digestive capacity)
7) Satwa (Pasychic state) 8) Oka (adaptations) 9) Vaya (age) 10) Bala (Strength)
**1) Dosha :-** (Its influence in the Selection of vasti) Vasti is given in Vata Predominent disease.
a) In dosha kshaya :- Brumhan, Balya, Varnya, uthkleshan Vasti should give.
b) In dosha Vruddhi :- Dosha hara,shodhan, Teekshna Vasti should give. c) Rasagatha dosha :- Langhan, paachan chikitsa. d) Raktha gatha dosaha :- Shaman, Varnya, Balya, Rakta Vasti. e) Mamsa gatha dosha :- Kshara, agni Karma, Lekhan Brumhan Vasti. f) medo gatha dosha :- Lekhana, Karshan, Vasti. g) Astigatha dosha : - Ghritha, Ksheera Vasti. h) Majjagatha dosha :- shaman, Brumhana Vasti. i) Shukra gatha dosha :- Vaajikaran Vasti. j) In Aama dosha vasti is contra indicated.
**Note :-** According to Rasa and other symptoms also Vasti can be planned.

## 2) Aushadhi - (Drugs).

Drug composition should be planned according to the diagnosis, strength of the disease, patient and digestive capacity etc.,

The drug should not be Aamata, heenata, Atimatra, Atisheeta, ati ushna, ati teekshna, ati mrudu, ati snigda, ati Ruksha, ati sandra and ati drava etc.,

## 3) Desha (Climates - influence).

a) Bhumi desha (jangala, Anupa, Sadaran)
b) Aatura (Patients body constituion)

365

### 4) Kala .

Vaman after 15 days Virechana, after 7 days Niruha, after 9th day Anuvasan.
**Vagbhat :-** After Virechan 7th day to 15th day Anuvasan then Niruha should give atrernatively

### 5) Satmya :- (Adaptability)

Niruha Vasti should give on empty stomach (after fully digested but not in hungry state).

### 6) Agni :- In mandagni Niruha Vasti is contraindicated.
### 7) Satwa :(Mind)

The dosage of drug or tolerance of pain during the therapy can be judged according to knowledge of pravara madyama and Avara satwa of thepatient.

8) Oka Saatmya ( Adaptations developed by habbit etc., ) By this the proper indications and selection of the drug can be assessed.

### 9) VAYAS (AGE)

Dosage, size of Vastiyantra, time and duration can be assesed.

### 10) Bala (Strength of the Patient).

Selection of type of the therapy dosage and duration can be assessed by the strength of the patient.

## DOSAGE OF NIRUHA VASTI.

| SI. | Age | Dosage in prasruthi | Dosage in tolas |
|---|---|---|---|
| 1. | 1 to 12 Years yearly 1/2 prasruthi increases | 1 Yr = 1/2 Prasruti, 12th Yr = 6 Prasruthi, | 4 Tola 48 Tola |
| 2. | 12 to 18 Years Yearly 1 Prasruthi Increase. | 18 th Year = 12 Prasruthi | 96 Tola |
| 3. | 18 to 70 Years | 12 Prasruthi | 96 Tolas |
| 4. | After 70 Years | 10 Prasruthi | 80 Tolas. |

The common Niruha dosage of an adult is 12 Prasruti = 96 Tolas.

### Pradaana Karma of Vasti :-
a) Vasti Pranidana
b) Vasti Pratyagamana - Nireekshan
c) samyak yoga, Asamyak Yoga etc.

### a) Vasti Pranidanam (Induction of Medicine).

1) Abhyanga (local and genral) 2) Swedan (Local and general) 3) Vasti Yantra Preparation and filling the medicine for induction. 4) Patient should lie down on leftside with left lower extremity is straight and right lower extremity flexed on knee and hip joint 5) Patient is asked to take deep breath during the induction of medicines. 6) Shivering of hands should be avoided as it may injure the anal region. 7) Quick Or slow induction of Vasti is not advisable

8) Total medicine should not introduce into Pakwashaya in order to avoid entry of Vayu into Pakwashaya which may produce pain. 9) Vasti tube should be pulled out immmediately after introduction of medicine. 10) Patient should remain lying in the same posture for 1/2 minute. 11) After that patient should take up utkatakassan to eliminate mala vegas.

## B) VASTI PRATYAAGAMANA KALA.

Duration of elimination of Vasti is known as Pratyagaman Kala, that is 1 Muhurtha (48 Minutes). If vasti does not come in 1 muhurtha the patient may die or get severe pain with following complications a) Kosta aadmana b) pakwashaya shoola c) Mutra shoola d) Vata Pratiloma e) Cardiac pain f) Vistambha g) Arati h) jwara.

**If Vasti doesnt come out intime. :-** 1) Teekshna vasti 2) phala varthi 3) Katisweda, 4) udara sweda 5) Producing fear complexion 6) Giving rechan

**Adequate features of vasti (samyak yoga) :-**

1) Natural Elimination of Vasti without extra stimulations (Prasrusta VitKatha). 2) Normal urination (prasrusta mutrata) 3) Normal elimination of Flattus (Prasrusta Vatata) 4) Elimination of Mala, Pitta, Kapha and Vata in Order. 5) Lightness in the body 6) Good appetite 7) Good taste in eating. 8) lightness in pakwashya, mutrashaya etc., 9) Control of the disease (ringa Nivruthi) 11) Improvement of health.

**In Adequate Features of Vasti (Asmyak Yoga )**

1) Severe pain in different parts. 2) Oedema 3) Rhinitis 4) Cutting pain at anal region. 5) nausea 6) Retention of Flattus 7) Retention of urine 8) Dyspnoea 9) Improper elimination of Vasti 10) Loss of taste 11) Heavyness of body.

**Features of Excessive Vasti (Ati Yog).**

1) Body pain 2) Debility 3) Tiredness (Klama) 4) Tremors (kampa) 5) Sleep mood 6) Giddiness 7) Hiccough 8) Mental disturbances (Unmada) 9) Drowsiness 10) Features of Virechan ati yoga.

# Post Vasti Regimen  (Vasti Pashchyath Karma )

1) After introduction of Niruha Vasti within one muhurtha Vasti vega has to come out with adequate features.

If the medicine only come out immediately, second Niruha vasti can be given, Even though adequate Features are not seen 3rd 4th 5th Niruha vasti should not give, that causes Pakwashaya shotha, so After 2nd Niruha Vasti sneha vasti should give, then only Niruha vasti can be given for the adequate features and health.

**2) Pathya.**

1) Rest 2) Warm Water bath.

3) Milk, dalsoup (Yoosha) and jangala mamsarasa should give according to the strength, digestive capacity and doshic condition of the patient.

**According ot Sushruth.**

a) in Vata dosha-Mamsa rasa b) Pitta dosha-Milk c) Kapha dosh -Yoosha should give.

**Note :-** 1) Light diet, (1/3 of normal diet ) should give. 2) In the same evening only anuvasan Vasti should give. The Following Activities should be avoided after Vasti karma.

1) Excessive sitting, standing, travelling and talking.

2) Avoid day sleeping, coitus, suppression of natural urges, Cold, sunlight, anxiety, anger, untimely food and incompatible food.

**Vasti Vyapad :- Complications of Vasti.**

a) Vasti Netra vyapath complications due to incorrect Vasti netra.

| | Vasti Netra dosha | Complications. |
|---|---|---|
| 1) | Smaller | Drug doesnt enter upto Pakwashaya |
| 2) | Lengthy | Spreads to deeper parts |
| 3) | Thin | Pain to rectum. |
| 4) | Thick | Irritation to rectum. |
| 5) | Destructed | Pain to rectum. |
| 6) | Improper adjoining of Neta with Putaka | medicine comes out side |
| 7) | Perforations. | Pain to rectum. |
| 8) | Irregular | Improper entry of Medicine. |

b) Vasti Putak Vyapad (Complications of Vasti Putak) :- Urinary bladder (of animal,) rubber bladder etc.,

| | Vasti Putkaa dosha | Vyapad. |
|---|---|---|
| 1) | Vishama Vasti | Medicine goes in other directions. |
| 2) | Mamsala Vasti | Bad smell produced in the bladder. |
| 3) | Chidra yuktha Vasti | leakage of medicine. |
| 4) | Sthoola Vasti | Difficulty in induction of Medicine, |
| 5) | jala Yuktha | leakage of Medicine. |
| 6) | Vatala Vasti | Foam Production in the Medicine. |
| 7) | Atisnigda Vasti | Slipping while induction of Medicine. |
| 8) | Ati Klinna Vasti | Difficulty for holding. |

## c) Vasti Pranetha Vyapad (Complications of Vasti)

due to untrained or unexperienced person who gives vasti).

1) Savaatha Vasti daan (If complete medicine is introduced without residue, air also enters and causes pain and discomfort in Anus and Pakwashaya. Pakwashaya Abhyanga, Mrudu Sweda to rectum may relieve the problem.

2) Drutha praneetha Vasti Vyapad.

quick and irrelavantly introducing and removing the Vasti Netra causes pain, discomfort, dysuria, rigidity and Lumbar pains, Vata hara chikitsa has to give.

### 3) Tiryak Pranidaan.

Improper introducing of Vasti netra, drugs doesnt enter properly so cannot get the adequate results.

### 4) Ulluptha Dattha Vasti :-

Vasti putaka should press carefully, at a time without gaping and pressure variations, If not leads to vata prakopa and need Vata hara Chikitsa

**5) Sa Kampa Vasti Daan:-**
Should not shake or move the hands during the drug administration.

**6) Ati Praneetha Vasti :-**
Introducing of Vasti netra into deeper levels, causes ulceration and pain in the rectum.

**7) Ati Bahya, Atimanda Datta Vasti :-**Introducing of Vasti netra superficially and slowly. The medicine cann't reach Pakwashaya properly.

**8) Ativega Datta Vasti:-** By Introducing vasti netra very quickly - Medicine enters more deeply and causes adverse reactions.

**Note :-** After the Vasti administration Patient Should relax by raising the Anal region by putting some pillow to prevent the back flow of vasti dravya, and other vatic dosorders.

**Other Complications of Vasti :-** 12 in number they are.
1) Ayoga 2) Atiyoga 3) Klama 4) Aadman 5) Hiccough 6) Hruthprapthi 7) urdwaprathi 8) Pravahika 9) Shiroaarthi 10) Angaarthi 11) Parikarthika 12) Parisrava.

# Anuvasan Vasti.

1) Anuvasan Vasti is contra indicated in Kapha predominent, medo dosha, Aama dosha and in shodhan indicated disorders. 2) In Hemantha, Shishira and Vasantha ruthu Anuvasan Vasti should give in day time, and in sharath, greeshma and Varsha rutu in early nights. 3) It is administered immediately after meals.

4)     In Kapha dosha     -     1 to 3 Vasti.
         In Pitta dosha      -     5 to 7 Vasti,
         In Vata dosha      -     9to 11 Vasti should give.

5) Except in Vata predominent diseases Anuvasan Vasti should accompany Niruha Vasti for adequate results. 6) After elimination of male matra vaga only Anavasan Vasti should give. 7) After drug administration, the drug can reside for 12 o 24 hours, if drug cannot come even after 24 hours Teekshna Vasti or phala Varthi should give for the elimination. of the drug. 8) Rest of the therapy is as like Niruha Vasti.

**Complication of Anuvasan Vasti:-**
1) Sneha Vata Aavrutha 2) Pitta Aavrutha 3) Kapha Aavruth 4) Anna Aaavrutha 5) Pureesha Aavruth 6) Complication of Vasti if given empty stomach.

# Uttara Vasti.

Vasti if given through urethra Or Vagina, is known as uttara vasti.
DOSAGE OF DRUG :- 1/2 Phala Or 2 Tola.
According to sushruth = 1 Prasruthi, but for Garbhashaya shodhan = 2 Prasruti

**Indications :-** in most of urinary, vaginal and uterine disorders
**Note :-** 1) In Ladies for Garbhashaya shodhan the vasti should give in Rutukala, after 4 days of menstrual cycle.
2) If the given medicine is Oil predominent, the rules of Anuvaasan should follow,if decoction predominent medicine is given, the rules of Niruha Vati should follow.

# DHOOMA PANA

1) It is a special therapy to treat Kaphaj disorders of shiro Gala nasa, Karna, Vaksha (Chest) and Deha (General). Ex :- Pratisyaya, Shirashoola, Galaroga, Mukha roga Kasa, Swasa etc.,

2) It is a Pashcyat Karma to Nasya and Gandoosha, to scrape the kapha dosha which is sticked to the srotas.

Taking of medicated smoke either through the mouth or Nose and releasing it through mouth is called Dhooma pana, It is very quick and effective treatment for Kapha roga.

**Classification :-**
**1) According to Charaka** - 3 Types they are.
    a) Prayogika Or shaman dhooma Pana.
    b) Virechanika Dhooma Pana c) Snehika Dhooma Pana
**2) According to Sushrutha :-** 5 Types they are
a) Prayogika b) Virechanika c) Snehika d) kasaghna e) Vamaneeya Dhooma pana
**3) According to Vagbhata :-** 3 types, they are
a) Snigdha Dhooma Pana (Vata hara)
b) Madyama Dhooma Pana (Vata Kapha haram)
c) Teekshna Dhooma Pana (kapha haram)
**4) According to Sarangdhara and Bhavamishra :-** 6 types they are
a) Shaman b) Virechan c) Brumhan d) kasahara e) Vamak f) Vrana Dhoopana.

**1) Prayogika Dhooma Pana - Or Shaman Dhooma Pana.**
    Eladigana dravyas except kusta and Tagaru should parste on 12" length, Shara Kanda which is covered with silk cloth, upto 8" level it should be dried in shade then shara kanda should be removed the 8" medicated varthi should use for dhooma pana.

**2) Snehika Dhooma Pana**
    Varthi should prepare with Erenda, devadaru, madooschista sarja ras guugulu varthi should prepared for Dhooma pana.
**3) Virechanika Dhooma Pana:-**
    Varthi should prepare with shiro Virechana drugs like vidanga and has to use for Dhooma pana.
**4) Kasaghna Dhooma Pana.**
    Dhooma Varthi should prepare with Bruhathi, Kantakari, Trikatu, Kasamarda, Hingu, Guduchi, Karkataka Shrungi.etc drugs.
**5) Vamaneeya Dhooma Pana :-**
    Dhooma Varthi should prepare with snayu, Twak, horns, bones, dried fish, meat and insects Or with Vamaka dravyas.
**6) Vrana Dhoopana Varthi** should prepare with Vrana ropana dravyas.

## Indicatios of Dhooma Panam :-

Shiro gurutwa, shirashoola, peenasa, Arthavabhedak, Karnashoola, Netra shoola, kasa, Swasa, hiccough, Galagrah, chaladantha, Mukhapaka, Puthi Vakthratha, karnaroga, nasa roga, Aruchi, Manyastamba, hanugraha, Kandu, Swarabheda, Galashundi, Upajihwak, Khalithya, Phalitha, Indraluptha, kshavathu, Tandra, moha, Atinidra etc.,

## Contra Indications of Dhooma Panam :-

Pitta prakopa, Raktha Prakopa, Raktha Pitta, Bala (children), Vrudha (Old), garbini, sosha, murcha, Brama, Trushna, Kshathaksheena, Ruksha gathra, Talusosha, Mukhasosha, Shoka, bhaya, krodha, daha, the persons who undergone snehapana, Vasti, Virechana etc., are not Indicated for dhooma panam.

## Dhooma Pana Yantra .

It is prepared with Gold Silver Copper Bross etc., metals, it is tube like structure to which dhooma varthi is attached. The length of Dhooma Pana Yantra is as follows :-

| | | |
|---|---|---|
| For Prayogika Dhooma | - | 48 " |
| Virechanika | - | 24 " |
| Snehika | - | 32 " |
| Varnak Kasaghna | - | 16 " |
| Vrana Dhoopana | - | 8 " |

## Dhooma Pana Vidhi :-

The patient should be relax without any tensions and should sit for dhooma pana . Though medicated smoke is taken through mouth or nose it should be released through the mouth only.

| Name of Dhooma | Route of Dhooma Pana |
|---|---|
| 1) Prayogika | Should take through nose. |
| 2) Snehika | Mouth and Nose. |
| 3) Virechanika | Nose |
| 4) Kasaghna | Mouth |
| 5) Vamak | Mouth |
| 6) Vrana Dhoopana | The smoke is exposed to Vrana. with dhooma netra. |

The smoke is taken 3 to 4 times upto Salivation, lacrimation and Nasal discharge.

## Time schedule for Dhooma Pana:-

A) According to charak 8 Times for prayogika dhooma they are
1) After bath 2) After meals 3) After Vaman 4) After sneeze 5) After tooth brushing 6) After nasya 7) After anjana 8) After sleeping
" 9 Times in each time smoke has to take (Slight break should give after 3 times)."

## b) Sushrutha's Description :-

12 Times - In general for 3 types of dhooma pana they are.
1) After sneezing 2) After brushing of teeth 3) After Nasya 4) After bath 5) After meals
6) After Vaman 7) After sleeping 8) After coitus. 9) After going to toilet 10) After laughing 11) After Anger 12) After surgery.
c) Vagbhata explained 8 times in general for dhooma pana they are.

a) After 1) Hungry 2) Yawning 3) Deficatin 4) Coitus 4) Surgery 6) Laugh 7) Brushing of teeth 8) Urination- Mrudu dhooma (Snehika dhooma Pana ) has to give

b) above 8 times and 9) at nights 10) After meals 11) After Nasya in Madyama dhooma

c) After sleeping Nasya Anjan bath and vaman, Teekshna dhooma has give .

## Samyakyoga Lakshanas of Dhooma Pana :-

1) Lightness in throat Chest and head. 2) Indria and hrudaya niirmalya. 3) Controle of the disease. 4) Sound sleep 5) Normal appetite

## Heena Yoga of Dhooma Pana :-

Improper Elimination of Kapha from throat, head, nose, and sinuses; heaviness of head, lazyness, voice problems (hoarsness) and Uncontrolled disease.

## Aityoga of Dhooma Pana :-

Burning sensation in throat, palate, nose, and head; thirst, dryness of oro-pharyngeal and laryngeal mucosa, Bleeding from mouth and nose, vertigo, delirium, debility, sensory nerve damage may cause the problems like deafness - blindness, anosmia, tastelessness and loss of sensation.

## Complications :-

1) Indriopaghatha (Blind, deaf, anosmia, loss of Sensation,speach problems. etc).
2) Bleeding disorders 3) Vertigo 4) Delirium
5) Raktha and pitta Complications.

## Uses of Dhooma Panam :-

Prayogika dhooma reduces Vata & Kapha disorders, snehika dhooma controls Vata disorders and Virechanika dhooma controls Kapha disroders.

The uses are Indria shuddi and drudatwa, Vak shuddhi, Mukha Shuddhi, Drusti prasadana, and strength to Kesha Smashru and dantha.

The person who takes Dhooma pana regularly get relief from Kasa Swas Arochaka, Mukhalep, Swarabhed, Mukha srava, Tandra, Nidra, Peenasa, Kshavathu, Shiroroga, Karnaroga, Akshi roga, hanu and Manya roga.

## RAKTHA MOKSHANA .

## Synonyms :-

Raktha Mokshana, Rakthanirharan, Rakthasravana,
Rakthaharan, Shonitha Mokshan, Asra Visruti

It is a blood letting process especially mentioned in the Raktha and Pitta dsorders. Charaka and his followers didnot include Raktha mokshan in Pancha karma But sushrutha added it in panchakarma. The other panchakarma measures are designed to eliminate vitiated doshas But Rakthamokshan aimed to eliminate raktha with pitta. It is a very quick and most Fruitful therapy among all But also causes more comlications if improperly handled.

372

**Features of Raktha.**

1) Visrata (Haemic smell due to pruthwi), 2) Dravata (Liquidity due to apa), 3) Raaga (Redness due to agni), 4) Shyandan (mobility due to Vayu), 5) Laghuta (Lightness due to Aakash),

The colour of normal Raktha is compared to the padmaka Laksha and Gunja and when it is vitiated by doshas it discolours in to other
Ex :- In Vata vitiation blackish red.

**Functions of Raktha :-**

1) Jeevana (Life,) 2) Balya (gives strength). 3) Aayushya (longetivity of life). 4) Dhathu pusti (Gives strength to dhatu) 5) Nourishes the mamsa dhatu 6) Promotes tectile sensation and other special senses. 7) Deha sthiratha and dharana (for proper body built). 8) jatharagni Preraka (Stimulates the agni). 9) Gives colour complexion to Skin. 10) It is the prime cause for all systems to regulate properly.

**Vitiating Factors of Raktha .**

1) Suppresing the natural urges (Vagavarodha). 2) By improper food and habits (midyaahara Vihara). 3) Mental disturbances (mano Klesha) 4) Abhighata (injuries) 5) Krimi (Worm infestation or infection) 6) Shrama (Physical strain) 7) Aatapa Sevana (Exposure to Sun Stroke). 8) Avashyaya ( Exposure to moist). 9) Agni Mandya 10) Ajeerna 11) Intake of Abhishyanda Padartha like dadhi, Kanji, Masha, tila, Madya, Kuluttha etc., 12) Adyashan (Intake of more bulk Food) 13) Ajeernashan (in take of un digested materials) 14) Sleeping immediately after meals. 15) In take Viruddhahara 16) In take of more oily, rough, Hot, Cool, Spicy, Salt, sour , Itmes 17) Not indulging Raktha Mokshan, in Sharat rutu - by above factors Raktha vitiates and causes Rakthaja Vyadhies.

**Note :-** If the vitiation of Raktha is not treated in time causes Raktha Pradoshaj Vyadhies like - Kusta, Visarpa, Swara kshaya, Pitica, mada, Vyvarnya, Kamala, Vata Raktha, Switra, kandu, Kotha, Raktha Pitta, Asrugdhara, Guda Paka, Upajihwak, Rakthatwak, Ratha netra, Raktha Mutrata, Arsha, Medhra Paka, Pleeha vruddhi, Gulma, Vidradi, Aruchi, Puthinasa, Aasya Dourgandhya, Upakusha, Mukha Paka, Asramandala, Pipasa, Gurgatra, Shirashoola, Swedan, Shareera dourgandhya, shiro roga, indraluptha, Mukha roga, Brama, murcha, Sanyasa, Kshudraroga and Charmaroga etc., in above diseases Raktha mokshana is the proper therapy.

**Contra Indication :-**

1) Sarvanga Shopha 2) Debility 3) Pregnancy 4) Sosha 5) Anaemia 6) Children 7) The Old 8) Patients of Pandu, Arsha, udara and Kshaya.

## Classification of Raktha Mokshan.

1) Shastra Krutha Visravana
(Blood letting with metalic instruments)
     a) pracchana (incisions) b) Sira Vyadana (Veine Puncutre)

2) Anushastra Krutha Visravana.
(Blood letting with other than metalic instruments).
     a) Shrunga (application of Cow's horn for aspiration)
     b) Jalauka (application of leeches).
     c) Alaabu (Application of Alaabu for Cupping)
     d) Ghati Yantra (Cupping glass application.)

## Raktha Mokshan Prayog Bheda :-

Indication of different types of Raktha Moksham, Based on Dosha Raktha and strength of the patient.

| Sl. No. | Name | Charak | Sushruta | Vagbhata. |
|---|---|---|---|---|
| 1) | Shrung | In Vata Vitiation | In Vata dosha<br><br>In Tawak Sthita vitiated Raktha, in Avagadha tama Raktha and in Weak Persons. | In vitiated vata pitta dosha (not in Kapha dosha).<br>In Twak sthita vitiated Raktha. |
| 2) | Jalauka | In Pitta Vitiation | In pitta Vitiation,in Avagadha raktha, graditha raktha and in very delicate persons. | Pitta dosha, graditha Raktha and in very delicate person. |
| 3) | Alaabu | In Kapha Vitiation | In Kapha vitation,In Avagdhatara raktha. in twak sthita vitiated Raktha and in delicate Persons | In Vata Kapha Vitation (not in pitta vitiation) and in Twak sthita Rakth dosha. |
| 4) | Sira Vyada | InSarvanga Raktha dosha | Sarvanga Raktha and in strong persons | Sarvanga Raktha dosha. |
| 5) | Pracchan | Sarvanga Raktha dosha | Sarvanga Raktha dosha (uttana raktha) and in strong persons. | Sarvang Raktha dosha (utthana) Pinditha raktha. |
| 6) | Ghatee Yantra | Gulma Chikitsa | ---- | Kapha Vata vitiation (not in Pitta vitiation) Twak Sthita Raktha dosha. |

## 1) Jalaukava Charana :-
(Leech Therapy).

Jalauka name is given for living in water, There are two types 1) Savisha 2) Nirvisha.

## 1) Savisha Jalauka :- 6 Types they are
1) Krishna 2) Karbura 3) Alagarda 4) Indraayudha 5) Samudrika 6) Goghandan : These are found in dirty water especially in Rainy season, not used in Chikitsa, if used causes Oedema, itching sensation unconsciousnes, Fever, Burning sensation, Vomiting, delirium and body pains etc.,

## 2) NIRVISHA JALAUKA ;- 6 types they are.
1) Kapila 2) Pingala 3) Shankha Mukhi 4) Mooshika 5) Pundareeka Mukha 6) Saavarika. These are found in pure water especially in sharath rutu and are indicated for treatment.

**Note :-** Male leeches used in severe conditions and female leeches used in mild conditions.

## Indications For Jalaukavacharan.
1) Delicate and Weak persons those cannot bear the pain 2) Ladies 3) Children 4) The Old 5) The Rich 6) Pitta and Raktha Vitations. 7) Avagadha Raktha 8) Gulma 9) Arsha 10) Vidradi 11) Kusta 12) Vata raktha 13) Gala roga 14) Netra roga 15) Visha damstra 16) Visarpa 17) Shiro roga.

Leeches should collect from fresh water in sharath rutu and kept in pot or copper vessel in water with required food items, the water should change once in a week.

## Purification of Jalauka ;- (Shodhana)
To activate the blood sucking capacity and Locomotion of leeches the following measures should be taken.

1) Adding haridra and Sarshapa Churna to the water where the leeches are kept, or 2) Application of Haridra and Sarshapa churna to the body for 48 minutes (muhurtha).

3) Again Jalaukas should kept in Kanj and lastly in water The leeches should catch after putting on Gloves and should apply to the affected area of the patient.

## Poorva Karma :-
1) Sneha Sweda Vaman and Virechana should do for body purification.
2) Local Oleation (Sneha) and fomentation (the area of leech application should be dry and rough for the proper grip).

3) Application of Honey, then by a small incision (Pracchana ) to the skin bleeding surface should create to attract the leeches for proper grip, then it should be covered with thin white cloth.

**Observation During Jalauka Vacharana :-**

1) Bending of the body and distention of central portion of the body during Raktha mokshana (Leeches suck only impure blood without irritative complicatins.)

2) Pulsation on jalauka is visible that indicates it is sucking the impure blood.

3) If Pain. irritation is experienced at the site that indicate leech is sucking pure blood so leech should be seperated from the site, for that saindhava lavana churna should sprinkle over the leech by that immediately the leech separates, after removal of the leech, two attendants are required one for the maagement of the patient and Another for themanagment of leech.

4) Leach should handle gently and blood vomiting should be carried out to theleech tosave from complications like " Inthimada" in which theleech lost blood sucking capacity or it may die. Once used leech cannot be used for 7 days.

5) The patient should be treated for bleeding complications at the site, so ghritha Or madhu lepa, seka, Bandana etc., Should be don according to the necessity.

## 2) Sira Vyadana :-

Certain diseases are not cured by sheeta, ushna, Ruksha, snigda, Chikitsa, they should be considered as Rakthaja Vyadhies and they should be managed by Sira Vyadana.

It is indicated in all Raktha pradoshaj vyadhies.

**Contra Indications :-**

Children, Old, pregnant Ladies, Timid, sensitive, delicate, debilitative people Tired, due To Excercise, sexual inter course, stress and strain. The persons who undergone Vaman, Virechan Vasti, impotent, kasa, Swasa, Sosha, jwara. Akshepaka Pakshaghata, upavasa, Trushna, murcha etc., patients are not indicated for Siravyadan.

**Sira Vyadana Kala :** (Time schedule)

In Rainy Season when there is clear sky without clouds, in Summer when there is cool climate, in winter when there is hot climate. (the climate should not be too hot Or cool) in emergency at any time sira vyadhana can be conducted with proper care.

**Instruments Used For Sira Vyadana. :-**

1) Kutharica Shastra 2) Vreehi mukha Shastra 3) Trikurcha 4) the other needed materials are cotton, thread, bandage material, Saindhava lavana, jathyadi ghritha etc. Raktha stambaka dravyas, Alabu, shrunga, Shalakas for Agni karma should kept ready with the doctor while doing sira vyada.

## Poorva Karma: -

Bahya and Abhyantara sneha Sweda has to do (Sarvanga Shodhana), Liquid and less diet has to give on the day.

## Pradhana Karma :-

The patient is asked to be relax for the therapy, Sira Vyadana is carried out either in sitting position Or in lying position by depending upon the site of the disease. By proper ligation the vessels should be pressed and exposed properly, with kutharika Shastra the skin on the lesion should be incised and vessels should be exposed, then with the help of vreehi mukha shastra veinepuncture has todo with perfect care and technique, 1/2 Yava pramana Vyadana in well exposed parts and 1 Yava pramana vyadana in partial exposed part (where tissue is more.) if proper sira is not identified the nearest sira has to be punctured, while puncturing the vein the doctor should be very careful about the complications.

## Features of Adequate Sira Vyadana :-

1) Bleeding has to stop it self. 2) Lightness of the body. 3) Remission of symptoms like pain. 4) Control of the disease. 5) Physical and mental peace.6) Normal apetite and sound sleep.

## Features of Inadequate Sira Vyadana :-

1) Swelling 2) Inflammation 3) Agravation of Symptoms 4) Burning Sensation 5) Itching sensation 6) hyperaemia of the site.

## Features of Excessive Sira Vyadana :-

1) Head ache (Shira Shoola ) 2) Thirst (Trushna ) 3) Loss of vision (Andhathwa) 4) Burning Sensation(Daha) 5) Hiccough 6) Dyspncea (Swasa) 7) Cough(Kasa) 8) Anaemia (Pandu) 9) Convulsions (Akshepaka) 10) Glaucoma (Adhimantha) 11) Cataract and refractive errors (Timira) 12) Emaciation of body (dhathu kshaya) 13) Mono plegia (ekanga Vata) 14) Paralysis (Pakshaghath) 15) Delirium (Mano Vibraman 16) Unconscious (Murcha) 17) Death.

## Management of Inadequate Sira Vyadana ;-

The veinepucture area should be rubbed with the powders of ushna veerya, vishyanda Kara dravya to allow bleeding Ex :- ela,Karpoora, Kusta, Tagaru, Devadaru, Chitraka, Vidanga, Trikatu, ghruha dhooma, Arka, karanja etc.,

## Management of In Excessive Sira Vyadana :-

The bleeding should control by 1) Sandhana (adjoining the edges of ulcer by suturing etc) 2) Skandana (By sprinking the powders of sheeta veerya dravya to arrest the bleeding 3) Pachanam (medical cautery, by dusting Kshara bhasma etc.) 4) Dahanam (Agni Karma, cauterisation), In addition to above methods oral remedies should also be given to compensate the blood loss.

**Note :-** Maximum 1 prasta bloodshould remove by Siravyadana, that to not in a single day (Weekly once for 3 to 4 times).

## Post Raktha Mokshana Regimen.

1) Patient should consume light, easily digestable, haematenic diet.

2) Patient should avoid intake of excess cold Or hot items, anger, coitus, day sleeping, incompatible diet, Excessive work, stress and strain. 3) The diet regimen should follow for a month.

## List of Avedya Sira. (Veins rejected for Veinepuncture).

Total veines 700 among them 98 (Su) ,100 (Vag) Siras are avedya they are as follows :-

| Part | No. of Siras | | No. of Vedya Siras. | |
|------|-------------|---|---------------------|---|
| 1) Limbs | 400 | | 16 | |
| 2) Pelvic region | 32 | 8 | | |
| 3) Flanks | 16 | | 4 | |
| 4) Dorsum | 24 | | 4 | |
| 5) Abdomen | 24 | | 4 | |
| 6) Chest | 40 | | 14 | |
| 7) Neck | 56 (Sushrutha), | 16 | Matruka | 8 |
| | 24 (Vagbhata) | | Manya | 2 |
| | | | Neela | 2 |
| | | | Krukatika | 2 |
| | | | Vidura | 2 |
| | | | | ---- |
| | | | | 16 |
| | | | | ---- |
| 8) Jaws | 16 | 2 | (Hanu Sandhi sthitha) | |
| 9) Tongue | 36 Sushrutha, | 4 | (Rasavaha | 2 |
| | 16 Vagbhata | | Vakpravartaka | 2 |
| | | | | – |
| | | | | 4 |
| 10) Nose | 24 Sushrutha | 5 | Aupanasika | 4 |
| | | | Talu | 1 |
| | | | | – |
| | | | | 5 |
| | | | | – |
| | 24 Vagbhata | 3 | Gandha Sevani | 2 |
| | | | Talu | 1 |
| | | | | – |
| | | | | 3 |
| | | | | – |

| | | | | |
|---|---|---|---|---|
| 11) Ear | 10 Sushrutha, 16 Vagbhata | 2 | Shabda Vahini | 2 |
| 12) Eyes | 38 (Sushrutha) | 9 | Apanga | 2 |
| | | | Keshanthak | 4 |
| | | | Aavartha | 2 |
| | | | Stapani | 1 |
| | | | | – |
| | | | | 9 |
| | | | | – |
| | 53 Vagbhata | 13 | Above | 9 |
| | | | Nimesha Kriya | 2 |
| | | | Unmesha Kriya | 2 |
| | | | | – |
| | | | | 13 |
| | | | | --- |
| 13) Temporal | 10 Sushrutha, 16 Vagbhata | 2 | Sankha Sandhi gatha. | |
| 14) Cranium | 12 | 8 | Uthkshepa | 2 |
| | | | Seemantha | 5 |
| | | | Adipathi | 1 |
| | | | | – |
| | | | | 8 |
| | | | | – |

## 3) Pracchana :-

It is metalic instrumental blood letting process, shastrapada, pada are synonyms, itis a special therapy aswellas poorva Karma to other therapies (of Raktha Mokshan) It is indicated to remove pinditha suptha raktha in twak (Accumulated impure blood subcutaneously).

This process resembles Lekhana Karma in which the superficial strait, parallel, very close, imaginary incisions should be done quickly in prathiloma direction, the proximal part of thelesion should be tied to arrest theblood flow for proper elimination of impure blood.

The incisions should not do at Marma sandhi asti and snayu.

### 4) Shrungavacharana :-

It is nonmetalic blood letting process in which 7 " cow horn is used to suck the impure blood by creating vaccum in thehorn, it is meant to treat the Vataj, Raktha Pradoshaj Vyadhies.

After performing poorva karm and precchana, the base of thorn should fix to the lesion without air leakage, then vaccum should be created in the cavity of horm from the root (Second end ) of horn, air should be sucked, by that vitiated raktha Ozes andcollects in the horm by negative pressure

## 5) Alabu :-

It is non metalic blood letting process in which Raktha harana is done on the principle of cupping (Like shrunga ) . it is used in Kaphaj Raktha pradoshaj vyadhies. Alabu removes vitiated Raktha From 12" Distance. Alabu may be elongated or rounded. Madhura Or Tiktha, but Tiktha alabu is only indicated for Raktha mokshana in theKapha vitation.

Alabu should be collected, dried, central part should be cleaned, after poorva karma and pracchana alabu should be fixed to thewound by creating vaccum in thealabu, precaution should take for air tight, because of the negative pressure created in the alabu vitiated raktha Oozes and collects in alabu.

### Ghatee Yantra :-

The Principle and method of application is as like alabu but charaka especially used it in Gulma vyadhi to separate gulma From the root.

## NASYA KARMA

### Introduction :-

Nasya Karma is an important therapy among panchakarma, for the management of the diseases of Shalakya tantra (E.N.T. - Eye - and dental disease) and other systemic disorders like Vata Vyadhi - Unmada, Apasmara, Moorcha, Kesha Vikara and pumsamana Karma etc.,.
i.e., - Nasya Karma is having not only local but also systemic effects.
**Note : -** It is the last step in pancha Karma Therapy.

### Defination of Nasya :-

it is a special and important therapy in which the medicine is administered through thenose,either in the form of powder, liquid, oil or smoke. So only it is known as Nasya and the process is known as Nasya karma.

### Importance of Nasya Karma :-

Nose is the only gate way of head to eliminate the doshas from the head Nasya karma is the process in which the drug is administered through the nose to treat the diseases So only it is having utmost importance in the management of disases of Shalakya tantra and also in other systemic dosriders. Like Vata Vyadhi etc.,

### Synomyms of Nasya :-

1) Nasya 2) Shrio Virechana 3) Moordha Virechan 4) Shiro Vireka 5) Pracchardha.

### List of different Words used For Nasya :-

1) Nasya 2) Navana 3) Nasta 4) Shiro Virchana nasya 5) Shiro Vireka 6) Pradamana Nasya 7) Dmapana Nasya 8) Avapeedana Nasya 9) Marsha Nasya 10) Pratimarsha nasya 11) Dhooma Nasya 12) Snehana Nasya 13) Shodhana Nasya 14) Stambana Nasya 15) Prayogika Dhooma Nasya 16) Virechanika Dhoom Nasya

17) Snehika Dhooma Nasya 18) Brumhana nasya 19) Tarpana Nasya 20) Rechana Nasya 21) Shamana Nasya 22) Karshana Nasya 23) Sanghya Prabhooak Nasya 24) Pracchardak 25) Choorna Nasya 26) Swarsa Nasya 27) Kashaya nasya 28) Sneha Nasya 29) Raktha Nasya 30) Ksheera Nasya etc.,

It is a type of samshodhana Karma administered through the Nasal passage. it comprises a variety of procedures with slight difference in the therapy, those are grouped as follows .

## CLASSIFICATION OF NASYA :

**I) By CHARAKA :-**    a) 5 types                    (C.S. Si-9-89 to 92)
                       b) 3 types

a)    1) Navana              Snehana Nasya
                             Shodhana Nasya
      2) Avapeedana          Shodhana Nasya
                             Stambana Nasya
      3) Dmapana Nsya        ----
      4) Dhooma Nasya        Prayogika Dhooma Nasya
                             Virechanika Dhooma Nasya
                             Snehika Dhooma Nasya,
      5) Pratimarsha Nasya   Snehan Nasya
                             Rechan Nasya.

b)    1) - Rechana Nasya 2) Tarpana Nasya 3) Shamana Nasya


**II    By Sushrutha :-**       a) 2 Types                **(S.S.Ci. 40-21)**
                                b) 5 Types
a)    1- Shiro Virechana Nasya 2) Snehan Nasya
b)    1) - Nasya 2) - Shiro Virechana Nasya 3) - Pratimarsha Nasya
      4) - Ava Peedan Nasya  5)  - Pradamana Nasya.


**III)    By Vagbhata :-**               3 Types      **(AH. SU. 20-2)**
      1) - Virechana Nasya  2) - Brumhana Nasya   3) - Shamana Nasya.


**IV)    By Kashyap :-**               2 Types      **(Ka.Si.AS, 2,40)**
      1) - Brumhana Nasya (Poorana Nasya ) 2) - Karshana Nasya.(Shodak)


**V)    By Sarangdhar :-**             2 Types      **(Sh. U. 8-2 11,24.)**

      1) - RechanNasya Or Karshan . a) Avapeedan b) Pradamana.
      2) - Snehan Nasya Or Brumhannasya. a) Marsha b) Pratimarsha.


**VI)    By Bhoja :-**               **2 types**      **S.S. Cl. 40-23**
      1) Prayogika Nasya    2) Snehika Nasya


**VII)    By Videha**               **2 Types**      **S.S. Cl. 40-44**
      1) Sanghya prabhodaka nasya   2) Stambak nasya

**VIII) Charaka Also Mentioned :-** 7 Types of Nasya based on the parts used they are :

1) Phala Nasya 2) Patra nasya 3) Moola nasya 4) Kanda Nasya 5) Puspa nasya 6) Niryasa nasya 7) Twak Nasya.

**IX) Drugs Can be used for Nasya in the Following Forms :-**
a) Churna Nasya b) Kalka Nasya c) Swarasa nasya d) Ksheera Nasya e) Kwatha Nasya f) Saara Nasya g) Udaka Nasya h) Dhooma Nasya i) Mamsarasa Nasya j) Tail Nasya k) Ghritha Nasya l) Madya Nasya m) Raktha Nasya etc.,

# DRUGS USED FOR NASYA

## According to Chark :-

Apamarga, Pippali, Maricha Vidanga, Shigru, Sarshapa, Tumburu, Jeerak, Ajamoda, Pilu, harenuka, Pruthweeka, Surasa, Swetha, Kutheruka, Phaninjaka, Shireesha, Lashun, Haridra, Daruharidra, Sauvarchalavana, SaindhavaLavan, Jyothishmathi, Shunthi, Gandeera, shallaki, Tejovathi, Ingudi, Dalcini, Varthaki, Ela, Sumukha, Gandeeraka, Kalmalaka, Parnasa, ghrungver, Mulak, Tarkari, Arka, Alerka, Kusta, nagadanthi, Vacha, Bhargee, Gavakshea, Awakpushpee, Vruchcnikali, Brahmes, ativisha, Lodhra Madanphala, Sapthaparna, Nimba, Devadaru, Agaru, Sarela, Hingu, Guduchi, Bruhati, Ikshavak.

## 2) Sushrutha :-

Pippali, Vidanga, Apamarga, Shigru, Sarshapa, Shirisha, Maricha, Kareera, Bimbi, Sweta parajitha, Kinihi, Vacha, Jyothishmati, Karanja, Arka, Alarka, Lashuna, Atisa, Shunti, Talisapatra, Tamala patra, Surasa,Arjaka, Indgudi Medha, Shrungi, Matulunga, Murangee, Pily, jathi, Sala Tada, madhuka, Laksha, Hingu, Lavana, Madya, Gomaya, Gomutra.

## 3) Vagbhata :-

Vidanga, Apamarga, Trikatu, Daruharidra,Ral, Shireesa, Bruhati, Maukasara, Saindhavalavana, Daruharidraghana. Ela, Bruhat Ela, Hingu.

**Common Drugs Used for Nasya :-** Suggested by Kasthure .

## Churnas

| | | |
|---|---|---|
| Katphala Churna, | Trikatu Churna | Katu Tumbee Churna |
| Swasakuthara, | Vata Vidwamsini | Pippali Churna |
| Maricha Churna Vidanga Churna | | etc., |
| **Tailas** Anutaila, | Shatbindu Tail | Jatyadi Taila |
| Padmakadi Taila, | Panchaguna Tail, | Vachadi Tail |
| Ghritha etc., | | |

## Indications of Nasya :-

1) Shira Stamb (stiff head ) 2) Manya stamba (Stiff neck) 3) Dantha Shoola (toothache) 4) Hanugraha (lockjaw) 5) Peenasa (Corrhyza) 6) Gala Shundika (uvulitis) 7) Kantha shaluka (Adenoids) 8) Shukra (Corneal opacities and ulcer) 9) Timira (Dimvision 10) Varthma roga (Eyelid disorders) 11) Vyanga (Pigmentation of face) 12) Upajihwak (Cyst of tongue) 13) greeva Stamba (neck rigidity ) 14) Skandha roga (disease of Shoulder) 15) Anga shoola (Body pains) 16) Mukha roga (Oropharyngeal diseases) 17) Karna roga (Ear diseases) 18) Nasa shoola (Pain in the nose) 19) Akshi Shoola. (Pain in the eye ) 20) Shira shoola (Headache) 21) Arditavata (Facial Paralysis) 22) Apatantrek (Vata Vyadhi) 23) Apatanak (Vata Vyadhi ) 24) Gala Ganda (Goitre) 25) Dantha harsha (teeth Sensitivity) 26) Chala Dantha (loose tooth & decay) 27) Netra raji (Hyperacmia of eye  ball) 3)) Vaak grah (Aphonia) 31) Gadga (Stammering 32) Amsa shoola (Shoulder pain 33) Krathana (alteration of Voice) 34) dantha Stamba (Rigidity of teath).

## CONTRA INDICATIONS Of NASYA

| Sl. No. | Contra Indicated Condition | Complications due to administration. |
|---|---|---|
| 1. | After meals if nasya is given leads | Kasa, Swasa, Pratishyaya, chardi etc., Kapha Vikara |
| 2. | InIndigestion " | -do- |
| 3. | After Sneha Pana " | |
| 4. | After Madya Pana " | Causes Netra Srava, Gala Srava. |
| 5. | After jala Pana " | Avila netra, Timira and shiroroga. |
| 6. | When Desire to drink water " | |
| 7. | After head (Shira Snana) " | Pratishyaya, netra Srava, Gala Srava.karna Shoola, Shira Kampa. Vata Vikar. |
| 8. | Hungry " | Vata Vitiation. |
| 9. | Thirsty " | Mukha sosha. |
| 10. | Tierd " | Pain Increases. |
| 11. | Made (Semi  Consciousness) " | |
| 12. | Moorcha (Un consciousness) " | Samgya nash. |
| 13. | Abhighatha (injury) " | Severe Pain. |
| 14. | After Coitus when debility, | |
| 15. | weakness if Present | Pain in Shira netra vaksha |
| 16. | After Exercise if debility Present | Shakha (Limbs) |
| 17. | Acute Fever (grieved) " | |
| 18. | Shoka (Grieved) " | Timira - fever Increases. |
| 19. | After purgation (Virechan) " | Vata Vitition-Indriyaabhighata |
| 20. | After Vasti " | Kapha Vitiation, Gurutwa, Kandu, Krimi roga. |

| 21. | For Pregnant Lady | " | Garbha Vikruthi |
| 22. | For suthika (just delivere Lady | " | Dhathu Kshaya. |
| 23. | Nava PrathiShyaya | " | Pratishyaya Agrevates. |
| 24. | Apatarpitha (Weak Personality) | " | Dhathu kshaya develops. |
| 25. | Bala (Children) | | |
| 26. | Vruddha (Old People) | " | |
| 27. | Swasa | " | Diseeses become more Complicated. |
| 28. | Kasa | " | |
| 29. | Raktha Pitta | " | Cause debility(dhathu Kahaya). |
| 30. | Vegavaroda | | |

**Note :-** Specific Nasya can be given in above contra indications
Ex:- Sangya Prabhodak nasya in Morrcha etc.,

## 1) Naavana Nasya :-

It is oneof themost improtant Nasya which can be easily administrable and more beneficial. it is a procession which the medicated Oil is droped in to nose with the help of cotton (Pichu) Or Ink Piller.it is equivalent to Sushrutas Snehan Nasya and Shiro Virechan Nasya so only. It can be mainly classified in to 2 types a)Snehan Nasya and 2) Shodhan Nasya.

## a) Indications of Snehana Navana Nasya :-

1) Vataja ShiroRoga 2) Dantha Paatha 3) Keshapaatha 4) Karna shoola 5) Karna kshweda 6) Timira, 7) Swedopa ghatha 8) Nasa Roga, 9) Mukha sosha 10) Apabahuka 11) Akala Valee phalitha. 12) Nera Varthma roga 13) Vata Pittaja mukha roga 14) Arditha vata 15) Vatahatha Varthma 16) Darunaka.

**Dosage :-** Heena Matra (minimum dose) 8-8 drops in each nostril madyama Matra (Moderate dose) 16-16 drops.
Uttema Matra (perfect dose). 32-32 drops.

## b) Indication of Shodhana Navana Nasya :-

1) Kapha Rogas 2) Talu roga 3) Gala roga 4) Shiro roga 5) Nasa roga 6) Mukha roga 7) Aruchi 8) Shiro gurutwa 9) Shira Shoola 10) Peenas 11) Arthava bhedak 12) Krumi 13) Pratishyaya 14) Apasmar 15) Gandhagyannash.

| **Dosage :-** | Minimum dose | 4-4 drops in each nostril |
| | Modern dose | 6-6 " |
| | Perfect dose | 8-8 " |

## Time Shedule :-

| 1) | Kapha Roga | - | Fore noon (Poorvahan) |
| 2) | Pitta roga | - | After noon (madyahna) |
| 3) | Vata Roga | - | Evening (Aparahna) |

**Note ;-** (It should be given before meals and in day time).

## Seasonal Time Schedule For healthy People.

In
| | |
|---|---|
| Sheeta rutu | madyahna (Noon) |
| Sharat, Vansat rutu | Poorvahna (Morning) |
| Greeshma Rutu | Aparahna (Evening) |
| Varsha rutu | Non Cloudy day nasya has to do |

## 2) Avapeedan Nasya :-

Medicated drops extracted from Aushada Kalka (Paste of Medicine) and is instilled into nose is called Avapeedan Nasya. it is of two types.

A)
1) Shodhana (Rechan)
2) Stambana (Raktha Stambana).

B)
Chakrapani.
| | |
|---|---|
| 1) Shodana | kapha rechan. |
| 2) Stambana | Raktha Stambana. |
| 3) Shaman | For controlling Vitiated doshas (in debilitated persons). |

## c) Dalhana

1) Sangya prabhodan - in murcha, Visha roga, Apasmar, moha etc.,
2) Stamban - in Raktha pitta.

## Indications :-

1) Vishaabhighatha 2) Sanyasa 3) Moorcha 4) Moha 5) Apasmara 6) Apatantrak 7) Mada 8) Shirobhedan 9) Krodha 10) Bhaya 11) Mano roga 12) Karshya 13) Bheeru. 14) Stree 15) Bala 16) Vruddha

**Dose :-**
| | |
|---|---|
| Heena matra | 4-4 Drops. |
| Madyama Matra | 6-6 Drops. |
| Utthama Matra | 8-8 Drops. |

## 3) Dmapana Or Pradhamana Nasya :-

It is shodhana nasya in which medicated powder is blowed in the nose with the helop of 6 " Lengthy tube Or inhaling the medicated powder sachet (2 Tola fine powder should be packed in thin cloth.)

**Dose :-** 3 mucchuti.

**Indication :-** 1) Mental diseases (unmada, apasmara) 2) Krumija Shira shoola 3) Poisonous cases.

## 4) Dhooma Nasya :-

Inhaling Or taking themedicated smoke Or Vapour through nose with the help of Nasya netra by closing the other nostril. It is of 3 types 1) Prayogika dhooma nasya Or Shaman dhooma Nasya (in Vata kapha disorders) 2) Viirechanika dhooma (in Kaphaj disorders) 3) Snehika dhooma Nasya (in Vataj disroders). inhaled smoke should not release through nose by that eye complications may arise. the lenght of Nasya netra for prayogika dhoom Nasya 36 Angula, for Virechanika dhooma nasya 24 angula and for snehika dhooma Nasya 32 angula. (For prayogika dhooma netra 40 angula according to Vagbhata.).

**Dose :-** 9 Times the smoke or Vapour should take by giving small break after 3 times i.e. 3-3-3 times.

## 1) Drugs For Prayogika Dhooma Nasya :-

Harenu, Priangu, Kesar, Chandan, ela, usheera, padmaka, jatamamsi, Guggulu, Agaru, Lodra, Sarjaras, Musta, Pancha Valkal Bark etc.,

## 2) For Snehika Dhooma Nasya :-

Vasa, Ghritha, Maducchista and jeevaneeya gana.

## 3) For Viirechanika Dhooma Nasya :-

Swetha aparajitha, malkangini, harital, manashila, Agaru, etc,,

## 5) Marsha nasya - Prathimarsha nasya :-

Medicated Oil is droped in to nostrils in marsha and pratimarsha nasya but there is dosage and following differences present in between them.

## COMPARATIVE STUDY OF MARSHA PRATIMARSHA NASYA :-

| Sl. No | Prati Marsha nasya | Marsha Nasya |
|--------|--------------------|--------------|
| 1. | Never Produce Dosha vitiation | 1) May produce dosha Vititation. |
| 2. | Dose 2 drops Bid | 2) Dose 6 to 10 drops (6 heena, 8 madyama, 10 drops utthama) |
| 3. | Indicated for all age groups and in all seasons. | 3) Age and Seasional restricitions present. |
| 4. | Consists of less Sneha dravya | 4) Consists of More Sneha dravyas. |
| 5. | No Complications | 5) Complications may arise. |
| 6. | Slow Action | Quick action. |
| 7. | Lesspotent | More Potent |
| 8. | Easy administration | Helper needed to put the drops in nose. |
| 9. | Preventive aswellas curative therapy | Only curative therapy. |
| 10. | Indicated in less vitiated diseases, cannot control the more severe disroders. | Control high vitiated diseases. |

**Note :-** Pratimarsha nasya can be droped with droper or by dipping the finger in theOil upto 2 inches level.

## Indications of Pratimarsha Nasya :-

| | Indication | Benifit. |
|--|-----------|----------|
| 1. | Early Morning | 1. Kapha Dosha which is accumulated at night is reduced. |
| 2. | After brushing of teeth | 2. Teeth becomes strengthy, and mouth become fresh. |
| 3. | While going out side from house | 3. Prevents dust and smoke allergy. |

| | | |
|---|---|---|
| 4. | After Excercise | 4. The debility. Or tiredness is removed. |
| 5. | After coitus | 5. -do- |
| 6. | After tiredness due to walking | 6. -do- |
| 7. | After Kavalagrah | 7. Vision improves. |
| 8. | After anjan | 8. -do- |
| 9. | After meals | 9, Sroto shuddhi, |
| 10. | After Vaman | 10. Kapha shaman and Taste improves. |
| 11. | After sleeping in day time | 11. Heaviness and other symptoms controlled and promotes mental Peace. |
| 12. | In the evening | 12. Gives sound sleep at night |
| 13. | After Urination. | Vision improves. |
| 14. | After defication | Vision Improves. |

## Nasya Vidhi :-

Before instilling the drops into nose the doctor has to concentrate on thefollowing points.

1. Age of the Patient.

a) Indication 8 to 80 Years. b) Dhooma Nasya 12 to 80 Years. c) Pratimarsha nasya for all age groups.

2. Season (Kala)

Nasya in indicated in pravrut rutu, sharath and vasantha.

a) In greeshma rutu     Before Noon. b) In sheeta rutu   Noon. c) Varsha rutu Non Cloudy day. Nasya has to give

3. Strength of the patient.

a) For average strength patient - madyama matra, b) Perfect strength patient  utthama matra, c) Less than average strength patient Heena matra drug should be given.

4   Strength of the disease.

It is important to prepare themedicine whether mrudu vereya Or Madhyama Or Teekshna Vereya depends uopn thestrength of thedisease.

5. Type of the nasya :-

Different types of Nasya are explained, among those, the doctor has to decide what should be suitable.

6. After fixation of type of nasya and its dose, the doctor has to concentrate on materials needed for the therapy.

a. Nasya Bhavaan :-

It is a special room which should free from direct blow of air and dust, it should be perfect with alll requirements needed for Nasya.

### b) Nasya Asana :-

For sitting as well as lying purpose chair and Bed are needed for giving Nasya. (The bed should be adjusting type to raise the foot part or to down the head part, for proper medication) .c. Nasya Aushadhies :- The medicines needed for poorva pradhana and paschyat Karma should be collected.

**d) Nasya Yantra :-**For 1) navanaNasya - Marsha Nasya and Pratimarsha Nasya- droppers Or karpasa Pitch should use. 2) For dhooma nasya different sizes fo Dhooma Nasya netras should use.3) For aVapeedana Nasya thin cloth should be kept to extract the swarasa for Nasya.4) For Pradamana nasya, 6 angula length tube should keep for blowing medicated powder into the nose.

Besides above material efficient assistants, spittoons pots, dressing material, medicines to control the complications, material for Kavala, Gandoosha, dhooma pana(for paschyat Karma ) and other minor accessories needed for proper administration of Nasya should be procured to achieve good result.

## DOSAGE OF DRUG IN DIFFERENT TYPES OF NASYA

| Sl. No. | Name of Nasya | Heena Matra | madhyam Matra | utthama matra |
|---|---|---|---|---|
| 1. | Navana Shaman Nasya | 8-8 drops in each nostril. | 16 -16 drops | 32 -32 drops. |
| 2. | Navan Shodhana Nasya | 4-4 drops in each nostril | 6-6 drops. | 8-8 drops. |
| 3. | Avapeedana nasya | 4-4 drops in each nostril | 6-6 drops | 8-8 drops. |
| 4. | Pratimarsha Nasya | 2-2 drops in each nostril | 2-2 drops | 2-2 drops |
| 5. | Marsha Nasya | 6-6 drops | 8-8 drops | 10-10 drops. |
| 6. | Pradaman nasya | 3 Mucchyuti (2 to 4 rati) | 3 Mucchyuti | 3 Mucchyuti |
| 7. | Dhuma Nasya | 9 times the smoke shoud be taken by slight gap after 3 times | | |

# DOSAGE OF NASYA ACCORDING TO SARANGA DHARA .

1.  Teekhshna Aushadi   -   1 Shana (24 Rati ) Powder, 8 drops Liquids.
2.  Hingu                -   1 Yava (1/2 Rati)
3.  Saindhava Lavan      -   1 Masha (6 Rati)
4.  Milk                 -   8 shana 64 drops.
5.  Water (medicated)    -   3 Tola.

## Preparation of Patient For Nasya Vidhi.

1.  Sneha Pana is contra indicated, if needed 3 days sneha has to give, 4th day gap then 5th day nasya has to give. 2) Vega Nivruthi (mala - Mutra etc.) 3) Meals has to take. 4) Dhooma Pana- to clear the kapha from mouth, nose and throat.5) Shiro abyanga with Dhanvatari tail, Kseerabala tail etc. 6) Mrudu Sweda (Tapa Sweda) on the Head, mouth, Nose, neck and throat to liquify the doshas. 7) Gentle massage on throat neck face and frontal region. 8) patient should lie down on Nasya shayga by resting the head down wards than the normal level by raising the chin upwards to expose the nasal cavity 9) With the help of Dhooma Nasya netra or dropper or karpasa pichu, themedicine has to instil in one nostril by raising the tip of the nose , and the patient at the same time another nostril has to close, and the patient should beinstructed not to swallow the medicine but should squeeze inside. 10) While instilling the drug it should not be to cool or hot, should not instil either qucik Or delayed. 11) While dropping themedicine the patient is warned not to talk, angry Or laugh. 12) During the process the eyes should be covered with cloth.

## Pashchyat Karma :-

1) Mrudu sweda on face, Neck and Frontal region. 2) Gentle massage of Head, Frontal region, shoulder, hands and legs. 3) If. salivation occurs, patient is asked tospit it is spittons and Nasal discharge in the other pots and lacrimation should clean with clean, cloth. 4) After Nasya Karma Patient should wait for 100 matra Kala then he is treated with Kavala Gandoosh and Dhooma Pana, to clear the Kapha dosha from throat and other srotas - finally Lukewarm water gargling is given to clean themouth. 5) Light diet, and warm water is given for drinking, bath etc.

## 6) Avoiding :-

Cold water, exposure to dust smoke and heat, head bath, intake of alcohol. anger, sleep, travelling and usage of oils

## Features of Adequate Nasya :-

1.  Lightness of body. 2) Sound sleep. 3) Lightness in the head 4) Sensorial Happiness (indria prasannata). 5) Mental happiness. 6) Control of the disease.

## Features of Inadequate Nasya :-

1) Heavyness of head and body. 2) itching sensation. 3) Uncontrolled disase. 4) excessive secretion from Nose, mouth and eyes. 5) Mental and sensorial disturubances.

**Features of Excessive Nasya :-**
       1) Head ache. 2) Delirium 3) Agravation of disease 4) Giddiness.
**Note :-** Nasya is given daily or alternate day for 7 days (Vagbhata), 21 days Or upto result (sushrutha).

**Adantages of Adequate Nasya :-**
1) Prevention of eye disease. 2) Prevention of ear diseases. 3 prevention of Nasal diseases. 4) Healthy hair. 5) Provides strength to scalp 6) provides happines. 7) Improves voice. 8) Improves senses. 9) Pleasent oral smell 10). Rasayana. 11). prevention of Akala Vali Phalitha. 12). Prevention of urdwa Jathru vikaras.

# NASYA YOGAS INDIFFERENT DISEASES

**a) Nasa Rogas.**
**I) a) In Vataj prastishyaya :-** Rohishadi yoga pradamaenNasya.

**In Pittaja Pratishyaya :-**
Patha, haridra, Daruharidra, moorwa, pippali, Jathipallava, danthi, tila taila (pakwa taila) nasya.

**3) In kaphaj Pratishaya :-**
       a) Bharangyadi taila Nasya (Bharangi, Madanphala, Tarkari, Tulasi, Gomutra, Laksha, Vacha, vidanga, Kusta, Pippali, Karanja, and Sarshapa taila - Palwa taila nasya).

       B) Manahshiladi Churna Pradaman nasya (Manahshila, Vacha, Trikatu, Vidanga, hingu, gugulu, Katu dravya. c) Trikatu, Saindhavalavana, Kutaja, jeeraka, Gomtra - nasyam. d) Baladi taila Nasyam (Bala, Atibala, Bruhati,Vidanga, Kantakari, Vishunkarantha, Mudgaparni, Rasna, Punarnava, Tila taila, (pakwa Taila) Nasyam.)

**4) In Sanni Pathaja Pratishyaya :-**
       a) Rasanjanadi tailam for Nasyam.
       (Rasanjana Ativisha, Musta, Bhadradaru, taila).
**5) In Rakthaja Pratishyaya :-**
a) Vidangadi Nasya b) Gomutra + gorochana Nasya
**6) In Apeenasa :-**
       a) Hingu Trikatu, kutaja, shivati, (Truna), Laksha, Tulasi, Katphala, vacha, Kusta, sarshapa, Vidanga, Karanjabeeja, Avapeedan nasya. b) Above drugs+ Gomutra Sarshapa taila (Pakwa Taila nasya).

**7) In Nasa Raktha Srava :-**
       **a)** Neela kamala, Gyrika, chandan, shankha, Sharkara jala- Nasyam.**b)** Amrasti, Samanga, Dhataki, Mocha rasa, Lodra - Nasya .**c)** Draksha swarasa Or Ikshurasa Or kseera Or doorva swarasa Or Dadima Pushapa rasam Or Yavasa Moola andLashuna swarasa Or vasa swarasa Or Babbula Patra Swarasa nasyam.**d)** Priyala Taila nasya.
**e)** Yastimadu Ghritha Nasya. **f)** Jathyadi taila nasya.**g)** padmakadi Taila Nasya.

8) **In Kshavathu :-**  a) Trikatu, Shigrubeeja, Vidanga, Pradaman Nasya.

9) **In Deepathi  :-**  a) Rasanjan nasya

10) **In Nasanaha :-**  a) Bala Taila Nasyam. b) Shatbindu taila Nasya.

11) **In Nasa Sosha :-** a) Ksheerisarpi Nasya b) Anutaila Nasya

B) **MukhaRogas :- 1) Danthavesta -** Kakolyadi ghritha Nasyam.

2) **Saushira :-**  Yastimadu, Lodra, uthphala, Bala, Sariva, agaru, chandana, gyrika, sharkara, the prepared oil is used for nasya.

3) **Dantha Nadi :-**  ksheeri Vruksha taila Nasya.

4) **Tundikeri :-**  Apamarga, Vishnu Krantha, Danthi, Vidanga, Saindhava Lavan, Tila, Taila, (Pakwa Taila0 nasya.

c) **Nasya In Shiro Rogas :-**

1) In Vataja shiro roga a) Nasya with Rasnadi taila (Rasna Laghu Panchmamoola - ksheera). b) Mayuradya ghritha Or maha mayuradya ghritha. c) Bala Madhuka Yastimadu vidari chandana uthphala Jeevaka Rushabhak Draksha Sharkara Kseera jangala Mamsa - Tailam for Nasyam. d) Varunadi Ghritam for nasyam. e) Ashwagandhadi ghritha Nasya f) Shatbindu taila nasyam.g) Baladi ghritha for Nasya.

2) **In Pittaj Shiro Roga :-**

1) Ghirtha Nasyam b) Yastimadu Chandana sariva sharkara milk Draksha, Madhuka and ghritha (pakwa) - for Nasya. c) Yastimadu Ksheera sarpi for Nasya. d) Ksheera Sarpi Nasyam. e) Kumkum Pushpa (Kesare) Sharkara ghritha for Nasya. f) Twak, Patra, Sharkara Tandulodak - Avappedan Nasya.

3) **In Krimija Shiro Roga.**

a) Twak, Danthi, Vyaghranaki, Vidanga, Nava mallika, Sarshapa, Karanja, Shireesha, Ashmantak, Bilva, haridra hingu, Phainjak, Apamarga, Yoothika, mutra, Taila (Pakwa) for Nasyam. b) Above compound as powder for pradaman nasya. c) Shigrubeeja Karanja Beeja Trikatu for Avapeedan Nasya. d) Nasyam with blood (shonitham). e) Teekshna Nsyam with Vidanga apamarga maricha etc., drugs grinded in Aja mutra etc.,

4) **Kaphaj Shir Shoola :-**

a) Shunti + Ksheera nasya b) Teekshna Nasya with Katphala churna Or Trikatu Churna etc., (Pradaman Nasya).

5) **In Shirashoola :-**

a) Aparajitha moola Or phala swarasa Nasya.

b) **Gudadi Nasya :-**

Guda, shunti, pipplai, saindhava lavan- ushnajala - Nasya is Shiro, Karna, Nasa and Mukha rogas.

c) **Narayan Taial, Anutaila, Mashadi Taila etc.,**

Bramhan taila used for Nasya in shiro rogas to give nourishment (Shaman Nasya).

## 6) In Surya Vartha & Anantha Vata.

a) Nasya with Apamarga Swarasa b) Milk c) Ghritha d) Navaneetha e) Katphala churna f) Trikatu g) Chakra marda beeja h) Brungaraj swarasa, Aja ksheera i) Milk+ Ghee nasya j) Kesara fry in ghee with Sharkara nasya has to give. k) Tulasi beeja Nasya l) Shireesha moola swarasa Nasya m) Rasona Swarasa Nasya n) Swetha aparajitha moola swarasa Nasya o) Gunja Moola Swarasa Nasya.

## 7) Arthavabheda :-

a) Vidangadi Nasya - Vidanga, Krishna tila should be grinded in aja Ksheera for Nasya. b) Ksheera + Sharkara.c) Vachadi Avapeedan Nasya :- Vacha Pippali Yastimadu Yava, should grinded with water and with Honey for Nasya. d) Shireesha moola and phala Avapeedani Nasya. e) Vamshi moola and Karpoora Avapeedan Nasya. f) Madhu + ChandanAvapeedan Nasya. g) Madhu + Manashila Avapeedan Nasya. h) shireesha Beeja, apamarga moola, Bidalavan, Avapeedan Nasya. i) Mruthika (From chuhlika) + maricha choorna. Pradaman nasya j) Madhu + Taila Nasya k) Sarshapa taila Nasya.

| | |
|---|---|
| **8) Darunaka :-** | Bringaraj taila Nasyam. |
| **9) Indraluptha :-** | Nimba taila nasyam. |
| **10) Phalithya :-** | a) Ksheera, Sahachara, taila, Brungaraja Swarasa, Tulasi, Tila taila, yastimadu (Taila Paka vidhi) oil is used for Nasya. |
| | b) Prapoundareekadi taila nasya (Amalaki, Tila taila, Prapaundareeka, pippali, chandan, Neelothphala, Yastimadu (Taila Vidhi) |

## c) Vibheetakadi Nasya :-

(Vibheetaki, Nimba, Gambhari, hareetaki, Lisoda
Gunja- Pakwa Taila- as pratimarsha Nasya.

## D) In Vata Vyadhies :- 1) Rasnadi ghritha 2) Ksheerabala taila 3) Baladi ghritha manda 4) Mashadi nasya. (Masha, Kaunchabeeja Rasna Bala erenda moola rohins Truna, Ashwaganda - Quatha should prepare,and add saindhava lavan Hingu for Kashaya Nasya.

## E) In Tandra And Nidra :-

1) Marichadi Nasya - Krishna maricha, Pippali, shunti, Kankola, saindhava lavana, lashuna, guugulu, Katphhala, vacha, saindhava lavan - Rohitha matsya - as pradaman Nasya.

2) Saindhavadi Nasya :- Saindhava lavan, maricha, sarshapa, kusta grinded in mutra and used as Nasya. )

## F) In Unmadaa and Apasmara :-

Madhuka saradi nasya - Madhuka, shuktha, pippali, vacha,maricha saindhav lavana and water as nasya.

## g) In Unmada :-
## 1) Lashunadi ghritha -

100 Lashuna, 30 hareetaki, 1 phala Trikatu, 1 prasta Go charma masi, 2 Aadaka ksheera, and mutra, 1 prastam Ghee, 1 Palam hingu, 2 Kudava Honey, ghritha has to prepare for Navana Nasya.

## 2) Vyoshadi Nasya:-
Trikatu Haridra, Daruharidra, Manjista, hingu, Sarshapa, shireesha beeja, Karanja, Vacha, Triphala ,Samanga, priyang, Sariva, Devadaru, should grind in Aja mutra for Nasya.

## 3) Shireeshadi Nasya .
Shireesha, maduka, Hingu, Lashuna ,Tagara, Vacha, Kusta, should grind in Aja mutra for Nasya.

## 4) Pradaman Nasya.
Mutra, pitta, Roma, Nakha, Charma, of Animals.

## H) Apasmara :-
1) Bharangi, Vacha, Nagadanthi Or Jyothishmathi, Nagadanthi, Or Sariva, Sireesha, Shatavari, should grind with mutra for Nasya.

2. Triphala, Trikatu, Devadaru, Yavakshara, Trivruth, Apamarga, Phaninjaka, Karanja, should grind in Aja mutra the prepared taila is used for Nasya.

3. Pippali, vuschikali, kusta, Pancha Lavana, Bharangi , pradaman, Nasya.

## I) Hikka :-
1)      Lashuna + Rasona Swaras. 2)  Chandana + Stanya. 3) Saindhava Lavana + Ghritha manda. 4) Sharkara + Shunti. for Nasya.

## J) Kshataja Kasa .
1) Ghritha + Ksheera Nasya

## K)      1) Vataja Kasa :- Rasnadi ghritha Nasya (Rasna, dashamool, shatavari, kulutha badariphal, yava, Aja mamsa - ghritha).

## L) Visha chikitsa :-
1) Shireesha Swarasa + Maricha - Nasya. 2) Shireesha Swarasa + Shigruchurna Nasya. 3) Amrutha + Shireesha Twak, Trikatu, Triphala + ghritha - Nasya.

## M) Kusta vyadhi :-
1) Vidanga churna Pradaman Nasya.

# DESCRIPTION OF E.N.T. INSTRUMENTS

Plate - I and Plate II

**1)     Oto scope - electrical**
        It is self illuminating aural speculum with magnifying Lenses and handle, it is used to examine external ear canal and tympanic membrane.

**2)     Aural speculum (Toynbee's)**
        It is used for examination of the external ear and tympanic membrane by pulling the pinna upwards backwards and Laterally in adults and downwards backwards and Laterally in children. speculum should insert upto cartilage and bony junction of external auditory canal.

**3)     Tuning fork (Hartmanns)**
        It is used to determine the type and quality of deafness (rinne's Webers tests etc).

**4)     Aural syringe :-**
        This is used to remove the unimpacted foreign bodies from the ear like wax dried discharge of otitis media etc. While using the instrument it should not introduce in side the lumen as it will obstruct the way of returning Fluids should not syringe forciful and should not direct the noizzle straight that may damage the tympanic membrane, so should direct preferably to wards the roof of the canal.

**5)     Eustachian Catheter (kramer's)**
        It is used for Eustachian catheterization for diagnostic (to know the patency of eustachian tube) and therapeutic purposes (to remove Eustachian blockage and to give medication in the middle ear.)

**6)     Siegle's Pneumatic speculum :-**
        It contains ear speculum with magnifying Lens, , which is attached to rubber bulb and rubber tube. It is useful to test the mobility of tympanic membrane. The speculum  is fitted in the ear canal and makes an air tight chamber, by pressing the rubber bulb mobility of tympanic membrane is observed through the magnifying lens of ear speculum.

7)     Sef retaining Haemostatic mastoid retractor (Weis lander's )
        It is used in the both cortical and radical mastoidectomy operations.

**8)     Mastoid Gouge (Jenkin's)**
        It is used in mastoidectomy operation, Both cortical and radical to explore the mastoid antrum and the mastoid air cells.

**9)** **Mac Ewen's Cell Seeker with Scoop :-**
It is used in mastoidectomy operation to explore the air cells and mastoid antrum with the seeker and to scoop out the pathological air cells with the scoop .

**10)** **Staecke's Guide :-**
It is used in radical mastoidectomy operation, it guides the surgeon to explore the aditus and antrum, protects the facial nerve and Leteral Semi circular canal from injury at the time of removing the bridge and enlarging the aditus.

**11)** **Myringotome (Daggett's)**
It is used in myringotomy which means incision of the tympanic membran for better drainage of pus from middle ear.

**12)** **Aural Snare (ballance's)**
It is used to cut the pedicle of the aural polyp. The number " O", steel wire is used in this snare.

**13)** **Lemperti's end-aural speculum :-**
This is used to during mastoidectomy operation to apply end- aural incision of Lempert.

**14)** **End-Aural retractor with the third blade (Lempert's)**
It is used to retract the incision lines in the mastoidectomy operation, through endaural route. the third blade is used to retract the temporal muscle and fascia away from the field of operation.

## Plate - III and IV

**1)** **Thudichum Nasal speculum :-**
It is used for Anterior Rhinoscopy (examination of the Anterior part of Nasal cavity )

**2)** **Posterior Rhinoscopic mirror (St. clair thomson's)**
It is used to examine in the posterior part of the nose and the Nasopharynx.

**3)** **Antrum washing Cannula (Rose's) :-**
It is used for giving wash to maxillary antrum on the 4th to 6th post operative day of I.N. A. (intra nasal antrostomy)

**4)** **Nasal foreign body hook. :-**
Used for removal of foreign bodies from the nose.

**5)** **Antral harpoon (Tilley's) : -**
It is used for making an artificial opening in the inferior meatus of the naso antral wall, in intra nasal antrostomy operation.

**6)** **Antral Rosette Burr (Tilley's )**
It is used for enlarging and smoothening the margin of the artificial opening made by the harpoon in I.N.A.

7)     **Antral trocar and Cannula (Tilley-Lichl-witz) :-**
It is used for washing the maxillary antrum in cases of maxillary sinusitis for diagnstic. and therapeutic purposes.

8)     Killian's mucoperichondrial Elevator with the thumb rest (Right and Left).

These instruments are used in submucous resection (S.M.R.) operation of septum for elevating the muco perichondrium of septum in deviated nasal septal disease.

9)     Long bladed Nasal speculum (Stclair Thomsons) It is used to Keep the elevated mucoperichondrium of either side, away from the bare septum during s.m.R. operation.

10)    **Ballenger's Swivel Knife :-**
It is used to cut a quadrangular piece of cartilage of septum in S.M.R. operation.

11)    **Luc's Forceps :-**
It is used in caldwell-luc's operation, SMR operation for tissue biopsy form oralcavity and oropharynx, INA operation and in dissection method of tonsillectomy

12)    **Negus Modification of (Glegg's ) Nasal snare :-**
It's function is to crush and avulge the polyp from its base. Number. 1 steel wire is used.

13)    **Bayonet shaped Bone Gouge (killian's)**
It is used to cut the bony thickening or spurs along the maxillary crest.

# PLATES V. VI VII AND VIII :-

1) Tongue depressor (Lack's)
It is used to depress the anterior 2/3 of tongue to visualise the oral caivty and oropharnx cleraly.

2)     **Laryngeal mirror**
A mirror with straight handle is larngeal mirror used for indirect laryngoscopy

3)     **Laryngeal forceps  (Mackenzie's )**
These are sharp and culting types of forceps, used to take biopsy from the larynx and Hypopharynx.

4)     **Tonsillar Haemostatic Clamp (Yorke's)**
It is used to stop reactionary and secodary haemorrhage in the post. operative coses of tonsillectomy.

**5)      Adenoid Cyrette with Cage (St clair thomsons )**
It is used to curette the adenoids.

**6)      Draffin's Bipods**

**7)      Boyle Davis mouth gag** - These are used (Draffins bipods Boyle Davis mouth gap ) in dissection method of tonsillectomy under gneral anaesthesia.

**8)      Tonsil holding Forceps (Denis Browne's ) :-**
It is used to hold the toinsil and to pull it medially in dissection method of tonsillectomy.

**9)      Tonsil dissector with pillar retractor (Beavis)** This instrument is used for blunt dissection of the tonsil from it's bed, retractor is used to bend the anterior pillar to explore any bleeding point and tonsillar tag just after tonsillectomy.

**10)      Tonsillar Snare (Eve's)**
It is used to crust and cut the lower pole of tonsil in dissection method of tonsillectomy - Number "2" steel wire is used in it.

**11)      Negus artery Forceps :-**
A pair of Artery forceps with curved end, is used at the time of applying ligatures of bleeding points in the tonsillar bed.

**12)      Knot - Tier and Ligature slipper (Negus) :-**
This is used for slipping the ligature beyond the curved tip of the artery forceps and also to tie the knots during an attempt to stop the bleeding points. during tonsillectomy operation by dissection method.

**13)      Tonsil Guillotines (Ballenger's)**
These are Used in tonsilectomy by Guillotine method

**14)      Doyen's Mouth gap :-**
This is used for opening the mouth during tonsillectomy by guillotine tecnique

**15)      Peritonsillar abscess drainage Forceps or Quinsy dilator (St Clair thomsons)**
These are used for draining a peritonsilar abscess.

**16)      Direct Larngoscope (chevalier Jackson's)**
It is used for direct visualisation of larynx, to remove foreign bodies, papilloma or benigngrowth or for biopsy.

**17)      Paterson's Forceps :-**
A long and narrow pair of Forceps which may be passsed through the endoscopes

1)      Cutting type for taking biopsy.

2)      Holding type to remove Foreign bodies.

**18)    Broncho Scope (Chevalier Jackson's) :-**

This instrument contains holes on either side near its distal end to keep air way patent for the ventilation of one lung during examination of the bronchus and bronchioles of the other lung.

**19)    Oesophagoscope (Nagus )**

It is used for direct visualisation of the oesophageal Lumen , for removal of foreign bodies, for taking biopsy, diagnosis of cardiospasm and for dilatation of benign stricture of Oesophagus etc.

**20)    Tracheal Dilator (Troussaeu's )**

It is used in traceostomy operation to dilate the tracheal incision for smooth introduction of the tracheostomy tube.

**21)    Sharp tracheal hook :-**

It is used in tracheostomy operation to fix the trachea during its incision .

**22)    Blunt tracheal hook :-**

It is used to retract the isthmus of thyroid gland during tracheostomy operation.

**23)    Bivalved Metalic Tracheostomy tube (fuller's) :-**

The outer tube contains two cusps so only called Bivalved, it never gets blocked by tracheo bronchial secretions, after introduction of inner tube through the outer one, the opening shuld be covered with a piece of Sterile gauze.

**24)    Head mirror :-**

It is fixed to the head, The bright light which is comming form the source. should be focussed properly on the concave mirror of head mirror and the converged reflected light should expose to the site and through the cetral perforation of the concave mirror the affected part should be examined .

**25)    Head Light :-**

This contain concave mirror with central hole and light source togetherly so easy for focussing and examination.

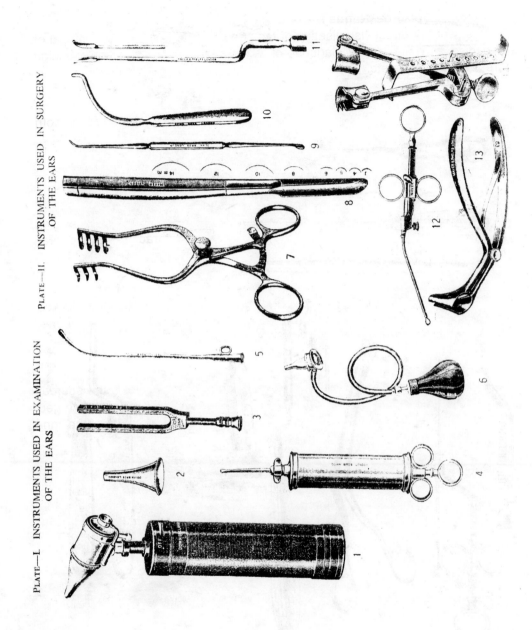

PLATE—I. INSTRUMENTS USED IN EXAMINATION OF THE EARS

PLATE—II. INSTRUMENTS USED IN SURGERY OF THE EARS

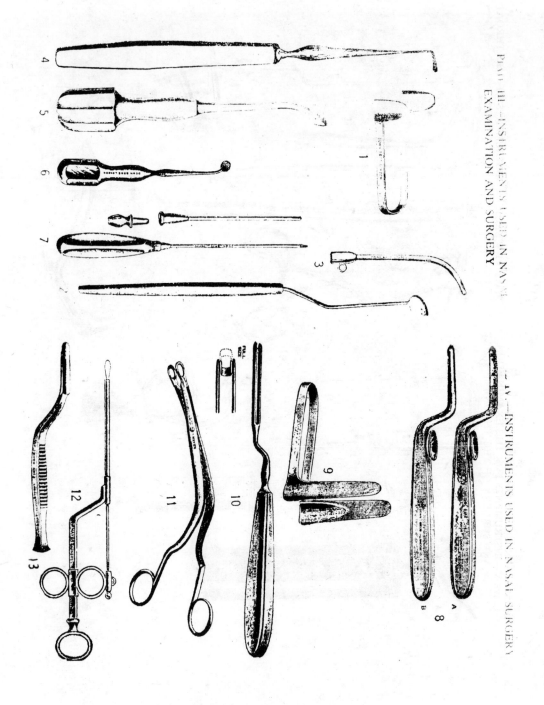

PLATE III.—INSTRUMENTS USED IN NAVAL EXAMINATION AND SURGERY

PLATE IV.—INSTRUMENTS USED IN NASAL SURGERY

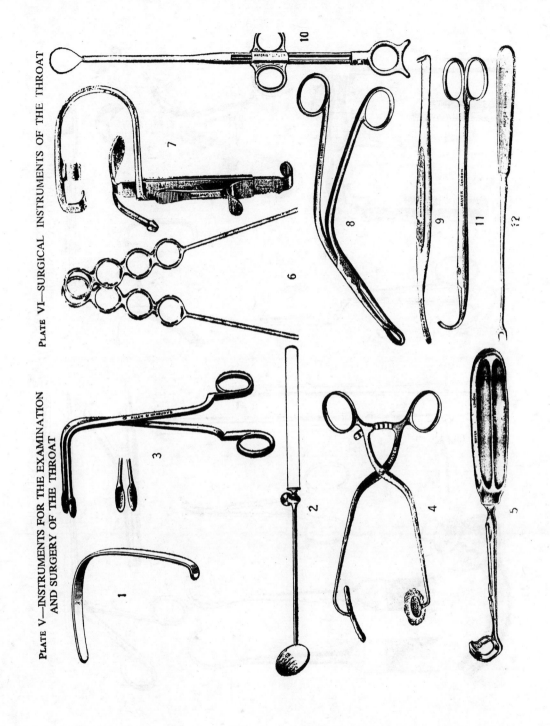

PLATE V.—INSTRUMENTS FOR THE EXAMINATION
AND SURGERY OF THE THROAT

PLATE VI.—SURGICAL INSTRUMENTS OF THE THROAT

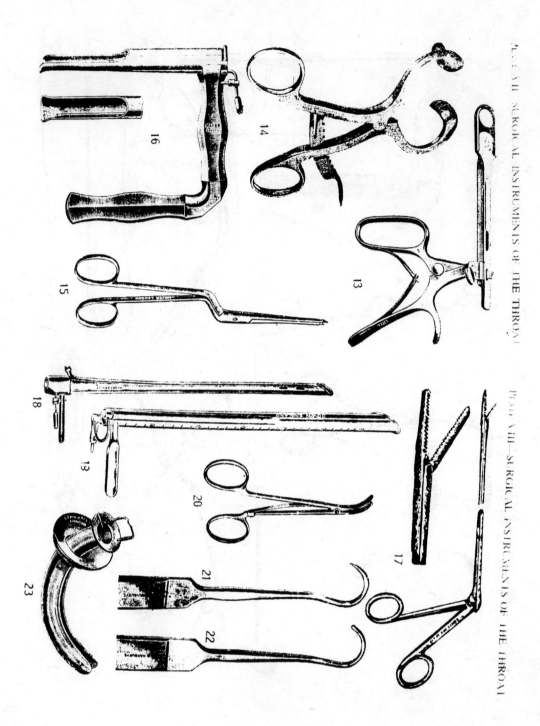

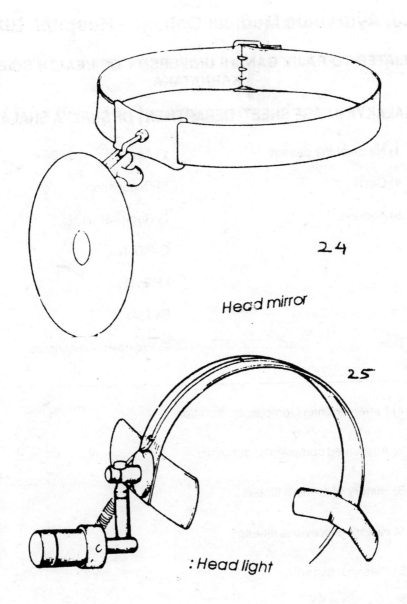

24

Head mirror

25

: Head light

# A MODEL CASE SHEET FOR SHALAKYA - II

## C.S.S.
# N.K.J. Ayurvedic Medical College - Hospital. BIDAR.

## AFFLIATED TO RAJIV GANDHI UNIVERSITY OF HEALTH SCIENCES KARNATAKA

## SHALAKYA II CASE SHEET- DEPARTMENT OF SHALYA SHALAKYA

I)   1) Name of the patient      2) Age     3) Sex

4) Caste      5) Occupation

6) Address      7) Registration No.

O.P.D. No.

I.P.D. No.

Bed No.

8.   Date      9) Provisional diagnosis.

---

II)   1) Patient's Chief Complaints, duration :

2) Associaed complaints, duration :

3) History of present illness :

4) History of previous illness :

5) Personal history :

6) Family history :

**III)**  **Asta sthana Pareeksha :-**

    1) Nadi                             2) Mutra

    3) Malam                          4) Jihwa

    5) Shabda                       6) sparsha

    7) Druk                           8) Akruthi

**IV)**  **Dasha - vidha pareeksha :-**

    1) Prakruthi                    2) Vikruthi

    2) Sara                          4) Samhanana

    5) Pramana                    6) Satmya

    7) Satwa                       8) Ahara Shakthi

    9) Vyayama Shakthi          10) Vayas.

**V)**  **Anga Pratyanga Pareeksha :-**

    1) Heart                        3) Liver

    2) Lungs                       4) Spleen

    Other :-

**VI)**  **Samsthanika - Pareeksha :-**  (Systemic Examination)

**VII)**  **Examination Nose :-**

    **1) Bahya Nasa :**
    a) Normal      (     )          b) Deformed     (           )
    c) Congenital Lesions :-
    d) Inflammatory Lesions :-
    e) Traumatic Lesions :-
    f) Operative lesions
    g) Others
    h) Description :-

2) **NASA PATALA (NASAL SEPTEM )**

a) Normal ( ) b) Deviated ( )
c) Description :-

3) **NASA GUHA (NASAL CAVITY )**
a) Normal b) Rhinitis . c) Atrophied. d) Hypertrophied. e) Furunculosis.
f) Crust formation, g) Occlusions. h) Nasal Polyp. i) Grandhi j) Arbuda.
k) Vidradi l) Bleeding m) Pain. n) Burning sensation. o) Itching snesation.
p) Sneezing. q) Nasal discharge its nature ..................
r) Swasa. 1) Normal, 2) obstructed Right side/Leftside .
s) Gandha gyanam 1) Normal 2) Absent 3) Altered 4) Reduced
5) Agravated.
t) Description.

4) **INSTRUMENTAL EXAMINATION - INVESTIGATIONS - REPORTS :-**

# VIII. Examination of EAR :-
### 1) BAHYA KARNA :
a) Normal ( ) b) Deformed ( )
c) Congenital Lesions :-
d) Inflammatory Lesions
e) Traumatic Lesions
f) Operative lesions.
g) Others.
h) Description :

2) **EXAMINATION OF EXTERNAL AUDITORY MEATUS :-**

a) Normal b) Wax. c) Foreign bodies. d) Inflammation e) Furunculosis.
f) Otitis Externa. g) Otomycosis. h) Trauma. i) Ear discharge, its nature .....
j) Otalgia 1) Local ( ) 2) Radiating ( ). 3) .
k) Polyp. l) Cyst. m) Tumours. n) Abscess. o) Fistula
p) Description :-

3) **Examination of Tympanic Membrane :-**
a) Normal b) Abnormal
c) Perforated i) Location ( ). 2) Size ( ) 3) Shape ( )
d) Discription

4) **Deafness :-** a) Conductive b) Sensori neural c) Mixed ( )
a) Tinnitus ( )b) Menier's Syndrome c) Vertigo ( ) d)

5) **INSTRUMENTAL EXAMINATION INVESTIGATIONS - REPORTS :-**
IX) **Others if any :**

**X)** **Examination of Shiras :-**
1) Normal
2) Shira shoola (Head ache)　　　　　(　　　)
a) Site of the pain :　　　　　b) Typeof pain :
c) Local pain :　　　　　d) Radiating pain
e) Continuous pain　　　　　f) Intermittent pain
g) Time of occurence　　　　　h) Time of agrevation
i) Durationof pain　　　　　j) Intensity of pain mild/ Severe
k) Reduce naturally　　　　　l) Reduce by medication.

3) Shirodaha ;　(　　)Shiro kandu :　(　　) 5) Shiro gurutwa : (　　)
6) Brama (　　) 7) Kapala Vikara　(　　) 8) Kesha Vikata　(　　)
9) Description :-
10) Investigations and reports :

# Examination of MUKHA :-

**XI)** **OSTA (Lips)**　　　Normal　　　(　　)
Akruthi (Shape)　　　Varna (Colour)
Parimana (size)　　　Vedana (pain)
Shotha (Oedema)　　　Kandu (itching)
Srava (Drava - Raktha - Puya - Pischila -)
Daha (burning sensation)　　　sputona (Cracking)
Discription :

**XII)** **Dantha Moola (Gums)**

Varana (colour)　　　Normal
Srava (Discharges)　　　shotha (Oedema)
Sosha　(atrophy)　　　Perforation.
Grandi　(Cyst)　　　Arbuda tumour
Shoola (pain)　　　Vidradi, abscess
　　　Daha (Buring Sensation).

**XII)** **DANTHA　(TEETH)**
　　　　　Normal (　　)
Akruthi (Sama - Vishama )　Varna (Colour )
Shoola (Pain )　Dantha Harsha (Sensitivity)
Sthithi (Sthira- chala)　(Sputana (cracking)
Dantha Chidra (Perforation)　Krimidantha (carees tooth)
Shotha (Oedema)　Gradhi (Cyst)
Arbuda (Tumour)　Vidradi (abscess)
Description :

**XIV)** **JIHWA (Tongue)**
Normal　　　Parimana (Size)　(　　)
Varna(Colour)　　　Akruthi (Shape)
Sputana (Cracking)　　　Vrana (ulceration)
Description :　　　Rasana (Taste

**XV) TALU (Palate)**

Varna (Colour)
Shoola (Pain)
Vrana (ulceration)
Description :-

Normal          (     )
Shotha (Oedema)
Sputana (Cracking)

**XVI) GALA (Throat)**

a) Varna (Colour)
Vedana (Pain)
Kandu (Itching)
Swara Vikar
Arbuda (Tumour)
Description :-

Normal          (     )
Shotha (Oedema)
Daha (burning)
Grandhi (Cysts)
Vidradi (abscess)

Instrumental Examination - Investigations - Report.

**XVII) Differential diagnosis :-**

**XVIII) Final Diagnosis.**

# XIX) Pancha Lakshana Nidanam :

1.      **Nidana :**

2.      **Poorva rupa :**

3.      **Rupam :**

4.      **Upashaya :**

5.      **Samprapthi :**

6.      **Dosha Vikruthi.**

7.      **Dushya Vikruthi**

8.      **Sroto Vikruthi**

9.      **Rogi bala**

10.     **Roga balam**

11.     **Sadhya Sadhyatha :**

XX)    A). ChiKitsaa Sutra :-

B) Pathya :

C) Apathya :

D) Aushada chikitsa :

I. Sthanika chikitsa

II) Saarva dehika chikitsa

## E)    Shastra Shikitsa

I. Poorva Karma

II. Pradhana karma

iii) Paschaat Karma

## XXI.   Result

## XXII)  Advises.

**Signature of Student**                    **Signature of the Lecture**

# BIBLIOGRAPHY

1.    Bruhattraya

2.    Laghutraya

3.    Basavarajeeya

4.    Chakradattha

5.    Hareetha Samhitha

6.    Vangasena

7.    Sachitra Shalakya by Dr. Ravindra Chandra Chaudari

8.    Shalakya tantra by Dr. Ramnath Dwivedi

9.    Shalakya tantra by Dr. Vishwanath Dwivedi

10.   Shalakya Tantra by Dr. K.V. Prabhakaram (Telugu)

11.   A Short Text book of ENT by maqbool

12.   A Short Text book of ENT by Bhargava

13.   A Short Text book of ENT by Barin Kumar Roy Chaudari

14.   A short Text book of ENT E.L.B.S Edition

15.   Fundamentals of ENT by SK. De